Functional Pain Syndromes

Mission Statement of IASP Press®

IASP brings together scientists, clinicians, health care providers, and policy makers to stimulate and support the study of pain and to translate that knowledge into improved pain relief worldwide. IASP Press publishes timely, high-quality, and reasonably priced books relating to pain research and treatment.

Functional Pain Syndromes:
Presentation and Pathophysiology

Editors

Emeran A. Mayer, MD

Departments of Medicine, Physiology and Psychiatry, David Geffen School of Medicine; Center for Neurobiology of Stress; and CURE: Digestive Diseases Research Center, UCLA, Los Angeles, California, USA

M. Catherine Bushnell, PhD

Department of Anesthesia and Faculty of Dentistry, Alan Edwards Centre for Research on Pain, McGill University, Montreal, Quebec, Canada; Department of Neurology and Neurosurgery, Montreal Neurological Institute, Montreal, Quebec, Canada

IASP PRESS® ◈ SEATTLE

Timely topics in pain research and treatment have been selected for publication, but the information provided and opinions expressed have not involved any verification of the findings, conclusions, and opinions by IASP®. Thus, opinions expressed in *Functional Pain Syndromes: Presentation and Pathophysiology* do not necessarily reflect those of IASP or of the Officers and Councilors.

No responsibility is assumed by IASP for any injury and/or damage to persons or property as a matter of product liability, negligence, or from any use of any methods, products, instruction, or ideas contained in the material herein. Because of the rapid advances in the medical sciences, the publisher recommends that there should be independent verification of diagnoses and drug dosages.

Library of Congress Cataloging-in-Publication Data

Functional pain syndromes : presentation and pathophysiology / editors,
Emeran A. Mayer, M. Catherine Bushnell.
    p. ; cm.
 Includes bibliographical references and index.
 Summary: "This book reviews the pathophysiology of functional pain
disorders, including irritable bowel syndrome, fibromyalgia, vulvodynia,
and interstitial cystitis, and considers the relationship of these
disorders with one another and with anxiety, depression, post-traumatic
stress disorder, and chronic fatigue syndrome. The authors also describe
treatment options, including antidepressants and psychological
therapies"--Provided by publisher.
 ISBN 978-0-931092-75-6 (pbk. : alk. paper)
1. Chronic pain. I. Mayer, Emeran A. II. Bushnell, M. Catherine,
1949- III. International Association for the Study of Pain.
 [DNLM: 1. Pain--complications. 2. Pain--physiopathology. 3.
Pain--therapy. WL 704 F979 2009]
 RB127.F86 2009
 616'.0472--dc22
                                    2009006751

Published by:
IASP Press®
International Association for the Study of Pain
111 Queen Anne Ave N, Suite 501
Seattle, WA 98109-4955, USA
Fax: 206-283-9403
www.iasp-pain.org

Printed in the United States of America

Contents

Contents

Emeran A. Mayer, MD, is Professor of Medicine, Physiology, and Psychiatry at the David Geffen School of Medicine at UCLA, Los Angeles, California, USA. He also serves as Co-Director of the CURE: Digestive Diseases Research Center and is Executive Director of the Center for Neurobiology of Stress. He is Associate Editor of *Gastroenterology* and has served on the editorial boards of the *American Journal of Gastroenterology*, *Clinical Gastroenterology and Hepatology* and the *American Journal of Physiology*. He is President of the Functional Brain Gut Research Group, 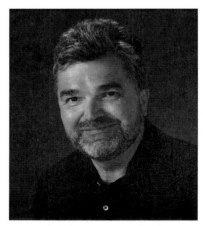 and serves as section head for neurogastroenterology on the Council of the American Gastroenterological Association. He has published many research papers and reviews, focusing particularly on basic and clinical aspects of visceral pain and on the interactions between the digestive system and the nervous system. He received his medical training at the Ludwig Maximilian University, Munich, Germany.

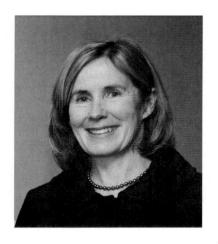 **M. Catherine Bushnell, PhD**, received her training in experimental psychology at the American University, Washington, DC, USA. She is Director of the Alan Edwards Centre for Research on Pain at McGill University in Montréal, Québec, Canada, where she also serves as Professor in the Faculty of Dentistry and as Harold Griffith Professor in the Department of Anesthesiology. She also serves as Adjunct Professor in the Department of Neurology and Neurosurgery at Montreal Neurological Institute. She is Editor-in-Chief of IASP Press and also serves on the editorial boards of *Pain Medicine*, *Clinical Journal of Pain*, *Journal of Neurophysiology*, and *European Journal of Pain*. She is a member of the Neuroscience Canada Science Advisory Council. In 2002, Dr. Bushnell received the Distinguished Career Award of the Canadian Pain Society, and in 2003 she received the Frederick Kerr Award for Basic Research in Pain from the American Pain Society. She has published many research papers, including studies of non-invasive imaging of pain and the neural correlates of psychological influences on pain.

Contributing Authors

Elie D. Al-Chaer, MS, PhD, JD *Center for Pain Research, Departments of Pediatrics, Internal Medicine-Gastroenterology, Neurobiology and Developmental Sciences, University of Arkansas for Medical Sciences, Little Rock, Arkansas, USA*

A. Vania Apkarian, PhD *Departments of Physiology, Anesthesia, and Surgery, and Lurie Cancer Center, Feinberg School of Medicine, Northwestern University, Chicago Illinois, USA*

Yitzchak M. Binik, PhD *Department of Psychology, McGill University, Montreal, Quebec, Canada*

Lori A. Birder, PhD *Department of Medicine, University of Pittsburgh School of Medicine, Pittsburgh, Pennsylvania, USA*

J. Douglas Bremner, MD *Departments of Psychiatry and Radiology, Emory University School of Medicine, Atlanta, Georgia, USA*

M. Catherine Bushnell, PhD *Department of Anesthesia, Faculty of Dentistry, and Alan Edwards Centre for Research on Pain, McGill University, Montreal, Quebec, Canada; Department of Neurology and Neurosurgery at Montreal Neurological Institute, Montreal, Quebec, Canada*

Paolo G. Camici, MD, FRCP, FESC, FACC, FAHA *National Heart and Lung Institute, Imperial College, London, United Kingdom*

Fernando Cervero, MD, PhD, DSc *Anesthesia Research Unit and Alan Edwards Centre for Research on Pain, McGill University, Montreal, Quebec, Canada*

Lin Chang, MD *Center for Neurobiology of Stress, David Geffen School of Medicine at UCLA, and VA Greater Los Angeles Healthcare System, Los Angeles, California, USA*

Christopher Chapple, MD, FRCS(Urol) *Department of Urology, Sheffield Teaching Hospitals NHS Trust, The Royal Hallamshire Hospital, Sheffield, United Kingdom*

Daniel J. Clauw, MD *Departments of Anesthesiology and Medicine, Chronic Pain and Fatigue Research Center, and Clinical and Translational Research, The University of Michigan, Ann Arbor, Michigan, USA*

Francis Creed, MD, FRCP, FRCPsych, FMedSci *Psychiatry Research Group, School of Medicine, University of Manchester, Manchester, United Kingdom*

Yves De Koninck, PhD *The Alan Edwards Centre for Research on Pain, McGill University, Montreal, Quebec, Canada; Robert-Giffard Research Center, Laval University, Quebec City, Quebec, Canada*

Douglas A. Drossman, MD *Center for Functional GI and Motility Disorders, Division of Gastroenterology and Hepatology, University of North Carolina, Chapel Hill, North Carolina, USA*

G.F. Gebhart, PhD *Department of Anesthesiology, Center for Pain Research, University of Pittsburgh, Pittsburgh, Pennsylvania, USA*

Randy Gollub, MD, PhD *Psychiatry Department, Athinoula A. Martinos Center for Biomedical Imaging, and GCRC Biomedical Imaging Core, Massachusetts General Hospital, Charlestown, Massachusetts, USA*

Wilfrid Jänig, Dr med *Institute of Physiology, University of Kiel, Kiel, Germany*

Jian Kong, MD, LicAc *Psychiatry Department and Athinoula A. Martinos Center for Biomedical Imaging, Massachusetts General Hospital, Charlestown, Massachusetts, USA*

Jeffrey M. Lackner, PsyD *University at Buffalo School of Medicine and Bio-medical Sciences, State University of New York, Buffalo, New York, USA*

Gudrun Lange, PhD *Pain and Fatigue Study Center, New Jersey Medical School, Newark, New Jersey, USA; War Related Illness and Injury Study Center, Veterans Affairs New Jersey Health Care System, East Orange, New Jersey, USA*

Kathleen C. Light, PhD *Department of Anesthesiology, Health Sciences Center, University of Utah, Salt Lake City, Utah, USA*

Jürgen Lorenz, Dr med *Hamburg University of Applied Sciences, Faculty of Life Sciences, Laboratory of Human Biology and Physiology, Hamburg, Germany*

R. Bruce Lydiard, PhD, MD *Psychiatry/Mental Health, Ralph H. Johnson VA Medical Center, Charleston, South Carolina, USA; Southeast Health Consultants, Mount Pleasant, South Carolina, USA*

William Maixner, DDS, PhD *Center for Neurosensory Disorders, University of North Carolina, Chapel Hill, North Carolina, USA*

Emeran A. Mayer, MD *Departments of Medicine, Physiology and Psychiatry, David Geffen School of Medicine, Center for Neurobiology of Stress, and CURE: Digestive Diseases Research Center, UCLA, Los Angeles, California, USA*

Lance M. McCracken, PhD *Centre for Pain Services, Royal National Hospital for Rheumatic Diseases and Centre of Pain Research, University of Bath, Bath, United Kingdom*

Andreas Meyer-Lindenberg, MD, PhD *Genes, Cognition and Psychosis Program, National Institute of Mental Health, National Institutes of Health, Bethesda, Maryland, USA; Central Institute of Mental Health, Mannheim, Germany*

Bruce D. Naliboff, PhD *Center for Neurobiology of Stress, Department of Psychiatry and Biobehavioral Sciences, David Geffen School of Medicine at UCLA, and Greater Los Angeles Healthcare System, Los Angeles, California, USA*

Vitaly Napadow, PhD, LicAc *Athinoula A. Martinos Center for Biomedical Imaging, Massachusetts General Hospital, Charlestown, Massachusetts, USA*

Benjamin H. Natelson, MD *Pain and Fatigue Study Center, Beth Israel Medical Center, Phillips Ambulatory Care Center, New York, New York, USA*

Jeanette Papp, PhD *Department of Human Genetics, David Geffen School of Medicine at UCLA, Los Angeles, California, USA*

Lukas Pezawas, Dr med *Genes, Cognition and Psychosis Program, National Institute of Mental Health, National Institutes of Health, Bethesda, Maryland, USA; Division of Biological Psychiatry, Medical University of Vienna, Vienna, Austria*

Ginger Polich, BA *Psychiatry Department, Massachusetts General Hospital, Charlestown, Massachusetts, USA*

Caroline F. Pukall, PhD *Department of Psychology, Queen's University, Kingston, Ontario, Canada*

Jamie L. Rhudy, PhD *Human Psychophysiology Laboratory, Department of Psychology, The University of Tulsa, Tulsa, Oklahoma, USA*

James P. Robinson, MD, PhD *Department of Rehabilitation Medicine, University of Washington, Seattle, Washington, USA*

Stuart D. Rosen, MA, MD, FRCP *National Heart and Lung Institute, Imperial College, London, United Kingdom*

Alan F. Schatzberg, MD *Department of Psychiatry and Behavioral Sciences, Stanford University School of Medicine, Stanford, California, USA*

Fergus Shanahan, MD, FRCP *Alimentary Pharmabiotic Centre, University College Cork, National University of Ireland, Cork, Ireland*

Eric Sobel, PhD *Department of Human Genetics, David Geffen School of Medicine at UCLA, Los Angeles, California, USA*

Robin Spiller, MD, FRCP *Nottingham Digestive Diseases Centre, Biomedical Research Unit, School of Medical and Surgical Sciences, Queen's Medical Centre, Nottingham, United Kingdom*

Irene Tracey, PhD *Centre for Functional Magnetic Resonance Imaging of the Brain, John Radcliffe Hospital, University of Oxford, Oxford, United Kingdom*

Charles J. Vierck, PhD *Department of Neuroscience and McKnight Brain Institute, University of Florida College of Medicine, Gainesville, Florida, USA*

Shelley A. Weaver, PhD *Quintiles, Parsippany, New Jersey, USA*

David A. Williams, PhD *Departments of Anesthesiology, Medicine, Psychiatry, and Psychology, and Chronic Pain and Fatigue Research Center, The University of Michigan, Ann Arbor, Michigan, USA*

Ji Zhang, MD, PhD *The Alan Edwards Centre for Research on Pain, McGill University, Montreal, Quebec, Canada*

Foreword

Few such widely expressed clinical problems are as poorly understood as those defined in this book as "functional" pain syndromes. Given the millions of people who suffer from these very difficult-to-manage problems, it is timely that our current knowledge of the overlapping comorbid conditions be described and explored for common mechanistic pathways that may account for the many conditions seen in these patients. Drs. Mayer and Bushnell are to be congratulated for bringing together an outstanding group of experts in each of their respective fields to provide a view of the current understanding of some of the most prevalent types of chronic pain conditions.

From a pathophysiological perspective, it is evident that we still have much to learn about the initiating stimuli and mechanisms of chronic persistent pain. It is clear that the central neural processing and consequent responses are distinct from those encountered in response to acute pain conditions. Very often, there is no identifiable stimulus for the pain perceived. It appears that a variety of afferent stimuli of either somatic or visceral origin can initiate this process, but neither the stimuli nor how the pain affect is sustained is known. Traditionally, in the absence of a scientific understanding of their disorders, patients are marginalized from meaningful professional care and treatment.

For patients, the effect of this marginalization can be devastating. Lacking a conventionally identifiable cause and easily measurable treatment outcomes, these multisystems illnesses are often viewed as illegitimate. Care by qualified clinicians becomes elusive. Long-suffering patients are vulnerable to offers of false hope, unnecessary procedures, and ineffective or even harmful treatments. Patients feel that they "fall through the cracks." They may be mismanaged and misdiagnosed, resulting in increased severity of their condition. The impact on quality of life strikes at every level—socially, financially, and educationally. The personal and financial costs extend to employers, insurers, an overburdened health care system, and society at large.

Multisystems illnesses have been part of the patient dialogue for decades. The voices of those who suffer from these confounding disorders have been heard through disease-specific patient organizations. Historically, it has been these patient organizations that have addressed the need to move the science forward in an interdisciplinary manner within their own organizations and through scientific meetings. Unfortunately, minimal efforts have been made within the professional community to conduct multidisciplinary research on these conditions and to educate clinicians on their reality and complexity. Hence, the care and treatment of individuals who present with one of these conditions, let alone two or more comorbid conditions, is segmented and unsystematic.

Although it is way past due that the pain and suffering of the millions of patients affected by these multisystems illnesses should be addressed, we are witnessing an increasing level of interest and enthusiasm on several fronts. Many patient advocacy groups are currently working together to bring attention to the need for research in an effort to better understand these illnesses. Responding to encouragement by advocacy groups, agencies of the National Institutes of Health have begun initiatives that encourage collaborative studies on these conditions. And, as is evidenced by this book, scientists and clinicians are coming together in an effort to better understand the potential interactions and relationships among these conditions.

We are heartened by these recent achievements, and we are determined to see the current momentum in this area not just be maintained but be accelerated. The improvement of the quality of health care and lives of millions of patients depends upon it.

Allen W. Cowley, Jr., PhD, Department of Physiology, Medical College of Wisconsin, Milwaukee, Wisconsin, USA

Terrie Cowley, BA, The TMJ Association, Milwaukee, Wisconsin, USA

Nancy J. Norton, BS, and *William F. Norton*, International Foundation for Functional Gastrointestinal Disorders, Milwaukee, Wisconsin, USA

Preface

In our current medical system, when a patient complains of physical pain or discomfort, and no physiological or "organic" cause for that pain can be identified, despite extensive diagnostic testing, the patient receives the diagnosis of a "functional" pain syndrome. If the pain is mainly referred to the abdomen and is associated with alterations in bowel habits, a diagnosis of irritable bowel syndrome is given; if the pain is widespread throughout the body, it is defined as fibromyalgia. As soon as the symptoms are attributed to dysfunction of a particular organ system (the urinary tract, digestive system, or joints), a new, symptom-based classification is assigned to a limited number of symptoms, and a particular syndrome is diagnosed. If no cause is found, many health care professionals will simply give a functional label, often implying that they do not believe that the patient really has anything seriously wrong. The vast majority of patients diagnosed with functional pain disorders are women, which only adds to the prejudice that these disorders are just varieties of neuroses or manifestations of excessive worrying.

Nevertheless, there now is a wealth of evidence that although such disorders may not express significant pathologies in the organs that are responsible for the primary symptoms, they are associated with substantial neurobiological, physiological, and sometimes anatomical changes in the central nervous system (CNS). In this perspective, the observed alterations in the periphery (upregulation of receptors and increased numbers of immune cells) can be explained as peripheral manifestations of chronically altered output from the CNS in the form of autonomic and neuro-endocrine activity. It remains to be determined what role the peripheral changes play in overall symptom presentation, and whether they are required to maintain alterations in bidirectional brain-body loops, providing altered feedback from the body to the brain.

Functional pain disorders such as irritable bowel syndrome, fibromyalgia, temporomandibular joint disorder, vulvodynia, and painful bladder syndrome/interstitial cystitis are now receiving much attention by researchers, but each syndrome is usually studied by subspecialist researchers as a separate entity, with funding coming from different institutes and other funding agencies Until recently, there has been minimal cross-talk between researchers engaged in these efforts, and little progress has occurred in the development of more effective therapies. However, accumulating evidence shows that these disorders have substantial comorbidity with each other and with other stress-related disorders such as chronic fatigue, post-traumatic stress disorder, disorders of mood and affect, and combat-related somatic symptoms (including the Gulf War syndrome). The link between pain and depression, for example, is almost impossible to sort out in terms of cause and effect. Patients diagnosed with depression often report pain, and patients diagnosed with chronic pain often report depression.

Similar pharmacological and nonpharmacological treatment strategies have been applied to many of these syndromes, and shared vulnerability factors in the form of gene polymorphisms and early life trauma have been identified. Recognizing these emerging shared features, and admitting the failure of the traditional subspecialist-focused approach in the development of cost-effective therapies, funding agencies have launched novel "roadmap" grant initiatives. A growing number of national and international meetings now feature symposia on the emerging unifying disease concept. This book is an attempt to integrate the exciting new findings from various disciplines in order to provide a unified picture of pain disorders that, separately, have been marginalized and trivialized by the medical community.

Experts in each disorder describe the essential features of some of the most common functional syndromes and were asked to emphasize both similarities and differences with other disorders. Despite a wide range of perspectives, many common themes have emerged through this approach. Chapters are organized according to disorders that are primarily somatic pain syndromes (fibromyalgia, chronic back pain, temporomandibular joint disorders, and vulvodynia), visceral pain syndromes (irritable bowel syndrome, chest pain, and painful bladder syndrome), and common comorbid non-pain syndromes (combat-related psychiatric syndromes, anxiety disorders, depression, somatization, and chronic fatigue). A number of chapters are devoted to identifying possible pathophysiological mechanisms contributing to the interrelated symptoms of these disorders. Other chapters address the influences of environment and genetic factors on functional pain syndromes and related disorders. Finally, treatment strategies, from pharmacological to cognitive-behavioral approaches and complementary therapies, are discussed as they apply to functional pain syndromes.

Finding a title for this book has proved problematic, highlighting the evolving nature of our understanding and conceptualization of these disorders. "Functional pain syndromes" (as opposed to "organic" disease) is a commonly applied term that encompasses the interrelated disorders described here. Nevertheless, this term has taken on a pejorative meaning, in that many health care professionals and laypersons believe it means that the pain is not real and the disorder is not serious. Many other names have been suggested to us, including "complex persistent pain disorders," "atypical pain syndromes," "idiopathic pain disorders," and "medically unexplained symptoms." Although these terms more clearly express the idea that there is a yet-to-be-identified cause of the pain, they are easily confused with terms applied to specific disorders, such as "complex regional pain syndrome" and "atypical facial pain."

As we were planning this volume, we were told by some colleagues that the time had not yet arrived for such a book, since scientists have not yet clearly identified the causes for the various disorders. However, it is now clear that there is a high comorbidity between these individual syndromes, that there are similar premorbid vulnerability factors (such as gene polymorphisms, female sex, and early life trauma) and similar trigger factors (including psychological and physical stressors), that there are similar abnormalities in CNS anatomy and function across conditions, and that many of these disorders can be associated with changes in cognitive function. Thus, we feel that the time has arrived to look at all functional pain disorders and other comorbid conditions together. Only by doing so we will be able to understand the myriad of environmental, genetic, and physiological conditions that lead to each chronic pain patient's unique pathology.

We would like to thank the many people who made this project possible, especially our chapter authors for volunteering their priceless time and expertise, and without whom this project would not have been possible. We also thank the IASP Press staff for their invaluable collaboration in designing, editing, and assembling the book. We hope this book will lead to a better appreciation of diverse pain syndromes that have remained a mystery, so that patients will receive the understanding and treatment they greatly need.

M. Catherine Bushnell, PhD
Emeran A. Mayer, MD

Part I

Somatic Pain Syndromes

Fibromyalgia

Daniel J. Clauw[a,b,e,f] and David A. Williams[a,b,c,d,e]

Departments of [a]Anesthesiology, [b]Medicine, [c]Psychiatry, and [d]Psychology, [e]Chronic Pain and Fatigue Research Center, and [f]Clinical and Translational Research, The University of Michigan, Ann Arbor, Michigan, USA

Overview

Fibromyalgia syndrome (FM) is a manifestation of chronic widespread pain (CWP) with a prevalence of 2% in the general population [118]. Clinically, individuals with FM present with a variety of physical symptoms, including widespread pain, fatigue, tenderness, sleep disturbance, decrements in physical functioning, and disruptions in psychological functioning (e.g., memory problems, concentration difficulties, diminished mental clarity, mood disturbances, and lack of well-being) [37,80,116,126]. Fibromyalgia occurs more frequently in females, and the comorbid overlap of the syndrome with related functional disorders is high [2,22]. Comorbidities may include temporomandibular disorder (TMD), irritable bowel syndrome (IBS), and chronic fatigue syndrome (CFS). Triggering of FM appears to require a genetic predisposition coupled with environmental stressors [19,30,31,47,57,109]. The maintenance of FM over time appears to be related to centrally mediated amplifications in the processing and integration of sensory, cognitive, and affective information, dysfunction in

endogenous noxious inhibitory systems, sleep disturbance, and dysautonomia [72,73,81,82,114]. Thus, it is likely that there are multiple dysregulated pathways by which a given individual develops the clinical picture
qualifying for the diagnosis of FM. The stance taken within this chapter
reflects our belief that there are indeed neurobiological underpinnings associated with FM. Moreover, we take the position that this constellation of
neurobiological processes is not unique to FM, but may partially account
for symptomatology in related conditions such as IBS, TMD, and CFS.

History of Fibromyalgia

Fibrositis, a term coined by Sir William Gowers in 1904, is the diagnostic
forerunner of fibromyalgia. Fibrositis was thought to be a common cause
of muscular pain; however, its association with "psychogenic rheumatism"
detracted from its broad clinical acceptance as a legitimate condition. The
current concept of fibromyalgia was established by Smythe and Moldofsky
in the mid-1970s [104]. The name change reflected the observation that
there was no inflammation (-*itis*) in the connective tissues of individuals
with this condition, but instead pain (-*algia*). These authors and others
characterized the most common tender points (regions of extreme tenderness in these individuals), and reported that patients with fibromyalgia
also had disturbances in deep and restorative sleep, along with other somatic complaints [83,124].

While there were no formal clinical criteria for FM, the American College of Rheumatology (ACR) developed research criteria to assist
methodologically in gaining a better understanding of the condition [119].
These criteria required that an individual have both a history of chronic
widespread pain (CWP), and the finding of at least 11 of a possible 18 tender points on examination. To date, these criteria have been invaluable in
facilitating a wealth of research on a select patient population.

The diagnostic emphasis upon tender points, however, has led to
the misperception that FM reflects a problem with the peripheral muscles
or specific pathophysiology associated with the tender points [22,125]. In
fact, it was not until investigators concluded that FM was not a condition
localized to peripheral damage or inflammation, and began to explore the

contribution of central neural mechanisms, that rapid advances occurred in the field. The shift from a peripheral focus to the inclusion of central mechanisms has been the key to better understanding not only of FM but of related conditions as well. For example, IBS was previously termed "spastic colitis," emphasizing local pathophysiology, until it was recognized that there was little "-*itis*" and that motility changes were not the only major pathological feature. Research on TMD has similarly begun including central mechanisms rather than focusing exclusively on abnormalities in the jaw. Interstitial cystitis/painful bladder syndrome is undergoing a similar "conversion."

Genetic Factors

Evidence exists for a strong familial component in the development of FM. First-degree relatives of individuals with FM display an eight-fold greater risk of developing FM than those in the general population [5]. Family members of individuals with FM are more tender than the family members of controls, irrespective of the presence of pain, and family members of individuals with FM are also much more likely to have other disorders related to FM such as IBS, TMD, headaches, and other regional pain syndromes [18,59,62]. This familial and personal coaggregation of conditions was originally termed *affective spectrum disorder* [58], and more recently *central sensitivity syndromes* or *chronic multisymptom illnesses* [38,127].

Specific genetic polymorphisms that are associated with a higher risk of developing fibromyalgia are starting to emerge. To date, the serotonin 5-HT2A receptor polymorphism T/T phenotype, as well as serotonin transporter, dopamine 4 receptor, and COMT (catecholamine *O*-methyl transferase) polymorphisms, are seen in higher frequency in individuals with FM [13,16,17,85]. All of the polymorphisms identified to date involve the metabolism or transport of monoamines, compounds that play a critical role in the human stress response. Ongoing research seeks to identify genetic polymorphisms and haplotypes associated with an increased likelihood of developing chronic regional or widespread pain as well as the tendency to augment the processing of sensory information.

Environmental Triggers

As with most illnesses purported to have genetic underpinnings, environmental factors play a prominent role in the triggering and maintenance of FM. Environmental "stressors" temporally associated with the development of fibromyalgia include physical trauma (especially involving the trunk), certain infections such as hepatitis C, Epstein Barr virus, parvovirus, and Lyme disease, and emotional stress. Of note, each of these stressors leads to CWP or fibromyalgia in only 5–10% of individuals who are exposed; the overwhelming majority of individuals who experience these same infections or other stressful events regain their baseline state of health [22].

Stress and Fibromyalgia

Disparate "stressors" can trigger or maintain the development of FM and related conditions; thus, the human stress response has been closely examined for a causative role. The human stress response is mediated primarily by the activity of the hypothalamus, with the release of corticotropin-releasing hormone, and by the locus-ceruleus-norepinephrine/autonomic (sympathetic) nervous system in the brainstem. Throughout history, these systems have been highly adaptive for identifying threats to survival; however, for some individuals, the stress response may be inappropriately triggered by an assortment of modern occurrences posing no or little actual threat to survival. Suboptimal triggering of the stress response unleashes a cascade of physiological responses more frequently than the body can tolerate [99].

Recent reviews regarding the role that "stressors" (both physical and psychosocial) play in adverse health outcomes in FM suggest that factors other than the intensity of the stressor are important. Female gender, worry over illness, expectation of illness chronicity, and inactivity or time off work following the stressor each increase the likelihood of developing pain or other somatic symptoms [77]. Naturally occurring catastrophic events such as earthquakes, floods, or fires are much *less* likely to lead to chronic somatic symptoms than similarly stressful events that are "man made" such as chemical spills, war [23], or being the victim in an auto accident [21]. Being exposed to a multitude of stressors simultaneously, or over a period of time, also may increase the likelihood of later somatic symptoms and or psychological sequelae. Personally relevant stressors appear to influence the symptoms of FM more saliently than global stressors. Two studies performed in the United States just before and after the terrorist attacks of September 11, 2001, serve as examples. In one study performed by Raphael and colleagues, no differences in FM pain complaints or other somatic symptoms were seen in residents of New York and New Jersey surveyed just before and then after the terrorist attacks on the World Trade Center [95]. A second study performed in the Washington, DC, region (near the Pentagon, the other site of attack) during the same time period found that individuals with fibromyalgia had no worsening of pain or other somatic symptoms following the attacks, compared to the days before [113]. Any flares in pain were more likely to be tied to personally relevant events and daily hassles [92].

Many studies have identified abnormalities in the hypothalamic-pituitary-adrenal (HPA) axis and the sympathetic nervous system in fibromyalgia and related conditions [4,25,29,32,73,94]. These studies often report either hypo- or hyperactivity of both the HPA axis and the sympathetic nervous system. These data have been difficult to interpret because the precise abnormality tends to vary from study to study. "Abnormal" HPA or autonomic function is typically found in a very small percentage of patients (while the abnormality is statistically significant, there is tremendous overlap between patients and controls).

Nearly all of the neuroendocrine studies have been cross-sectional, with only inferential support for the HPA or autonomic dysfunction found in fibromyalgia being causative of the pain and other symptoms. In two recent studies examining HPA function in fibromyalgia, McLean et al. showed that salivary cortisol levels covaried with pain levels, and that cerebrospinal fluid (CSF) levels of corticotropin-releasing hormone were more closely related to an individual's pain level or an early life history of trauma than to their status as an individual with FM or a healthy control [78,79]. Most previous studies of HPA and autonomic function in fibromyalgia failed to control for pain levels or for a previous history of trauma, post-traumatic stress disorder, or other comorbid disorders that could affect HPA or autonomic dysfunction.

Heart rate variability at baseline and in response to tilt table testing has been evaluated in patients with fibromyalgia as a surrogate measure of autonomic function. Consistent and reproducible findings support the notion that individuals have a lower baseline heart rate variability than do controls (in three cross-sectional studies by two different groups) [24,25,73]. Lower heart rate variability is suggestive of poor cardiovagal tone. Moreover, recent findings also suggest that aberrations in heart rate variability may predispose to fibromyalgia symptoms [46,74,75], possibly identifying patients at risk. Heart rate variability was found to normalize following exercise therapy, suggesting that the findings might be an epiphenomenon due in part to deconditioning [36].

Augmented Pain and Sensory Processing

Fibromyalgia is defined in part by tenderness, and considerable work has been focused on understanding the nature of the tenderness experienced by patients. One of the earliest findings in this regard was that the tenderness in fibromyalgia is not in fact confined to tender points; rather, it extends throughout the entire body [50,117]. Tender point counts are influenced by concurrent distress [48,115,117], the rate by which pressure increases when assessing tender points, and whether the stimulus pressure is controlled by the patient or a staff member [60,90]. An additional biasing factor is whether tenderness is assessed using an ascending delivery of pressure or one that is random. Ascending stimuli are highly predictable, and expectations for pain and personal motivation for tolerating pain can confound the assessment of tenderness [88,89, 91]. Studies using random pressure stimuli support the notion that these measures of pressure pain threshold are less influenced by levels of distress [90]. Studies of tender point count also suggest that pressure pain thresholds at any four points in the body were highly correlated with the average tenderness at all 18 tender points and four "control points" (the thumbnail and forehead) [91]. These latter findings suggest that generalized tenderness may be a marker of FM. Finer distinctions (e.g., active and control points) may not be as relevant.

Generalized Sensory Augmentation in Fibromyalgia

In addition to reporting heightened sensitivity to pressure stimuli, individuals with FM also judge other types of stimuli applied to the skin are as being more painful or noxious. For example, they may show a decreased threshold to heat [40,44,66,88], cold [65,66], and electrical stimuli [8] and increased sensitivity to hypertonic saline muscle infusion [120]. Increased sensitivity does not appear to be limited to the somatosensory system but appears to occur with audition and olfaction as well. Gerster and colleagues demonstrated that individuals with FM display a low noxious threshold to auditory tones, a finding that has undergone several replications [43,76]. These early audition studies used ascending measures of auditory threshold; they were subject to the same biases previously mentioned for ascending pressure stimuli. A recent study by Geisser and colleagues used the "random staircase" paradigm to assess auditory threshold in individuals with FM [41]. This study found comparably low thresholds to both types of stimuli. The notion that fibromyalgia and related syndromes might represent biological amplification of all sensory stimuli has significant support from functional imaging studies suggesting that the insula is the most consistently hyperactive cortical region. This region has been noted to play a critical role in sensory integration, with the posterior insula serving a purer sensory role, and the anterior insula being associated with the emotional processing of sensations [27,28,106].

Specific Mechanisms Associated with Low Pain Threshold in Fibromyalgia

Two different specific pathogenic mechanisms have been posited as contributing to lowered pain thresholds in individuals with FM: (1) a reduction of descending analgesic activity, and (2) hyperactivity of excitatory afferent systems.

Attenuated Diffuse Noxious Inhibitory Controls

In healthy humans and laboratory animals, application of an intense painful stimulus for 2 to 5 minutes produces generalized whole-body analgesia. This analgesic effect, termed "diffuse noxious inhibitory controls" (DNIC), has been consistently observed to be attenuated or absent in groups of FM patients, compared to healthy controls [61,66,70,71]. Wilder-Smith and colleagues have shown similar findings in IBS [112]. While attenuated DNIC is not found in all individuals with fibromyalgia or IBS, it is considerably more common in patients than in controls.

The DNIC response in humans is believed to be partly mediated by descending opioidergic and serotonergic-noradrenergic pathways. In fibromyalgia, the accumulating data suggest that opioidergic activity is either normal or increased, given that levels of enkephalins in the CSF are roughly twice as high in FM as in healthy controls [9]. In response to the introduction of carfentanil, PET data similarly show that baseline μ-opioid receptor binding is decreased in multiple pain-processing regions in the brains of FM patients, consistent with what would be expected if there were an increased release of endogenous opioids in FM, leading to high baseline occupancy of the receptors [55].

An intact endogenous opioidergic analgesic system is consistent with the anecdotal clinical experience that opioids are generally ineffective analgesics in patients with FM. In contrast, studies have shown the opposite for serotonergic and noradrenergic activity in FM. Research has found that the principal metabolite of norepinephrine, 3-methoxy-4-hydroxyphenethylene (MPHG), is lower in the CSF of FM patients [98]. Similarly patients with FM were shown to have reduced serum levels of serotonin and its precursor, L-tryptophan, as well as reduced levels of the principal serotonin metabolite, 5-HIAA, in their CSF [98,128]. Further evidence for this mechanism comes from treatment studies finding that nearly any type of compound that simultaneously raises both serotonin and norepinephrine (e.g., tricyclics, duloxetine, milnacipran, or tramadol) will have efficacy in treating FM [6,7,11,42].

Excitatory Afferent Systems

In animal models, central sensitization is associated with excitatory amino acid and substance P hyperactivity [121–123]. In FM, four independent studies have shown that individuals with FM have approximately threefold higher CSF concentrations of substance P, when compared with normal controls [14,97,108,110]. Other chronic pain syndromes, such as osteoarthritis of the hip and chronic low back pain, have also been associated with elevated substance P levels. Interestingly, once elevated, substance P levels do not appear to change dramatically, and they do not rise in response to acute painful stimuli. Thus, high substance P appears to be a biological marker for the presence of chronic pain.

Glutamate is a prominent excitatory neurotransmitter within the central nervous system, and in FM, CSF levels of glutamate are twice as high as in controls [100]. Moreover, a recent study using proton spectroscopy demonstrated that the glutamate levels within the insula of individuals with FM fluctuated in response to changes in clinical and experimental pain [54,56].

Cortical Representation of Pain Processing in Fibromyalgia

Functional neural imaging enables investigators to visualize how the brain processes the sensory experience of pain. Functional magnetic resonance imaging (fMRI), single photon emission computed tomography (SPECT), positron emission tomography (PET), and proton spectroscopy are the most commonly used methods in studies of FM.

Single-Photon-Emission Computed Tomography

SPECT was the first functional neuroimaging technique to be used in fibromyalgia. SPECT imaging involves the introduction into the participant's bloodstream of radioactive compounds, which then decay over time, providing a window for viewing neural activity. The first studies using SPECT imaging in individuals with FM found decreased blood flow in both the caudate and the thalamus compared to age- and education-matched healthy controls [68,84]. Subsequent SPECT studies using a more sensitive radioligand, ^{99m}Tc-ECD (technetium-ethyl cysteinate dimer), found hyperperfusion in FM within the somatosensory cortex and hypoperfusion in the anterior and posterior cingulate, the amygdala, the medial frontal and parahippocampal gyrus, and the cerebellum [51,52]. One longitudinal treatment trial used SPECT imaging to assess changes in neurocortical regional blood flow following administration of amitriptyline in 14 FM patients [3]. After 3 months of treatment, increased blood flow was observed in the bilateral thalamus and the basal ganglia. These data suggest that amitriptyline may normalize the decreased blood flow in these regions, perhaps reducing pain perception.

Functional Magnetic Resonance Imaging

The first study to use fMRI in fibromyalgia patients was performed by Gracely et al. In this study, 16 individuals with FM and 16 matched controls were exposed to painful pressures while being scanned [49]. Individuals with FM exhibited increased neurocortical activations in the primary and secondary somatosensory cortex, the insula, and the anterior cingulate, all regions commonly associated with pain processing in healthy normal subjects during painful stimuli. Of interest, however, was that these activations occurred in response to pressure stimuli that were much milder than those used to elicit cortical activity in healthy controls. Healthy controls required nearly twice as much pressure stimulation to evoke cortical activity in pain-processing regions. Similar findings have been identified in FM in response to heat stimuli [26].

Positron Emission Tomography

PET has been used in several studies in fibromyalgia. In the first such study, Yunus and colleagues did not identify any differences in regional cerebral blood flow between fibromyalgia patients and controls [129]. However, Wood and colleagues used PET to show that attenuated dopaminergic activity may be playing a role in pain transmission in fibromyalgia [120]. Recently, Harris and colleagues showed evidence of decreased μ-opioid receptor availability (possibly due to increased release of endogenous μ-opioids) in fibromyalgia [55].

Structural Abnormalities in Fibromyalgia

Although a few studies have found mild abnormalities in the skeletal muscles of fibromyalgia patients, these findings have been inconsistent and may be indicative of deconditioning [10,33,39]. A few studies suggest subtle differences in cortical or subcortical brain structure in individuals with this condition. P31-spectroscopy has been used to examine muscle metabolism in fibromyalgia, but the results are conflicting: one study comparing sedentary controls to FM found no differences, and the other found lower adenosine triphosphate levels among individuals with FM [87,103]. Studies suggest that the tenderness in fibromyalgia is not confined to just the muscle; therefore, most investigators have concluded that primary muscle disease is not a likely cause of the pain associated with fibromyalgia.

Some data suggest that a subset of individuals with fibromyalgia may have abnormalities involving small sensory nerves in the skin, indicative of a small-fiber neuropathy [20,63]. Data are also emerging to suggest subtle abnormalities in brain structure in fibromyalgia [67,105]. Thus, if there are structural abnormalities or damage to tissues in fibromyalgia, the best evidence for appears to implicate neural tissues.

Sleep and Activity in Fibromyalgia

In addition to pain, problems with sleep, fatigue, and poor physical function are common in FM. One of the earliest biological findings in fibromyalgia was that selective sleep deprivation produces FM-like symptoms in healthy individuals. These findings have been replicated by several groups [83,86]. However, the EEG abnormalities that were noted in this first study and initially thought to be a marker for fibromyalgia, so-called alpha intrusions, have subsequently been found to be present in normal controls and in individuals with other conditions [15,34]. More recent findings from polysomnography suggest that sleep abnormalities that are more characteristic of FM include fewer sleep spindles, an increase in cyclic alternating pattern rate, upper airway resistance syndrome, and poor sleep efficiency [69,96,101,102]. Curiously, sleep abnormalities rarely correlate with other symptoms in FM, and many investigators believe that identifying and treating specific sleep disorders often seen in FM patients (such as obstructive sleep apnea, upper airway resistance, and restless leg or periodic limb movement syndromes) do not necessarily lead to improvements in the core symptoms of FM.

Physical functional status is characteristically lower in FM than in many other medical conditions including chronic obstructive pulmonary disease. While self-report is most commonly used to assess physical functional status, actigraphy or the use of wrist-watch-like movement accelerometers can provide a more objective assessment of when and how much individuals are being active [64].

Kop and colleagues demonstrated that although patients with FM have physical functioning scores nearly two standard deviations below the population average on the Medical Outcomes Study 36-item Short-Form Health Survey, they have the same average activity level as a group of sedentary controls. The difference between FM and healthy controls appears to be that individuals with FM have much lower peak activity levels, suggesting that the problems in FM are due to an inability to rise to the intermittent demands of day-to-day life rather than limitations in overall functioning.

Comorbid Psychiatric Factors

In addition to neurobiological mechanisms, comorbid psychiatric factors can influence symptom expression in many individuals with FM. The rate of current psychiatric comorbidity in patients with FM may be as high as 30% to 60% in tertiary care settings, and the rate of lifetime psychiatric disorders may be even higher [12,35,59]. Depression and anxiety disorders are most commonly seen. However, these rates may be artifactually elevated by virtue of the fact that most of these studies have been performed in tertiary care centers; population-based or community-based studies have substantially lower rates of psychiatric conditions [1,111].

In contrast to early assumptions that FM was simply a variant of depression, neuroimaging data suggest that the pain of FM is experienced independently of depression status. Giesecke et al. explored the relationship between depression and enhanced evoked pain sensations in FM patients qualifying as having both pain and depression and in a sample of individuals with FM without depression. Augmented sensory activity was observed in pain-processing regions for both groups of individuals, suggesting that depression is not responsible for the pain of FM. Additional activity within the anterior insula and amygdala were noted in the FM group with comorbid depression. These data are consistent with other evidence in the pain field that suggests that different regions of the brain are preferentially responsible for processing the sensory intensity versus affective aspects of pain sensation [93].

Behavioral and Psychosocial Factors

Population-based studies have demonstrated that the relationship between pain and distress is complex and that distress can be both a cause and a consequence of pain. As pain persists, individuals begin to function less well in their various roles. They may have difficulties with spouses or children, and with work inside or outside the home, which can exacerbate symptoms and lead to behavioral changes that in the long term prove contrary to healthy adaptation. Examples include isolation, cessation of pleasurable activities, and reductions in activity and exercise. In the worst cases, patients become involved with disability and compensation systems, which mitigates against improvement [53].

The influence of psychological factors is quite different from the influences of psychiatric illnesses. The latter are almost always negative, whereas psychological influences occur naturally and can influence symptoms either positively or negatively. Several groups have attempted to identify subgroups of individuals with FM, and each has included psychosocial factors in the grouping rationale [45,107]. One of these studies examined how differential degrees of affective, behavioral, cognitive, or functional status and hyperalgesia interact to produce subgroups of patients that would potentially have differential responses to treatment. Three subgroups were identified. The first comprised approximately half of the patients; this subgroup had mild levels of depression and anxiety, had normal cognition regarding pain, and were mildly tender (although tender enough to meet the ACR criteria). The second subgroup, representative of a "tertiary care" sample, were slightly more tender, and they displayed high levels of negative affect and maladaptive cognitions such as external locus of pain control and catastrophizing. The third subgroup, perhaps the most interesting, included individuals who were the most tender, but with no negative psychological or cognitive factors and some positive cognitive elements such as internal locus of control. This group may be thought of as "resilient" individuals, with positive psychological and cognitive factors "buffering" the neurobiological factors leading to pain and other symptoms in FM.

Conclusions

The condition known as fibromyalgia has for many years suffered from a lack of clinical credibility, a lack of consensus regarding the underlying pathophysiology, a research definition but no clinical definition, and inconsistencies in assessment. Many of these deficiencies are changing as more rigorous scientific methods borrowed largely from the general chronic pain literature are being applied to FM. Recent studies are revealing multiple dysregulated neurobiological systems underlying the pain and suffering of individuals with FM. Some, but not all, of the neurobiological underpinnings of FM are also seen in other conditions characterized by persistent pain such as IBS, chronic pelvic pain, and TMD. While these other pain conditions are more regional, it is likely that FM is a prototypic example of these other conditions advancing to become more global or systemic in nature. Future work is needed to gain a better understanding of the interplay between genetic predisposition and the behavioral and environmental factors that interact to produce FM and related conditions.

References

[1]   Aaron LA, Bradley LA, Alarcon GS, Alexander RW, Triana-Alexander M, Martin MY, Alberts KR. Psychiatric diagnoses in patients with fibromyalgia are related to health care-seeking behavior rather than to illness. Arthritis Rheum 1996;39:436–45.
[2]   Aaron LA, Burke MM, Buchwald D. Overlapping conditions among patients with chronic fatigue syndrome, fibromyalgia, and temporomandibular disorder. Arch Intern Med 2000;160:221–7.
[3]   Adiguzel O, Kaptanoglu E, Turgut B, Nacitarhan V. The possible effect of clinical recovery on regional cerebral blood flow deficits in fibromyalgia: a prospective study with semiquantitative SPECT. South Med J 2004;97:651–5.

[4]   Adler GK, Kinsley BT, Hurwitz S, Mossey CJ, Goldenberg DL. Reduced hypothalamic-pituitary and sympathoadrenal responses to hypoglycemia in women with fibromyalgia syndrome. Am J Med 1999;106:534–43.

[5]   Arnold LM, Hudson JI, Hess EV, Ware AE, Fritz DA, Auchenbach MB, Starck LO, Keck PE, Jr. Family study of fibromyalgia. Arthritis Rheum 2004;50:944–52.

[6]   Arnold LM, Keck PEJ, Welge JA. Antidepressant treatment of fibromyalgia. A meta-analysis and review. Psychosomatics 2000;41:104–13.

[7]   Arnold LM, Lu Y, Crofford LJ, Wohlreich M, Detke MJ, Iyengar S, Goldstein DJ. A double-blind, multicenter trial comparing duloxetine with placebo in the treatment of fibromyalgia patients with or without major depressive disorder. Arthritis Rheum 2004;50:2974–84.

[8]   Arroyo JF, Cohen ML. Abnormal responses to electrocutaneous stimulation in fibromyalgia. J Rheumatol 1993;20:1925–31.

[9]   Baraniuk JN, Whalen G, Cunningham J, Clauw DJ. Cerebrospinal fluid levels of opioid peptides in fibromyalgia and chronic low back pain. BMC Musculoskel Disord 2004;5:48.

[10] Bennett RM, Jacobsen S. Muscle function and origin of pain in fibromyalgia. Baillieres Clin Rheumatol 1994;8:721–46.

[11] Bennett RM, Kamin M, Karim R, Rosenthal N. Tramadol and acetaminophen combination tablets in the treatment of fibromyalgia pain: a double-blind, randomized, placebo-controlled study. Am J Med 2003;114:537–45.

[12] Boissevain MD, McCain GA. Toward an integrated understanding of fibromyalgia syndrome. I. Medical and pathophysiological aspects. Pain 1991;45:227–38.

[13] Bondy B, Spaeth M, Offenbaecher M, Glatzeder K, Stratz T, Schwarz M, de Jonge S, Kruger M, Engel RR, Farber L, Pongratz DE, Ackenheil M. The T102C polymorphism of the 5-HT2A-receptor gene in fibromyalgia. Neurobiol Dis 1999;6:433–9.

[14] Bradley LA, Alberts KR, Alarcon GS, Alexander MT, Mountz JM, Wiegent DA, Liu HG, Blalock JE, Aaron LA, Alexander RW, San Pedro EC, Martin MY, Morell AC. Abnormal brain regional cerebral blood flow and cerebrospinal fluid levels of substance P in patients and non-patients with fibromyalgia. Arthritis Rheum 1996;39(9S):1109.

[15] Branco J, Atalaia A, Paiva T. Sleep cycles and alpha-delta sleep in fibromyalgia syndrome. J Rheumatol 1994;21:1113–7.

[16] Buskila D. Genetics of chronic pain states. Best Pract Res Clin Rheumatol 2007;21:535–47.

[17] Buskila D, Cohen H, Neumann L, Ebstein RP. An association between fibromyalgia and the dopamine D4 receptor exon III repeat polymorphism and relationship to novelty seeking personality traits. Mol Psychiatry 2004;9:730–1.

[18] Buskila D, Neumann L, Hazanov I, Carmi R. Familial aggregation in the fibromyalgia syndrome. Semin Arthritis Rheum 1996;26:605–11.

[19] Buskila D, Neumann L, Vaisberg G, Alkalay D, Wolfe F. Increased rates of fibromyalgia following cervical spine injury. A controlled study of 161 cases of traumatic injury. Arthritis Rheum 1997;40:446–52.

[20] Caro XJ, Winter EF, Dumas AJ. A subset of fibromyalgia patients have findings suggestive of chronic inflammatory demyelinating polyneuropathy and appear to respond to IVIg. Rheumatology (Oxford) 2008;47:208–11.

[21] Chrousos GP, Gold PW. The concepts of stress and stress system disorders. Overview of physical and behavioral homeostasis. JAMA 1992;267:1244–52.

[22] Clauw DJ, Chrousos GP. Chronic pain and fatigue syndromes: Overlapping clinical and neuroendocrine features and potential pathogenic mechanisms. Neuroimmunomodulation 1997;4:134–53.

[23] Clauw DJ, Engel CC, Jr., Aronowitz R, Jones E, Kipen HM, Kroenke K, Ratzan S, Sharpe M, Wessely S. Unexplained symptoms after terrorism and war: an expert consensus statement. J Occup Environ Med 2003;45:1040–8.

[24] Cohen H, Buskila D, Neumann L, Ebstein RP. Confirmation of an association between fibromyalgia and serotonin transporter promoter region (5-HTTLPR) polymorphism, and relationship to anxiety-related personality traits. Arthritis Rheum 2002;46:845–7.

[25] Cohen H, Neumann L, Shore M, Amir M, Cassuto Y, Buskila D. Autonomic dysfunction in patients with fibromyalgia: Application of power spectral analysis of heart rate variability. Semin Arthritis Rheum 2000;29:217–27.

[26] Cook DB, Lange G, Ciccone DS, Liu WC, Steffener J, Natelson BH. Functional imaging of pain in patients with primary fibromyalgia. J Rheumatol 2004;31:364–78.

[27] Craig AD. Interoception: the sense of the physiological condition of the body. Curr Opin Neurobiol 2003;13:500–5.

[28] Craig AD. Human feelings: why are some more aware than others? Trends Cogn Sci 2004;8:239–41.

[29] Crofford LJ, Pillemer SR, Kalogeras KT, Cash JM, Michelson D, Kling MA, Sternberg EM, Gold PW, Chrousos GP, Wilder RL. Hypothalamic-pituitary-adrenal axis perturbations in patients with fibromyalgia. Arthritis Rheum 1994;37:1583–92.

[30] Culclasure TF, Enzenauer RJ, West SG. Post-traumatic stress disorder presenting as fibromyalgia. Am J Med 1993;94:548–9.

[31] Dailey PA, Bishop GD, Russell IJ, Fletcher EM. Psychological stress and the fibrositis/fibromyalgia syndrome. J Rheumatol 1990;17:1380–5.

[32] Demitrack MA, Crofford LJ. Evidence for and pathophysiologic implications of hypothalamic-pituitary-adrenal axis dysregulation in fibromyalgia and chronic fatigue syndrome. Ann NY Acad Sci 1998;840:684–97.

[33] Drewes AM, Andreasen A, Schroder HD, Hogsaa B, Jennum PJ. Pathology of skeletal muscle in fibromyalgia: a histo-immuno-chemical and ultrastructural study. Br J Rheumatol 1993;32:479–83.

[34] Drewes AM, Svendsen L. Quantification of alpha-EEG activity during sleep in fibromyalgia: A study based on ambulatory sleep monitoring. J Musculoskel Pain 1994;2:33–53.

[35] Epstein SA, Kay GG, Clauw DJ, Heaton R, Klein D, Krupp L, Kuck J, Leslie V, Masur D, Wagner M, Waid R, Zisook S. Psychiatric disorders in patients with fibromyalgia. A multicenter investigation. Psychosomatics 1999;40:57–63.

[36] Figueroa A, Kingsley JD, McMillan V, Panton LB. Resistance exercise training improves heart rate variability in women with fibromyalgia. Clin Physiol Funct Imaging 2008;28:49–54.

[37] Forseth KO, Gran JT. Management of fibromyalgia: what are the best treatment choices? Drugs 2002;62:577–92.

[38] Fukuda K, Nisenbaum R, Stewart G, Thompson WW, Robin L, Washko RM, Noah DL, Barrett DH, Randall B, Herwaldt BL, Mawle AC, Reeves WC. Chronic multisymptom illness affecting Air Force veterans of the Gulf War. JAMA 1998;280:981–8.

[39] Geel SE. The fibromyalgia syndrome: Musculoskeletal pathophysiology. Semin Arthritis Rheum 1994;23:347–53.

[40] Geisser ME, Casey KL, Brucksch CB, Ribbens CM, Appleton BB, Crofford LJ. Perception of noxious and innocuous heat stimulation among healthy women and women with fibromyalgia: association with mood, somatic focus, and catastrophizing. Pain 2003;102:243–50.

[41] Geisser ME, Gracely RH, Giesecke T, Petzke FW, Williams DA, Clauw DJ. The association between experimental and clinical pain measures among persons with fibromyalgia and chronic fatigue syndrome. Eur J Pain 2007;11:202–7.

[42] Gendreau RM, Thorn MD, Gendreau JF, Kranzler JD, Riberio S, Gracely R.H., Williams DA, Mease PJ, McLean SA, Clauw DJ. The efficacy of milnacipran in patients with fibromyalgia. J Rheumatol 2005; 32:1975–85.

[43] Gerster JC, Hadj-Djilani A. Hearing and vestibular abnormalities in primary fibrositis syndrome. J Rheumatol 1984;11:678–80.

[44] Gibson SJ, Littlejohn GO, Gorman MM, Helme RD, Granges G. Altered heat pain thresholds and cerebral event-related potentials following painful CO_2 laser stimulation in subjects with fibromyalgia syndrome. Pain 1994;58:185–93.

[45] Giesecke T, Williams DA, Harris RE, Cupps TR, Tian X, Tian TX, Gracely RH, Clauw DJ. Subgrouping of fibromyalgia patients on the basis of pressure-pain thresholds and psychological factors. Arthritis Rheum 2003;48:2916–22.

[46] Glass JM, Lyden A, Petzke F, Clauw D. The effect of brief exercise cessation on pain, fatigue, and mood symptom development in healthy, fit individuals. J Psychosom Res 2004;57:391–8.

[47] Goldenberg DL. Fibromyalgia and its relation to chronic fatigue syndrome, viral illness and immune abnormalities. J Rheumatol Suppl 1989;19:91–3.

[48] Gracely RH, Grant MA, Giesecke T. Evoked pain measures in fibromyalgia. Best Pract Res Clin Rheumatol 2003;17:593–609.

[49] Gracely RH, Petzke F, Wolf JM, Clauw DJ. Functional magnetic resonance imaging evidence of augmented pain processing in fibromyalgia. Arthritis Rheum 2002;46:1333–43.
[50] Granges G, Littlejohn G. Pressure pain threshold in pain-free subjects, in patients with chronic regional pain syndromes, and in patients with fibromyalgia syndrome. Arthritis Rheum 1993;36:642–6.
[51] Guedj E, Cammilleri S, Colavolpe C, Taieb D, de Laforte C, Niboyet J, Mundler O. Predictive value of brain perfusion SPECT for ketamine response in hyperalgesic fibromyalgia. Eur J Nucl Med Mol Imaging 2007;34:1274–9.
[52] Guedj E, Taieb D, Cammilleri S, Lussato D, de Laforte C, Niboyet J, Mundler O. 99mTc-ECD brain perfusion SPECT in hyperalgesic fibromyalgia. Eur J Nucl Med Mol Imaging 2007;34:130–4.
[53] Hadler NM. If you have to prove you are ill, you can't get well. The object lesson of fibromyalgia. Spine 1996;21:2397–400.
[54] Harris RE, Clauw DJ. How do we know that the pain in fibromyalgia is "real"? Curr Pain Headache Rep 2006;10:403–7.
[55] Harris RE, Clauw DJ, Scott DJ, McLean SA, Gracely RH, Zubieta JK. Decreased central mu-opioid receptor availability in fibromyalgia. J Neurosci 2007;27:10000–6.
[56] Harris RE, Sundgren PC, Pang Y, Hsu M, Petrou M, Kim SH, McLean SA, Gracely RH, Clauw DJ. Dynamic levels of glutamate within the insula are associated with improvements in multiple pain domains in fibromyalgia. Arthritis Rheum 2008;58:903–7.
[57] Hazlett RL, Haynes SN. Fibromyalgia: a time-series analysis of the stressor-physical symptom association. J Behav Med 1992;15:541–58.
[58] Hudson JI, Goldenberg DL, Pope HGJ, Keck PEJ, Schlesinger L. Comorbidity of fibromyalgia with medical and psychiatric disorders. Am J Med 1993;92:363–7.
[59] Hudson JI, Hudson MS, Pliner LF, Goldenberg DL, Pope HGJ. Fibromyalgia and major affective disorder: A controlled phenomenology and family history study. Am J Psychiatry 1985;142:441–6.
[60] Jensen K, Andersen HO, Olesen J, Lindblom U. Pressure-pain threshold in human temporal region. Evaluation of a new pressure algometer. Pain 1986;25:313–23.
[61] Julien N, Goffaux P, Arsenault P, Marchand S. Widespread pain in fibromyalgia is related to a deficit of endogenous pain inhibition. Pain 2005;114:295–302.
[62] Kato K, Sullivan PF, Evengard B, Pedersen NL. Chronic widespread pain and its comorbidities: a population-based study. Arch Intern Med 2006;166:1649–54.
[63] Kim SH, Kim DH, Oh DH, Clauw DJ. Characteristic electron microscopic findings in the skin of patients with fibromyalgia—preliminary study. Clin Rheumatol 2008;27:407–11.
[64] Kop WJ, Lyden A, Berlin AA, Ambrose K, Olsen C, Gracely RH, Williams DA, Clauw DJ. Ambulatory monitoring of physical activity and symptoms in fibromyalgia and chronic fatigue syndrome. Arthritis Rheum 2005;52:296–303.
[65] Kosek E, Ekholm J, Hansson P. Sensory dysfunction in fibromyalgia patients with implications for pathogenic mechanisms. Pain 1996;68:375–83.
[66] Kosek E, Hansson P. Modulatory influence on somatosensory perception from vibration and heterotopic noxious conditioning stimulation (HNCS) in fibromyalgia patients and healthy subjects. Pain 1997;70:41–51.
[67] Kuchinad A, Schweinhardt P, Seminowicz DA, Wood PB, Chizh BA, Bushnell MC. Accelerated brain gray matter loss in fibromyalgia patients: premature aging of the brain? J Neurosci 2007;27:4004–7.
[68] Kwiatek R, Barnden L, Tedman R, Jarrett R, Chew J, Rowe C, Pile K. Regional cerebral blood flow in fibromyalgia: single-photon-emission computed tomography evidence of reduction in the pontine tegmentum and thalami. Arthritis Rheum 2000;43:2823–33.
[69] Landis CA, Lentz MJ, Rothermel J, Buchwald D, Shaver JL. Decreased sleep spindles and spindle activity in midlife women with fibromyalgia and pain. Sleep 2004;27:741–50.
[70] Lautenbacher S, Rollman GB. Possible deficiencies of pain modulation in fibromyalgia. Clin J Pain 1997;13:189–96.
[71] Leffler AS, Hansson P, Kosek E. Somatosensory perception in a remote pain-free area and function of diffuse noxious inhibitory controls (DNIC) in patients suffering from long-term trapezius myalgia. Eur J Pain 2002;6:149–59.

[72] Martinez-Lavin M. Dysfunction of the autonomic nervous system in chronic pain syndromes. In: Wallace DJ, Clauw DJ, editors. Fibromyalgia and other central pain syndromes. Philadelphia: Lippincott Williams and Wilkins; 2005. pp 81–8.

[73] Martinez-Lavin M, Hermosillo AG, Rosas M, Soto ME. Circadian studies of autonomic nervous balance in patients with fibromyalgia: a heart rate variability analysis. Arthritis Rheum 1998;41:1966–71.

[74] McBeth J, Jones K. Epidemiology of chronic musculoskeletal pain. Best Pract Res Clin Rheumatol 2007;21:403–25.

[75] McBeth J, Silman AJ, Gupta A, Chiu YH, Ray D, Morriss R, Dickens C, King Y, Macfarlane GJ. Moderation of psychosocial risk factors through dysfunction of the hypothalamic-pituitary-adrenal stress axis in the onset of chronic widespread musculoskeletal pain: findings of a population-based prospective cohort study. Arthritis Rheum 2007;56:360–71.

[76] McDermid AJ, Rollman GB, McCain GA. Generalized hypervigilance in fibromyalgia: Evidence of perceptual amplification. Pain 1996;66:133–44.

[77] McLean SA, Clauw DJ. Predicting chronic symptoms after an acute "stressor"—lessons learned from 3 medical conditions. Med Hypotheses 2004;63:653–8.

[78] McLean SA, Williams DA, Groner KH, Ambrose K, Lyden A, Gracely RH, Crofford LJ, Geisser ME, Biswas P, Clauw DJ. Naturalistic evaluation of cortisol secretion and symptoms in fibromyalgia and healthy controls. Arthritis Rheum 2005;52:3660–9.

[79] McLean SA, Williams DA, Stein PK, Harris RE, Lyden AK, Whalen G, Park KM, Liberzon I, Sen A, Gracely RH, Baraniuk JN, Clauw DJ. Cerebrospinal fluid corticotropin-releasing factor concentration is associated with pain but not fatigue symptoms in patients with fibromyalgia. Neuropsychopharmacology 2006;31:2776–82.

[80] Mease PJ, Clauw DJ, Arnold LM, Goldenberg DL, Witter J, Williams DA, Simon LS, Strand CV, Bramson C, Martin S, Wright TM, Littman B, Wernicke JF, Gendreau RM, Crofford LJ. Fibromyalgia syndrome. J Rheumatol 2005;32:2270–7.

[81] Moldofsky H. Sleep, neuroimmune and neuroendocrine functions in fibromyalgia and chronic fatigue syndrome. Adv Neuroimmunol 1995;5:39–56.

[82] Moldofsky H. Sleep and pain. Sleep Med Rev 2001;5:385–96.

[83] Moldofsky H, Scarisbrick P, England R, Smythe H. Musculoskeletal symptoms and non-REM sleep disturbance in patients with "fibrositis syndrome" and healthy subjects. Psychosom Med 1975;37:341–51.

[84] Mountz JM, Bradley LA, Modell JG, Alexander RW, Triana-Alexander M, Aaron LA, Stewart KE, Alarcon GS, Mountz JD. Fibromyalgia in women. Abnormalities of regional cerebral blood flow in the thalamus and the caudate nucleus are associated with low pain threshold levels. Arthritis Rheum 1995;38:926–38.

[85] Offenbaecher M, Bondy B, de Jonge S, Glatzeder K, Kruger M, Schoeps P, Ackenheil M. Possible association of fibromyalgia with a polymorphism in the serotonin transporter gene regulatory region. Arthritis Rheum 1999;42:2482–8.

[86] Older SA, Battafarano DF, Danning CL, Ward JA, Grady EP, Derman S, Russell IJ. The effects of delta wave sleep interruption on pain thresholds and fibromyalgia-like symptoms in healthy subjects; correlations with insulin-like growth factor I. J Rheumatol 1998;25:1180–6.

[87] Park JH, Phothimat P, Oates CT, Hernanz-Schulman M, Olsen NJ. Use of P-31 magnetic resonance spectroscopy to detect metabolic abnormalities in muscles of patients with fibromyalgia. Arthritis & Rheumatism 1998;41:406–13.

[88] Petzke F, Clauw DJ, Ambrose K, Khine A, Gracely RH. Increased pain sensitivity in fibromyalgia: effects of stimulus type and mode of presentation. Pain 2003;105:403–13.

[89] Petzke F, Gracely RH, Khine A, Clauw DJ. Pain sensitivity in patients with fibromyalgia (FM): Expectancy effects on pain measurements. Arthritis & Rheumatism 1999;42:S342.

[90] Petzke F, Gracely RH, Park KM, Ambrose K, Clauw DJ. What do tender points measure? Influence of distress on 4 measures of tenderness. J Rheumatol 2003;30:567–74.

[91] Petzke F, Khine A, Williams D, Groner K, Clauw DJ, Gracely RH. Dolorimetry performed at 3 paired tender points highly predicts overall tenderness. J Rheumatol 2001;28:2568–9.

[92] Pillow DR, Zautra AJ, Sandler I. Major life events and minor stressors: identifying mediational links in the stress process. J Pers Soc Psychol 1996;70:381–94.

[93] Price DD. Psychological and neural mechanism of the affective dimension of pain. Science 2000;288:1769–72.
[94] Qiao ZG, Vaeroy H, Morkrid L. Electrodermal and microcirculatory activity in patients with fibromyalgia during baseline, acoustic stimulation and cold pressor tests. J Rheumatol 1991;18:1383–9.
[95] Raphael KG, Natelson BH, Janal MN, Nayak S. A community-based survey of fibromyalgia-like pain complaints following the World Trade Center terrorist attacks. Pain 2002;100:131–9.
[96] Rizzi M, Sarzi-Puttini P, Atzeni F, Capsoni F, Andreoli A, Pecis M, Colombo S, Carrabba M, Sergi M. Cyclic alternating pattern: a new marker of sleep alteration in patients with fibromyalgia? J Rheumatol 2004;31:1193–9.
[97] Russell IJ, Orr MD, Littman B, Vipraio GA, Alboukrek D, Michalek JE, Lopez Y, MacKillip F. Elevated cerebrospinal fluid levels of substance P in patients with the fibromyalgia syndrome. Arthritis Rheum 1994;37:1593–601.
[98] Russell IJ, Vaeroy H, Javors M, Nyberg F. Cerebrospinal fluid biogenic amine metabolites in fibromyalgia/fibrositis syndrome and rheumatoid arthritis. Arthritis Rheum 1992;35:550–6.
[99] Sapolsky RM. Why stress is bad for your brain. Science 1996;273:749–50.
[100] Sarchielli P, Di Filippo M, Nardi K, Calabresi P. Sensitization, glutamate, and the link between migraine and fibromyalgia. Curr Pain Headache Rep 2007;11:343–51.
[101] Sarzi-Puttini P, Rizzi M, Andreoli A, Panni B, Pecis M, Colombo S, Turiel M, Carrabba M, Sergi M. Hypersomnolence in fibromyalgia syndrome. Clin Exp Rheumatol 2002;20:69–72.
[102] Sergi M, Rizzi M, Braghiroli A, Sarzi PP, Greco M, Cazzola M, Andreoli A. Periodic breathing during sleep in patients affected by fibromyalgia syndrome. Eur Respir J 1999;14:203–8.
[103] Simms RW, Roy SH, Hrovat M, Anderson JJ, Skrinar G, LePoole SR, Zerbini CA, de Luca C, Jolesz F. Lack of association between fibromyalgia syndrome and abnormalities in muscle energy metabolism. Arthritis Rheum 1994;37:794–800.
[104] Smythe HA, Moldofsky H. Two contributions to understanding of the "fibrositis" syndrome. Bull Rheum Dis 1977;28:928–31.
[105] Sundgren PC, Petrou M, Harris RE, Fan X, Foerster B, Mehrotra N, Sen A, Clauw DJ, Welsh RC. Diffusion-weighted and diffusion tensor imaging in fibromyalgia patients: a prospective study of whole brain diffusivity, apparent diffusion coefficient, and fraction anisotropy in different regions of the brain and correlation with symptom severity. Acad Radiol 2007;14:839–46.
[106] Tracey I, Mantyh PW. The cerebral signature for pain perception and its modulation. Neuron 2007;55:377–91.
[107] Turk DC, Okifuji A, Sinclair JD, Starz TW. Pain, disability, and physical functioning in subgroups of patients with fibromyalgia. J Rheumatol 1996;23:1255–62.
[108] Vaeroy H, Helle R, Forre O, Kass E, Terenius L. Elevated CSF levels of substance P and high incidence of Raynaud phenomenon in patients with fibromyalgia: new features for diagnosis. Pain 1988;32:21–6.
[109] Waylonis GW, Perkins RH. Post-traumatic fibromyalgia. A long-term follow-up. Am J Phys Med Rehabil 1994;73:403–12.
[110] Welin M, Bragee B, Nyberg F, Kristiansson M. Elevated Substance P levels are contrasted by a decrease in met-enkephalin-arg-phe levels in CSF from fibromyalgia patients. J Musculoskel Pain 1995;3:4.
[111] White KP, Nielson WR, Harth M, Ostbye T, Speechley M. Does the label "fibromyalgia" alter health status, function, and health service utilization? A prospective, within-group comparison in a community cohort of adults with chronic widespread pain. Arthritis Rheum 2002;47:260–5.
[112] Wilder-Smith CH, Robert-Yap J. Abnormal endogenous pain modulation and somatic and visceral hypersensitivity in female patients with irritable bowel syndrome. World J Gastroenterol 2007;13:3699–704.
[113] Williams DA, Brown SC, Clauw DJ, Gendreau RM. Self-reported symptoms before and after September 11 in patients with fibromyalgia. JAMA 2003;289:1637–8.
[114] Williams DA, Gracely RH. Biology and therapy of fibromyalgia. Functional magnetic resonance imaging findings in fibromyalgia. Arthritis Res Ther 2006;8:224.
[115] Wolfe F. The relation between tender points and fibromyalgia symptom variables: evidence that fibromyalgia is not a discrete disorder in the clinic. Ann Rheum Dis 1997;56:268–71.

[116] Wolfe F, Hawley DJ. Psychosocial factors and the fibromyalgia syndrome. Z Rheumatol 1998;57 Suppl 2:88–91.
[117] Wolfe F, Ross K, Anderson J, Russell IJ. Aspects of fibromyalgia in the general population: Sex, pain threshold, and fibromyalgia symptoms. J Rheumatol 1995;22:151–6.
[118] Wolfe F, Ross K, Anderson J, Russell IJ, Hebert L. The prevalence and characteristics of fibromyalgia in the general population. Arthritis Rheum 1995;38:19–28.
[119] Wolfe F, Smythe HA, Yunus MB, Bennett RM, Bombardier C, Goldenberg DL, Tugwell P, Campbell SM, Abeles M, Clark P. The American College of Rheumatology 1990 Criteria for the Classification of Fibromyalgia. Report of the Multicenter Criteria Committee. Arthritis Rheum 1990;33:160–72.
[120] Wood PB, Patterson JC, Sunderland JJ, Tainter KH, Glabus MF, Lilien DL. Reduced presynaptic dopamine activity in fibromyalgia syndrome demonstrated with positron emission tomography: a pilot study. J Pain 2007;8:51–8.
[121] Woolf CJ. Windup and central sensitization are not equivalent. Pain 1996;66:105–8.
[122] Woolf CJ, Thompson SW. The induction and maintenance of central sensitization is dependent on N-methyl-D-aspartic acid receptor activation; implications for the treatment of post-injury pain hypersensitivity states. Pain 1991;44:293–9.
[123] Xu XJ, Dalsgaard CJ, Wiesenfeld-Hallin Z. Spinal substance P and N-methyl-D-aspartate receptors are coactivated in the induction of central sensitization of the nociceptive flexor reflex. Neuroscience 1992;51:641–8.
[124] Yunus M, Masi AT, Calabro JJ, Miller KA, Feigenbaum SL. Primary fibromyalgia (fibrositis): Clinical study of 50 patients with matched normal controls. Semin Arthritis Rheum 1981;11:151–71.
[125] Yunus MB. Towards a model of pathophysiology of fibromyalgia: aberrant central pain mechanisms with peripheral modulation. J Rheumatol 1992;19:846–50.
[126] Yunus MB. Symptoms and signs of fibromyalgia syndrome: an overview. In: Wallace DJ, Clauw DJ, editors. Fibromyalgia and other central pain syndromes. Philadelphia: Lippincott Williams & Wilkins; 2005. pp 125–32.
[127] Yunus MB. Central sensitivity syndromes: a new paradigm and group nosology for fibromyalgia and overlapping conditions, and the related issue of disease versus illness. Semin Arthritis Rheum 2008;37:339–52.
[128] Yunus MB, Dailey JW, Aldag JC, Masi AT, Jobe PC. Plasma tryptophan and other amino acids in primary fibromyalgia: a controlled study. J Rheumatol 1992;19:90–4.
[129] Yunus MB, Young CS, Saeed AS, Aldag JC. Positron emission tomography (PET) imaging of the brain in fibromyalgia syndrome (FMS). Arthritis Rheum 1997;40(9S):970.

Correspondence to: Daniel J. Clauw, MD, Department of Anesthesiology, 24 Frank Lloyd Wright Drive, Lobby M, University of Michigan, Ann Arbor, MI 48106, USA. Email: dclauw@med.umich.edu.

Low Back Pain

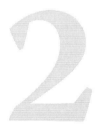

James P. Robinson[a] and A. Vania Apkarian[b]

[a]Department of Rehabilitation Medicine, University of Washington, Seattle, Washington, USA;
[b]Departments of Physiology, Anesthesia, and Surgery, and Lurie Cancer Center, Feinberg School of Medicine, Northwestern University, Chicago, Illinois, USA

Low back pain is a common scourge in Western societies and seems to be a prevalent problem worldwide [42,46,63]. In this chapter, we discuss whether such pain should be considered a straightforward consequence of injury/dysfunction of the spine, or the result of more complex processes involving nervous system processing of sensory information.

Low Back Pain: Definitions and Distinctions

Some clarification of the descriptive term "low back pain" is needed. For purposes of a case definition, it is usually defined as pain involving the lumbar region or the gluteal region. At the outset, it is important to distinguish among several different disorders that are associated with low back pain. Some have nothing to do with the spine; for example, endometriosis and pancreatic carcinoma can cause referred pain to the low back.

Among conditions that are thought to involve intrinsic pathology of the lumbar spine, three categories can be distinguished. First, pain can be secondary to a specific, well-characterized disorder of the spine;

examples include vertebral body fractures and metastatic lesions. Sciatica is the second category of intrinsic spinal disorder. By definition, patients with sciatica experience pain radiating into one or both of their legs, and they may not be aware of significant back pain. However, sciatica is classified as a low back disorder because it is almost always a result of pathology in the lumbar spine. The final, and most enigmatic category, is nonspecific LBP (NSLBP). Patients with nonspecific LBP experience pain in the lumbar, lumbosacral, or gluteal regions, and physicians believe that the pain stems from intrinsic spinal pathology. However, as discussed below, it has been exceedingly difficult to identify the pathology underlying NSLBP. The underwhelming results of attempts to characterize the pathophysiological basis of NSLBP have led some to speculate that the condition might have more in common with functional syndromes such as fibromyalgia than with orthopedic conditions such as a torn anterior cruciate ligament in the knee.

Another important distinction is between acute (short-term) LBP and chronic LBP that seriously disrupts a patient's life. Although perhaps 80% of the U.S. population experience episodes of LBP during their lives [37], most of them recover well from their episodes. For these people, episodic LBP represents a nuisance, but not a major health problem. Other individuals experience LBP over extended periods of time, but are able to go on with their lives despite their symptoms [94,96]. Some individuals, however, develop persistent LBP that seriously interferes with major life activities such as working. This chapter will focus on chronic, disabling LBP for two practical reasons. First, LBP becomes a serious health problem only when it is chronic and causes prolonged disability. Second, most attempts to understand the biology of LBP are carried out in patients who are developing or have developed chronic, disabling LBP.

Conceptual Models for Nonspecific Low Back Pain

The End-Organ Dysfunction Model

Most researchers who study NSLBP and most clinicians who treat the problem assume that the symptoms reflect structural abnormalities (lesions) in the lumbar spine due to some combination of injuries and degenerative changes. The fundamental premise of this model is that patients feel back pain because of a nociceptive focus in the spine. Thus, the pain experiences of patients represent normal functioning of the nervous system in the context of tissue injury/dysfunction.

Altered Nervous System Processing Models

We are not aware of any publications that articulate alternatives to the end-organ dysfunction model and compare them with that model. However, we believe it is appropriate to group these alternatives under the general rubric "altered nervous system processing models." The fundamental premise in these models is that patients with NSLBP suffer from alterations in nervous system encoding or processing of sensory information, rather than from ongoing injury or dysfunction in some structure in the lumbar spine. While various altered nervous system processing models share a rejection of the straightforward link between pathology in the end organ (the lumbar spine) and the experience of pain, they differ in the alternative path postulated.

These alternatives include the following: (1) Chronic LBP starts with a structural lesion focus in the spine, but the nociceptive barrage associated with this condition leads to sensitization of the central nervous system (CNS). Thus, over time, the pain that a patient experiences becomes autonomous from the structural lesion that initially subserved it. (2) Nociceptive input from other areas of the body might cause a generalized sensitization of the CNS. This model implies that a patient's experience of chronic LBP has its origins in a structural lesion with nociception, but that the offending lesion might be located in some other part of the body. (3) The key factor underlying LBP might be heightened susceptibility to pain, because of either genetic factors or a variety of psychological traits.

Domains of Evidence

In this chapter, we review evidence that bears on the plausibility of these two models (or classes of models) to explain NSLBP. The evidence falls into several domains. Although the evidence within each domain (except the last) is not determinative, it at least provides support for one model or the other. The following domains are considered: (1) the presence of a distinct event that causes symptoms; (2) symptoms correlate with a well-defined, characteristic biological abnormality; (3) genetics; (4) co-occurrence with other pain syndromes; (5) co-occurrence with emotional dysfunction; (6) evidence of abnormal functioning in the nervous system; (7) response to treatment.

The Presence of a Distinct Event That Causes Symptoms

The end-organ dysfunction model is most plausible when a person's symptoms can be traced back to a distinct injury involving overwhelming mechanical forces. Examples include an individual who falls with her arm outstretched and sustains a Colles fracture of the wrist, or the running back in football whose knee is twisted as he is tackled and sustains a tear of the anterior cruciate ligament of the knee. In contrast, NSLBP that develops insidiously, in the absence of injury, would at least suggest some variants of the altered nervous system processing model.

A striking feature of NSLBP is that it often begins in the absence of a definable biomechanical load [22]. The absence of any characteristic mechanical trauma at the time when LBP starts does not necessarily negate the end-organ dysfunction model. For example, it might be appropriate to construe NSLBP as a repetitive strain or cumulative trauma disorder, similar to disorders that are seen in the upper extremities. From this perspective, NSLBP is viewed as being caused by mechanical loads put on the spine, but not necessarily by the load that immediately preceded the onset of symptoms. However, the fact that NSLBP frequently starts in the absence of any definable mechanical load raises the possibility that altered nervous system processing is the primary problem in NSLBP, whereas mechanical loads and structural lesions may have little to do with the symptoms that patients experience.

Correlation of Symptoms with a Well-Defined, Characteristic Biological Abnormality

A primary goal in characterizing any medical disorder is to find a biological abnormality that is characteristic of the disorder and correlates well with subjective indicators of the disorder. Examples abound, such as serum glucose level for diabetes, an S3 and cardiomegaly for left ventricular failure, and so on. Conversely, if no biological indicator can be found that correlates with symptoms of a disorder, the possibility emerges that patients reporting the symptoms are suffering from something other than end-organ dysfunction.

Nonspecific LBP has been an enigma precisely because the symptoms patients report are only loosely correlated with indices of biological pathology in the lumbar spine. Specialists in musculoskeletal medicine typically rely primarily on imaging studies to understand the symptoms of the patients they evaluate. For patients with NSLBP, imaging studies have focused primarily on intervertebral disks and facet joints. It is beyond the scope of this chapter to review the hundreds of studies that have been performed to determine the associations between abnormalities demonstrated in imaging studies of these structures and LBP. One of the many challenges in reviewing this literature is that multiple imaging modalities have been used on the lumbar spine, including plain X-rays, computed tomography scans, myelograms, magnetic resonance imaging (MRI) scans, bone scans, and single photon emission computed tomography (SPECT) scans. Moreover, physicians have evolved in their thinking about the findings considered to be significant on these scans. For example, radiologists who interpreted lumbar MRI scans during the 1980s routinely commented on indices of disk degeneration, such as disk dessication and disk space narrowing, and clinicians widely assumed that these radiographic findings identified individuals with diskogenic pain. However, in 1988, Modic and colleagues [69] studied changes in the vertebral bodies above and below degenerated disks. There is evidence that the "Modic" changes identified by these authors are more closely associated with NSLBP symptoms than are changes in the appearance of intervertebral disks [57]. Thus, the search for visible evidence of structural abnormalities that can account for NSLBP is by no means over.

Results to date, however, have been discouraging with respect to the significance of abnormalities in disks and facet joints. Historically, there has been a tendency for research to identify an anatomical finding that might be clinically significant for LBP patients, only to be followed by research showing a high prevalence of the finding in asymptomatic individuals [15,50,52,98], along with the inability of the putative finding to predict low back symptoms in longitudinal studies [18,19,23]. Reasonable conclusions from the abundant evidence now available are that: (a) degenerative changes in lumbar intervertebral disks and facet joints are highly prevalent in individuals with and without LBP; (b) these changes increase as a function of the age of the individuals, and (c) associations between abnormalities in these structures and symptoms are modest.

Another approach to diagnosing structural pathology in the spine uses pain provocation and palliation techniques [16,17,28,47]. The basic logic underlying this approach is that a pain generator can be identified on the basis of a patient's responses to interventions designed to provoke pain (e.g., by injection of hypertonic saline) or to palliate pain (by injection of a local anesthetic). A well-studied example of this general approach is provocative diskography, in which patients' responses of to intradiskal injections of contrast dye (to provoke pain as well as to define the anatomy of a disk) and local anesthetic are used to infer whether a particular disk is playing a major role in clinical pain [28].

Two approaches involving pain provocation and palliation have been used to determine whether lumbar facet joints play a significant role in the pain of patients with LBP. One approach is to inject a joint suspected to be the source of a patient's pain with a local anesthetic (with or without an accompanying corticosteroid) [61]. The other, designated "medial branch block," is to inject the sensory nerves that innervate a suspected facet joint [65].

Whereas the clinical significance of abnormalities noted on imaging studies can be evaluated by determining the prevalence of the findings in asymptomatic individuals, the significance of results from provocative/palliative procedures is more difficult to determine. In principle, one might rely on face validity and assert that if a patient reports substantial relief of his or her typical LBP following injection of a facet joint, it proves that the facet joint was the generator of the pain. However, this analysis is challenged by the high placebo response rate to anesthetic injections in the spine [10,21,25,26,64,88], and it is generally not accepted by clinicians or researchers. A more persuasive argument for the significance of pain provocation/palliation procedures is the demonstration that when structures diagnosed by these procedures are treated, patients reliably demonstrate long-term clinical improvement. For example, if a facet joint is believed to be the cause of a patient's symptoms, it can be treated by a facet neurotomy, which involves radiofrequency ablation of the sensory nerves from the joint. If such treatment reliably leads to long-term symptomatic improvement, it would strengthen the hypothesis that the suspected facet joint was in fact the pain generator for that patient. As discussed below, there is some evidence for effectiveness of facet neurotomies in carefully selected LBP patients.

In summary, attempts to identify pain generators in patients with NSLBP via anatomical studies or pain provocation/palliation techniques have met with some success. Some observers emphasize the difficulty of achieving specific diagnoses in these patients, but in doing so they typically either give no substantiating evidence [101] or hearken back to opinions stated in a publication from 1982 [97] as evidence of the difficulty of achieving specific diagnoses in NSLBP [79]. We are not aware of any serious attempt to estimate the percentage of NSLBP patients for whom specific structural diagnoses can be achieved on the basis of currently available imaging and pain provocation/palliation procedures. It is almost certainly the case, however, that attempts to identify a pain generator to account for the symptoms of patients with NSLBP often fail. These failures raise the possibility that the pain reported by the patients is not closely associated with a structural lesion in the spine.

Genetics and Low Back Pain

Genetic research could in principle support either the end-organ dysfunction model or the altered nervous system models. If, for example, research demonstrated a genetic basis for degeneration of the spine, and the degenerative changes were closely associated with LBP symptoms, the evidence would support an end-organ dysfunction model (although it would focus on host "resistance" rather than on environmental insults). Conversely, evidence that pain sensitivity has a genetic basis would tend to support the hypothesis that LBP is largely the result of heightened pain sensitivity.

Research in monozygotic and dizygotic twins has shown that disk degeneration, as measured by MRI scan, is strongly influenced by genetic factors, with heritability ranging from 51% [12] to 74% [83]. Other research has shown that an increased risk of disk degeneration is associated with various polymorphisms, including the Trp2 tryptophan allele [48], two alleles of the interleukin-1 gene family [90], and polymorphisms of the vitamin D receptor gene [56]. In the aggregate, these studies support the conclusion that genetic factors strongly affect a structure in the spine that is thought to subserve LBP, whereas environmental stressors have a surprisingly weak effect [11].

In terms of the issues addressed in this chapter, the above findings are consistent with the end-organ dysfunction model, but they do not provide conclusive evidence for it. The problem is that although disk degeneration is thought to be a major contributor to back pain, multiple studies have found only weak associations to support such a premise. Not surprisingly, evidence for a genetic basis for LBP has been less clearcut than evidence for a genetic basis for disk degeneration. Battie et al. [12] note that various studies have shown that genetic factors account for anywhere between 0% and 57% of the variance in back pain reporting. In their study, Battie et al. used statistical modeling to infer the extent to which disk degeneration and reported LBP reflected shared genetic influences. Their data supported the conclusion that "disk degeneration is one pathway through which genes influence back pain problems" (p. 278), but they noted that the majority of variance in reported back pain could not be explained on the basis of either genetic factors or the environmental factors that they investigated.

While research demonstrating a genetic basis for degeneration of an important structure in the spine supports the end organ dysfunction model of NSLBP, other genetic research supports the conclusion that pain perception and pain sensitivity are influenced by genetic factors. Since this research is reviewed in another chapter, it will not be summarized here. Suffice it to say that genetic evidence cuts both ways with respect to the appropriateness of the end-organ dysfunction model versus models of altered nervous system functioning.

Co-occurrence with Other Pain Syndromes

The end-organ injury model suggests that LBP should occur independently of any other painful condition. A patient with LBP obviously might have some other painful disorders, such as chronic headaches. However, the frequency of co-occurrence of LBP and chronic headaches should be no more than the joint probability of occurrence of two independent events: i.e., p(LBP + headaches) = p(LBP) × p(headaches). In contrast, some versions of the altered nervous system model imply that people who suffer from chronic LBP are predisposed to painful disorders. Thus, in a cohort of LBP patients, one would expect to find other painful disorders (e.g., headaches, neck pain, fibromyalgia, TMD, and abdominal pain) to occur disproportionately. Research generally supports the hypothesis that individuals with LBP are at higher risk than others to report additional chronic pain syndromes, including neck pain [55], TMJD [99], arthritis and headaches [95].

The covariation between LBP and other pain syndromes is more consistent with altered nervous system processing models than with the end-organ dysfunction model. This point is made in an article by Croft et al. [30], who state: "One explanation [for the co-variation] is an underlying generalized vulnerability to chronic pain. Theories and empirical data about central pain and pain processing, and about the plastic memory of the nervous system for pain operating independently of the initial site of nociceptive stimulus, together provide relevant mechanisms for the epidemiological observations. The implication is that these processes will always produce an association between any two chronic pain syndromes stronger than the estimate derived from their separate occurrence rates." (p. 237).

Co-occurrence with Emotional Dysfunction

The end-organ dysfunction model emphasizes mechanical and biological causes of NSLBP rather than psychological ones. The model thus implies that prior to the onset of their pain, LBP patients should be indistinguishable from the general public with respect to psychiatric dysfunction. Of course, individuals who develop a painful condition that negatively affects their ability to function in important social roles, they would be at risk for secondary psychiatric problems such as anxiety or depressive disorders. Thus, evidence that people with NSLBP subsequently develop emotional distress is compatible with the end-organ dysfunction model. In contrast, at least some versions of the altered nervous system model invoke psychological vulnerabilities as a key causal factor in chronic LBP. Thus, the demonstration of increased premorbid psychiatric dysfunction among patients with chronic LBP would support the altered nervous system model.

Evidence regarding premorbid psychological functioning in individuals with functional pain syndromes is discussed in several chapters of this volume, and therefore will not be summarized in any detail here. A cursory review of this literature, however, reveals evidence to support the significance of these premorbid factors. For example, recent epidemiological studies have found that the risk of LBP is increased among individuals who have experienced stressful events or psychological dysfunction during childhood and early adulthood. Specific predictors have included adverse circumstances or dysfunctional behavior on the part of participants' parents (unemployment, divorce, or substance abuse), physical abuse, frightening experiences, prolonged hospitalizations, moderate to high levels of reported psychological distress, and a history of emotional or behavioral disorders [58,71]. Also, there is evidence that psychosocial factors in the workplace—such as job satisfaction, perceived control over work demands and job insecurity—influence the occurrence and/or duration of episodes of LBP [13,41,60].

However, premorbid psychological distress and psychosocial stressors are only modestly associated with subsequent LBP, and they do not stand out as predictors in comparison to multiple other factors. Rubin [82] summarizes the situation as follows: "The risk factors for the development of spine pain are multidimensional, with physical attributes, socioeconomic status, general medical health and psychological state, and occupational environmental factors all playing a role in contributing to the risk for experiencing pain" (p. 367).

Thus, while research data support the view that psychological dysfunction and psychosocial stressors increase the risk of LBP, they do not provide overwhelming evidence for the importance of these factors.

Evidence of Abnormal Functioning in the Nervous System

Prior to reviewing the human evidence regarding the role of the CNS in LBP, it is helpful to look at the basic science work regarding peripheral and central plasticity following peripheral inflammatory and neuropathic injuries. This is a vast topic and the information available continues to expand. Here we only attempt to review the general observations in an effort to clarify the notions of end-organ dysfunction or altered nervous system processing regarding LBP symptoms.

There is ample evidence that sustained peripheral injury, be it inflammatory or neuropathic, causes local reorganization of nociceptive and non-nociceptive afferents. Depending on the type of injury, different afferent fiber types begin expressing novel Na^+ channels, neuropeptides, cytokines, and many other chemicals. These substances lead to preferential changes in excitability of afferents to external (painful and nonpainful) stimuli and also to changes in resting membrane properties, such that nociceptors that in healthy tissue are usually silent and are only activated with proper stimuli can now generate spontaneous action potentials and become contributors to perception of pain in the absence of external stimuli [3,39,49,54,100]. Physiologically, the sum total of such changes in responsiveness of peripheral afferents can be viewed as the end-organ dysfunction. The very simple fact that LBP patients point to their back as the source of the pain may be construed as evidence for end-organ dysfunction, but the counterexample is patients with various phantom pain sensations for body parts that are completely missing, indicating that central processes in the absence of an end organ still may give rise to pains localized to specific body parts. On the other hand, simple everyday observations regarding changes in levels of LBP by body repositioning, by hot or cold presses, or other manipulations of the site where the pain is felt (clinical procedures that are reviewed below) provide some evidence that the end organ is probably involved in LBP.

The spinal cord dorsal horn is the first relay and central processing site for nociception, and basic science studies provide ample evidence for plasticity in afferent input processing in various animal models for persistent pain [3,39,49,54,100]. Overall, the evidence points to increased gain for nociceptive signaling, which may affect specific spinocephalad pathways, depending on the type of peripheral injury. These studies also indicate that descending modulatory circuitry is fundamentally involved in this change of nociceptive gain. Thus, the animal studies point to increased gain in both the periphery and the spinal cord for chronic pain models.

Given that descending modulatory circuits integrate supraspinal cortical and subcortical information, changes in properties of descending modulation point to the role of cortical influences on the spinal cord processing of nociception, and evidence is in fact accumulating in this direction. Studies in rodents now show that manipulating local circuitry in the anterior cingulate, amygdala, insula, and medial prefrontal cortex modulates pain behavior and also changes response properties of spinal cord nociceptors, and further show that in various neuropathic or inflammatory conditions, response properties in multiple supraspinal regions are also modified [6,51,53,73]. This circuitry must play a role in the mechanisms by which learned behavior can modify responses to painful stimuli, and reciprocally pain experiences induce changes in behavior and learning and memory, sometimes causing fear, anxiety, and depression.

Yet even at the level of the spinal cord circuitry, there are clear signs of specialization between elements involved in acute nociception and others subserving hyperalgesia and allodynia. When procedures are performed in experimental animals to selectively destroy nociceptive neurons located in lamina I of the spinal dorsal horn, which express the receptor for substance P, and many of which project supraspinally, then neither inflammation nor neuropathy leads to full expression of hyperalgesia [66]. On the other hand, the animals' responses to acute noxious stimuli are not altered. Thus, these neurons seem important for the development of hyperalgesia, but not essential for acute pain.

Consistent and complementary to these results are studies from Sandkühler's laboratory, where spinal cord long-term potentiation (LTP) and depression (LTD)—forms of enhancement or depression of synaptic inputs—have been studied for nociceptive inputs. The results demonstrate that distinct frequency stimulation of afferents can cause LTP on specific dorsal horn cells with specific supraspinal targets [84]. There is also evidence that inflammatory and neuropathic injuries differentially affect expression of various neuropeptides and related receptors in the spinal cord, and at least in neuropathic conditions spinal cord neurons undergo apoptosis [39]. Animal behavioral studies now convincingly demonstrate the influence of genetics on pain behavior as well [70]. With this overview of the animal evidence regarding peripheral and central nervous system involvement in chronic pain, we will try to map the observations in humans with LBP and discuss the extent to which current evidence favors peripheral versus central events underlying this clinical condition.

Non-invasive brain imaging techniques provide direct access to the brain, and patients with LBP have now been studied with a variety of such approaches. The bulk of the evidence in this area comes from the laboratory of one of the authors of this chapter, and as a result the evidence remains limited and awaits validation by other investigators. Still, for almost 10 years patients' brain properties have been studied and various abnormalities observed. These abnormalities can be divided into three categories: functional, anatomical, and cognitive.

Functional Abnormalities

Even though one can question whether any of the animal models approximate LBP, and especially NSLBP, and keeping in mind that the details of peripheral and spinal cord plasticity are dependent on the specifics of the injury giving rise to pain behavior, the simplest expectation in LBP is enhanced nociceptive transmission from the periphery to supraspinal targets. Unfortunately, the electrophysiological properties of nociceptive afferents and of spinal cord neurons in humans with LBP remain unavailable for scientific observation, although there are hints that this limitation may soon be overcome. Non-invasive human brain imaging techniques, on the other hand, have made the rest of the CNS accessible for observation. As the spinothalamic pathway is commonly assumed to be the primary nociceptive signaling system in the CNS, then the cortical regions it subserves should indicate enhanced activity either for spontaneous pain or for various external painful, and even nonpainful, stimuli in LBP.

Only one study has demonstrated enhanced activity for spinothalamic representation [43]. The investigators examined brain activity for

pressure pain applied to the thumbnail and contrasted the results of patients with NSLBP with those of fibromyalgia patients and healthy subjects. In one set of experiments, the investigators contrasted brain activity for equal pressure stimuli. They observed that both groups of patients
reported higher pain perception and demonstrated activation of more
brain areas than the controls. When the experiment was conducted using stimuli that produced comparable pain perceptions across the three
groups, and thus were of lower intensity in the patients, then brain activity
was not different among groups [43]. In another similar study, thermal
pain was studied on the hand in NSLBP patients and contrasted to healthy
subjects. With this stimulus modality, no differences in brain activity were
observed, although stimulus or perception matching procedures were less
rigorous [32]. Thus, mechanical but not thermal pain perception may be
enhanced in NSLBP. Underlying mechanisms for this difference remain
obscure, and trivial explanations cannot be discounted, such as subjects'
increased attention to the modality and the influence of spontaneous pain
on other sensory modalities. Nevertheless, the result can also be construed
as pointing to the notion of central disposition for enhanced pain, at least
for pressure. Importantly, the brain regions where activity was higher in
NSLBP were the same regions responding to more intense stimuli in the
control subjects, suggesting that this activity is a pure increase in gain of
the system rather than a new representation.

A consistent brain activity pattern has been observed for acute
experimental painful stimuli in healthy subjects [2,77]. Multiple studies
(with the exception of the Giesecke et al. report [43]) indicate that instead of enhancement of brain regions identified for acute pain (assumed
to represent spinothalamic inputs), there is decreased activity in many
characteristic regions in response to noxious stimuli [2,31,76]. Furthermore, regions that cannot be considered part of the spinothalamic inputs
seem to show increased activity, mainly prefrontal cortical areas and related subcortical structures [2]. Thus, there seems to be a decrease in gain
in brain regions involved in acute pain and an increase in gain in areas
outside this representation. These changes could occur anywhere from
the dorsal horn to the cortex, although a spinal cord change in gain can
achieve the observed results most directly, with decreased transmission

through spinothalamic neurons and increased transmission through nociceptive nonspinothalamic pathways. The rest of this section discusses the evidence regarding these notions.

Ongoing spontaneous pain is a characteristic and common complaint of LBP patients. Recent evidence indicates that the perceived magnitude of this spontaneous pain fluctuates at the scale of seconds to minutes, with temporal characteristics that distinguish LBP from other chronic pain conditions [35]. When brain activity is examined for these spontaneous fluctuations of LBP, the only brain area that is observed to be activated is the medial prefrontal cortex (mPFC) [7]. When brain activity for thermal painful stimuli is examined in the same LBP patients, applied to the back at the LBP site, activity in the brain is completely different and closely matches that observed for acute pain in healthy subjects (Fig. 1).

The mPFC is a highly complex region, most elaborated in primates and especially in humans, and it is thought to be fundamentally involved in top-down modulation of behavior. Accordingly, one explanation of the difference between spontaneous pain and thermal pain representation would be that the former is mainly driven by emotional centers of the brain while the latter is a result of activating the end organs. This explanation is weakened by the observation that when spontaneous pain is increasing, the brain activity pattern closely corresponds to the pattern for thermal pain. Therefore, the argument advanced in the study is that a transient signal generated by the end organ invades the cortex, where it is then maintained and perpetuated in the mPFC, where the percept becomes more emotional and more self-referential [7]. Moreover, the mPFC activity is coupled with activation of the basal ganglia, amygdala, medial thalamus, and brainstem, which suggests that spinocephalad pathways outside of the spinothalamic tract are preferentially involved in sustained spontaneous LBP. Importantly, the activity observed in mPFC could explain the intensity of LBP experienced by the participants at a confidence level higher than 80%.

These results are reminiscent of the observations regarding the role of lamina I neurons expressing receptors for substance P, as well as the differential potentiation of spinal cord nociceptors with distinct frequency stimulation of peripheral nociceptive afferents described above.

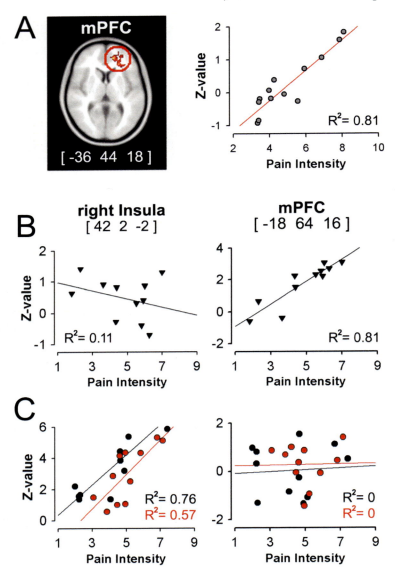

Fig. 1. The brain region identified as best correlated to intensity of back pain is distinct from that for thermal pain [7]. (A) The medial prefrontal cortex (mPFC) is the region best correlated to intensity of pain. The regression shows the relationship of the region to back pain intensity in each patient studied. (B) The graph again demonstrates that the mPFC activity best correlates to each patient's intensity of back pain, identified in a new group of patients, while activity in the right insula does not correlate with this parameter. (C) The right insula, but not the mPFC, correlates best to the thermal painful stimuli applied either to the patients or to a group of normal healthy subjects.

These findings imply that spontaneous pain of LBP involves a transient activation of the spinothalamic pathway (activation that is sustained for the duration of thermal painful stimuli in both LBP and in healthy subjects) and a novel, more sustained activation of pathways that access the amygdala, basal ganglia, and mPFC. Curiously, the transient activation when spontaneous LBP is increasing involves the insula, and the size of insular activation tightly and positively correlates with the number of years the patients have had LBP. This insular activity, again with a confidence level of more than 80%, reflects the duration of LBP.

Therefore, the two fundamental properties of LBP, namely its intensity and its duration, are directly observed in the brain activity of these patients. What are the mechanisms underlying this reorganization of pain representation in LBP? Can we rule out that the observed activity is a consequence of living, and coping, with LBP for a long number of years? Moreover, as soon as the end-organ input ceases, would these activity patterns revert to those of the healthy brain? These questions cannot be answered by functional imaging studies, although the evidence of insular activity reflecting duration of LBP suggests that pain duration is playing an important role in the observed brain activity.

The involvement of the end organ in LBP is suggested in a recent functional MRI (fMRI) study, where LBP patients used a 5% lidocaine patch on the affected site to control back pain [9]. The treatment did decrease intensity of spontaneous LBP, which was reflected in decreased mPFC activity. Although the mechanism by which lidocaine patches produce pain relief is uncertain [38,44], research to date supports the conclusion that they exert a local effect by blocking Na^+ channels in sensory afferents in the region where the patch is applied. Thus, the findings of Baliki et al. [9] support the conclusions that mPFC activity reflects the intensity of low back pain, and that it is modulated by end-organ input, or at least by input from afferents close to the end organ.

Even when LBP patients perform a simple, everyday motor-attentional task where their performance matches that of normal subjects, brain activity differs between the two groups [8]. In this case, however, the difference is only observed for negative activations; that is, the brain state is different when the subjects are not doing anything but is matched when they are engaged in the task. The result demonstrates that the brain of LBP patients is never truly at rest, with the presence of the pain distorting the properties and connectivity pattern of the resting brain in a complicated manner that is not yet understood. Are these changes simply a reflection of the presence of spontaneous LBP, and would the brain revert to normal when the pain is properly treated? At this stage we do not have the answers.

Anatomical Abnormalities

Evidence that the brain may be abnormal in individuals with LBP was first noted in a study that measured the local concentrations of various brain metabolites [45]. The authors noted a decreased concentration of N-acetyl-aspartate (a marker for neuronal density) in the dorsolateral prefrontal cortex (DLPFC), and suggested that the region may be undergoing atrophy in LBP. A subsequent automated anatomical morphometric study confirmed this observation and showed that both the DLPFC and thalamus show gray matter atrophy in cases of LBP [5]. This general observation—decreased brain regional gray matter in chronic pain—has now been confirmed by a number of studies from various laboratories and for a variety of other clinical pain conditions (Figs. 2 and 3). For LBP, the extent of atrophy could be linked to the number of years the patients were living with the condition, suggesting that at least part of the process is a consequence of the persistence of LBP. Importantly, this study had a patient group large enough to be subdivided into one group with NSLBP and another with radicular LBP. The investigators showed that atrophy in the DLPFC was significantly greater in the group with radicular LBP. The observed regional brain atrophy is reminiscent of the apoptosis seen in animal models of neuropathic pain [3,87]. On the other hand, multiple other mechanisms may also explain the result. It remains unclear to what extent these changes are due to neuronal damage or death or simply to local changes in connectivity or relative changes in sizes of neurons or glia. Most importantly, it is not clear whether these changes are reversible, and whether they reflect causes or consequences of LBP. It is noteworthy that extrapolating the whole neocortical brain size in LBP to a pain duration of zero (i.e., prior

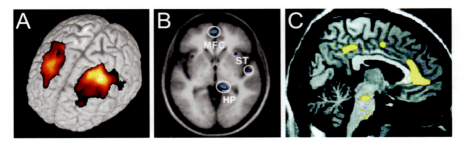

Fig. 2. Brain atrophy in three different clinical populations indicates unique patterns of atrophy. (A) In chronic back pain, atrophy is mainly in the bilateral dorsolateral prefrontal cortex. (B) In fibromyalgia, atrophy is in the medial prefrontal cortex (MFC) as well as in more posterior regions (adapted from Kuchinad et al. [57]). (C) In tension headache, atrophy is seen in the medial prefrontal cortex, in more posterior cingulate regions, and in the brainstem (adapted from Schmidt-Wilcke et al. [86]).

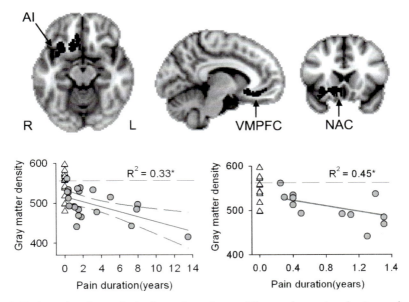

Fig. 3. Brain regional atrophy is shown in patients with complex regional pain syndrome (CRPS). Twenty-two patients were contrasted to 22 age- and gender-matched healthy subjects. Decreased gray matter is seen in a single region in the right hemisphere extending from the anterior insula (AI) to the ventromedial prefrontal cortex (VMPFC). Left graph indicates that the extent of gray matter decrease in CRPS (circles) is correlated to the duration of living with the condition. Triangles are matched healthy controls. The dashed line shows the mean gray matter density in the healthy subjects. The right graph shows the dependence of pain duration for CRPS patients living with pain for less than 1.5 years, and their respective matched healthy controls. (Figure adapted from Geha et al. [40].)

to onset of LBP) indicates that the brain size is still below that of normal subjects, suggesting a predisposing factor.

The gray matter atrophy in LBP could also be linked to the brain activity observed in these patients. Multiple studies indicate that the DLP-FC and mPFC inhibit each other, and this inhibition could be demonstrated for spontaneous pain in LBP [7]. Therefore, it could be hypothesized that the extent of atrophy of the DLPFC is linked to the amount of activity in the mPFC. Because mPFC activity strongly correlates to the intensity of pain, one could then state that the DLPFC atrophy contributes to the increased mPFC activity and thus also to the intensity of LBP.

One approach for clarifying mechanisms of atrophy is to study its relationship to white matter connectivity. This approach was recently applied in patients with complex regional pain syndrome (CRPS) [40]. The study first demonstrates that brain regional atrophy is also seen in CRPS, but the brain regions involved are distinct from those of LBP. More importantly, it shows that gray matter atrophy is coupled with decreases in white matter connectivity, especially over long-distance connections, as well as with target-specific increased white matter connectivity. Therefore, the study shows specific rewiring of the brain in clinical chronic pain. Again, however, we do not know the extent to which this rewiring is a consequence of or a predisposing factor for the clinical pain. In contrast to the LBP brain atrophy study, where the shortest duration of LBP included in the study was 2 years (as a precaution to ensure that all cases were chronic), in the CRPS study the patients recruited had CRPS for more than 3 months. When these data are examined over the whole group or just for the patients who had CRPS for less than 1.2 years, one sees that the dependence of regional atrophy on pain duration is much higher for the subgroup with shorter duration (Fig. 3), where in fact there seems to be a very steep decrease in gray matter density in the first 6 months. This finding suggests an initial atrophy process that then stabilizes, implying a direct link between brain atrophy and the onset of CRPS. The observation is reminiscent of the time course seen for apoptosis in the spinal cord in animals with experimental neuropathic injury, where cell death occurs within a fixed time window after injury (about 20 days in rats) and then occurs at a slower rate afterwards [40].

Cognitive Abnormalities

The brain abnormalities seen in LBP provide specific hypotheses for cognitive deficits that may be studied in these patients. The atrophy in the DLPFC and the activity in the mPFC suggest that LBP is more of an emotional state and that such patients may become less sensitive to other emotional stimuli, given the distraction that LBP would impose. Investigators tested this possibility using an emotional decision-making task and found that LBP patients were impaired on the task in proportion to the intensity of their pain [4]. Moreover, the activity of the insula was also observed to be abnormal in LBP. The insula is known to be a primary gustatory region, and when LBP patients were tested for gustation, they showed better abilities in taste perception than normal subjects [89]. Therefore, LBP patients exhibit specific cognitive abnormalities that can be linked to their brain activity and brain morphological abnormalities.

It is remarkable that brain activity, morphology, and cognitive abnormalities can be linked to each other in LBP, and that these abnormalities can be tightly correlated to the intensity and duration of LBP. These correlations are far stronger than correlations between pain intensity and evidence of end-organ pathology, as demonstrated by imaging studies or pain provocation/palliation studies. However, these are only correlations, and causative evidence awaits future longitudinal studies.

Response to Treatment

Medicine is a practical profession. For conditions that are not life threatening, patients expect medical treatment to ease their suffering and improve the quality of their lives. Thus, the ultimate practical validation of any model of a medical disorder is the ability of treatment based on that model to help patients who suffer from the disorder.

The end-organ dysfunction model has dominated research on the treatment of spine conditions in general, and NSLBP in particular. The research that is most relevant to the present chapter involves treatment directed toward intervertebral disks and facet joints in the lumbar spine.

The literature on treatments directed toward diskogenic pain is vast and often contradictory. It is beyond the scope of this chapter to review this literature in depth. Broadly speaking, such treatments can be divided into three groups: spinal fusion, disk replacement surgery, and less invasive therapies such as intradiskal electrothermal therapy (IDET). Within each category, there are many specific procedures. For example, spinal fusion techniques include posterolateral fusions, transforaminal fusions, anterior fusions, and circumferential fusions. The procedures can be performed with a variety of kinds of instrumentation.

In general, case series and prospective cohort studies have supported the effectiveness of all three approaches. For example, Andersson et al. [1] reported on 33 studies of spinal fusion for diskogenic pain. On average, patients in these studies reported a 50% reduction in pain, 42% improvement in the Oswestry Disability Index, and 46% improvement in the Medical Outcomes Study 36-item Short-Form Health Survey (SF-36). In 18 studies of IDET, the authors found 51%, 14%, and 36% improvement on these three indices, respectively.

In contrast, randomized controlled trials (RCTs) have yielded less impressive results. In the case of spinal fusion, RCTs have compared surgery to rehabilitative care. Mirza and Deyo [68] recently reviewed relevant studies and concluded that the evidence to date suggests that the results of spinal fusion are not any better than those of well-designed rehabilitation programs. A recent study by Carragee et al. [24] raised significant questions about the efficacy of spinal fusion based on diskography-demonstrated diskogenic pain. They compared the effects of surgical intervention for carefully selected cohorts of patients with diskography-demonstrated diskogenic pain to ones with unstable spondylolisthesis, a well-accepted structural lesion of the spine. The percentage of excellent results among the spondylolisthesis cohort was 72%; in contrast, only 27% of diskogenic patients had excellent results.

The first artificial disk to receive approval by the Food and Drug Administration (FDA) for use in the United States was the Charite disk. In an RCT performed in order to receive FDA approval, the effectiveness of the Charite disk was compared to that of anterior interbody fusion in 304 patients [14]. At 24-month follow-up, patients treated with the Charite disk expressed higher levels of satisfaction than ones treated with spinal fusion, and were comparable in level of disability. A later RCT was performed on the Pro-Disk-L [102]. It demonstrated superior outcomes compared to circumferential fusions. At this point, the most conservative judgment of artificial disks is that they produce clinical results comparable to those of spinal fusions. It should be noted, however, that knowledge about artificial disks is rapidly expanding. Multiple artificial disks—including the Maverick, the Flexicore, and the Kineflex [101]—have recently been developed and are undergoing clinical trials.

Two RCTs have been performed on IDET. In both instances, a genuine IDET procedure was compared to a sham procedure. One of the studies demonstrated modest benefit for IDET [75]; the other found no difference between the IDET group and the control group [36].

An abundant literature describes treatments directed toward pain originating from facet joints. Although intra-articular injections of facet joints with local anesthetics and steroids have the potential to produce long-term symptom relief, the treatment that has received the most attention is medial branch neurotomy (often described as facet neurotomy). In this procedure, sensory nerves emanating from a target facet joint are destroyed with a thermal lesion (usually by heating them via radiofrequency waves). Studies without control groups suggest that between 35% and 80% of patients report substantial pain relief approximately 1 year after a lumbar facet neurotomy [34,85].

A recent review by Boswell et al. [20] identified eight RCTs on facet neurotomies, of which only two met stringent methodological criteria [62,93]. Both of these studies demonstrated therapeutic benefit from facet neurotomies for up to 1 year. Based on their review of the RCTs and of several less-well designed studies, Boswell et al. concluded that there is moderate evidence for short- and long-term pain relief from lumbar facet neurotomy. A recent RCT by Nath et al. [72], which was not included in the Boswell et al. review, showed a significant benefit from lumbar facet neurotomy.

Overall, the literature on treatments directed toward diskogenic pain and pain mediated by facet joints in the lumbar spine is voluminous, heterogeneous, and difficult to summarize. On balance, it appears that there is some evidence for efficacy of the procedures that have been studied, in particular disk arthroplasty, spinal fusion, IDET, and facet neurotomy. It is important to note, however, that in studies with relatively good methodology, recruitment of patients is very selective. For example, in the study by Nath et al., 376 patients were initially evaluated for inclusion, but only 40 ended up undergoing facet neurotomy. Thus, even though procedures directed toward diskogenic pain and facet joint pain can claim to be successful, they appear to be relevant to only a minority of patients with chronic NSLBP.

Treatment studies can also support models that attribute LBP to altered nervous system functioning. For example, if one accepts the premise that CNS sensitization is a form of neuropathic pain [29,78,81], the hypothesis that CNS sensitization plays a major role in LBP suggests that antidepressants and anticonvulsants should be helpful. The hypothesis that psychological distress and poor coping strategies are major contributors to LBP suggests that psychological therapies should be helpful.

A recent comprehensive review [27] found some evidence to support the efficacy of tricyclic antidepressants in the treatment of LBP. An earlier review [91] concluded that there was evidence of modest benefit from both tricyclic and tetracyclic antidepressants. In contrast, a recent Cochrane Collection review [92] determined that there was no evidence of benefit for these antidepressants in the treatment of LBP. A reasonable conclusion from these contradictory reviews is that the benefits for LBP patients from antidepressants are modest at best.

As far as anticonvulsants are concerned, a review by Chou and Huffman [27] found evidence for effectiveness of gabapentin in the treatment of radiculopathy, and one study found topiramate to be effective in treating a mixed group of patients with chronic LBP that included both cases of NSLBP and radiculopathies. There was no convincing evidence for benefit from anticonvulsants in patients with NSLBP.

There is also evidence that psychological therapies can benefit patients with chronic LBP. This conclusion is supported by a comprehensive Cochrane collection review [74] and by a more recent systematic review [80]. However, psychological therapies, like antidepressant medications and anticonvulsants, appear to have only modestly beneficial effects on LBP patients. Certainly, they cannot be construed as curative. Another caveat is that studies demonstrating the benefits of these therapies are generally short in duration (typically lasting several weeks). There are essentially no data on long-term outcomes of the therapies.

In summary, there is some evidence to support the efficacy of treatments based on the end-organ dysfunction model and also of treatments based on various models attributing LBP to altered nervous system functioning. However, the results of these treatments are far from overwhelming. As a broad index of how far we have to go in the treatment of LBP, Martin et al. [67] examined U.S. survey data in the to estimate the costs and benefits of spine care in 1997 and 2005. They estimated that the cost of spine care increased 65% in the 8-year interval. However, patients with spine problems reported worse mental health, physical functioning, work/school limitations, and social limitations in 2005 compared with 1997. These somber findings are consistent with the widely held perception among clinicians that LBP tends to be refractory to treatment. In essence, neither advocates of the end-organ dysfunction model nor proponents of the altered nervous system processing models can claim to have proven their case on the basis of the effectiveness of treatments based on their models.

Conclusions

This chapter has contrasted the end-organ injury/dysfunction model of NSLBP with various alternatives that can be grouped as models stressing altered nervous system processing. In our view, there is significant evidence to support the end-organ injury/dysfunction model. At the same time, it is evident that attempts to diagnose and treat NSLBP on the basis of this model often fail. Moreover, psychological research and recent investigations of neurophysiological processes in chronic pain highlight the fact that the pain of many patients with NSLBP depends not only on the "signal" of a structural lesion in the spine, but also on the "noise" introduced by altered nervous system processing.

In particular, brain imaging studies emphasize the fact that from the viewpoint of the brain, LBP is a far more homogeneous entity than has been assumed when viewed from the perspective of end-organ injury/dysfunction. The brain imaging studies summarized above imply that the central reorganization that seems to accompany LBP is more stereotypical, and as a result it may be a more dominant factor in the condition. Given that the central component repeatedly shows up as correlated to the duration and intensity of the condition, the implication is that the symptoms of patients with NSLBP may be controlled more efficiently by manipulations that target the central processes rather than the end organ. Moreover, the likelihood of reverting central organization back to its normal state by blocking the end-organ signal seems remote, given the recent evidence that the anatomy of the brain is changing, and especially given the axonal connectivity between brain regions, where atrophy is observed in patients with chronic pain.

The relative importance of structural lesions versus altered nervous system processing almost certainly varies from patient to patient. At one extreme, there are undoubtedly patients whose NSLBP is appropriately construed as a fairly direct consequence of a structural lesion in the spine. At the other extreme are patients who have essentially no spine pathology, but experience pain primarily because of alterations in nervous system processing. It is likely that most patients with NSLBP are somewhere between these poles—their symptoms result from various combinations of structural lesions plus alterations in nervous system processing. Here we should emphasize the results from animal studies that have convincingly demonstrated that persistent pain induced by end-organ damage induces central reorganization that may not be reversible.

A key limitation in discussions of the end-organ injury/dysfunction model and various alternatives to it is that research studies on models of NSLBP tend to occur in isolation. We are not aware of any comprehensive attempts to compare and contrast these models conceptually, or to compare them with respect to empirical validation. A few studies have been published [23,33] on the significance of psychological versus orthopedic indices in LBP. We are not aware of research comparing the significance of orthopedic indicators versus indicators of altered sensory processing as evidenced by fMRI phenomena. A multitude of questions could be examined. For example, do LBP patients with accentuated activity in the mPFC respond differently to spine surgery from ones without such activity? Does accentuated mPFC activity normalize after NSLBP patients receive treatment that leads to clinical improvement?

Given the lack of communication among proponents of different models of NSLBP and the multiple gaps in research, we are not in a position to give a definitive answer to the question of whether NSLBP can best be construed as a straightforward consequence of end-organ injury/dysfunction, or as the result of more complex processes related to altered nervous system functioning. We hope we have achieved the more modest goals of describing alternative models of NSLBP, pointing out the need for further conceptual analysis of these models, discussing the types of research that bear on the validity of various models, and encouraging dialogue among researchers who conceptualize NSLBP in different ways.

References

[1]   Andersson GB, Mekhail NA, Block JE. Treatment of intractable discogenic low back pain. A systematic review of spinal fusion and intradiscal electrothermal therapy (IDET). Pain Physician 2006;9:237–48.
[2]   Apkarian AV, Bushnell MC, Treede RD, Zubieta JK. Human brain mechanisms of pain perception and regulation in health and disease. Eur J Pain 2005;9:463–84.
[3]   Apkarian AV, Scholz J. Shared mechanisms between chronic pain and neurodegenerative disease. Drug Discov Today Dis Mech 2006;3:319–26.
[4]   Apkarian AV, Sosa Y, Krauss BR, Thomas PS, Fredrickson BE, Levy RE, Harden RN, Chialvo DR. Chronic pain patients are impaired on an emotional decision-making task. Pain 2004;108:129–36.
[5]   Apkarian AV, Sosa Y, Sonty S, Levy RM, Harden RN, Parrish TB, Gitelman DR. Chronic back pain is associated with decreased prefrontal and thalamic gray matter density. J Neurosci 2004;24:10410–15.
[6]   Baliki M, Al-Amin HA, Atweh SF, Jaber M, Hawwa N, Jabbur SJ, Apkarian AV, Saade NE. Attenuation of neuropathic manifestations by local block of the activities of the ventrolateral orbito-frontal area in the rat. Neuroscience 2003;120:1093–104.
[7]   Baliki MN, Chialvo DR, Geha PY, Levy RM, Harden RN, Parrish TB, Apkarian AV. Chronic pain and the emotional brain: specific brain activity associated with spontaneous fluctuations of intensity of chronic back pain. J Neurosci 2006;26:12165–73.
[8]   Baliki MN, Geha PY, Apkarian AV, Chialvo DR. Beyond feeling: chronic pain hurts the brain, disrupting the default-mode network dynamics. J Neurosci 2008;28:1398–403.
[9]   Baliki MN, Geha PY, Jabakhanji R, Harden N, Schnitzer TJ, Apkarian AV. A preliminary fMRI study of analgesic treatment in chronic back pain and knee osteoarthritis. Mol Pain 2008;4:47.
[10] Barnsley L, Lord S, Bogduk N. Comparative local anaesthetic blocks in the diagnosis of cervical zygapophysial joint pain. Pain 1993;55:99–106.
[11] Battie MC, Videman T. Lumbar disc degeneration: epidemiology and genetics. J Bone Joint Surg Am 2006;88(Suppl 2):3-9.
[12] Battie MC, Videman T, Levalahti E, Gill K, Kaprio J. Heritability of low back pain and the role of disc degeneration. Pain 2007;131:272–80.
[13] Bigos SJ, Battie MC, Spengler DM, Fisher LD, Fordyce WE, Hansson T, Nachemson AL, Zeh J. A longitudinal, prospective study of industrial back injury reporting. Clin Orthop Relat Res 1992;21–34.
[14] Blumenthal S, McAfee PC, Guyer RD, Hochschuler SH, Geisler FH, Holt RT, Garcia R Jr, Regan JJ, Ohnmeiss DD. A prospective, randomized, multicenter Food and Drug Administration investigational device exemptions study of lumbar total disc replacement with the CHARITE artificial disc versus lumbar fusion: part I: evaluation of clinical outcomes. Spine 2005;30:1565–75.

[15] Boden SD, Davis DO, Dina TS, Patronas NJ, Wiesel SW. Abnormal magnetic-resonance scans of the lumbar spine in asymptomatic subjects. A prospective investigation. J Bone Joint Surg Am 1990;72:403–8.

[16] Bogduk N. Practice guidelines: spinal diagnostic treatment procedures. San Francisco: International Spine Intervention Society, 2004. Pain Med 2005;6:139–42.

[17] Bogduk N, Long DM. Percutaneous lumbar medial branch neurotomy: a modification of facet denervation. Spine 1980;5:193–200.

[18] Boos N, Semmer N, Elfering A, Schade V, Gal I, Zanetti M, Kissling R, Buchegger N, Hodler J, Main CJ. Natural history of individuals with asymptomatic disc abnormalities in magnetic resonance imaging: predictors of low back pain-related medical consultation and work incapacity. Spine 2000;25:1484–92.

[19] Borenstein DG, O'Mara JW, Jr., Boden SD, Lauerman WC, Jacobson A, Platenberg C, Schellinger D, Wiesel SW. The value of magnetic resonance imaging of the lumbar spine to predict low-back pain in asymptomatic subjects: a seven-year follow-up study. J Bone Joint Surg Am 2001;83-A:1306–11.

[20] Boswell MV, Colson JD, Sehgal N, Dunbar EE, Epter R. A systematic review of therapeutic facet joint interventions in chronic spinal pain. Pain Physician 2007;10:229–53.

[21] Carragee EJ, Alamin TF, Carragee JM. Low-pressure positive discography in subjects asymptomatic of significant low back pain illness. Spine 2006;31:505–9.

[22] Carragee E, Alamin T, Cheng I, Franklin T, Hurwitz E. Does minor trauma cause serious low back illness? Spine 2006;31:2942–9.

[23] Carragee EJ, Alamin TF, Miller JL, Carragee JM. Discographic, MRI and psychosocial determinants of low back pain disability and remission: a prospective study in subjects with benign persistent back pain. Spine J 2005;5:24–35.

[24] Carragee EJ, Lincoln T, Parmar VS, Alamin T. A gold standard evaluation of the "discogenic pain" diagnosis as determined by provocative discography. Spine 2006;31:2115–23.

[25] Carragee EJ, Tanner CM, Khurana S, Hayward C, Welsh J, Date E, Truong T, Rossi M, Hagle C. The rates of false-positive lumbar discography in select patients without low back symptoms. Spine 2000;25:1373–80.

[26] Carragee EJ, Tanner CM, Yang B, Brito JL, Truong T. False-positive findings on lumbar discography. Reliability of subjective concordance assessment during provocative disc injection. Spine 1999;24:2542–7.

[27] Chou R, Huffman LH. Medications for acute and chronic low back pain: a review of the evidence for an American Pain Society/American College of Physicians clinical practice guideline. Ann Intern Med 2007;147:505–14.

[28] Cohen SP, Larkin TM, Barna SA, Palmer WE, Hecht AC, Stojanovic MP. Lumbar discography: a comprehensive review of outcome studies, diagnostic accuracy, and principles. Reg Anesth Pain Med 2005;30:163–83.

[29] Crofford LJ. The relationship of fibromyalgia to neuropathic pain syndromes. J Rheumatol Suppl 2005;75:41–5.

[30] Croft P, Dunn KM, Von Korff M. Chronic pain syndromes: you can't have one without another. Pain 2007;131:237–8.

[31] Derbyshire SW. Meta-analysis of thirty four independent samples studied using PET reveals a significantly attenuated central response to noxious stimulation in clinical pain patients. Curr Rev Pain 1999;3:265–80.

[32] Derbyshire SW, Jones AK, Creed F, Starz T, Meltzer CC, Townsend DW, Peterson AM, Firestone L. Cerebral responses to noxious thermal stimulation in chronic low back pain patients and normal controls. Neuroimage 2002;16:158–68.

[33] Don AS, Carragee E. A brief overview of evidence-informed management of chronic low back pain with surgery. Spine J 2008;8:258–65.

[34] Dreyfuss P, Halbrook B, Pauza K, Joshi A, McLarty J, Bogduk N. Efficacy and validity of radiofrequency neurotomy for chronic lumbar zygapophysial joint pain. Spine 2000;25:1270–7.

[35] Foss JM, Apkarian AV, Chialvo DR. Dynamics of pain: fractal dimension of temporal variability of spontaneous pain differentiates between pain states. J Neurophysiol 2006;95:730–6.

[36] Freeman BJ, Fraser RD, Cain CM, Hall DJ, Chapple DC. A randomized, double-blind, controlled trial: intradiscal electrothermal therapy versus placebo for the treatment of chronic discogenic low back pain. Spine 2005;30:2369–77.

[37] Frymoyer JW. Back pain and sciatica. N Engl J Med 1988;318:291–300.

[38] Gammaitoni AR, Alvarez NA, Galer BS. Safety and tolerability of the lidocaine patch 5%, a targeted peripheral analgesic: a review of the literature. J Clin Pharmacol 2003;43:111–17.

[39] Gardell LR, Vanderah TW, Gardell SE, Wang R, Ossipov MH, Lai J, Porreca F. Enhanced evoked excitatory transmitter release in experimental neuropathy requires descending facilitation. J Neurosci 2003;23:8370–9.

[40] Geha PY, Baliki MN, Harden RN, Bauer WR, Parrish TB, Apkarian AV. The brain in chronic CRPS pain: abnormal gray-white matter interactions in emotional and autonomic regions. Neuron 2008;60(4):570–81

[41] Ghaffari M, Alipour A, Farshad AA, Jensen I, Josephson M, Vingard E. Effect of psychosocial factors on low back pain in industrial workers. Occup Med (Lond) 2008;58:341–7.

[42] Ghaffari M, Alipour A, Jensen I, Farshad AA, Vingard E. Low back pain among Iranian industrial workers. Occup Med (Lond) 2006;56:455–60.

[43] Giesecke T, Gracely RH, Grant MA, Nachemson A, Petzke F, Williams DA, Clauw DJ. Evidence of augmented central pain processing in idiopathic chronic low back pain. Arthritis Rheum 2004;50:613–23.

[44] Gimbel J, Linn R, Hale M, Nicholson B. Lidocaine patch treatment in patients with low back pain: results of an open-label, nonrandomized pilot study. Am J Ther 2005;12:311–19.

[45] Grachev ID, Fredrickson BE, Apkarian AV. Abnormal brain chemistry in chronic back pain: an in vivo proton magnetic resonance spectroscopy study. Pain 2000;89:7–18.

[46] Gureje O, Von Korff M, Simon GE, Gater R. Persistent pain and well-being: a World Health Organization study in primary care. JAMA 1998;280:147–51.

[47] Hancock MJ, Maher CG, Latimer J, Spindler MF, McAuley JH, Laslett M, Bogduk N. Systematic review of tests to identify the disc, SIJ or facet joint as the source of low back pain. Eur Spine J 2007;16:1539–50.

[48] Higashino K, Matsui Y, Yagi S, Takata Y, Goto T, Sakai T, Katoh S, Yasui N. The alpha2 type IX collagen tryptophan polymorphism is associated with the severity of disc degeneration in younger patients with herniated nucleus pulposus of the lumbar spine. Int Orthop 2007;31:107–11.

[49] Hunt SP, Mantyh PW. The molecular dynamics of pain control. Nat Rev Neurosci 2001;2:83–91.

[50] Jarvik JJ, Hollingworth W, Heagerty P, Haynor DR, Deyo RA. The longitudinal assessment of imaging and disability of the back (LAID back) study: baseline data. Spine 2001;26:1158–66.

[51] Jasmin L, Rabkin SD, Granato A, Boudah A, Ohara PT. Analgesia and hyperalgesia from GABA-mediated modulation of the cerebral cortex. Nature 2003;424:316–20.

[52] Jensen MC, Brant-Zawadzki MN, Obuchowski N, Modic MT, Malkasian D, Ross JS. Magnetic resonance imaging of the lumbar spine in people without back pain. N Engl J Med 1994;331:69–73.

[53] Johansen JP, Fields HL. Glutamatergic activation of anterior cingulate cortex produces an aversive teaching signal. Nat Neurosci 2004;7:398–403.

[54] Julius D, Basbaum AI. Molecular mechanisms of nociception. Nature 2001;413:203–10.

[55] Kaaria S, Solovieva S, Leino-Arjas P. Associations of low back pain with neck pain: a study of industrial employees with 5-, 10-, and 28-year follow-ups. Eur J Pain 2008; Epub Jun 19.

[56] Kawaguchi Y, Kanamori M, Ishihara H, Ohmori K, Matsui H, Kimura T. The association of lumbar disc disease with vitamin-D receptor gene polymorphism. J Bone Joint Surg Am 2002;84:2022–8.

[57] Kjaer P, Korsholm L, Bendix T, Sorensen JS, Leboeuf-Yde C. Modic changes and their associations with clinical findings. Eur Spine J 2006;15:1312–19.

[58] Kopec JA, Sayre EC. Stressful experiences in childhood and chronic back pain in the general population. Clin J Pain 2005;21:478–83.

[59] Kuchinad A, Schweinhardt P, Seminowicz DA, Wood PB, Chizh BA, Bushnell MC. Accelerated brain gray matter loss in fibromyalgia patients: premature aging of the brain? J Neurosci 2007;27:4004–7.

[60] Lee H, Wilbur J, Kim MJ, Miller AM. Psychosocial risk factors for work-related musculoskeletal disorders of the lower-back among long-haul international female flight attendants. J Adv Nurs 2008;61:492–502.

[61] Leonardi M, Pfirrmann CW, Boos N. Injection studies in spinal disorders. Clin Orthop Relat Res 2006;443:168–82.

52 J.P. Robinson and A.V. Apkarian

[62] Lord SM, Barnsley L, Wallis BJ, McDonald GJ, Bogduk N. Percutaneous radio-frequency neurotomy for chronic cervical zygapophyseal-joint pain. N Engl J Med 1996;335:1721–6.
[63] Louw QA, Morris LD, Grimmer-Somers K. The prevalence of low back pain in Africa: a systematic review. BMC Musculoskelet Disord 2007;8:105.
[64] Manchikanti L, Pampati V, Fellows B, Bakhit CE. The diagnostic validity and therapeutic value of lumbar facet joint nerve blocks with or without adjuvant agents. Curr Rev Pain 2000;4:337–44.
[65] Manchikanti L, Singh V, Falco FJ, Cash KA, Pampati V. Lumbar facet joint nerve blocks in managing chronic facet joint pain: one-year follow-up of a randomized, double-blind controlled trial: Clinical Trial NCT00355914. Pain Physician 2008;11:121–32.
[66] Mantyh PW, Rogers SD, Honore P, Allen BJ, Ghilardi JR, Li J, Daughters RS, Lappi DA, Wiley RG, Simone DA. Inhibition of hyperalgesia by ablation of lamina I spinal neurons expressing the substance P receptor. Science 1997;278:275–9.
[67] Martin BI, Deyo RA, Mirza SK, Turner JA, Comstock BA, Hollingworth W, Sullivan SD. Expenditures and health status among adults with back and neck problems. JAMA 2008;299:656–64.
[68] Mirza SK, Deyo RA. Systematic review of randomized trials comparing lumbar fusion surgery to nonoperative care for treatment of chronic back pain. Spine 2007;32:816–23.
[69] Modic MT, Steinberg PM, Ross JS, Masaryk TJ, Carter JR. Degenerative disk disease: assessment of changes in vertebral body marrow with MR imaging. Radiology 1988;166:193–9.
[70] Mogil JS, Ritchie J, Sotocinal SG, Smith SB, Croteau S, Levitin DJ, Naumova AK. Screening for pain phenotypes: analysis of three congenic mouse strains on a battery of nine nociceptive assays. Pain 2006;126:24–34.
[71] Mustard CA, Kalcevich C, Frank JW, Boyle M. Childhood and early adult predictors of risk of incident back pain: Ontario child health study 2001 follow-up. Am J Epidemiol 2005;162:779–86.
[72] Nath S, Nath CA, Pettersson K. Percutaneous lumbar zygapophysial (Facet) joint neurotomy using radiofrequency current, in the management of chronic low back pain: a randomized double-blind trial. Spine 2008;33:1291–7.
[73] Neugebauer V, Li W, Bird GC, Han JS. The amygdala and persistent pain. Neuroscientist 2004;10:221–34.
[74] Ostelo RW, van Tulder MW, Vlaeyen JW, Linton SJ, Morley SJ, Assendelft WJ. Behavioural treatment for chronic low-back pain. Cochrane Database Syst Rev 2005;(1):CD002014
[75] Pauza KJ, Howell S, Dreyfuss P, Peloza JH, Dawson K, Bogduk N. A randomized, placebo-controlled trial of intradiscal electrothermal therapy for the treatment of discogenic low back pain. Spine J 2004;4:27–35.
[76] Peyron R, Laurent B, Garcia-Larrea L. Functional imaging of brain responses to pain: a review and meta-analysis. Neurophysiol Clin 2000;30:263–88.
[77] Price DD. Psychological and neural mechanisms of the affective dimension of pain. Science 2000;288:1769–72.
[78] Price DD, Staud R. Neurobiology of fibromyalgia syndrome. J Rheumatol Suppl 2005;75:22–8.
[79] Reichenbach S, Katz JN. When East meets West: comments on 'Back pain as a communicable disease'. Int J Epidemiol 2008;37:74–6.
[80] Robinson JP, Leo R, Wallch J, McGough E, Schatman M. Rehabilitative treatment for chronic pain. In: Stannard C, Kalso E, Ballantyne J, editors. Evidence-based chronic pain management. Oxford: Blackwell Publishing; 2008.
[81] Rowbotham MC. Is fibromyalgia a neuropathic pain syndrome? J Rheumatol Suppl 2005;75:38–40.
[82] Rubin DI. Epidemiology and risk factors for spine pain. Neurol Clin 2007;25:353–71.
[83] Sambrook P.N., MacGregor A.J., Spector T.D. Genetic influences on cervical and lumbar disc degeneration: a magnetic resonance imaging study in twins. Arthritis Rheum 1999;42:366–72.
[84] Sandkühler J. Understanding LTP in pain pathways. Mol Pain 2007;3:9.
[85] Schaerer JP. Radiofrequency facet rhizotomy in the treatment of chronic neck and low back pain. Int Surg 1978;63:53–9.
[86] Schmidt-Wilcke T, Leinisch E, Straube A, Kampfe N, Draganski B, Diener HC, Bogdahn U, May A. Gray matter decrease in patients with chronic tension type headache. Neurology 2005;65:1483–6.

[87] Scholz J, Broom DC, Youn DH, Mills CD, Kohno T, Suter MR, Moore KA, Decosterd I, Coggeshall RE, Woolf CJ. Blocking caspase activity prevents transsynaptic neuronal apoptosis and the loss of inhibition in lamina II of the dorsal horn after peripheral nerve injury. J Neurosci 2005;25:7317–23.

[88] Schwarzer AC, Aprill CN, Derby R, Fortin J, Kine G, Bogduk N. The false-positive rate of uncontrolled diagnostic blocks of the lumbar zygapophysial joints. Pain 1994;58:195–200.

[89] Small DM, Apkarian AV. Increased taste intensity perception exhibited by patients with chronic back pain. Pain 2006;120:124–30.

[90] Solovieva S, Lohiniva J, Leino-Arjas P, Raininko R, Luoma K, la-Kokko L, Riihimaki H. Intervertebral disc degeneration in relation to the COL9A3 and the IL-1ss gene polymorphisms. Eur Spine J 2006;15:613–9.

[91] Staiger TO, Gaster B, Sullivan MD, Deyo RA. Systematic review of antidepressants in the treatment of chronic low back pain. Spine 2003;28:2540–5.

[92] Urquhart DM, Hoving JL, Assendelft WW, Roland M, van Tulder MW. Antidepressants for nonspecific low back pain. Cochrane Database Syst Rev 2008(1):CD001703

[93] Van Kleef M, Barendse GA, Kessels A, Voets HM, Weber WE, de LS. Randomized trial of radiofrequency lumbar facet denervation for chronic low back pain. Spine 1999;24:1937–42.

[94] Von Korff M. Studying the natural history of back pain. Spine 1994;19:2041S–6.

[95] Von Korff M, Crane P, Lane M, Miglioretti DL, Simon G, Saunders K, Stang P, Brandenburg N, Kessler R. Chronic spinal pain and physical-mental comorbidity in the United States: results from the national comorbidity survey replication. Pain 2005;113:331–9.

[96] Von Korff M, Deyo RA, Cherkin D, Barlow W. Back pain in primary care. Outcomes at 1 year. Spine 1993;18:855–62.

[97] White AA, III, Gordon SL. Synopsis: workshop on idiopathic low-back pain. Spine 1982;7:141–9.

[98] Wiesel SW, Tsourmas N, Feffer HL, Citrin CM, Patronas N. A study of computer-assisted tomography. I. The incidence of positive CAT scans in an asymptomatic group of patients. Spine 1984;9:549–51.

[99] Wiesinger B, Malker H, Englund E, Wanman A. Back pain in relation to musculoskeletal disorders in the jaw-face: a matched case-control study. Pain 2007;131:311–9.

[100] Woolf CJ, Salter MW. Plasticity and pain: role of the dorsal horn. In: McMahon SB, Koltzenburg M, editors. Textbook of pain. New York: Churchill-Livingstone; 2006. p. 91–105.

[101] Zeller JL. Artificial spinal disk superior to fusion for treating degenerative disk disease. JAMA 2006;296:2665–7.

[102] Zigler J, Delamarter R, Spivak JM, Linovitz RJ, Danielson GO III, Haider TT, Cammisa F, Zuchermann J, Balderston R, Kitchel S, et al. Results of the prospective, randomized, multicenter Food and Drug Administration investigational device exemption study of the ProDisc-L total disc replacement versus circumferential fusion for the treatment of 1-level degenerative disc disease. Spine 2007;32:1155–62.

Correspondence to: A. Vania Apkarian, PhD, Department of Physiology, 5-120 Ward Building, Northwestern University, Feinberg School of Medicine, 303 East Chicago Ave, Chicago IL, 60611, USA. Email: a-apkarian@northwestern.edu.

Temporomandibular Joint Disorders

William Maixner

Center for Neurosensory Disorders, School of Dentistry, University of North Carolina, Chapel Hill, North Carolina, USA

Complex persistent pain conditions include the most prevalent of all painful conditions, such as temporomandibular joint disorder (TMJD), headache conditions, fibromyalgia, irritable bowel syndrome, interstitial cystitis, chronic pelvic pain, whiplash-associated disorders, and vulvar vestibulitis. The worldwide prevalence of these conditions, also known as functional pain syndromes, is 15–20% for adults [4]. World Health Organization surveys show that approximately 1 in 10 primary care patients develops a persistent pain condition within 12 months; approximately 50% of those who develop such a condition do not recover within 12 months [23].

TMJD is characterized by spontaneous pain and jaw-function-induced pain in the muscles of mastication and the temporomandibular joint. TMJD is among the most common functional pain syndromes, with a prevalence estimate ranging from 3% to 15% for Western populations [14,29]. Most studies have found that TMJD, like other functional pain syndromes, is 1.5–2 times more prevalent in women in the community setting. The prevalence of TMJD varies across the lifespan. Prevalence appears to peak in the reproductive years (20 to 45 years of age), although both young children and elderly adults can also suffer from TMJD. Few studies have examined the incidence of painful TMJD, but the outcomes of recent studies provide evidence for an annual incidence rate of 2–4% for onset of the condition and approximately 0.1% for development of chronic TMJD [13,14,52]. Longitudinal studies have shown substantial variations in the time course of myofascial TMJD, with 31% of cases persisting over a 5-year period, 33% going into remission, and 36% recurring [47].

It has become increasing evident that TMJD is not a unitary or "isolated" disorder, but in fact is a multifactorial disorder that is frequently associated with other functional pain syndromes, including (but

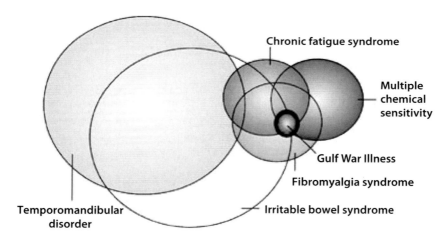

Primary Diagnosis	Percentage of Overlap with Secondary Condition				
	FMS	CFS	IBS	TMJD	MCS
FMS	NA	70	32–80	75	55
CFS	35–70	NA	58–92	20	41–67
IBS	32–65	58–92	NA	32–65	ND
TMJD	13–18	20	64	NA	ND
MCS	33–55	30	ND	ND	NA

Fig. 1. Degree of overlap of various syndromes with a secondary condition (adapted from Dadabhoy and Clauw [7]). Abbreviations: FMS: fibromyalgia syndrome; CFS: chronic fatigue syndrome; IBS: irritable bowel syndrome; MCS: multiple chemical sensitivity; NA: not applicable; ND: not determined; TMJD: temporomandibular joint disorder.

not limited to) fibromyalgia syndrome, irritable bowel syndrome, chronic headache, interstitial cystitis, chronic pelvic pain, chronic tinnitus, whiplash, and vulvar vestibulitis [7,11] (see Fig. 1). Many of these conditions tend to cluster as comorbid conditions characterized by a complaint of pain as well as a mosaic of abnormalities in motor function, autonomic balance, neuroendocrine function, and sleep.

Individual variations in the molecular pathways that affect pain sensitivity and psychological status may produce the heterogenous signs and symptoms that aggregate into *clusters* of phenotypically distinct subgroups of patients, on the basis of different sets of genetic and environmental causes (Fig. 2) [11,12,36]. As shown in Fig. 1, many functional pain syndromes overlap and are proposed to share some common pathways or mechanisms of pathology [7,9,59,70,72,76–80]. Consistent with

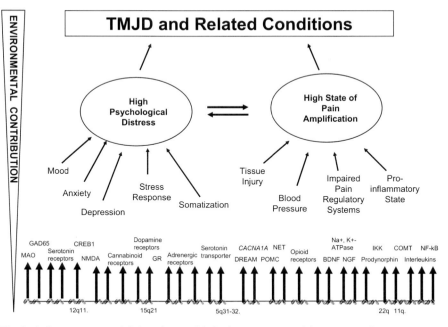

Fig. 2. A descriptive model that depicts likely determinants of the onset and maintenance of TMJD and related disorders. These factors are determined by both genetic variability and environmental events that determine an individual's psychological profile and pain amplification status. These two primary domains are interactive and influence the risk of pain onset and persistence. Likely modifiers of the interaction between genetic and environmental factors include sex and ethnicity. Adapted from Diatchenko et al. [11].

the heuristic model presented in Fig. 2, the majority of individuals suffering from functional pain syndromes demonstrate a state of pain amplification and psychological distress [1,3,21,37,60,64,80] (for a review, see
Diatchenko et al. [11]). Importantly, there is substantial individual variability in the relative contribution of pain amplification and psychological phenotypes to functional pain syndromes, resulting in considerable
heterogeneity in the signs and symptoms seen in patients. The resulting
pattern of causative genetic and environmental factors that contribute
to conditions such as TMJD demonstrates the need to develop mecha-
nism-based treatments for TMJD and other functional pain syndromes
[11,12,56].

Pain Amplification: A Determinant of Onset and Persistence of TMJD and Related Syndromes

A few studies have sought to prospectively identify risk factors or risk determinants that are associated with or mediate the onset and maintenance
of functional pain syndromes. A well-established predictor of onset is the
presence of another chronic pain condition, characterized by a state of
pain amplification [65]. Additionally, widespread pain is a risk indicator
for dysfunction associated with painful TMJD and for lack of response to
treatment [48]. Recently, we demonstrated that individuals who are more
sensitive to noxious stimuli are significantly more likely to develop painful
TMJD than those who are less sensitive (risk ratio = 2.7) [52]. The outcomes of several cross-sectional studies also suggest that a substantial percentage of patients with functional pain syndromes, including TMJD [33–
36,51], IBS [26,64,68,69,71], fibromyalgia [3,22,54,55], migraine headache
[27,31,67], and VVS [32,45] are influenced by a state of pain amplification
(for review, see Yunus [76–78]). A recent review on this topic by Yunus
[76] notes that a common feature in a large percentage of patients with
such syndromes is enhanced pain sensitivity (see Table I). These findings
suggest that pain amplification, and the associated processes that mediate
pain transmission and modulation, represent key factors in maintaining
these syndromes.

Table I
Number of studies (and total number of patients examined) that report an increase in pain sensitivity across nociceptive modalities and across functional pain syndromes

Stimulus	Number of Studies (Total Number of Patients Examined)							
	FM	CFS	IBS	TTH	Migraine	TMJD	MPS/RSTPS	PD
Pressure (somatic)	15 (580)			4 (178)	3 (117)	2 (42)	9 (462)	1 (20)
Pressure (rectal)			26 (822)					
Heat (somatic)	12 (480)		2 (21)	1 (50)	3 (117)	3 (76)	3 (137)	2 (42)
Heat (rectal)			1 (46)					
Cold (somatic)	8 (255)		1 (33)		1 (41)		2 (184)	
Electric (cutaneous)	4 (61)		1 (12)				2 (36)	
Electric (i.m.)	2 (41)	1 (23)					2 (36)	1 (10)
Electric (spinal reflex)	2 (107)		1 (14)	1 (40)			1 (27)	
Electric (rectal)			2 (21)					
Ischemic	1 (60)					2 (72)		
Hypertonic saline	2 (41)					1 (22)	1 (11)	
Auditory stimulus	1 (20)		1 (15)		1 (65)			

Abbreviations: CFS = chronic fatigue syndrome, FM = fibromyalgia syndrome, IBS = irritable bowel syndrome, i.m. = intramuscular, MPS = myofascial pain syndrome, PD = primary dysmenorrhea, RSTPS = regional soft tissue pain syndrome, TMJD = temporomandibular joint disorders, TTH = tension-type headache.

Enhanced pain perception experienced by patients with functional pain syndromes may result from a dysregulation in peripheral and central systems that produce dynamic, time-dependent changes in the excitability and response characteristics of neuronal and glial cells. This dysregulation probably contributes to changes in mood and in motor, autonomic, and neuroendocrine responses as well as altered pain perception (Fig. 2)

[11,33,36,58,66]. However, not all functional pain syndrome patients exhibit pain amplification [21]. While the majority of TMJD patients show enhanced sensitivity to ischemic pain [34], approximately 25% show no change in ischemic pain perception relative to controls (Maixner and Fillingim, unpublished observation). These findings strongly support the view that there are individual variations in the factors that contribute to pain sensitivity and create the clusters of signs and symptoms observed in functional pain syndromes [21,50,50,59–61]. There is a primary research need to identify and examine the heterogeneity of pain perception in large populations of patients with functional pain syndromes and to identify specific phenotypic factors that permit the identification of unique clusters of patients. The molecular mechanisms that differentiate these clusters of patients and contribute to pain amplification also require examination.

Psychological Distress as a Determinant of Functional Pain Syndromes

Heightened psychological distress represents another domain of risk factors for functional pain syndromes (Fig. 2). Patients with these syndromes have elevated depression, anxiety [5,60,63], and perceived stress [1] relative to pain-free controls. Somatization, which is the tendency to report numerous physical symptoms in excess of that expected from physical examination [16], is associated with more than a twofold increase in TMJD incidence, with decreased improvement in TMJD facial pain after 5 years [43] and increased pain following treatment [38]. Somatization is also highly associated with widespread pain, with the number of muscle sites painful to palpation [73], and with the progression from acute to chronic TMJD [19]. In a first-of-its-kind prospective study on 244 initially TMJD-free females, we found that somatization, anxiety, depression, and perceived stress represent significant risk factors for TMJD onset (with significant risk ratios ranging from 2.1 to 6.0) [52]. These results suggest that somatization, negative affect/mood, and environmental stress independently or jointly contribute to the risk of onset and maintenance of functional pain syndromes. However, as in the case of pain amplification, there are clusters of patients with functional pain syndromes who manifest patterns of psychological distress. It is likely that there are large populations or clusters of patients with functional pain syndromes who share some (but not all) psychological factors. There is a research need to examine the heterogeneity of shared and unique psychological factors in large populations of patients with functional pain syndromes.

Genetic Variations Influencing Pain Amplification and Psychological Distress

Pain sensitivity and psychological distress are influenced by several genetic variants that mediate the activity of biological pathways (Fig. 2). Thus, when coupled with environmental factors such as physical or emotional stress, individual polymorphic variations in genes coding for key protein regulators of these pathways interact to produce a phenotype that is vulnerable to functional pain syndromes. The commonality of pain amplification and psychological distress in most patients with these syndromes may explain why there is so much comorbidity among patients. However, there must also be additional biological or psychological factors in addition to pain amplification and psychological distress that determine which specific functional pain syndromes will develop in an individual patient.

Both clinical and experimental pain perception are influenced by genetic variants [13,39,41,42]. (For a recent comprehensive review, see Diatchenko et al. [12].) The relative importance of genetic versus environmental factors in human pain perception is becoming clearer, with heritability for pain perception across several experimental modalities reported to range from 22% to 60% [41,42]. Several recent studies have also established a genetic association with a variety of psychological traits and disorders that influence risk of developing functional pain syndromes. Twin studies show that 30–50% of individual variability in the risk to develop an anxiety disorder is due to genetic factors [20]. The heritability of unipolar depression is also remarkable, with estimates ranging from 40% to 70% [30]. Moreover, normal variations in these psychological traits show substantial heritability [2,15,18].

With advances in high-throughput genotyping methods, the number of genes associated with pain sensitivity and complex psychological disorders such as depression, anxiety, stress response, and somatization has increased exponentially. A few examples of the genes associated with these traits include genes expressing catechol-*O*-methyltransferase *(COMT)* [10,13,24,52], adrenergic receptor β_2 *(ADRB2)* [9], the serotonin transporter *(5-HTT)* [6,20,25], cyclic AMP-response element binding protein 1 [81], monoamine oxidase A [8], GABA-synthetic enzyme [53], D_2 dopamine receptors [28], glucocorticoid receptors [74], interleukins 1β and 1α [75], Na+, K+-ATPase, and voltage-gated calcium channels [17].

The gene encoding COMT, an enzyme involved in catechol and estrogen metabolism, has been implicated in the onset of TMJD [13,52]. Three common haplotypes of the human *COMT* gene are associated with pain sensitivity and with the likelihood of developing TMJD. Haplotypes associated with heightened pain sensitivity produce lower COMT activity. It has also been reported that the haplotype associated with increased pain sensitivity is associated with an increased likelihood and greater symptom severity in a Spanish, but not a Mexican, cohort of fibromyalgia patients [62]. The inhibition of COMT activity has functional consequences and heightens pain sensitivity and proinflammatory cytokine release in animal models via activation of $\beta_{2/3}$-adrenergic receptors [40,57]. Consistent with these observations, we have also reported that three major haplotypes of the human gene *ADRB2* are strongly associated with the risk of developing TMJD [9].

Because it is highly likely that functional pain syndromes share common underlying pathophysiological mechanisms, it is expected that a set of functional genetic variants are associated with comorbid functional pain syndromes and related signs and symptoms. For example, a common single nucleotide polymorphism (SNP) in codon 158 ($val_{158}met$) of *COMT* is associated with pain ratings, μ-opioid system responses [46], TMJD risk [13,52], and development of fibromyalgia [24], as well as with addiction, cognition disorders, and common affective disorders [44]. Common polymorphisms in the promoter of the *5-HTT* gene are associated with depression, stress-related suicidality [6], anxiety [20], somatization, and TMJD risk [25]. It is likely that there are several genes that exhibit such pleiotropic effects, which interact to contribute to specific quantitative phenotypic traits or factors that combine to form specific clusters.

On the other hand, a defining feature of common complex phenotypes is that no single genetic locus contains alleles that are necessary or sufficient to produce a complex disease or disorder. A substantial percentage of the variability observed with complex clinical phenotypes can be explained by genetic polymorphisms that are relatively common (i.e., greater than 10%) in the population, although the phenotypic penetrance of these common variants is frequently not very high [49]. Thus, the varied clinical phenotypes associated with functional pain syndromes most likely result from interactions between many genetic variants of multiple genes. As a result, interactions among these distinct variants produce a wide range of clinical signs and symptoms, such that not all patients show the same broad spectrum of abnormalities in pain amplification and psychological distress.

Furthermore, environmental factors also play a crucial role in gene penetrance in multifactorial complex diseases. For example, functional polymorphism in the promoter region of the *5-HTT* gene is associated with the influence of stressful life events on depression, providing evidence of a gene-by-environment interaction, in which an individual's response to environmental insult is moderated by his or her genetic makeup [6]. There is a need for future research that seeks to identify phenotypic factors and population clusters and to identify the molecular profiles that underlie the phenotypic factors and clusters of patients with functional pain syndromes.

Since each individual patient will experience unique environmental exposures and possess unique genetic antecedents to vulnerability to functional pain syndromes, the most efficient way to identify genetic markers for these syndromes is to analyze the interactive effects of polymorphic variants of multiple functionally related candidate genes. The complex interaction between these polymorphic variants will yield several unique subtypes of TMJD patients who are susceptible to a variety of similar syndromes. The documentation that multiple genetic pathways and environmental factors interact to produce a diverse set of syndromes in TMJD patients, with persistent pain as a primary symptom, will enable the development of new algorithms and methods of diagnosing, classifying, and treating patients with TMJD and related syndromes. There is a need to provide new knowledge that substantiates the view that functional pain syndromes overlap with respect to two intermediate phenotypes—pain amplification and psychological distress—and that distinctions between the syndromes (in defining symptoms) are related to differences in genes and environmental influences that modify pain amplification and psychological distress. This heuristic model implies that variations between patients with the same syndrome (e.g., TMJD) may be due to different combinations of genes (or environmental influences) that lead to similar, but not identical, phenotypes. A primary research goal for the future is to distinguish between genes, psychological traits, and environmental exposures that are common to multiple functional pain syndromes versus those that are unique to specific syndromes.

Conclusions

There is growing evidence that functional pain syndromes, such as TMJD, are associated with both physical factors (e.g., trauma or infection) and psychological triggers (e.g., psychological or emotional stress), which, in susceptible individuals, initiate pain amplification and psychological distress. However, each individual has a different likelihood of developing these conditions. This probability is defined by a complex interaction between the individual's genetic background and the extent of exposure to specific environmental events. Elucidation of the physiological and psychological factors that contribute to and maintain pain amplification and psychological distress, as well as greater insight into the underlying genetic factors, will substantially contribute to our understanding of the mechanisms that evoke painful sensations in patients with functional pain syndromes. Moreover, there is a considerable need to develop methodologies that permit the subclassification or clustering of individual patients with functional pain syndromes based on specific phenotypic factors or traits and associated genetic variations, which will permit better diagnoses and inform individually based treatments. The future investigation of the pathways of vulnerability associated with TMJD and related syndromes requires an interdisciplinary approach by accomplished pain clinicians, pain researchers, psychophysiologists, molecular and cellular geneticists, biostatisticians, and epidemiologists who collectively are able to work in a cohesive manner to identify the psychological and physiological risk factors, and the associated genetic polymorphisms, that influence pain amplification and psychological profiles in study participants diagnosed with functional pain disorders.

Acknowledgments

I would like to thank the outstanding group of investigators and patients who have assisted me with this work over the last several years. I'm much indebted and appreciative of your contributions. This work was supported by NIH grants DE07509, NS045685, DE16558 and NS41670. Dr. William Maixner is a cofounder, officer, and equity shareholder in Algynomics, Inc.

References

[1]   Beaton RD, Egan KJ, Nakagawa-Kogan H, Morrison KN. Self-reported symptoms of stress with temporomandibular disorders: comparisons to healthy men and women. J Prosthet Dent 1991;65:289–93.

[2]   Bouchard TJ Jr, McGue M. Genetic and environmental influences on human psychological differences. J Neurobiol 2003;54:4–45.

[3]   Bradley LA, McKendree-Smith NL. Central nervous system mechanisms of pain in fibromyalgia and other musculoskeletal disorders: behavioral and psychologic treatment approaches. Curr Opin Rheumatol 2002;14:45–51.

[4]   Brennan F, Carr DB, Cousins M. Pain management: a fundamental human right. Anesth Analg 2007;105:205–21.

[5]   Broderick JE, Junghaenel DU, Turk DC. Stability of patient adaptation classifications on the multidimensional pain inventory. Pain 2004;109:94–102.

[6]   Caspi A, Sugden K, Moffitt TE, Taylor A, Craig IW, Harrington H, McClay J, Mill J, Martin J, Braithwaite A, et al. Influence of life stress on depression: moderation by a polymorphism in the 5-HTT gene. Science 2003;301:386–9.

[7]   Dadabhoy D, Clauw DJ. Therapy insight: fibromyalgia—a different type of pain needing a different type of treatment. Nat Clin Pract Rheumatol 2006;2:364–72.

[8]   Deckert J, Catalano M, Syagailo YV, Bosi M, Okladnova O, Di Bella D, Nothen MM, Maffei P, Franke P, Fritze J, et al. Excess of high activity monoamine oxidase A gene promoter alleles in female patients with panic disorder. Hum Mol Genet 1999;8:621–4.

[9]   Diatchenko L, Anderson AD, Slade GD, Fillingim RB, Shabalina SA, Higgins TJ, Sama S, Belfer I, Goldman D, Max MB, et al. Three major haplotypes of the beta2 adrenergic receptor define psychological profile, blood pressure, and the risk for development of a common musculoskeletal pain disorder. Am J Med Genet B Neuropsychiatr Genet 2006;141:449–62.

[10] Diatchenko L, Nackley AG, Slade GD, Bhalang K, Belfer I, Max MB, Goldman D, Maixner W. Catechol-O-methyltransferase gene polymorphisms are associated with multiple pain-evoking stimuli. Pain 2006;125:216–24.

66 W. Maixner

[11] Diatchenko L, Nackley AG, Slade GD, Fillingim RB, Maixner W. Idiopathic pain disorders: pathways of vulnerability. Pain 2006;123:226–30.
[12] Diatchenko L, Nackley AG, Tchivileva IE, Shabalina SA, Maixner W. Genetic architecture of human pain perception. Trends Genet 2007;23:605–13.
[13] Diatchenko L, Slade GD, Nackley AG, Bhalang K, Sigurdsson A, Belfer I, Goldman D, Xu K, Shabalina SA, Shagin D, et al. Genetic basis for individual variations in pain perception and the development of a chronic pain condition. Hum Mol Genet 2005;14:135–43.
[14] Drangsholt MT, LeResche L. Temporomandibular disorder pain. In: Crombie IK, Croft PR, Linton SJ. Epidemiology of pain. Seattle: IASP Press, 1999. p. 203–33.
[15] Eid M, Riemann R, Angleitner A, Borkenau P. Sociability and positive emotionality: genetic and environmental contributions to the covariation between different facets of extraversion. J Pers 2003;71:319–46.
[16] Escobar JI, Burnam MA, Karno M, Forsythe A, Golding JM. Somatization in the community. Arch Gen Psychiatry 1987;44:713–18.
[17] Estevez M, Gardner KL. Update on the genetics of migraine. Hum Genet 2004;114:225–35.
[18] Exton MS, Artz M, Siffert W, Schedlowski M. G protein beta3 subunit 825T allele is associated with depression in young, healthy subjects. Neuroreport 2003;531–33.
[19] Garofalo JP, Gatchel RJ, Wesley AL, Ellis E. Predicting chronicity in acute temporomandibular joint disorders using the research diagnostic criteria. J Am Dent Assoc 1998;129:438–47.
[20] Gordon JA, Hen R. Genetic approaches to the study of anxiety. Annu Rev Neurosci 2004;27:193–222.
[21] Gracely RH, Geisser ME, Giesecke T, Grant MA, Petzke F, Williams DA, Clauw DJ. Pain catastrophizing and neural responses to pain among persons with fibromyalgia. Brain 2004;127:835–43.
[22] Granges G, Littlejohn G. Pressure pain threshold in pain-free subjects, in patients with chronic regional pain syndromes, and in patients with fibromyalgia syndrome. Arthritis Rheum 1993;36:642–46.
[23] Gureje O, Von Korff M, Simon GE, Gater R. Persistent pain and well-being: a World Health Organization study in primary care. JAMA 1998;280:147–51.
[24] Gursoy S, Erdal E, Herken H, Madenci E, Alasehirli B, Erdal N. Significance of catechol-O-methyltransferase gene polymorphism in fibromyalgia syndrome. Rheumatol Int 2003;23:104–7.
[25] Herken H, Erdal E, Mutlu N, Barlas O, Cataluk O, Oz F, Guray E. Possible association of temporomandibular joint pain and dysfunction with a polymorphism in the serotonin transporter gene. Am J Orthod Dentofacial Orthop 2001;120:308–13.
[26] Kanazawa M, Palsson OS, Thiwan SI, Turner MJ, van Tilburg MA, Gangarosa LM, Chitkara DK, Fukudo S, Drossman DA, Whitehead WE. Contributions of pain sensitivity and colonic motility to IBS symptom severity and predominant bowel habits. Am J Gastroenterol 2008;103:2550–61.
[27] Kitaj MB, Klink M. Pain thresholds in daily transformed migraine versus episodic migraine headache patients. Headache 2005;45:992–8.
[28] Lawford BR, McD YR, Noble EP, Kann B, Arnold L, Rowell J, Ritchie TL. D2 dopamine receptor gene polymorphism: paroxetine and social functioning in posttraumatic stress disorder. Eur Neuropsychopharmacol 2003;13:313–20.
[29] LeResche L. Epidemiology of temporomandibular disorders: implications for the investigation of etiologic factors. Crit Rev Oral Biol Med 1997;8:291–305.
[30] Lesch KP. Gene-environment interaction and the genetics of depression. J Psychiatry Neurosci 2004;29:174–84.
[31] Lipton RB, Bigal ME, Ashina S, Burstein R, Silberstein S, Reed ML, Serrano D, Stewart WF, American Migraine Prevalence Prevention Advisory Group. Cutaneous allodynia in the migraine population. Ann Neurol 2008;63:148–58.
[32] Lowenstein L, Vardi Y, Deutsch M, Friedman M, Gruenwald I, Granot M, Sprecher E, Yarnitsky D. Vulvar vestibulitis severity: assessment by sensory and pain testing modalities. Pain 2004;107:47–53.
[33] Maixner W. Myogenous temporomandibular disorder: a persistent pain condition associated with hyperalgesia and enhanced temporal summation of pain. In: Brune K, Handwerker HO, editors. Hyperalgesia: molecular mechanisms and clinical implications. Seattle: IASP Press; 2004. p. 373–86.

[34] Maixner W, Fillingim R, Booker D, Sigurdsson A. Sensitivity of patients with painful temporo-mandibular disorders to experimentally evoked pain. Pain 1995;63:341–51.

[35] Maixner W, Fillingim R, Sigurdsson A, Kincaid S, Silva S. Sensitivity of patients with painful tem-poromandibular disorders to experimentally evoked pain: evidence for altered temporal summa-tion of pain. Pain 1998;76:71–81.

[36] Maixner W, Sigurdsson A, Fillingim R, Lundeen T, Booker D. Regulation of acute and chronic orofacial pain. In: Fricton JR, Dubner RB. Orofacial pain and temporomandibular disorders. New York: Raven Press; 1995. p. 85–102.

[37] McBeth J, Macfarlane GJ, Benjamin S, Silman AJ. Features of somatization predict the on-set of chronic widespread pain: results of a large population-based study. Arthritis Rheum 2001;44:940–6.

[38] McCreary CP, Clark GT, Oakley ME, Flack V. Predicting response to treatment for temporoman-dibular disorders. J Craniomandib Disord 1992;6:161–9.

[39] Mogil JS. The genetic mediation of individual differences in sensitivity to pain and its inhibition. Proc Natl Acad Sci 1999;96:7744–51.

[40] Nackley AG, Tan KS, Fecho K, Flood P, Diatchenko L, Maixner W. Catechol-O-methyltransfer-ase inhibition increases pain sensitivity through activation of both beta2- and beta3-adrenergic receptors. Pain 2007;128:199–208.

[41] Nielsen CS, Stubhaug A, Price DD, Vassend O, Czajkowski N, Harris JR. Individual differences in pain sensitivity: genetic and environmental contributions. Pain 2008;136:21–9.

[42] Norbury TA, MacGregor AJ, Urwin J, Spector TD, McMahon SB. Heritability of responses to painful stimuli in women: a classical twin study. Brain 2007;130:3041–9.

[43] Ohrbach R, Dworkin SF. Five-year outcomes in TMD: relationship of changes in pain to changes in physical and psychological variables. Pain 1998;74:315–26.

[44] Oroszi G, Goldman D. Alcoholism: genes and mechanisms. Pharmacogenomics 2004;2005:1037–48.

[45] Pukall CF, Binik YM, Khalife S, Amsel R, Abbott FV. Vestibular tactile and pain thresholds in women with vulvar vestibulitis syndrome. Pain 2002;96:163–75.

[46] Rakvag TT, Klepstad P, Baar C, Kvam TM, Dale O, Kaasa S, Krokan HE, Skorpen F. The Val-158Met polymorphism of the human catechol-O-methyltransferase (COMT) gene may influ-ence morphine requirements in cancer pain patients. Pain 2005;116:73–8.

[47] Rammelsberg P, LeResche L, Dworkin S, Mancl L. Longitudinal outcome of temporomandibular disorders: a 5-year epidemiologic study of muscle disorders defined by research diagnostic crite-ria for temporomandibular disorders. J Orofac Pain 2003;17:9–20.

[48] Raphael KG, Marbach JJ. Widespread pain and the effectiveness of oral splints in myofascial face pain. J Am Dent Assoc 2001;132:305–16.

[49] Risch NJ. Searching for genetic determinants in the new millennium. Nature 2000:847–56.

[50] Rudy TE, Turk DC, Zaki HS, Curtin HD. An empirical taxometric alternative to traditional clas-sification of temporomandibular disorders. Pain 1989;36:311–20.

[51] Sarlani E, Greenspan JD. Evidence for generalized hyperalgesia in temporomandibular disorders patients. Pain 2003;102:221–6.

[52] Slade GD, Diatchenko L, Bhalang K, Sigurdsson A, Fillingim RB, Belfer I, Max MB, Goldman D, Maixner W. Influence of psychological factors on risk of temporomandibular disorders. J Dent Res 2007;86:1120–5.

[53] Smoller JW, Rosenbaum JF, Biederman J, Susswein LS, Kennedy J, Kagan J, Snidman N, Laird N, Tsuang MT, Faraone SV, et al. Genetic association analysis of behavioral inhibition using candi-date loci from mouse models. Am J Med Genet 2001;105:226–35.

[54] Staud R. New evidence for central sensitization in patients with fibromyalgia. Curr Rheumatol Rep 2004;6:259.

[55] Staud R, Vierck CJ, Mauderli AP, Robinson ME, Cannon RI, Price DD. Evidence for abnormal central pain processing in patients with fibromyalgia syndrome. Arthritis Rheum 2000;43:S172–S172.

[56] Svensson P, Graven-Nielsen T. Craniofacial muscle pain: review of mechanisms and clinical manifestations. J Orofac Pain 2001;15:117–45.

[57] Tan KS, Nackley AG, Satterfield K, Maixner W, Diatchenko L, Flood PM. Beta2 adrenergic re-ceptor activation stimulates pro-inflammatory cytokine production in macrophages via PKA- and NF-kappaB-independent mechanisms. Cell Signal 2007;19:251–60.

[58] Thieme K, Rose U, Pinkpank T, Spies C, Turk DC, Flor H. Psychophysiological responses in patients with fibromyalgia syndrome. J Psychosom Res 2006;61:671–9.

[59] Thieme K, Turk DC. Heterogeneity of psychophysiological stress responses in fibromyalgia syndrome patients. Arthritis Res Ther 2006;8:R9.

[60] Thieme K, Turk DC, Flor H. Comorbid depression and anxiety in fibromyalgia syndrome: relationship to somatic and psychosocial variables. Psychosom Med 2004;66:837–44.

[61] Turk DC, Rudy TE. Toward an empirically derived taxonomy of chronic pain patients: integration of psychological assessment data. J Consult Clin Psychol 1988;56:233–8.

[62] Vargas-Alarcon G, Fragoso JM, Cruz-Robles D, Vargas A, Vargas A, Lao-Villadoniga JI, Garcia-Fructuoso F, Ramos-Kuri M, Hernandez F, Springall R, et al. Catechol-O-methyltransferase gene haplotypes in Mexican and Spanish patients with fibromyalgia. Arthritis Res Ther 2007;9:R110.

[63] Vassend O, Krogstad BS, Dahl BL. Negative affectivity, somatic complaints, and symptoms of temporomandibular disorders. J Psychosom Res 1995;39:889–99.

[64] Verne GN, Price DD. Irritable bowel syndrome as a common precipitant of central sensitization. Curr Rheumatol Rep 2002;4:322–8.

[65] Von Korff M, Dworkin SF, Le Resche L, Kruger A. An epidemiologic comparison of pain complaints. Pain 1988;32:173–83.

[66] Watkins LR, Milligan ED, Maier SF. Glial proinflammatory cytokines mediate exaggerated pain states: implications for clinical pain. Adv Exp Med Biol 2003;521:1–21.

[67] Weissman-Fogel I, Sprecher E, Granovsky Y, Yarnitsky D. Repeated noxious stimulation of the skin enhances cutaneous pain perception of migraine patients in-between attacks: clinical evidence for continuous sub-threshold increase in membrane excitability of central trigeminovascular neurons. Pain 2003;104:693–700.

[68] Whitehead WE, Engel BT, Schuster MM. Irritable bowel syndrome: physiological and psychological differences between diarrhea-predominant and constipation-predominant patients. Dig Dis Sci 1980;25:404–13.

[69] Whitehead WE, Holtkotter B, Enck P, Hoelzl R, Holmes KD, Anthony J, Shabsin HS, Schuster MM. Tolerance for rectosigmoid distention in irritable bowel syndrome. Gastroenterology 1990;98:1187–92.

[70] Whitehead WE, Palsson O, Jones KR. Systematic review of the comorbidity of irritable bowel syndrome with other disorders: what are the causes and implications? Gastroenterology 2002;122:1140–56.

[71] Whitehead WE, Palsson OS. Is rectal pain sensitivity a biological marker for irritable bowel syndrome: psychological influences on pain perception. Gastroenterology 1998;115:1263–71.

[72] Whitehead WE, Palsson OS, Levy RR, Feld AD, Turner M, Von Korff M. Comorbidity in irritable bowel syndrome. Am J Gastroenterol 2007;102:2767–76.

[73] Wilson L, Dworkin SF, Whitney C, LeResche L. Somatization and pain dispersion in chronic temporomandibular disorder pain. Pain 1994;57:55–61.

[74] Wust S, Van Rossum EF, Federenko IS, Koper JW, Kumsta R, Hellhammer DH. Common polymorphisms in the glucocorticoid receptor gene are associated with adrenocortical responses to psychosocial stress. J Clin Endocrinol Metab 2004;89:565–73.

[75] Yu YW, Chen TJ, Hong CJ, Chen HM, Tsai SJ. Association study of the interleukin-1 beta (C-511T) genetic polymorphism with major depressive disorder, associated symptomatology, and antidepressant response. Neuropsychopharmacology 2003;28:1182–5.

[76] Yunus MB. Fibromyalgia and overlapping disorders: the unifying concept of central sensitivity syndromes. Semin Arthritis Rheum 2007;36:339–56.

[77] Yunus MB. Role of central sensitization in symptoms beyond muscle pain, and the evaluation of a patient with widespread pain. Best Pract Res Clin Rheumatol 2007;21:481–97.

[78] Yunus MB. Central sensitivity syndromes: a new paradigm and group nosology for fibromyalgia and overlapping conditions, and the related issue of disease versus illness. Semin Arthritis Rheum 2008;37:339–52.

[79] Zolnoun D, Hartmann K, Lamvu G, As-Sanie S, Maixner W, Steege J. A conceptual model for the pathophysiology of vulvar vestibulitis syndrome. Obstet Gynecol Surv 2006;61:395–401;quiz 423.

[80] Zolnoun DA, Rohl J, Moore CG, Perinetti-Liebert C, Lamvu GM, Maixner W. Overlap between orofacial pain and vulvar vestibulitis syndrome. Clin J Pain 2008;24:187–91.

[81] Zubenko GS, Maher B, Hughes HB III, Zubenko WN, Stiffler JS, Kaplan BB, Marazita ML. Ge-
      nome-wide linkage survey for genetic loci that influence the development of depressive disorders
      in families with recurrent, early-onset, major depression. Am J Med Genet 2003;123B:1–18.

Correspondence to: William Maixner, DDS, PhD, Director, Center for Neurosensory Disorders, Room 2111, Old Dental Building, University of North Carolina, Chapel Hill, NC 27599-7455, USA. Email: bill_maixner@dentistry.unc.edu.

Vulvodynia

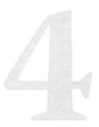

Caroline F. Pukall[a] and Yitzchak M. Binik[b]

[a]Department of Psychology, Queen's University, Kingston, Ontario, Canada;
[b]Department of Psychology, McGill University, Montreal, Quebec, Canada

Vulvodynia (i.e., chronic vulvar pain) affects 16% of women in the general population [34], negatively affecting their psychosocial function and quality of life [3]. Despite its high prevalence and detrimental effects, vulvodynia has only recently received systematic attention from health professionals, researchers, and funding agencies. In addition, a comprehensive, pain-based classification of vulvodynia has recently been proposed by the International Society for the Study of Vulvovaginal Disease (ISSVD).

The ISSVD defines vulvodynia as non-medically explained vulvar pain and categorizes different subtypes according to pain location [46]. *Generalized* vulvodynia refers to pain that affects the entire vulvar area, whereas *localized* vulvodynia refers to pain in a specific vulvar area (e.g., the clitoris). These two types of vulvar pain are then characterized according to the temporal pattern of the pain. The pain can be provoked, unprovoked, or both, with provoked pain resulting from sexual or nonsexual activities.

This chapter will focus on the two most common subtypes of vulvodynia, provoked vestibulodynia (PVD), formerly termed *vulvar vestibulitis syndrome,* and generalized vulvodynia (GVD). PVD affects 12% of premenopausal women in the general population, whereas GVD has been estimated to affect 6–7% of women, primarily those over the age of 30 years [34]. It is possible that the lower prevalence rate for GVD relative to PVD has led to a paucity of empirical literature on this condition. Although one research group has systematically published multiple methodologically acceptable articles on GVD (e.g., [32]), most one-time studies suffer from numerous methodological problems and are based on small and potentially unrepresentative samples. Review articles (e.g., [57]) reflect this scarcity of information, and virtually all reach a similar conclusion: that little is known about GVD and more research is necessary. This situation is frustrating for clinicians, researchers, and patients alike.

Clinical Characteristics and Pathophysiology

Provoked Vestibulodynia

Provoked vestibulodynia refers to provoked pain localized to the vulvar vestibule (i.e., vaginal entrance). The most common presenting symptom of PVD is that of entry dyspareunia (i.e., pain during sexual intercourse), frequently described as burning and/or sharp [6]. Some women report pain since their first vaginal penetration attempt (i.e., primary PVD), whereas others report that the pain developed after a period of pain-free sexual intercourse (i.e., secondary PVD).

When a patient describes symptoms similar to those of PVD, a thorough clinical examination is recommended [28] because the diagnosis of PVD is made only in the absence of relevant visible findings. Thus, the clinician must exclude all infectious, inflammatory, neoplastic, and neurological disorders [46]. The cotton-swab test should be performed to determine the specific location of the hypersensitivity. This test is the standard gynecological diagnostic test for PVD, and it consists of the palpation of various vulvar sites, including the vestibule, with a cotton swab. If the patient reports pain during vestibular palpation, then the diagnosis of PVD is confirmed. Although the cotton-swab test can be performed in a variety of ways, the palpation of the vestibular sites should be conducted in a randomized order to prevent sensitization [56]. An instrument called a vulvalgesiometer can be used to quantify the amount of pressure needed to elicit a pain response [59].

Given that the diagnosis of PVD is not derived from a specific pathophysiological condition, there are probably multiple etiologies for this condition. Local, systemic, and central factors have been suggested.

Local Factors

Initial studies suggested that inflammation of the vestibular mucosa was responsible for the pain (e.g., [17]); however, more recent investigations have not supported a direct role for inflammation in PVD (e.g., [9]). Thus, researchers have examined the tissue for other signs of abnormalities and have reported findings such as an increase in vanilloid receptor VR1 expression [77] and an increased proliferation of nerve fibers (e.g., [12,13]) in PVD versus control samples. Some suggest that the proliferation can be induced by mast cells, which may trigger nerve growth factor and heparanase, potentially in response to an allergen [13]. In addition, some authors have suggested that early injury to the vestibule due to mechanical trauma (e.g., early age of first tampon use and sexual intercourse [5,34]) or due to changes in the bacterial and hormonal milieu (resulting from, for example, repeated yeast infections or the early use of hormonal contraceptives [3,4,14,42]) can potentially lead to hyperinnervation of the area. Indeed, early alterations to tissue can lead to its hyperinnervation and concomitant hypersensitivity, as has been shown in the wounded hindpaw model in young rats compared to adult rats [20]. The heightened sensitivity in the vestibules of women with PVD has been demonstrated in several controlled psychophysical investigations with various forms of stimulation (e.g., [11,41,55]).

Although the precise source of the hyperinnervation in PVD is not known, the increase in pain sensitivity might lead to hypertonicity (i.e., increased muscle tension) of the surrounding area [64], as has been suggested in chronic neck pain [38] and fibromyalgia [48]. The hypertonicity could lead to an increase in pain perception, contributing to the cycle of pain. In line with this suggestion, surface electromyographic (EMG) recordings of the pelvic floor in women with PVD demonstrate abnormalities as compared to those of non-affected women [27]; EMG abnormalities have also been found in patients with temporomandibular joint disorders [40]. Additional abnormalities in the pelvic floor of women with PVD have also been demonstrated in superficial (but not deep) pelvic floor muscles [63], indicating that hypertonicity most likely plays a role in the maintenance, but not in the development, of the pain.

Systemic Factors

Hormonal factors have been proposed to play a role in PVD. For example, early menarche and dysmenorrhea have been associated with an increased risk of PVD [5,34]). Moreover, studies indicate that women who start using oral contraceptives at an early age have an increased risk of developing PVD [5,14], because prolonged exposure to progestins may render the vestibular mucosa more sensitive to pain [10]. Although these findings support the partial role of hormones in PVD, the exact mechanisms involved are unknown.

Gerber and colleagues [26] conducted a series of studies examining genetic factors in women with PVD and found that these women have a genetic profile consistent with the increased production of the pro-inflammatory cytokine interleukin-1β, leading to a severe and prolonged inflammatory response. These authors further indicated that some women with PVD may have difficulty terminating this exaggerated response. Similar processes have been found to contribute to chronic inflammation in individuals with inflammatory bowel disease [16].

Central Factors

Researchers have investigated brain morphology and function. One team examined gray matter density in women with and without PVD [68]. Results indicate that women with PVD exhibit significant increases in gray matter density in areas implicated in pain modulation (e.g., the basal ganglia and parahippocampal gyrus). Increases in gray matter density have been demonstrated in several chronic pain conditions (such as chronic back pain [67]). In addition, Pukall and colleagues [58] used functional magnetic resonance imaging (fMRI) to investigate neural activation patterns in women with and without PVD during painful vestibular stimulation. Results indicated increases in neural activation in women with PVD, a pattern often found in patients with other syndromes causing hypersensitivity (e.g., irritable bowel syndrome [7]). Overall, these neural changes suggest that PVD may be mediated by abnormalities in the central nervous system.

Generalized Vulvodynia

Some experts suggest that GVD is best conceptualized as a neuropathic pain process [21] resulting from injury to the sensory system such as from surgery, sporting activities, or childbirth [70]. However, the etiology of GVD remains elusive, and the pain most likely results from a variety of sources. In general, the pathophysiological hypotheses concerning the pain mechanisms of GVD are quite similar to those for PVD. As such, it is not at all clear whether to conceptualize GVD and PVD on a continuum or as distinct problems. Three small studies empirically addressed this issue [22,43,61], but they reached different conclusions.

Provoked Vestibulodynia, Generalized Vulvodynia, and Comorbid Pain Disorders

Sadownik [65] reported that approximately 55% of women with vulvar pain complaints either suspected they had or were diagnosed with another chronic pain condition, such as pelvic pain, bowel conditions, or bladder problems. However, this study did not verify the diagnoses, and the vulvodynia group appeared to have additional vulvar complaints (e.g., itching) that could potentially rule out the diagnosis of vulvodynia. Complicating the issue of comorbidity is that dyspareunia, the main complaint in PVD, has been associated with many pain disorders, such as chronic pelvic pain (CPP), interstitial cystitis (IC), and irritable bowel syndrome (IBS). Whether the dyspareunia is reflective of "true" PVD is unknown in most cases; however, dyspareunia (if it is not explicitly described as "deep") will be discussed in relation to other pain problems. Moreover, although a handful of studies have focused on PVD and self-reported comorbid conditions, even less is known about GVD and coexisting diagnoses. Further, PVD could overlap with GVD, and PVD has been considered to be difficult to distinguish in terms of pain characteristics from vaginismus (a condition in which vaginal penetration is very difficult or impossible due to high levels of fear and muscle tension). Information in the realm of dyspareunia, PVD, and GVD is discussed below in relation to other chronic pain conditions; however, systematic and empirical investigations are needed in order to clarify these relationships.

Chronic Pelvic Pain and Interstitial Cystitis

Chronic pelvic pain and vulvodynia are sometimes categorized together under the label of chronic pelvic pain syndrome (CPPS) [47], with some authors referring to vulvodynia as "vulvar CPPS" [66]. Despite the attempt to combine these two diagnoses, it is clear that the pain locations differ. The pain of CPP usually occurs in the lower abdomen and pelvis, whereas the pain of vulvodynia is restricted to the vulvar (i.e., external genital) area. Pain descriptors and severity also differ, with women with CPP reporting more severe pain than women with vulvar pain [32]. Despite these differences, a major complaint of women with CPP is that of dyspareunia, with one study reporting a comorbidity rate of 41% in women with CPP as compared to 14% of women without CPP in a random sample in the United Kingdom [84]. In addition, an online study of women with vulvar pain reported that 13% had received a diagnosis of CPP in the past [29]. Thus, it appears as if a constellation of vulvar and pelvic conditions may occur together in some women. Indeed, some authors propose that several gynecological factors can lead to an increased risk of developing CPP [39], including bladder conditions such as IC [66].

Interstitial cystitis, characterized by urinary urgency, frequency, and dysuria, often in combination with pelvic pain, is cited as a possible cause of CPP and is frequently comorbid with it (e.g., [30]). IC is also usually associated with dyspareunia (e.g., [51,80]). Further, of all possible pain conditions, IC is the one that most frequently co-occurs with PVD in the published literature, with one paper stating that PVD is the seventh most common IC-associated condition [2]. Although the prevalence of the co-occurrence of the two disorders is not known, clinical studies indicate that 25% of IC sufferers complain of vulvar pain [69] and that 11–32% of PVD/vulvar pain sufferers report having IC [29,44]. It is theorized that IC and PVD co-occur because of a defect in the epithelium of the urogenital sinus, from which the bladder, lower vagina, and vestibule develop [25]. However, one study examining whether epithelial defects and evidence of immunofluorescence typically found in IC patients were present in women with PVD had mixed findings: while positive immunofluorescence was found in women with PVD, Van Gieson staining revealed no evidence of alterations or defects [71]. Despite these ambiguous findings, several case reports [25,69,74] link the two conditions. Moreover, one recently published study comparing IC-affected women with (51%) and without vulvodynia (49%) found that those with IC and vulvodynia had significantly higher levator muscle pain ratings in response to pressure and a greater number of lifetime pelvic surgeries than women with IC alone; the groups did not differ on numerous other demographic variables, medical history, or abuse history [52]. Although the procedures used to diagnose vulvodynia in this study were not typical of the clinical or research literature, the study indicates some parallels between the two conditions.

Irritable Bowel Syndrome

Irritable bowel syndrome, characterized by abdominal pain, distension, and abnormal bowel habits, is frequently associated with CPP (e.g., [79]) and dyspareunia (e.g., [23,53,81]). An online study of women reporting vulvar pain problems indicated that 35% of them had also received a diagnosis of IBS [29]. More recently, two studies found a significant association between vulvodynia and IBS [3,4].

Other Pain Disorders

A high percentage of more than 400 women with vulvar pain reported having received diagnoses of fibromyalgia (21%), temporomandibular joint disorder (19%), and chronic fatigue syndrome (11%) in an online study [29]; however, this study was uncontrolled, all diagnoses were self-reported, and many women reported vulvar pain problems other than PVD or GVD. Vulvodynia has not been reported to co-occur with back pain in any study thus far, but dyspareunia has been associated with back pain (e.g., [31,72]).

Prevalence surveys of vulvodynia have found that affected women were significantly more likely than controls to report chronic medical conditions, including chronic fatigue syndrome and fibromyalgia [3,4]. Women with PVD also report significantly more pain-related complaints (e.g., dysmenorrhea) than non-affected women [19,54,55]. Interestingly, during a tender point examination (typically used to diagnose fibromyalgia and consisting of the manual palpation of nine bilateral body areas), women with PVD reported significantly more painful tender points than age- and contraceptive-matched control participants [54]. Although women with PVD did not meet the criteria for fibromyalgia, they tended to report more widespread pain than control women. Consistent with these results, other studies have demonstrated that women with PVD are more sensitive to various forms of painful stimulation (e.g., pressure or heat) over nongenital body areas, such as the deltoid muscle and forearm (e.g., [55]). Increases in sensitivity have also been reported outside the main area of pain complaint in other pain problems, such as migraine (e.g., [15]). These results support the idea that both peripheral and central nervous system factors play a role in PVD.

Affective Characteristics in Vulvodynia

Any chronic pain condition can lead to, or exacerbate, psychological symptoms. Affected individuals may become highly anxious about their pain and engage in avoidance behaviors [78]; heightened anxiety has been demonstrated in vulvodynia patients (e.g., [1]) as well as in women with IC [60] and CPP (e.g., [36]). Heightened fear of pain during sexual intercourse has been documented in women with IC [52], and women with PVD report more fear of genital pain compared to nongenital pain [50]. Some affected women avoid or discontinue sexual activity altogether (e.g., [3]) and demonstrate more defensive behaviors in a gynecological examination than control women [63], indicating that the fear affects both self-report responses and behavioral reactions. Findings from studies of back pain patients who scored high on measures of pain-related anxiety and fear indicate that they also report high levels of attention to pain sensations [18]; a similar hypervigilance to pain-related stimuli has been demonstrated in women with PVD [50].

Unfortunately, this pattern of increased fear, attention, and avoidance is related to higher scores on measures of disability and psychological distress, including depression [45]. Heightened levels of depression—although not clinical depression per se—have also been reported in women with vulvodynia, with case-control studies indicating that vulvodynia is associated with a higher prevalence of depressive symptoms as compared with non-affected women [3,4].

High scores in pain catastrophizing (the tendency to focus on pain and to evaluate one's ability to deal with it in a negative manner) also appear to be related to high levels of psychological distress and disability [76]. Women with PVD catastrophize more about their vulvar pain as compared with their most distressing, regularly experienced nonvulvar pain [55]. Perhaps the high level of catastrophizing in women with vulvodynia partially accounts for the findings of lowered quality of life and problems with sexual function [3].

Further research is needed in the area of psychosocial function in women with vulvodynia, specifically in the area of intimate relationships and partner characteristics, because such variables have been proven important in chronic pain conditions (e.g., [35,73]). It is possible that the extent of the pain in terms of location and temporal pattern may play a role in differential psychosocial impact. For example, one important potential difference between GVD and PVD is the extent of psychosocial interference. Sexual intercourse is the major provoking stimulus for women with PVD, and interference with sexual response and its sequelae are the major effects. Women with PVD are able to cope in a variety of ways, ranging from avoidance of sexuality to bearing the pain to please their partners [29]. The task for women with GVD is much more difficult because their vulvar pain typically lasts longer and is temporally unpredictable. In addition to interfering with sexuality, GVD is much more likely to interfere with activities of daily living. It is therefore not surprising to find several reports emphasizing the psychosocial distress of women with GVD [1,75,82]. Moreover, preliminary research supports the idea that different forms of vulvar and pelvic pain syndromes may entail different psychosocial effects. One study indicated that women with CPP exhibit higher levels of pain catastrophizing and are more likely to have experienced sexual abuse than women with vulvodynia [8].

The topic of childhood victimization as a specific contributor to vulvodynia has received mixed support, with most studies finding no differences between affected and non-affected participants (e.g., [62]). However, a recent epidemiological study indicated that childhood physical or sexual abuse by a primary family member may play a role in vulvodynia [33]. These and other predisposing factors should be further examined.

Discussion

Evidence has accumulated on potential local, systemic, and central factors in vulvodynia. Mechanisms such as central sensitization or wind-up could perhaps explain the progression of the vulvar pain in PVD to an increase in body-wide sensitivity [83]. However, no prospective studies have examined this progression, and it is therefore difficult to determine which type of pain starts first or if they both develop in tandem. Another factor may play a role in the increase in widespread sensitivity: Gerber et al. [26] proposed that the genetic profile found in women with PVD might trigger inflammatory events in other parts of the body, resulting in an overall increase in sensitivity to pain. This hypothesis may be supported by authors stating that the origin of all pain is inflammation and the inflammatory response [49]; however, this explanation remains to be empirically tested. Further, studies examining brain morphology and function suggest that the pain may be modulated by abnormalities in the central nervous system [58,68].

It is likely that multiple factors at each of these levels play a role, interacting with psychosocial processes to worsen or ameliorate the pain experience (e.g., [37]). In relation to PVD, Zolnoun et al. [83] proposed that physical factors (e.g., injury to the vulva or increased pelvic floor muscle tension), a state of pain amplification (e.g., an intense and prolonged inflammatory response or peripheral and central sensitization), and high levels of psychological distress (e.g., depression or anxiety) interact with each other to produce the pain of PVD. Similar to this proposed model is one offering the involvement of "limbic-associated pelvic pain" in CPP, in which a psychosocial stressor leads to alterations in the pain pathways of the central nervous system [24].

Although the topic of vulvodynia, its pathophysiological mechanisms, and the associated affective characteristics have only recently received systematic attention, a large amount of knowledge has amassed over the past 10–15 years. The knowledge base, however, is not sufficient at this point to offer a comprehensive model concerning the development and maintenance of vulvar pain. Certainly, pain-based pathophysiological mechanisms play a role, and investigations of other factors are emerging and expanding the existing literature.

References

[1]   Aikens JE, Reed BD, Gorenflo DW, Haefner HK. Depressive symptoms among women with vulvar dysesthesia. Am J Obstet Gynecol 2003;189:462–6.
[2]   Alagiri M, Chottiner S, Slade D, Hanno P. Interstitial cystitis: unexplained associations with other chronic disease and pain syndromes. Urol 1997;49(Suppl 5A):52–7.
[3]   Arnold LD, Bachmann GA, Rosen R, Kelly S, Rhoads GG. Vulvodynia: characteristics and associations with comorbidities and quality of life. Obstet Gynecol 2006;107:617–24.
[4]   Arnold LD, Bachmann GA, Rosen R, Rhoads GG. Assessment of vulvodynia symptoms in a sample of US women: a prevalence survey with a nested case control study. Am J Obstet Gynecol 2007;196:128e1–6.
[5]   Bazin S, Bouchard C, Brisson J, Morin C, Meisels A, Fortier M. Vulvar vestibulitis syndrome: an exploratory case-control study. Obstet Gynecol 1994;783:47–50.
[6]   Bergeron S, Binik YM, Khalifé S, Pagidas K, Glazer HI. Reliability and validity of the diagnosis of vulvar vestibulitis syndrome. Obstet Gynecol 2001;98:45–51.
[7]   Bernstein CN, Frankenstein UN Rawsthorne P, Pitz M, Summers R, McIntyre MC. Cortical mapping of visceral pain in patients with GI disorders using functional magnetic resonance imaging. Am J Gastroenterol 2002;97:319–27.
[8]   Bodden-Heinrich R, Küppers V, Beckmann M, Özörnek MH, Rechenberger I, Bender HG. Psychosomatic aspects of vulvodynia: comparison with the chronic pelvic pain syndrome. J Reprod Med 1999;44:411–6.
[9]   Bohm-Starke N, Falconer C, Rylander E, Hilliges M. The expression of cyclooxygenase 2 and inducible nitric oxide synthase indicates no active inflammation in vulvar vestibulitis. Acta Obstet Gynecol Scand 2001;80:638–44.
[10] Bohm-Starke N, Johannesson U, Hilliges M, Rylander E, Torebjörk E. Decreased mechanical pain threshold in the vestibular mucosa of women using oral contraceptives. J Reprod Med 2004;49:888–92.
[11] Bohm-Starke N, Hilliges M, Brodda-Jansen G, Rylander E, Torebjörk E. Psychophysical evidence of nociceptor sensitization in vulvar vestibulitis syndrome. Pain 2001;94:177–83.
[12] Bohm-Starke N, Hilliges M, Falconer C, Rylander E. Increased epithelial innervation in women with vulvar vestibulitis syndrome. Gynecol Obstet Invest 1998;46:256–60.
[13] Bornstein J, Cohen Y, Zarfati S, Sela S, Ophir E. Involvement of heparanase in the pathogenesis of localized vulvodynia. Int J Gynecol Pathol 2008;27:136–41.
[14] Bouchard C, Brisson J, Fortier M, Morin C, Blanchette C. Use of oral contraceptives and vulvar vestibulitis: a case-control study. Am J Epidemiol 2002;156:254–61.
[15] Burstein R, Yarnitsky D, Goor-Aryeh F, Ransil BJ, Bajwa ZH. An association between migraine and cutaneous allodynia. Ann Neurol 2000;47:614–24.
[16] Casini-Raggi V, Kam L, Chong YJ, Fiocchi C, Pizarro TT, Cominelli F. Mucosal imbalance of IL-1 and IL-1 receptor antagonist in inflammatory bowel disease: a novel mechanism of chronic intestinal inflammation. J Immunol 1995;154:2434–40.

82   C.F. Pukall and Y.M. Binik

[17] Chaim W, Meriwether C, Gonik B, Qureshi F, Sobel JD. Vulvar vestibulitis subjects undergoing surgical intervention: a descriptive analysis and histopathological correlates. Eur J Obstet Gynecol Reprod Biol 1996;68:165–8.
[18] Crombez G, Vlaeyen JWS, Heuts PHTG, Lysens R. Pain-related fear is more disabling than pain itself: evidence on the role of pain-related fear in chronic back pain disability. Pain 1999;80:329–39.
[19] Danielsson I, Eisemann M, Sjöberg I, Wikman M. Vulvar vestibulitis: a multi-factorial condition. Br J Obstet Gynecol 2001;108:456–61.
[20] De Lima J, Alvares D, Hatch DJ, Fitzgerald M. Sensory hyperinnervation after neonatal skin wounding: effect of bupivacaine sciatic nerve block. Br J Anaest 1999;83:662–4.
[21] Edwards L. New concepts in vulvodynia. Am J Obstet Gynecol 2003;189:S24–S30.
[22] Edwards L. Subsets of vulvodynia: overlapping characteristics. J Reprod Med 2004;49:883–7.
[23] Fass R, Fullerton S, Naliboff B, Hirsh T, Mayer EA. Sexual dysfunction in patients with irritable bowel syndrome and non-ulcer dyspepsia. Digestion 1998;59:79–85.
[24] Fenton BW. Limbic associated pelvic pain: a hypothesis to explain the diagnostic relationships and features of patients with chronic pelvic pain. Med Hypotheses 2007;69:282–6.
[25] Fitzpatrick CC, DeLancey JOL, Elkins TE, McGuire EJ. Vulvar vestibulitis and interstitial cystitis: a disorder of urogenital sinus-derived epithelium? Obstet Gynecol 1993;81:860–2.
[26] Gerber S, Bongiovanni AM, Ledger WJ, Witkin SS. Interleukin-1B gene polymorphism in women with vulvar vestibulitis syndrome. Eur J Obstet Gynecol Reprod Biol 2003;107:74–7.
[27] Glazer HI, Rodke G, Swencionis C, Hertz R, Young AW. Treatment of vulvar vestibulitis syndrome with electromyographic biofeedback of pelvic floor musculature. J Reprod Med 1995;40:283–90.
[28] Goldstein A, Pukall CF. Provoked vestibulodynia. In: Goldstein AT, Pukall CF, Goldstein I, editors. Female sexual pain disorders: evaluation and management. Oxford: Blackwell Publishing; in press.
[29] Gordon AS, Panahian-Jand M, McComb F, Melegari C, Sharp S. Characteristics of women with vulvar pain disorders: responses to a web-based survey. J Sex Marital Ther 2003;29(Suppl):45–58.
[30] Grace VM, Zondervan KT. Chronic pelvic pain in New Zealand: prevalence, pain severity, diagnoses and use of health services. Aust N Z J Public Health 2004;28:369–75.
[31] Gürel H, Gürel SA. Dyspareunia, back pain, and chronic pelvic pain: the importance of this pain complex in gynecological practice and its relation with grandmultiparity and pelvic relaxation. Gynecol Obstet Invest 1999;48:119–22.
[32] Haefner HK, Khoshnevisan MH, Bachman JE, Flowe-Valencia HD, Green CR, Reed BD. Use of the McGill Pain Questionnaire to compare women with vulvar pain, pelvic pain, and headaches. J Reprod Med 2000;45:665–71.
[33] Harlow BL, Stewart EG. Adult-onset vulvodynia in relation to childhood violence victimization. Am J Epidemiol 2005;161:871–80.
[34] Harlow BL, Wise LA, Stewart EG. Prevalence and predictors of chronic lower genital tract discomfort. Am J Obstet Gynecol 2001;185:545–50.
[35] Johansen AB, Cano A. A preliminary investigation of affective interaction in chronic pain couples. Pain 2007;132 (suppl 1):S86–S95.
[36] Kaya B, Unal S, Onzeli Y, Gursoy N, Tekiner S, Kafkasli A. Anxiety, depression and sexual dysfunction in women with chronic pelvic pain. Sex Relationship Ther 2006;21:187–96.
[37] Keefe FJ, Rumble ME, Scipio CD, Giordano LA, Perri LM. Psychological aspects of persistent pain: current state of the science. J Pain 2004;5:195–211.
[38] Larsson R, Öberg PA, Larsson SE. Changes of trapezius muscle blood flow and electromyography in chronic neck pain due to trapezius myalgia. Pain 1999;79:45–50.
[39] Latthe P, Mignini L, Gray R, Hills R, Khan K. Factors predisposing women to chronic pelvic pain: systematic review. BMJ 2006;332:749–55.
[40] Liu ZJ, Yamagata K, Kasahara Y, Ito G. Electromyographic examination of jaw muscles in relation to symptoms and occlusion of patients with temporomandibular joint disorders. J Oral Rehab 1999;26:33–47.
[41] Lowenstein L, Vardi Y, Deutsch M, Friedman M, Gruenwald I, Granot M, Sprecher E, Yarnitsky D. Vulvar vestibulitis severity: assessment by sensory and pain testing modalities. Pain 2004;107:47–53.

[42] Mann MS, Kaufman RH, Brown D, Adam E. Vulvar vestibulitis: significant clinical variables and treatment outcome. Obstet Gynecol 1992;79:122–5.

[43] Masheb RM, Lozano-Blanco, Kohorn EI, Minkin MJ, Kerns RD. Assessing sexual function and dyspareunia with the Female Sexual Function Index (FSFI) in women with vulvodynia. J Sex Marital Ther 2004;30:315–24.

[44] McCormack WM. Two urogenital sinus syndromes: interstitial cystitis and focal vulvitis. J Reprod Med 1990;35:873–6.

[45] McCracken LM, Zayfert C, Gross RT. The Pain Anxiety Symptoms Scale: Development and validation of a scale to measure fear of pain. Pain 1992;50:67–73.

[46] Moyal-Barracco M, Lynch PJ. 2003 terminology and classification of vulvodynia: a historical perspective. J Reprod Med 2004;49:772–7.

[47] Newman DK. Pelvic disorders in women: chronic pelvic pain and vulvodynia. Ostomy Wound Management 2000;46:48–54.

[48] Offenbächer M, Stucki G. Physical therapy in the treatment of fibromyalgia. Scand J Rheumatol Suppl 2000;113:78–85.

[49] Omoigui S. The biochemical origin of pain: the origin of all pain is inflammation and the inflammatory response. Part 2 of 3. Inflammatory profile of pain syndromes. Med Hypotheses 2007;69:1169–78.

[50] Payne KA, Binik YM, Amsel R, Khalifé S. When sex hurts, anxiety and fear orient attention towards pain. Eur J Pain 2005;9:427–36.

[51] Peters K, Girdler B, Carrico D, Ibrahim I, Diokno A. Painful bladder syndrome/interstitial cystitis and vulvodynia: a clinical correlation. Int Urogynecol J Pelvic Floor Dysfunct 2008;19:665–9.

[52] Peters KM, Killinger KA, Carrico D, Ibrahim IA, Diokno AC, Graziottin A. Sexual function and sexual distress in women with interstitial cystitis: a case-control study. Urol 2007;70:543–7.

[53] Prior A, Wilson K, Whorwell PJ, Faragher EB. Irritable bowel syndrome in the gynecological clinic. Digestive Dis Sci 1989;34:1820–4.

[54] Pukall CF, Baron M, Amsel R, Khalifé S, Binik YM. Tender point examination in women with vulvar vestibulitis syndrome. Clin J Pain 2006;22:601–9.

[55] Pukall CF, Binik YM, Khalifé S, Amsel R, Abbott FV. Vestibular tactile and pain thresholds in women with vulvar vestibulitis syndrome. Pain 2002;96:163–75.

[56] Pukall CF, Payne KA, Binik YM, Khalifé S. Pain measurement in vulvodynia. J Sex Marital Ther 2003;29(Suppl):111–120.

[57] Pukall CF, Smith KB, Chamberlain SM. Provoked vestibulodynia. Womens Health 2007;3:583–92.

[58] Pukall CF, Strigo IA, Binik YM, Amsel R, Khalifé S, Bushnell MC. Neural correlates of painful genital touch in women with vulvar vestibulitis syndrome. Pain 2005;115:118–27.

[59] Pukall CF, Young RA, Roberts MJ, Sutton KS, Smith KB. The vulvalgesiometer as a device to measure genital pressure-pain threshold. Physiol Measurement 2007;28:1543–50.

[60] Rabin C, O'Leary A, Neighbors C, Whitmore K. Pain and depression experienced by women with interstitial cystitis. Women Health 2000;31:67–81.

[61] Reed BD, Gorenflo DW, Haefner H. Generalized vulvar dysesthesia vs. vestibulodynia: are they distinct diagnoses? J Reprod Med 2003;48:858–64.

[62] Reissing ED, Binik YM, Khalifé S, Cohen D, Amsel R. Etiological correlates of vaginismus: sexual and physical abuse, sexual knowledge, sexual self-schema, and relationship adjustment. J Sex Marital Ther 2003;29:47–59.

[63] Reissing ED, Binik YM, Khalifé S, Cohen D, Amsel R. Vaginal spasm, pain, and behavior: an empirical investigation of the diagnosis of vaginismus. Arch Sex Beh 2004;33:5–17.

[64] Rosenbaum TY. Pelvic floor involvement in male and female sexual dysfunction and the role of pelvic floor rehabilitation in treatment: a literature review. J Sex Med 2007;4:4–13.

[65] Sadownik LA. Clinical profile of vulvodynia patients: a prospective study of 300 patients. J Reprod Med 2000;45:679–84.

[66] Sand PK. Chronic pain syndromes of gynecologic origin. J Reprod Med 2004;49:230–4.

[67] Schmidt-Wilke T, Leinisch E, Ganssbauer S, Draganski B, Bogdahn U, Altmeppen J, May A. Affective components and intensity of pain correlate with structural differences in gray matter in chronic back pain patients. Pain 2006;125:89–97.

[68] Schweinhardt P, Kuchinad A, Pukall CF, Bushnell MC. Increased gray matter density in young women with chronic vulvar pain. Pain 2008; in press.

[69] Selo-Ojeme DO, Paranjothy S, Onwude JL. Interstitial cystitis coexisting with vulvar vestibulitis in a 4-year-old girl. Int Urogynecol J 2002;13:261–2.
[70] Stewart E. Vulvodynia: diagnosing and managing generalized dysesthesia. OBG Management 2001;13:48–57.
[71] Stewart EG, Berger BM. Parallel pathologies? Vulvar vestibulitis and interstitial cystitis. J Reprod Med 1997;42:131–4.
[72] Sobhgol SS, Charndabee SMA. Rate and related factors of dyspareunia in reproductive age women: a cross-sectional study. Int J Impotence Res 2007;19:88–94.
[73] Stroud MW, Turner JA, Jensen MP, Cardenas DD. Partner responses to pain behaviors are associated with depression and activity interference among persons with chronic pain and spinal cord injury. J Pain 2006;7:91–9.
[74] Tarr G, Selo-Ojme DO, Onwude JL. Coexistence of vulvar vestibulitis and interstitial cystitis. Acta Obstet Gynecol Scand 2003;82:969.
[75] Tribó MJ, Andión O, Ros S, Gilaberte M, Gallardo F, Toll A, Ferrán M, Bulbena A, Pujol RM, Banos JE. Clinical characteristics and psychopathological profile of patients with vulvodynia: an observational and descriptive study. Dermatol 2008;216:24–30.
[76] Turner J, Jensen M, Warms C, Cardenas D. Catastrophizing is associated with pain intensity, psychological distress, and pain-related disability among individuals with chronic pain after spinal cord injury. Pain 2002;98:127–34.
[77] Tympanidis P, Casula M, Yiangou Y, Terenghi G, Dowd P, Anand P. Increased vanilloid receptor VR1 innervation in vulvodynia. Eur J Pain 2004;8:129–33.
[78] Vlaeyen JWS, Linton SJ. Fear-avoidance and its consequences in chronic musculoskeletal pain: a state of the art. Pain 2000;85:317–32.
[79] Walker EA, Gelfand AN, Gelfand MD, Green C, Katon WJ. Chronic pelvic pain and gynecological symptoms in women with irritable bowel syndrome. J Psychosom Obstet Gynecol 1996;17:39–46.
[80] Whitmore K, Siegel JF, Kellogg-Spadt S. Interstitial cystitis/painful bladder syndrome as a cause of sexual pain in women: a diagnosis to consider. J Sex Med 2007;4:720–7.
[81] Whorwell PJ, McCallum M, Creed FH, Roberts CT. Non-colonic features of irritable bowel syndrome. Gut 1986;27:37–40.
[82] Wylie K, Hallam-Jones R, Harrington C. Psychological difficulties within a group of patients with vulvodynia. J Psychosom Obstet Gynecol 2004;25:257–65.
[83] Zolnoun D, Hartmann K, Lamvu G, As-Sanie S, Maixner W, Steege J. A conceptual model for the pathophysiology of vulvar vestibulitis syndrome. Obstet Gynecol Surv 2006;61:395–401.
[84] Zondervan KT, Yudkin PL, Vessey MP, Jenkinson CP, Dawes MG, Barlow DH, Kennedy SH. Chronic pelvic pain in the community: symptoms, investigations, and diagnoses. Am J Obstet Gynecol 2001;184:1149–55.

Correspondence to: Caroline F. Pukall, PhD, Department of Psychology, Queen's University, Kingston, Ontario, Canada K7L 3N6. Tel: 1-613-533-3200; fax: 1-613-533-2499; email: caroline.pukall@queensu.ca.

Part II

Visceral Pain Syndromes

Irritable Bowel Syndrome and Related Functional Disorders

Lin Chang[a,b] and Douglas A. Drossman[c]

[a]Center for Neurobiology of Stress, David Geffen School of Medicine at UCLA, Los Angeles, California, USA; [b]VA Greater Los Angeles Healthcare System, Los Angeles, California, USA; [c]Center for Functional GI and Motility Disorders, Division of Gastroenterology and Hepatology, University of North Carolina, Chapel Hill, North Carolina, USA

Functional gastrointestinal (GI) disorders are chronic or recurrent conditions that cannot be explained by structural abnormalities of the GI tract. According to the recently updated Rome III diagnostic criteria, there are 27 adult and 17 pediatric functional GI disorders [39]. Irritable bowel syndrome (IBS) is the most common and most extensively studied of these disorders. The key symptom required for the diagnosis of IBS is abdominal pain [99], which is associated with increased health care utilization and has been shown to independently predict severity [87,153] and health-related quality of life [154]. IBS commonly overlaps with other pain-associated functional GI disorders such as functional dyspepsia, with symptoms referred to the gastroduodenal region (i.e., the epigastric area); functional gall bladder and sphincter of Oddi disorder, localized to the right upper quadrant; and functional abdominal pain, which is chronic or severe pain unrelated to changes in bowel habit. These disorders exist in the absence of any organic, systemic, or metabolic disease that is likely to explain the symptoms [160]. In addition, IBS commonly coexists with other chronic functional pain disorders including fibromyalgia, interstitial cystitis, and temporomandibular joint disorder (TMD) [175]. This overlap suggests shared underlying pathophysiological mechanisms in the central nervous system (CNS). The pathophysiology of IBS is complex and multidetermined, and it may vary among individuals or in the same individual over time. In the absence of reliable biomarkers, the diagnosis remains based on symptom criteria, as symptoms are what bring patients to their doctors. Treatment response is assessed by patient-reported outcomes. In the future, biomarkers may evolve that can identify specifically treatable subsets of this disorder, and which may relate to disease severity. Treatment consists of both pharmacological and nonpharmacological approaches, whose efficacy is variable depending on the nature of the condition and method of treatment. This chapter will provide an overview of IBS and a review of the coexistence of this disorder with other pain and symptom-based syndromes.

Epidemiology and Definition of Irritable Bowel Syndrome

Definition, Prevalence, and Impact

Irritable bowel syndrome is defined as a functional bowel disorder in which there is abdominal pain or discomfort associated with defecation or a change in bowel habit [98]. IBS is subtyped based on predominant bowel habit: IBS with constipation (IBS-C), with diarrhea (IBS-D), and with a mixed pattern (IBS-M) [98]. The subtype classifications are based on the prevalence of altered stool form (e.g., loose/watery stools or hard, lumpy stools) [98]. IBS is estimated to affect approximately 10–20% of adults and adolescents worldwide [59,98,139]. Varying gender and cultural factors—including differences in health care seeking, access to medical care, and diagnostic practices—may influence the wide range of these rates [76]. In the United States, IBS accounts for 12% of diagnoses made by primary care physicians and 28% of diagnoses made by gastroenterologists (41% if other functional GI disorders are included) [110]. The peak prevalence is between the ages of 20 and 30 years, although patients typically seek treatment for IBS between the ages of 30 and 50 years; the prevalence of the syndrome declines after age 55 [41,71]. There is a decrease in reporting frequency among older individuals, particularly in women [55]. However, the majority of individuals with IBS symptoms do not seek health care for their GI symptoms.

The economic burden of the disease has been estimated to be $1.6 to 10 billion in direct costs and $19.2 billion in indirect costs [142,162]. A recent systematic review evaluated 18 studies from the United States and United Kingdom that measured the costs associated with IBS. Calculated for the year 2002, the total direct cost estimates per patient per year ranged from U.S. $348 to $8750, and indirect costs ranged from U.S. $355 to $3344 [102]. In a more recent study of primary care and gastroenterology clinic patients seen at a managed care organization, mean total annual costs for health care averaged $5049 for IBS [122]. While most persons with IBS do not consult a physician, there are still between 2.4 and 3.5 million physician visits annually for IBS in the United States. When Levy and colleagues measured the medical care costs of IBS in a large health maintenance organization, the total costs of care in the index year were almost 50% higher in patients with IBS compared to non-IBS controls [95]. Most of the extra health care costs in IBS patients were not directly related to care for IBS or other lower GI problems but rather involved non-GI-related problems. This finding is consistent with the reported observations of the comorbidity of IBS with other disorders.

One of the main components of indirect costs associated with IBS is the reduction in work productivity that has been reported. In the previously mentioned systematic review, the average number of days off work per year because of IBS was found to range between 8.5 and 21.6 [102]. A naturalistic multicenter study was conducted in Canada to assess the impact of IBS treatments on work productivity, health-related quality of life, and resource utilization in 1,555 patients with physician-diagnosed IBS symptoms [125]. Work productivity was assessed with the Work Productivity and Activity Impairment questionnaire (WPAI) [135]. Patients reported 5.6% work absenteeism, 31.4% presenteeism (impairment at work), and 34.6% overall work productivity loss, equivalent to 13.8 hours lost productivity per 40-hour work week. In a longitudinal IBS registry from eight U.S. centers, clinical factors associated with IBS-related absenteeism and presenteeism were assessed in 170 study subjects. The number of non-GI comorbidities and overall IBS severity independently predicted absenteeism [152]. Taken together, these studies show that IBS patients incur greater health care costs, use more health care resources, and have decreased work productivity due to a variety of symptoms that are not limited to the digestive system.

Sex and Gender Differences in Clinical Presentation

Most population-based studies have found women to be at least twice as frequently affected as men, with prevalence ratios ranging from 2 to 3:1 [41,76,140]. However, some studies, particularly those conducted in Asian countries, have failed to show a sex difference [59,76]. It is unclear whether this difference relates to gender or sociocultural differences in symptom re-porting or in the true prevalence. Women with IBS are more likely to have IBS-C [143,145,163], abdominal bloating with visible abdominal distension [28], and greater symptom severity than men with IBS [33,167]. They also report more extraintestinal symptoms, greater impact of symptoms on daily life, and lower quality of life [33,146,167]. In addition, it appears that female sex is a risk factor for the development of post-infectious IBS [120].

Evidence suggests that several factors may contribute to sex- and gender-related differences in IBS. These factors include sex differences in visceral hypersensitivity, autonomic tone, neuroimmune function, hor-monal influences, cognitive response to pain, gender role, and report-ing bias [27]. In retrospective and prospective studies, women with IBS report greater GI symptom severity at the time of menses than healthy women [65,69,73,75,173]. However, while some studies report an effect of menstrual cycle phase on IBS symptoms, other studies do not. Increased abdominal pain and bloating and changes in stool form and frequency have been reported at the time of menses compared to at other menstrual cycle phases [65,69,73]. Furthermore, increased GI symptoms in women with IBS just prior to and during menses are associated with evidence of visceral hypersensitivity to rectal balloon distension [69,73]. Limited evidence suggests that fluctuations in ovarian hormones may be associ-ated with increased reporting of GI symptoms at the time of menses. A well-designed prospective study evaluated GI and non-GI symptoms over the menstrual cycle in women with IBS and in healthy women. Women with IBS-C reported more constipation starting in the early luteal phase (when estrogen and progesterone levels are high) and continuing into the premenses phase, whereas women with IBS-D reported looser stools relatively later in the cycle during the premenses and menses phases (when estrogen and progesterone levels fall) [65].

Sex-related differences may also affect responses to both psychological and pharmacological therapy. In a study conducted in 250 treatment-refractory IBS patients in the United Kingdom, women with IBS demonstrated an overall greater improvement in treatment response (52% vs. 33%) and better long-term outcome with hypnotherapy compared to men with IBS [57]. Pharmacological treatment responses may also differ by sex. Women may have a more robust response to serotonergic agents, such as alosetron and tegaserod, than men [24,79,113,121,172]. In the case of tegaserod, this finding may be partly due to the small number of men with IBS-C studied. It is conceivable that women with IBS are more responsive to certain types of treatment such as hypnotherapy and pharmacological agents that exert their benefit due to inhibitory effects in brain regions of the central homeostatic network. These regions, such as the dorsal anterior cingulate cortex (dACC) [133] and amygdala [10], are more abnormally activated in women than in men with IBS in response to visceral events. In the case of pharmacological agents, sex differences in pharmacokinetics may help explain differences in treatment response in women and men with IBS. For example, pharmacokinetic analyses have confirmed that alosetron clearance is 28% lower in women, resulting in approximately 30–50% higher concentrations in women compared to men for a given dose [81].

Comorbidity with Other Disorders

There has been growing scientific interest in the association of the functional GI disorders with other medical or psychiatric conditions. For example, IBS can co-occur with other functional GI disorders such as functional dyspepsia or functional heartburn; with somatic syndromes such as fibromyalgia, chronic fatigue, or TMD; or with psychiatric syndromes such as post-traumatic stress disorder (PTSD), Axis I anxiety or depressive disorders, or somatization disorder [175]. Also, the term "so-matization" can be used descriptively for patients who report many symp-toms. Comorbidities among the functional GI disorders may be explained by known pathophysiological associations such as altered motility, auto-nomic dysfunction, and visceral hypersensitivity. However, the association of IBS and other functional GI disorders with other somatic or psychiatric symptoms or disorders requires a different understanding.

Functional GI Disorders

The association of IBS with other functional GI and non-GI disorders is shown in Table I [119,136,175]. Functional dyspepsia is currently defined as the presence of symptoms thought to originate in the gastroduodenal region, in the absence of structural disease that is likely to explain the symp-toms (which can be ruled out by tests including upper endoscopy). Current-ly diagnosed using the Rome III symptom-based criteria, functional dys-pepsia has been subgrouped into two more distinctively defined disorders: (1) postprandial distress syndrome characterized by meal-induced dyspep-tic symptoms (early satiation and postprandial fullness) and (2) epigastric

Table I
Comorbidity of related gastrointestinal (GI) and non-GI disorders
with irritable bowel syndrome (IBS)

Disorder	Prevalence of IBS in the Disorder (%)	Prevalence of the Disorder in IBS (%)
Gastrointestinal Disorders [136,175]		
Gastroesophageal reflux disease [119]	31–71	28–80
Functional dyspepsia [161]	28–47	28–57
Other Somatic Disorders [136,175]		
Fibromyalgia	32–77	28–65
Chronic fatigue syndrome	35–92	14*
Chronic pelvic pain	29–79	35*
Dysmenorrhea or premenstrual syndrome	50*	10–18
Temporomandibular joint disorder	64*	16*
Interstitial cystitis	30.2*	

* Based on results of only one study.

pain syndrome characterized by pain or burning in the epigastrium [160]. Heartburn (a burning sensation in the epigastrium that radiates retrosternally) is not thought to be a symptom that arises primarily from the gastroduodenum, and it has moderate specificity for gastroesophageal reflux disease (GERD). Therefore, it is excluded from the definition of functional dyspepsia, although it can occur simultaneously [160]. The high overlap between IBS and upper-GI syndromes suggests a unifying explanation such as motor and sensory dysfunction.

Interestingly, IBS-C patients report upper abdominal symptoms more commonly than do IBS-D patients [143,161]. Symptoms referred to the upper-GI tract are more prevalent in IBS-C than IBS-D. These symptoms include early satiety (56.7% vs. 33.9%) [143], fullness (63.2% vs. 38.5%) [143], and abdominal pain (36.8% vs. 24.4%) [161]. In addition to reporting more coexistent upper-GI symptoms, IBS-C patients more commonly complain of extraintestinal symptoms such as musculoskeletal symptoms and impairments in sleep, appetite, and sexual function [143]. These findings suggest that there may be differences in autonomic and perceptual responses to viscerosomatic stimuli or in psychological factors such as symptom reporting between the two subtypes.

Symptom Reporting and Comorbidity with Non-GI Disorders

Historically, studies show that patients with IBS may report extraintestinal symptoms such as fatigue [103,176], muscle pain or stiffness [66,86,103,176], headache [103,176], sleep disturbances [51,65,169], sexual dysfunction [52], and alterations in mood such as anxiety and depression [65,66,94]. Some non-GI symptoms such as urinary urgency, muscle stiffness, and altered taste and smell are reported more frequently in women with IBS than men [86]. In fact, in IBS patients, the prevalence of the following somatic syndromes is also high[1]: fibromyalgia (32.5%; range, 28–65%),

---

[1] We define a *symptom* as an unmeasurable feeling or departure from normal function that is experienced and reported by the patient, which may or may not indicate the presence of a somatic or psychiatric disorder. Examples include headache, sadness, abdominal pain, or early satiety. A *syndrome* or *disorder* is a collection of symptoms or dysfunctions that cluster together across individuals to define a classified medical or psychiatric disorder. Examples include migraine headache, PTSD, IBS, and functional dyspepsia. Syndromes are often diagnosed using predefined criteria such as the DSM-IV classification system for psychiatry and the Rome criteria for functional GI disorders.

chronic fatigue syndrome (14%), chronic pelvic pain (35%), and TMD (16%). The presence of coexistent extraintestinal symptoms is also quite common, even when diagnostic criteria for specific medical conditions are not met. For example, a patient may have urinary urgency or myalgias but not fulfill criteria for interstitial cystitis or fibromyalgia, respectively. Notably, the prevalence of psychiatric symptoms and disorders—including anxiety and depressive disorders, PTSD, and somatization disorders—in IBS patients in the clinic and the tertiary care referral population ranges from 40% to 60%, which is increased compared to healthy controls [94].

Many of the studies reporting these comorbidities come from re-ferral practices where IBS patients with more severe disorders are seen. However, the prevalence of comorbid symptoms and disorders are not the same for all patients. Rather, they exist on a continuum, depending on the health care setting within which the patients are seen (e.g., general population, primary care, referral settings) or the severity of the underly-ing condition. Twenty-five years ago a large survey found that the number of non-GI symptoms reported increased from one in healthy subjects to two in individuals with IBS who never sought health care to three among IBS patients who had seen a physician [141]. Over the next decade, studies confirmed that symptom reporting frequency correlates with psychoso-cial difficulties and with the severity of the disorder and is more frequent in referral practices than in primary care or among patients with IBS not seeing physicians [43,78,149]. Similar observations occur with other dis-orders including fibromyalgia [150,151], chronic fatigue syndrome, and other somatic syndromes [32,156].

Fig. 1 demonstrates this relationship graphically for IBS. The pro-portion of individuals with mild, moderate, and severe symptoms is rep-resented by the size of the triangle. Individuals with more severe IBS are less common and are usually seen in referral centers. Moving toward the right of the triangle, as the illness becomes more severe, there are greater psychosocial disturbances including abuse history and poorer coping, and concurrently there is an increase in symptom reporting [42,45].

These observations were further clarified by the publication of a re-port from the National Institute of Medicine entitled "Gulf War and health: physiologic, psychologic and psychosocial effects of deployment-related

Peripheral and Brain-Gut Influences on Severity in IBS

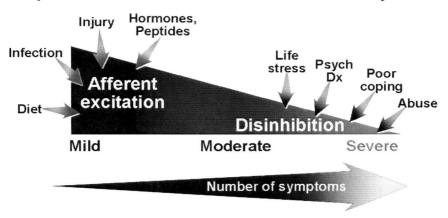

Fig. 1. Graphic demonstration of the prevalence of mild, moderate, and severe irritable bowel syndrome (IBS) based on the size of the triangle. As seen on the right side, individuals with more severe IBS are of lower frequency and are seen to have greater psychosocial disturbances including abuse history and poorer coping, and concurrently there is an increase in symptom reporting.

stress" [106]. The report portrayed a strong relationship between soldiers being deployed to a war zone where there was traumatic exposure including injury, witnessing mutilation, or caring for dead bodies and the ensuing development of medical and psychological symptoms and syndromes. In fact, clusters of several medical symptoms were noted, such as "Gulf War Syndrome" (which includes IBS, chronic fatigue, and chemical sensitivity syndrome), and in addition PTSD and cognitive impairments. The associations of anxiety, abuse, and the increased tendency to report somatic symptoms (i.e., somatization) has been described under the category of affective spectrum disorder [62,70].

Thus, it is now believed that the psychological effects of abuse or wartime exposure may produce disruption in central pain modulation systems and in brain circuits at the interface of emotion and pain [137]. Similarly, patients with IBS and fibromyalgia have shown altered activation in the dACC in response to visceral and somatic stimuli, respectively [25,108,170]. This change leads to a lowering of sensation thresholds, with a loss of the brain's ability to "filter" bodily sensations. The result is an increase in physical and psychological symptoms and syndromes (such as IBS, fibromyalgia, headache, and joint pains) which has been variably described as "somatization," comorbidities, or just "extraintestinal" functional GI symptoms [107].

Symptoms, Diagnosis, and Evaluation

The diagnosis of IBS is currently based on symptom criteria, and most recently is based on the Rome III criteria (Table II) [98]. The differential diagnosis for the symptoms of IBS is quite broad and includes organic, structural GI diseases such as inflammatory bowel disease, colon cancer, and celiac disease; endocrine disorders such as thyroid disease; and gynecological conditions such as endometriosis and ovarian cancer. However,

Table II
Rome III criteria for the diagnosis of irritable bowel syndrome

These criteria must be fulfilled for the last 3 months, with symptom onset at least 6 months prior to diagnosis:

Recurrent abdominal pain or discomfort* at least 3 days per month in the last 3 months that is associated with two or more of the following:

- Improvement with defecation
- Onset associated with a change in stool frequency
- Onset associated with a change in stool form (appearance)

Source: [98].
*Discomfort means an uncomfortable sensation that is not described as pain.

the use of the symptom-based diagnostic criteria, evaluation for alarm signs or "red flags" (e.g., blood in the stool, unintentional weight loss, or a family history of colon cancer or inflammatory bowel disease), and exclusion of celiac disease in some populations is sufficient to make the diagnosis of IBS [21,98].

Current evidence suggests that a battery of diagnostic tests is not necessary because the prior probability of another disease (with the exception of celiac disease) in the population of patients presenting with the symptoms of IBS is low. The value of ordering other less routine tests in IBS has also been studied, and in general these tests are not favored [21,99]. Colon cancer surveillance has demonstrated that the prevalence of colon cancer in IBS patients is 1/10 that in the general population [21]. This low prevalence is most likely due to the fact that IBS patients undergo colon screening examinations more frequently and at an earlier age than the general population.

Pathophysiology

The pathophysiology of IBS is complex, multifactorial, and varies across individuals or in the same individual over time. Increasing evidence shows that brain-gut interactions are altered in IBS patients, resulting in abnormal GI motility, enhanced visceral perception, and dysregulated autonomic, neuroendocrine, and neuroimmune function (Fig. 2). A network of brain regions that is consistently activated in response to nonpainful and painful visceral and somatic afferent stimuli is termed the homeostatic afferent processing network [105]. This network includes the insula, dACC, thalamus, and parabrachial nucleus [105]. Activation of this network can

Brain-Gut Interactions

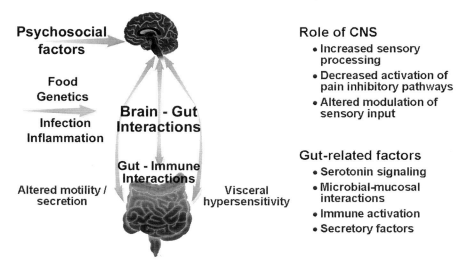

Psychosocial factors

Food
Genetics

Infection
Inflammation

Brain - Gut Interactions

Gut - Immune Interactions

Altered motility / secretion

Visceral hypersensitivity

Role of CNS
- Increased sensory processing
- Decreased activation of pain inhibitory pathways
- Altered modulation of sensory input

Gut-related factors
- Serotonin signaling
- Microbial-mucosal interactions
- Immune activation
- Secretory factors

Fig. 2. Brain-gut interactions are important in modulating gastrointestinal function in health and disease. Various factors can affect brain-gut interactions at a central (CNS) and peripheral level, resulting in changes in gut motility and secretion, visceral perception, and neuroimmune function. The central and peripheral abnormalities within the brain-gut axis that have been studied in irritable bowel syndrome (IBS) are shown.

affect arousal, emotion, pain modulation, central autonomic regulation of GI motility, and secretory function, with important consequences for the development of symptoms that involve both alterations in perception and autonomic responses to visceral events.

Enhanced Visceral Perception

Visceral sensations are transmitted from the gut via visceral afferent nerves to the brain, which perceives their painful and nonpainful characteristics. Enhanced perception of visceral stimuli, either as a result of increased activation of visceral afferent pathways or as central amplification of normal visceral input, has emerged as an important concept in IBS. Altered perception in IBS may result from at least two types of processes: (1) hyperalgesia, which results from peripheral sensitization or altered descending pain modulation; and (2) a cognitive process of hypervigilance toward aversive events arising from the viscera [117]. In experimental studies conducted in patients with functional GI disorders including IBS and functional dyspepsia, visceral perception has been most often assessed using the barostat, a computerized distension device that measures smooth muscle tone and visceral perception (e.g., sensory thresholds and/or ratings) to balloon distension in the GI tract. Many laboratories have demonstrated decreased sensory thresholds to colonic distension in IBS patients compared to healthy individuals [109,117,130,174]. Furthermore, it has also been shown that visceral hypersensitivity is not limited to the colon and rectum in IBS but also involves regions of the small intestine and the esophagus [1,165]. Barostat studies have suggested that visceral hypersensitivity may be a "biological marker" for IBS [35,109]. Bouin et al. [13] suggested that rectal pain thresholds measured by the barostat may help confirm the diagnosis of IBS as well as discriminate IBS from other causes of abdominal pain. He found that rectal pain thresholds were lower in IBS patients compared to healthy controls, and patients with painless constipation and functional dyspepsia. At a level of 40 mm Hg, the sensitivity of rectal barostat to identify IBS patients from normal and non-IBS subjects was found to be 95.5% with a specificity of 71.8%. The positive predictive value was calculated to be 85.4%, while the negative predictive value was 90.2% [13]. However, in a recent study by

Camilleri and colleagues [19] conducted in 116 IBS patients (predominantly women) and 41 healthy women, only 11.3%, 18.1%, and 16% of all IBS patients had increased sensory ratings for gas, urgency, and pain, respectively, at random-phasic distensions of 36 mm Hg above baseline operating pressure.

Thus, while barostat studies arguably offer the best current technology for measurement of visceral perception, the readouts (pain threshold or sensory ratings) are subjectively determined, and findings are not consistently abnormal in all IBS patients. Variability in barostat studies may be partly due to a number of factors that affect barostat measurements of visceral perception in IBS. These include the sex of the individual [29], predominant bowel habit [143,179], psychological factors and stress [36,38,128] and food ingestion [18,147].

Altered Central Modulation of Perception of Visceral Stimuli

Studies using positron emission tomography (PET) or functional magnetic resonance imaging (fMRI) show that the brain activation patterns elicited in response to intestinal distension are different in IBS patients than in controls. The mechanisms for the enhanced brain response in IBS patients are thought to involve increased peripheral signaling from the gut, amplification of a normal intestinal signal during transmission from the gut to the brain, or amplification of the signal within the brain itself [3].

Comparisons of brain activation in IBS patients and healthy individuals have recently been reviewed [105,134]. A more comprehensive review of studies conducted in IBS can also be found in Chapter 18 by Lorenz and Tracey. Key findings reported in brain imaging studies in IBS include the following: (1) While there are similar areas of brain activation in IBS and healthy control subjects, activation is altered in several areas including regions of the homeostatic afferent network such as the insula, thalamus, dACC, amygdala, and prefrontal cortex. (2) Altered brain activation to intestinal stimulation has been demonstrated in IBS patients vs. controls to subliminal distension pressures [84], aversive distension pressures [108,116,177], and anticipation of a noxious but undelivered stimulus [11,115,116]. (3) Variable, and sometimes contradictory, brain activation patterns have been reported in IBS that may be due in part to different experimental paradigms and methods of analysis [105,134]. (4) Brain activation in IBS can be affected by the sex of the individual [114], by a history of sexual or physical abuse [137], and by comorbid fibromyalgia [25].

Autonomic Nervous System Dysfunction

The autonomic nervous system (ANS) modulates and coordinates GI motility, secretion of water and electrolytes, and immune function. A number of abnormal motor patterns have been reported in patients with IBS, but they have limited diagnostic value because many of the techniques are not standardized, the indications have not been clearly defined, the correlation between symptoms and alterations is poor, findings are inconsistent between studies, and therapeutic options are limited [80]. There are various types of motility procedures, including scintigraphic gastric emptying and GI transit measurements, intestinal manometry, and barostat testing. Some are invasive and of limited availability. Motility has usually been measured during basal conditions and in response to various forms of stimulation such as food, bile salts, hormones, and neuropeptides as well as psychological stress. Motor abnormalities provoked by these stimuli are more prominent in functional GI disorders than during basal conditions [80].

Gut transit refers to the time taken for food or other material to pass through the GI tract and is a clinically relevant measure of GI function, primarily related to GI motility and secretion [80]. IBS-D patients have been shown to have accelerated gut transit compared to controls and occasionally to IBS-C patients [20,58,67,72,168]. The majority of IBS-C patients have transit times within normal range. In a recent study using scintigraphic measurement of GI transit, colon transit was abnormal in 32% of IBS patients, which included 46% of IBS-D patients with accelerated transit, 16% of IBS-C patients with delayed transit, and 14% of IBS-M patients with accelerated transit and 3% with delayed transit [19].

Previous studies utilizing various methods to measure systemic ANS function in IBS patients have shown inconsistent results, possibly due to differences in sample characteristics, assessment parameters, and conditions under which measurements were taken. However in response to stress, the balance of the sympathetic nervous system and parasympathetic nervous system shifts such that the former increases while the latter decreases. As measured by heart rate variability, which is a commonly used technique to measure cardioautonomic tone, a pattern of increased ratio of sympathetic to parasympathetic tone has been reported in IBS patients compared to controls [164]. Notably, this pattern of ANS dysregulation has been reported more often in men with IBS [164] compared to women with IBS, and in women with IBS-C with moderate to high disease severity. [16]

Hypothalamic-Pituitary-Adrenal Axis Function

As a key stimulator of the stress response, corticotropin-releasing factor (CRF) is found in brain regions, including the paraventricular nucleus, the central nucleus of the amygdala, and hindbrain regions, and in the periphery, including the gut, skin, adrenal glands, and placenta [5]. Hypothalamic CRF release results in the release of adrenocorticotropin from the pituitary gland, which then acts on the adrenal cortex to release cortisol into the bloodstream. The hypothalamic-pituitary-adrenal (HPA) axis is a highly dynamic system with an intrinsic diurnal and pulsatile rhythm that can be stimulated under certain conditions (e.g., infection, sleep deprivation, or psychological stress). Although few studies have evaluated basal and stimulated levels of HPA axis hormones, most support an enhanced HPA axis responsiveness in IBS without psychiatric comorbidity. Studies in IBS patients have measured basal [12,30,64] and stimulated HPA axis hormone levels in response to a meal [49], hormone challenge [12,37,54], or mental stress [36,48,128]. Three studies reported basal free cortisol levels in IBS patients, finding either elevated [30, 64] or blunted [12] levels. It is important to note that the patient group in the latter study was comprised of patients with functional GI disorders with a high prevalence of psychiatric comorbidity. Most, but not all, studies examining stimulated HPA axis hormone levels have demonstrated normal to increased HPA axis responses in IBS patients compared to controls [12,36,37,48,49,54,128]. Reactivity of the HPA axis to a stressor may be variable and is dependent on the salience of the stressor to the respective individual. It has been suggested that elevated HPA axis responses may be a reflection of a history of traumatic early life events, rather than a specific marker for a given disorder such as depression, or PTSD [63]. However, this suggestion has not been specifically studied in IBS. In addition, the relationship between HPA axis hormones and IBS symptoms or inflammatory or immune markers in the gut remains unclear and requires further study. Overall, studies have not found a relationship between HPA axis response and IBS symptoms.

It is likely that the non-HPA axis CRF pathways play a more prominent role in the clinical symptoms of IBS. Increasing preclinical evidence supports the notion that central and/or peripheral CRF_1 receptors are involved in stress-related anxiogenic behavior, activation of colonic secretory and motor function, and visceral hypersensitivity [100]. However, only a limited number of studies have evaluated the effects of CRF or CRF-receptor antagonists in IBS. In humans, systemic administration of CRF has also been associated with increased rectal sensitivity in healthy controls [90], and with increased colonic motility in IBS patients compared to controls [54]. Administration of a nonselective CRF antagonist reduced increases in colonic motility, abdominal pain, and anxiety ratings to electrical stimulation in the rectum in IBS patients but not in controls [138]. These studies support a physiological role of CRF in GI motility and perception that may be altered in IBS and suggest that a CRF-receptor antagonist may be an effective therapeutic agent for IBS.

Increased Immune Markers

It has been hypothesized that IBS patients or a subset of such patients have a compromised ability to downregulate the inflammatory response to infection and that this alteration may result in increased proinflammatory cytokines levels or an increase in EC cells [6]. Increased cellular infiltrate in the colonic mucosa and lamina propria has been reported in a subset of individuals who develop IBS-like symptoms after an enteric infection ("post-infectious IBS") [47] and in unselected IBS patients [6,22,124]. However, it is not entirely clear whether these findings are truly pathophysiological mechanisms related to gut function and IBS symptoms or whether they represent an epiphenomenon. Recent studies argue that peripheral immune changes are related to IBS symptoms.

Barbara and colleagues [6] reported increased numbers of mucosal mast cells residing near nerves and found a significant correlation between the vicinity of mast cells to nerves and both the severity and frequency of abdominal pain and discomfort. More recently, Barbara et al. [7] found that levels of mast cell mediators (tryptase and histamine) and prostaglandin E_2 were increased in the colonic mucosa of IBS patients vs. controls. Mucosal supernatants from colonic biopsies of IBS patients markedly enhanced the firing of mesenteric nerves and stimulated mobilization of Ca^{+2} in dorsal root ganglia neurons in rats. Excitation of dorsal root ganglia was inhibited by histamine H_1 blockade and serine protease inactivation [7]. In a complementary study by Gecse and colleagues [56], supernatants from fecal samples of IBS-D patients had threefold increases in total fecal serine protease activity compared to healthy controls. Serine proteases are signaling molecules that activate protease-activated receptors, which can modulate GI function including motility, permeability, sensation, and inflammation [56]. Administration of the fecal supernatants from IBS-D patients into the colon of mice was associated with allodynia and increased colonic paracellular permeability. In contrast, some studies argue against a predominant role of colonic mucosal immune activation in IBS symptomatology. In a randomized, placebo-controlled trial evaluating the efficacy of prednisolone in postinfectious IBS, prednisolone treatment was associated with a significant decrease in lamina propria lymphocytes compared to placebo. However, this change was not associated with any significant treatment-related improvement in abdominal pain, diarrhea, or bowel frequency or urgency [46]. While the pro-inflammatory cytokine profile in the blood has been reported to be higher in IBS patients compared to controls [37,96,123], colonic mucosal cytokine expression is normal to decreased in IBS-D patients compared to controls [30]. While the latter finding needs to be confirmed in larger samples, these studies suggest alterations in serum, but not gut, cytokine levels. Serum cytokine levels do not necessarily reflect levels or expression of various cytokines in the gut mucosa but may depend on activated immunocytes in the spleen or liver [118]. Furthermore, elevated levels of pro-inflammatory serum cytokines such as interleukin-6 have been reported during somatic stress, in depression, and even with intense exercise [17,101]. Therefore, they may not be related to mucosal immune activation, but rather reflect the effects of stress or comorbid psychiatric conditions.

Genetic Factors

Growing evidence supports a genetic component in the etiology of IBS. Familial clustering studies have demonstrated an increased odds ratio of having a first-degree relative with abdominal pain or bowel troubles [97] or IBS [74] in patients with IBS. Most, but not all, twin studies support a genetic contribution to the development of IBS [8,88,93,111,112]. However, studies suggest that environmental factors such as social learning [93] and early adverse life events such as restricted fetal growth [8] can increase the risk of developing IBS. In an interesting, recently published study using data collected from 44,897 individuals in the Swedish Twin Registry, a strong association was found between chronic widespread pain, a cardinal symptom of fibromyalgia, and other pain-related disorders including IBS, joint pain, and headache. Additionally, the researchers found that unmeasured genetic and family environmental factors were likely to mediate these associations [77].

In summary, the pathophysiology of IBS is complex and multifactorial and cannot be explained by a single mechanism. Central and peripheral factors as well as vulnerability factors can influence the development of IBS and affect symptom exacerbations.

Treatment of Irritable Bowel Syndrome

Treatment of IBS consists of general measures, pharmacotherapy, and nonpharmacological approaches. Medications approved by the U.S. Food and Drug Administration (FDA) for the treatment of IBS are limited due to a number of factors including a perceived higher risk-over-benefit ratio. [23] However, some medications that have been approved by the FDA for other indications have shown variable efficacy in IBS and are often used in clinical practice. In addition, patients often are treated using nonpharmacological approaches or may seek out alternative treatments on their own to control their symptoms. Treatment of IBS will be briefly reviewed, and the reader is referred to several recent comprehensive reviews of IBS treatment [99,104,155,171].

General Guidelines

Patient-Provider Relationship

An effective patient-provider relationship has been associated with improved health status and increased efficiency of care [157] and is essential in the successful management of IBS. In order to establish an effective and interactive relationship with patients, health care providers should obtain a medical history through a patient-centered interview, conduct a cost-efficient investigation including a physical examination, and provide a clear explanation of IBS and the patient's symptoms that takes into consideration the patient's beliefs. They should address the patient's expectations, involve the patient in the treatment, and establish a long-term relationship with the patient [39]. Recognition of stressors or other inciting factors associated with symptoms is vitally important since stress can exacerbate IBS symptoms and reduce chances of disease remission [9,26,39].

Diet

Between 20% and 65% of patients report that their IBS symptoms are triggered by food. However, studies to support the relationship between diet, specifically food allergies or food intolerances, and IBS symptoms are limited [60,126,148]. Not to be ignored is the fact that eating a meal in general has physiological consequences (e.g., gastric distension, release of neuropeptides, and increased gut transit) that could produce or exacerbate symptoms. Foods commonly associated with food intolerance include foods rich in carbohydrates, fatty foods, milk, wheat, eggs, nuts, shellfish, and soybeans. Although exclusion diets as treatment for IBS have shown some benefit, ranging from 15% to 71%, additional studies are necessary to determine if food avoidance is an effective treatment for IBS [126,180]. Given that food intolerances are common among IBS patients and may result in diarrhea, bloating, and abdominal pain, the recommendation to eat frequent smaller meals may not only be diagnostic by discerning whether the problem is food specific or relates to eating in general, but may also be therapeutic.

Pharmacotherapy Directed at the Predominant Symptom

Selection of the best drug to treat IBS is often based on the patient's predominant and most bothersome symptom and on the severity of IBS (mild, moderate, or severe). As mentioned above, only a few drugs have been approved specifically for the treatment of IBS. Others used off-label in the treatment of IBS have been approved for other conditions such as functional constipation, fibromyalgia, or depression, which often coexist with IBS. These agents act on targets within the brain-gut axis (Fig. 3) with central and/or peripheral effects. This section will focus more on centrally acting therapies that are used not only in IBS but in other chronic pain disorders.

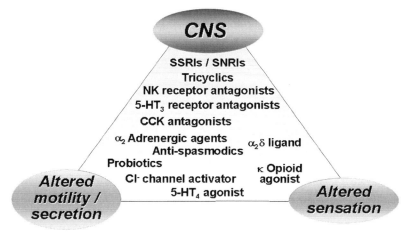

Fig. 3. Various pharmacological agents that are currently available or in development for the treatment of irritable bowel syndrome (IBS) include centrally and peripherally acting agents. They are shown in proximity to the specific targeted effect they exert, whether it is by modulating the central nervous system (CNS), by improving gastrointestinal motility and secretion, or by acting as an analgesic agent. SSRIs = selective serotonin reuptake inhibitors; SNRIs = serotonin norepinephrine reuptake inhibitors; NK = neurokinin; 5-HT = serotonin.

Treatments for IBS-C

The treatments used primarily for IBS-C patients are peripherally acting agents that enhance GI motility and secretion and thus improve stool frequency and consistency. These include fiber and bulking agents, laxatives, lubiprostone, and to a lesser extent, the selective 5-hydroxytryptamine-4 (5-HT$_4$) agonist tegaserod.

Bulking agents and laxatives. These agents can improve stool frequency and stool consistency in patients with constipation, but there is insufficient evidence to determine if they are beneficial in providing global relief of IBS symptoms [15,131]. Unlike chronic constipation, where obtaining laxation is the treatment goal, the relief of abdominal pain, which is presumably related to enhanced visceral perception, is the hallmark for a clinical response in IBS.

Tegaserod. Tegaserod is a 5-HT$_4$ partial agonist that was approved by the FDA for the treatment of IBS-C in women and the treatment of chronic idiopathic constipation in men and women under the age of 65, based on multicenter randomized, placebo-controlled studies demonstrating its efficacy [50,79,113]. However, tegaserod is currently only available in the United States for emergency use and must be requested from the FDA because of concerns of cardiovascular ischemic events associated with its use [53].

Lubiprostone. Lubiprostone is a specific chloride channel (CIC-2) activator in the GI tract and is FDA-approved for the treatment of IBS-C in women and for chronic idiopathic constipation in men and women. Two 12-week double-blind, randomized, placebo-controlled studies of lubiprostone at 8 µg twice daily in adults with IBS-C demonstrated a significant improvement in overall response and individual symptoms of constipation [40]. The efficacy of lubiprostone may be more robust for bowel habits than for pain.

Treatments for IBS-D

Antidiarrheals. Although the efficacy of antidiarrheals has not been specifically studied in IBS, this class of drugs is often used as a first-line treatment for diarrhea in IBS-D, particularly for mild to moderate symptoms. Loperamide is a peripherally acting opioid receptor agonist that improves diarrhea symptoms, including stool consistency and bowel frequency and urgency [4]; it can useful in IBS-D, particularly if given prophylactically.

Alosetron. One of the most effective agents for IBS-D is alosetron, which is a 5-HT$_3$ receptor antagonist currently FDA approved for the treatment of severe IBS-D in women. Blockade of 5-HT$_3$ receptors by alosetron has peripheral actions (slowing intestinal transit, decreasing chloride and water secretion, and increasing rectal compliance) and central actions (reducing visceral perception) [10,61]. High-quality studies have demonstrated the efficacy of alosetron in women with more severe symptoms including urgency [82,89,91]. However, due to concerns about ischemic colitis and serious complications of constipation with alosetron, the medication is available only under a restricted use program by the FDA for the treatment of severe IBS-D in women who have failed to respond to conventional therapy.

Treatments for Gas and Bloating

Two classes of pharmacological therapies that have been shown to provide relief of gas and bloating in limited studies are antibiotics (e.g., rifaximin [127, 144]) and probiotics [132]. Large, multicenter, high-quality trials are needed to sufficiently determine the efficacy of these peripherally acting agents in IBS.

Other Agents

Antispasmodics

Antispasmodics are often in used in clinical practice to help relieve abdominal pain in IBS patients. Two meta-analyses evaluated the efficacy of antispasmodics in randomized, controlled clinical trials in IBS [92,129]. Overall, smooth-muscle relaxants improved the global rating of symptoms and reduced pain in patients with IBS [129], but only octylonium bromide was found to be effective in IBS when low-quality studies were excluded [92].

Antidepressants

Antidepressants are increasingly used for a variety of reasons relating to improvement in abdominal pain and discomfort, treatment of associated psychological comorbidities, including anxiety and depression (depression is often treated with higher dosages), and on occasion for improvement of stool symptoms.

Tricyclic antidepressants (TCAs). TCAs are often used in chronic pain disorders including fibromyalgia, interstitial cystitis, and migraine headaches. Although their efficacy has been studied in IBS, TCAs are not FDA approved for the treatment of IBS. A systematic review of seven randomized clinical trials conducted in 2002, which were assessed to be of low quality, found evidence that TCAs may decrease abdominal pain, although their effects may be limited [15]. In 2003, a randomized, placebo-controlled trial in 431 women with functional bowel disorders (87.2% had IBS) evaluated the efficacy and safety of desipramine [44]. The study found that desipramine was not significantly more efficacious than placebo in the intention-to-treat analysis, but the effect was significant in the per-protocol analysis (i.e., only in those who completed the study). Treatment was more beneficial for those with moderate symptoms, abuse history, no depression, and IBS-D symptoms. TCAs are frequently initiated at low doses at bedtime and gradually increased as tolerated. An effective physician-patient relationship is important in helping the patient to stay on the medication to achieve an optimal treatment response during the first week or two when side effects are most problematic.

Selective serotonin reuptake inhibitors (SSRIs). SSRIs are increasingly prescribed as treatment for IBS patients; however, they are not FDA approved for use in IBS, nor are they particularly effective for treatment of abdominal pain or discomfort. Only a limited number of randomized, controlled trials are available on which to make conclusions about the efficacy of SSRIs. Several studies have evaluated the efficacy of these agents in patients with IBS, but they have enrolled relatively small numbers of patients. Limited evidence has shown that SSRIs may improve overall well-being, symptom frequency, and, less often, abdominal pain in IBS [34,158,159,166]. However, these drugs can be used to reduce anxiety associated with the symptoms, to augment the pain relief benefit of low-dose TCAs in some cases, and to reduce anxiety-related behaviors such as agoraphobia or obsessiveness surrounding the bowel symptoms. High-quality studies in larger patient samples are needed to evaluate the efficacy of SSRIs in IBS and determine if SSRIs can relieve IBS symptoms irrespective of their effects on mood.

Serotonin-norepinephrine reuptake inhibitors (SNRIs). More recently, because of their combined noradrenergic and serotonergic effect, these agents are being increasingly used for painful medical conditions. They do not have the same degree of antihistaminic or anticholinergic effects as the TCAs. The main side effect for duloxetine is nausea. Venlafaxine requires higher dosages to achieve noradrenergic effects and hence pain reduction. The effect of venlafaxine on colonic sensorimotor function was studied in healthy humans. Compared to placebo, venlafaxine decreased colonic compliance and reduced fasting and postprandial tone. Additionally, it was associated with a lower increase in sensation scores for pain per unit change in distension pressure, particularly at the higher pressures [31]. No studies to date have been done in IBS, but studies with SNRIs show benefit in fibromyalgia. Two randomized, placebo-controlled trials have demonstrated that duloxetine is superior to placebo in decreasing pain, global symptom severity, and functional impairment [2]. The beneficial effect of duloxetine on pain reduction was found to be independent of secondary improvement in mood.

Gabapentin and Pregabalin

Gabapentin and pregabalin are centrally acting agents that have been used to treat neuropathic pain, fibromyalgia, and epilepsy. Gabapentin is an analogue of the inhibitor neurotransmitter γ-aminobutyric acid (GABA), and pregabalin is a second-generation $\alpha_2\delta$ ligand that is structurally related to GABA but does not act on GABA receptors. Both act on $\alpha_2\delta$ subunits of voltage-gated calcium channels on nerve terminals, resulting in decreased depolarization and release of excitatory neurotransmitters such as glutamate, norepinephrine, substance P, and calcitonin gene-related peptide [68]. The effect of gabapentin [85] and pregabalin [68] on visceral perceptual thresholds to rectal balloon distension was assessed in two separate randomized, placebo-controlled trials in IBS patients. Both studies demonstrated small but significant increases in perceptual thresholds to nonpainful sensations and pain (i.e., decreased perception) with gabapentin and pregabalin compared to placebo. Adverse events that were most commonly reported with both medications were dizziness and somnolence. Clinical trials with larger samples are needed to determine if these drugs have efficacy in relieving the clinical symptoms of IBS, particularly abdominal pain.

Nonpharmacological Therapies

There are several psychological treatments for which there is convincing evidence of efficacy. This approach is more extensively reviewed in Chapter 23 by Lackner and McCracken. The best evidence is for cognitive-behavioral therapy (CBT), which is a short-term, goal-oriented form of psychotherapy that focuses on the role that thoughts play in determining behaviors and emotional responses [14,44,83], and for gut-directed hypnotherapy [178], which is hypnosis that is directed toward relaxation and control of intestinal motility by repeated suggestion of control over symptoms, followed by ego-strengthening. These therapies can be used in patients with various predominant symptom patterns.

Conclusion

Irritable bowel syndrome is a common GI disorder frequently diagnosed by primary care providers, gastroenterologists, and other health care providers. While this condition is defined and characterized by abdominal pain and altered bowel habits, when the symptoms are more severe, a proportion of individuals with IBS also report upper-GI symptoms and extraintestinal symptoms that are often due to a coexistence with other conditions. Brain-gut alterations, which are associated with dysregulations in adaptive systems, including pain modulatory pathways, with ANS function, and with neuroendocrine and neuroimmune function, are likely to be of key importance in IBS pathophysiology. Comorbidity occurs as the illness becomes more severe, with greater psychosocial disturbances and symptom reporting, and is likely mediated by dysregulations in CNS circuits concerned with pain, emotion, and autonomic responses. Treatment of IBS is limited, although various pharmacological and nonpharmacological approaches are used. Selection of pharmacological therapies is usually based on the predominant symptom and its severity. Drugs used to treat altered bowel habits in IBS are typically peripherally acting agents. The medications that appear to be more effective in treating pain and other symptoms in moderate to severe cases are centrally acting and have also shown efficacy in conditions that commonly coexist with IBS.

Acknowledgment

Dr. Chang has served as a consultant for Albireo, Forest, Ironwood, McNeil, Prometheus, Salix, Synergy, Takeda, and Tioga and has received research grant support from GlaxoSmithKline, Prometheus, and Rose Pharma. Dr. Drossman has been a consultant for Takeda, Sucampo, McNeil, Wyeth, Ironwood, Salix, and Tioga over the past year. He has received research funds from Takeda, McNeill, and Astra Zeneca.

References

[1]   Accarino AM, Azpiroz F, Malagelada JR. Symptomatic responses to stimulation of sensory pathways in the jejunum. Am J Physiol 1992;263:G673–G7.

[2]   Arnold LM, Pritchett YL, D'Souza DN, Kajdasz DK, Iyengar S, Wernicke JF. Duloxetine for the treatment of fibromyalgia in women: pooled results from two randomized, placebo-controlled clinical trials. J Womens Health (Larchmt) 2007;16:1145–56.

[3]   Azpiroz F, Bouin M, Camilleri M, Mayer EA, Poitras P, Spiller RC. Mechanisms of hypersensitivity in IBS and functional disorders. Neurogastroenterol Motil 2007;19:62–88.

[4]   Baker DE. Loperamide: a pharmacological review. Rev Gastroenterol Disord 2007;7 Suppl 3:S11–8.

[5]   Bale TL, Vale WW. CRF and CRF receptors: Role in stress responsivity and other behaviors. Annu Rev Pharmacol Toxicol 2004;44:525–57.

[6]   Barbara G, Stanghellini V, De Giorgio R, Cremon C, Cottrell GS, Santini D, Pasquinelli G, Morselli-Labate AM, Grady EF, Bunnett NW, Collins SM, Corinaldesi R. Activated mast cells in proximity to colonic nerves correlate with abdominal pain in irritable bowel syndrome. Gastroenterology 2004;126:693–702.

[7]   Barbara G, Wang B, Stanghellini V, De Giorgio R, Cremon C, Di Nardo G, Trevisani M, Campi B, Geppetti P, Tonini M, Bunnett NW, Grundy D, Corinaldesi R. Mast cell-dependent excitation of visceral-nociceptive sensory neurons in irritable bowel syndrome. Gastroenterology 2007;132:26–37.

[8]   Bengtson MB, Ronning T, Vatn MH, Harris JR. Irritable bowel syndrome in twins: genes and environment. Gut 2006;55:1754–9.

[9]   Bennett EJ, Tennant CC, Piesse C, Badcock CA, Kellow JE. Level of chronic life stress predicts clinical outcome in irritable bowel syndrome. Gut 1998;43:256–61.

[10] Berman SM, Chang L, Suyenobu B, Derbyshire SW, Stains J, FitzGerald L, Mandelkern M, Hamm L, Vogt B, Naliboff BD, Mayer EA. Condition-specific deactivation of brain regions by 5-HT3 receptor antagonist alosetron. Gastroenterology 2002;123:969–77.

[11] Berman SM, Naliboff BD, Suyenobu B, Labus JS, Stains J, Ohning G, Kilpatrick L, Bueller JA, Ruby K, Jarcho J, Mayer EA. Reduced brainstem inhibition during anticipated pelvic visceral pain correlates with enhanced brain response to the visceral stimulus in women with irritable bowel syndrome. J Neurosci 2008;28:349–59.

[12] Bohmelt AH, Nater UM, Franke S, Hellhammer DH, Ehlert U. Basal and stimulated hypothalamic-pituitary-adrenal axis activity in patients with functional gastrointestinal disorders and healthy controls. Psychosom Med 2005;67:288–94.

[13] Bouin M, Plourde V, Boivin M, Riberdy M, Lupien F, Laganiere M, Verrier P, Poitras P. Rectal distension testing in patients with irritable bowel syndrome: sensitivity, specificity, and predictive values of pain sensory thresholds. Gastroenterology 2002;122:1771–7.

[14] Boyce PM, Talley NJ, Balaam B, Koloski NA, Truman G. A randomized controlled trial of cognitive behavior therapy, relaxation training, and routine clinical care for the irritable bowel syndrome. Am J Gastroenterol 2003;98:2209–18.

[15] Brandt LJ, Bjorkman D, Fennerty MB, Locke GR, Olden K, Peterson W, Quigley E, Schoenfeld P, Schuster M, Talley N. Systematic review on the management of irritable bowel syndrome in North America. Am J Gastroenterol 2002;97:S7–S26.

[16] Cain KC, Jarrett ME, Burr RL, Hertig VL, Heitkemper MM. Heart rate variability is related to pain severity and predominant bowel pattern in women with irritable bowel syndrome. Neurogastroenterol Motil 2007;19:110–8.

[17] Calcagni E, Elenkov I. Stress system activity, innate and T helper cytokines, and susceptibility to immune-related diseases. Ann NY Acad Sci 2006;1069:62–76.

[18] Caldarella MP, Milano A, Laterza F, Sacco F, Balatsinou C, Lapenna D, Pierdomenico SD, Cuccurullo F, Neri M. Visceral sensitivity and symptoms in patients with constipation- or diarrhea-predominant irritable bowel syndrome (IBS): effect of a low-fat intraduodenal infusion. Am J Gastroenterol 2005;100:383–9.

[19] Camilleri M, McKinzie S, Busciglio I, Low PA, Sweetser S, Burton D, Baxter K, Ryks M, Zinsmeister AR. Prospective study of motor, sensory, psychologic, and autonomic functions in patients with irritable bowel syndrome. Clin Gastroenterol Hepatol 2008;6:772–81.

[20] Cann PA, Read NW, Brown C, Hobson N, Holdsworth CD. Irritable bowel syndrome: relationship of disorders in the transit of a single solid meal to symptom patterns. Gut 1983;24:405–11.

[21] Cash BD, Schoenfeld P, Chey WD. The utility of diagnostic tests in irritable bowel syndrome patients: A systematic review. Am J Gastroenterol 2002;97:2812–9.

[22] Chadwick VS, Chen W, Shu D, Paulus B, Bethwaite P, Tie A, Wilson I. Activation of the mucosal immune system in irritable bowel syndrome. Gastroenterology 2002;122:1778–83.

[23] Chang L. The trials and tribulations of drug development for functional gastrointestinal disorders. Neurogastroenterol Motil 2008;20 Suppl 1:130–8.

[24] Chang L, Ameen VZ, Dukes GE, McSorley DJ, Carter EG, Mayer EA. A dose-ranging, phase II study of the efficacy and safety of alosetron in men with diarrhea-predominant IBS. Am J Gastroenterol 2005;100:115–23.

[25] Chang L, Berman S, Mayer EA, Suyenobu B, Derbyshire S, Naliboff B, Vogt B, FitzGerald L, Mandelkern MA. Brain responses to visceral and somatic stimuli in patients with irritable bowel syndrome with and without fibromyalgia. Am J Gastroenterol 2003;98:1354–61.

[26] Chang L, Drossman DA. Optimizing patient care: the psychological interview in irritable bowel syndrome. Clin Perspectives 2002;5:336–42.

[27] Chang L, Heitkemper MM. Gender differences in irritable bowel syndrome. Gastroenterology 2002;123:1686–701.

[28] Chang L, Lee OY, Naliboff B, Schmulson M, Mayer EA. Sensation of bloating and visible abdominal distension in patients with irritable bowel syndrome. Am J Gastroenterol 2001;96:3341–7.

[29] Chang L, Naliboff BD, Labus JS, Schmulson M, Lee OY, Olivas TI, Stains J, Mayer EA. Effect of sex on perception of rectosigmoid stimuli in irritable bowel syndrome. Am J Physiol Regul Integr Comp Physiol 2006;291:R277–R84.

[30] Chang L Sundaresh S, Elliott J, Anton PA, Baldi P, Licudine A, Mayer M, Vuong T, Hirano M, Naliboff BD, Ameen VZ, Mayer EA Dysregulation of the hypothalamic-pituitary-adrenal (HPA) axis in irritable bowel syndrome. Neurogastroenterol Motil 2008; in press.

[31] Chial HJ, Camilleri M, Ferber I, Delgado-Aros S, Burton D, McKinzie S, Zinsmeister AR. Effects of venlafaxine, buspirone, and placebo on colonic sensorimotor functions in healthy humans. Clin Gastroenterol Hepatol 2003;1:211–8.

[32] Clauw DJ, Chrousos GP. Chronic pain and fatigue syndromes: Overlapping clinical and neuroendocrine features and potential pathogenic mechanisms. Neuroimmunomodulation 1997;4:134–53.

[33] Coffin B, Dapoigny M, Cloarec D, Comet D, Dyard F. Relationship between severity of symptoms and quality of life in 858 patients with irritable bowel syndrome. Gastroenterol Clin Biol 2004;28 11–5.

[34] Creed F, Fernandes L, Guthrie E, Palmer S, Ratcliffe J, Read N, Rigby C, Thompson D, Tomenson B, North of England IBSRG. The cost-effectiveness of psychotherapy and paroxetine for severe irritable bowel syndrome. Gastroenterology 2003;124:303–17.

[35] Delvaux M, Louvel D, Lagier E, Scherrer B, Abitbol JL, Frexinos J. The kappa agonist fedotozine relieves hypersensitivity to colonic distension in patients with irritable bowel syndrome. Gastroenterology 1999;116:38–45.

[36] Dickhaus B, Mayer EA, Firooz N, Stains J, Conde F, Olivas TI, Fass R, Chang L, Mayer M, Naliboff BD. Irritable bowel syndrome patients show enhanced modulation of visceral perception by auditory stress. Am J Gastroenterol 2003;98:135–43.

[37] Dinan TG, Quigley EM, Ahmed SM, Scully P, O'Brien S, O'Mahony L, O'Mahony S, Shanahan F, Keeling PW. Hypothalamic-pituitary-gut axis dysregulation in irritable bowel syndrome: plasma cytokines as a potential marker? Gastroenterology 2006;130:304–11.

[38] Dorn SD, Palsson OS, Thiwan SI, Kanazawa M, Clark WC, van Tilburg MA, Drossman DA, Scarlett Y, Levy RL, Ringel Y, Crowell MD, Olden KW, Whitehead WE. Increased colonic pain sensitivity in irritable bowel syndrome is the result of an increased tendency to report pain rather than increased neurosensory sensitivity. Gut 2007;56:1202–9.

[39] Drossman DA. The functional gastrointestinal disorders and the Rome III process. Gastroenterology 2006;130:1377–90.

[40] Drossman DA, Chey W, Panas R, Wahle A, Scott C, Ueno R. Lubiprostone significantly improves symptom relief rates in adults with irritable bowel syndrome and constipation (IBS-C): data from two twelve-week, randomized, placebo-controlled double-blind trials. Gastroenterology 2007;132:2586–7.

[41] Drossman DA, Li Z, Andruzzi E, Temple R, Talley NJ, Thompson WG, Whitehead WE, Janssens J, Funch-Jensen P, Carazziari E, Richter JE, Koch GG. U.S. householder survey of functional gastrointestinal disorders. Prevalence, sociodemography and health impact. Dig Dis Sci 1993;38:1569–80.

[42] Drossman DA, Li Z, Leserman J, Toomey TC, Hu YJ. Health status by gastrointestinal diagnosis and abuse history. Gastroenterology 1996;110:999–1007.

[43] Drossman DA, McKee DC, Sandler RS, Mitchell CM, Cramer EM, Lowman BC, Burger AL. Psychosocial factors in the irritable bowel syndrome. A multivariate study of patients and non-patients with irritable bowel syndrome. Gastroenterology 1988;95:701–8.

[44] Drossman DA, Toner BB, Whitehead WE, Diamant NE, Dalton CB, Duncan S, Emmott S, Proffitt V, Akman D, Frusciante K, et al. Cognitive-behavioral therapy versus education and desipramine versus placebo for moderate to severe functional bowel disorders. Gastroenterology 2003;125:19–31.

[45] Drossman DA, Whitehead WE, Toner BB, Diamant N, Hu YJ, Bangdiwala SI, Jia H. What determines severity among patients with painful functional bowel disorders? Am J Gastroenterol 2000;95:974–80.

[46] Dunlop SP, Jenkins D, Neal KR, Naesdal J, Borgaonker M, Collins SM, Spiller RC. Randomized, double-blind, placebo-controlled trial of prednisolone in post-infectious irritable bowel syndrome. Aliment Pharmacol Ther 2003;18:77–84.

[47] Dunlop SP, Jenkins D, Neal KR, Spiller RC. Relative importance of enterochromaffin cell hyperplasia, anxiety, and depression in postinfectious IBS. Gastroenterology 2003;125:1651–9.

[48] Elsenbruch S, Lovallo WR, Orr WC. Psychological and physiological responses to postprandial mental stress in women with the irritable bowel syndrome. Psychosom Med 2001;63:805–10.

[49] Elsenbruch S, Orr WC. Diarrhea- and constipation-predominant IBS patients differ in postprandial autonomic and cortisol responses. Am J Gastroenterol 2001;96:460–6.

[50] Evans BW, Clark WK, Moore DJ, Whorwell PJ. Tegaserod for the treatment of irritable bowel syndrome and chronic constipation. Cochrane Database Syst Rev 2007;CD003960.

[51] Fass R, Fullerton S, Diehl DL, Mayer EA. Sleep disturbance (SD) in patients with functional bowel disorders (FBD). Gastroenterology 1995;108:A596.

[52] Fass R, Fullerton S, Naliboff B, Hirsh T, Mayer EA. Sexual dysfunction in patients with irritable bowel syndrome and non-ulcer dyspepsia. Digestion 1998;59:79–85.

[53] Food and Drug Administration. Zelnorm (tegaserod maleate) information. 2008. Available at: www.fda.gov/cder/drug/infopage/zelnorm/default.htm.

[54] Fukudo S, Nomura T, Hongo M. Impact of corticotropin-releasing hormone on gastrointestinal motility and adrenocorticotropic hormone in normal controls and patients with irritable bowel syndrome. Gut 1999;42:845–9.

[55] Garcia Rodriguez LA, Ruigcmez A, Wallander MA, Johansson S, Olbe L. Detection of colorectal tumor and inflammatory bowel disease during follow-up of patients with initial diagnosis of irritable bowel syndrome. Scand J Gastroenterol 2000;35:306–11.

[56] Gecse K, Roka R, Ferrier L, Leveque M, Eutamene H, Cartier C, Ait-Belgnaoui A, Rosztoczy A, Izbeki F, Fioramonti J, Wittmann T, Bueno L. Increased faecal serine protease activity in diarrhoeic IBS patients: a colonic lumenal factor impairing colonic permeability and sensitivity. Gut 2008;57:591–9.

[57] Gonsalkorale WM, Miller V, Afzal A, Whorwell PJ. Long-term benefits of hypnotherapy for irritable bowel syndrome. Gut 2003;52:1623–9.

[58] Gorard DA, Libby GW, Farthing MJ. Effect of a tricyclic antidepressant on small intestinal motility in health and diarrhea-predominant irritable bowel syndrome. Dig Dis Sci 1995;40:86–95.

[59] Gwee KA. Irritable bowel syndrome in developing countries: a disorder of civilization or colonization? Neurogastroenterol Motil 2005;17:317–24.

[60] Halpert A, Dalton CB, Palsson O, Morris C, Hu Y, Bangdiwala S, Hankins J, Norton N, Drossman D. What patients know about irritable bowel syndrome (IBS) and what they would like to know. National Survey on Patient Educational Needs in IBS and development and validation of the Patient Educational Needs Questionnaire (PEQ). Am J Gastroenterol 2007;102:1972–82.

[61] Harris LA CL. Alosetron: an effective treatment for diarrhea-predominant irritable bowel syndrome. Womens Health 2007;3:15–27.

[62] Harter MC, Conway KP, Merikangas KR. Associations between anxiety disorders and physical illness. Eur Arch Psychiatry Clin Neurosci 2003;253:313–20.

[63] Heim C, Newport DJ, Bonsall R, Miller AH, Nemeroff CB. Altered pituitary-adrenal axis responses to provocative challenge tests in adult survivors of childhood abuse. Am J Psychiatry 2001;158:575–81.

[64] Heitkemper M, Jarrett M, Cain K, Shaver J, Bond E, Woods NF, Walker E. Increased urine catecholamines and cortisol in women with irritable bowel syndrome. Am J Gastroenterol 1996;91:906–13.

[65] Heitkemper MM, Cain KC, Jarrett ME, Burr RL, Hertig V, Bond EF. Symptoms across the menstrual cycle in women with irritable bowel syndrome. Am J Gastroenterol 2003;98:420–30.

[66] Hillila MT, Siivola MT, Farkkila MA. Comorbidity and use of health-care services among irritable bowel syndrome sufferers. Scand J Gastroenterol 2007;42:799–806.

[67] Horikawa Y, Mieno H, Inoue M, Kajiyama G. Gastrointestinal motility in patients with irritable bowel syndrome studied by using radio-opaque markers. Scand J Gastroenterol 1999;34:1190–5.

[68] Houghton LA, Fell C, Whorwell PJ, Jones I, Sudworth DP, Gale JD. Effect of a second-generation alpha2delta ligand (pregabalin) on visceral sensation in hypersensitive patients with irritable bowel syndrome. Gut 2007;56:1218–25.

[69] Houghton LA, Lea R, Jackson N, Whorwell PJ. The menstrual cycle affects rectal sensitivity in patients with irritable bowel syndrome but not healthy volunteers. Gut 2002;50:471–4.

[70] Hudson JI, Mangweth B, Pope HG, Jr., De Col C, Hausmann A, Gutweniger S, Laird NM, Biebl W, Tsuang MT. Family study of affective spectrum disorder. Arch Gen Psychiatry 2003;60:170–7.

[71] Hungin AP, Whorwell PJ, Tack J, Mearin F. The prevalence, patterns and impact of irritable bowel syndrome: An international survey of 40,000 subjects. Aliment Pharmacol Ther 2003;17:643–50.

[72] Hutchinson R, Notghi A, Smith NB, Harding LK, Kumar D. Scintigraphic measurement of ileocaecal transit in irritable bowel syndrome and chronic idiopathic constipation. Gut 1995;36:585–9.

[73] Jackson NA, Houghton LA, Whorwell PJ, Currer B. Does the menstrual cycle affect anorectal physiology? Dig Dis Sci 1994;39:2607–11.

[74] Kalantar JS, Locke GR, 3rd, Zinsmeister AR, Beighley CM, Talley NJ. Familial aggregation of irritable bowel syndrome: a prospective study. Gut 2003;52:1703–7.

[75] Kane SV, Sable K, Hanauer SB. The menstrual cycle and its effect on inflammatory bowel disease and irritable bowel syndrome: a prevalence study. Am J Gastroenterol 1998;93:1867–72.

[76] Kang JY. Systematic review: the influence of geography and ethnicity in irritable bowel syndrome. Aliment Pharmacol Ther 2005;21:663–76.

[77] Kato K, Sullivan PF, Evengard B, Pedersen NL. Chronic widespread pain and its comorbidities: a population-based study. Arch Intern Med 2006;166:1649–54.

[78] Katon W, Lin E, Von Korff M, Russo J, Lipscomb P, Bush T. Somatization: a spectrum of severity. Am J Psychiatry 1991;148:34–40.

116   L. Chang and D.A. Drossman

[79] Kellow J, Lee OY, Chang FY, Thongsawat S, Mazlam MZ, Yuen H, Gwee KA, Bak YT, Jones J, Wagner A. An Asia-Pacific, double blind placebo controlled, randomised study to evaluate the efficacy, safety, and tolerability of tegaserod in patients with irritable bowel syndrome. Gut 2003;52:671–6.
[80] Kellow JE, Azpiroz F, Delvaux M, Gebhart GF, Mertz H, Quigley EMM, Smout AJPM. Principles of applied neurogastroenterology: Physiology/motility-sensation. In: Drossman DA, Corazziari E, Delvaux M, Spiller RC, Talley NJ, Thompson WG, Whitehead WE, editors. Rome III: the functional gastrointestinal disorders. McLean, VA: Degnon Associates; 2006. pp 89–160.
[81] Koch KM, Palmer JL, Noordin N, Tomlinson JJ, Baidoo C. Sex and age differences in the pharmacokinetics of alosetron. Br J Clin Pharmacol 2002;53:238–42.
[82] Krause R, Ameen V, Gordon SH, West M, Heath AT, Perschy T, Carter EG. A randomized, double-blind, placebo-controlled study to assess efficacy and safety of 0.5 mg and 1 mg alosetron in women with severe diarrhea-predominant IBS. Am J Gastroenterol 2007;102:1709–19.
[83] Lackner JM, Jaccard J, Krasner SS, Katz LA, Gudleski GD, Holroyd K. Self-administered cognitive behavior therapy for moderate to severe irritable bowel syndrome: clinical efficacy, tolerability, feasibility. Clin Gastroenterol Hepatol 2008;6;899–906.
[84] Lawal A, Kern M, Sidhu H, Hofmann C, Shaker R. Novel evidence for hypersensitivity of visceral sensory neural circuitry in irritable bowel syndrome patients. Gastroenterology 2006;130:26–33.
[85] Lee KJ, Kim JH, Cho SW. Gabapentin reduces rectal mechanosensitivity and increases rectal compliance in patients with diarrhoea-predominant irritable bowel syndrome. Aliment Pharmacol Ther 2005;22:981–8.
[86] Lee OY, Mayer EA, Schmulson M, Chang L, Naliboff B. Gender-related differences in IBS symptoms. Am J Gastroenterol 2001;96:2184–93.
[87] Lembo A, Ameen VZ, Drossman DA. Irritable bowel syndrome: toward an understanding of severity. Clin Gastroenterol Hepatol 2005;3:717–25.
[88] Lembo A, Zaman M, Jones M, Talley NJ. Influence of genetics on irritable bowel syndrome, gastro-oesophageal reflux and dyspepsia: a twin study. Aliment Pharmacol Ther 2007;25:1343–50.
[89] Lembo AJ, Olden KW, Ameen VZ, Gordon SL, Heath AT, Carter EG. Effect of alosetron on bowel urgency and global symptoms in women with severe, diarrhea-predominant irritable bowel syndrome: analysis of two controlled trials. Clin Gastroenterol Hepatol 2004;2 675–82.
[90] Lembo T, Plourde V, Shui Z, Fullerton S, Mertz H, Tache Y, Sytnik B, Munakata J, Mayer EA. Effects of the corticotropin-releasing factor (CRF) on rectal afferent nerves in humans. Neurogastroenterol Motil 1996;8:9–18.
[91] Lembo T, Wright RA, Bagby B, Decker C, Gordon S, Jhingran P, Carter E, Lotronex Investigator T. Alosetron controls bowel urgency and provides global symptom improvement in women with diarrhea-predominant irritable bowel syndrome. Am J Gastroenterol 2001;96:2662–70.
[92] Lesbros-Pantoflickova D, Michetti P, Fried M, Beglinger C, Blum AL. Meta-analysis: The treatment of irritable bowel syndrome. Aliment Pharmacol Ther 2004;20:1253–69.
[93] Levy RL, Jones KR, Whitehead WE, Feld SI, Talley NJ, Corey LA. Irritable bowel syndrome in twins: Heredity and social learning both contribute to etiology. Gastroenterology 2001;121:799–804.
[94] Levy RL, Olden KW, Naliboff BD, Bradley LA, Francisconi C, Drossman DA, Creed F. Psychosocial aspects of the functional gastrointestinal disorders. Gastroenterology 2006;130:1447–58.
[95] Levy RL, Von Korff M, Whitehead WE, Stang P, Saunders K, Jhingran P, Barghout V, Feld AD. Costs of care for irritable bowel syndrome patients in a health maintenance organization. Am J Gastroenterol 2001;96:3122–9.
[96] Liebregts T, Adam B, Bredack C, Roth A, Heinzel S, Lester S, Downie-Doyle S, Smith E, Drew P, Talley NJ, Holtmann G. Immune activation in patients with irritable bowel syndrome. Gastroenterology 2007;132:913–20.
[97] Locke GR 3rd, Zinsmeister AR, Talley NJ, Fett SL, Melton LJ 3rd. Familial association in adults with functional gastrointestinal disorders. Mayo Clin Proc 2000;75:907–12.
[98] Longstreth GF, Thompson WG, Chey WD, Houghton LA, Mearin F, Spiller RC. Functional bowel disorders. Gastroenterology 2006;130:480–91.
[99] Longstreth GF, Thompson WG, Chey WD, Houghton LA, Mearin F, Spiller RC. Functional bowel disorders. In: Drossman DA, Corazziari E, Delvaux M, Spiller RC, Talley NJ, Thompson WG, Whitehead WE, editors. Rome III: the functional gastrointestinal disorders. McLean, VA: Degnon Associates; 2006. pp 487–556.

[100] Martinez V, Taché Y. CRF1 receptors as a therapeutic target for irritable bowel syndrome. Curr Pharm Des 2006;12:4071–88.

[101] Mastorakos G, Ilias I. Interleukin-6: a cytokine and/or a major modulator of the response to somatic stress. Ann NY Acad Sci 2006;1088:373–81.

[102] Maxion-Bergemann S, Thielecke F, Abel F, Bergemann R. Costs of irritable bowel syndrome in the UK and US. Pharmacoeconomics 2006;24:21–37.

[103] Maxton DG, Morris J, Whorwell PJ. More accurate diagnosis of irritable bowel syndrome by the use of 'non-colonic' symptomatology. Gut 1991;32:784–6.

[104] Mayer EA. Clinical practice. Irritable bowel syndrome. N Engl J Med 2008;358:1692–9.

[105] Mayer EA, Naliboff BD, Craig AD. Neuroimaging of the brain-gut axis: From basic understanding to treatment of functional GI disorders. Gastroenterology 2006;131:1925–42.

[106] Mayeux RDD, Basham KK, Bromet EJ, Burke GL, Charney DS, et al. Gulf war and health: physiologic, psychologic, and psychosocial effects of deployment-related stress. Washington, DC: National Academies Press; 2008.

[107] Mayeux RDD, Basham KK, Bromet EJ, Burke GL, Charney DS, et al. The stress response. In: Mayeux R DD, Basham KK, Bromet EJ, Burke GL, Charney DS, et al. Gulf war and health: physiologic, psychologic, and psychosocial effects of deployment-related stress. Washington, DC: National Academies Press; 2008. p. 49–74.

[108] Mertz H, Morgan V, Tanner G, Pickens D, Price R, Shyr Y, Kessler R. Regional cerebral activation in irritable bowel syndrome and control subjects with painful and nonpainful rectal distension. Gastroenterology 2000;118:842–8.

[109] Mertz H, Naliboff B, Munakata J, Niazi N, Mayer EA. Altered rectal perception is a biological marker of patients with irritable bowel syndrome. Gastroenterology 1995;109:40–52.

[110] Mitchell CM, Drossman DA. Survey of the AGA membership relating to patients with functional gastrointestinal disorders. Gastroenterology 1987;92:1282–4.

[111] Mohammed I, Cherkas LF, Riley SA, Spector TD, Trudgill NJ. Genetic influences in irritable bowel syndrome: a twin study. Am J Gastroenterol 2005;100:1340–4.

[112] Morris-Yates A, Talley NJ, Boyce PM, Nandurkar S, Andrews G. Evidence of a genetic contribution to functional bowel disorder. Am J Gastroenterol 1998;93:1311–7.

[113] Müller-Lissner SA, Fumagalli I, Bardhan KD, Pace F, Pecher E, Nault B, Ruegg P. Tegaserod, a 5-HT(4) receptor partial agonist, relieves symptoms in irritable bowel syndrome patients with abdominal pain, bloating and constipation. Aliment Pharmacol Ther 2001;15:1655–66.

[114] Naliboff BD, Berman S, Chang L, Derbyshire SWG, Suyenobu B, Vogt BA, Mandelkern M, Mayer EA. Sex-related differences in IBS patients: central processing of visceral stimuli. Gastroenterology 2003;124:1738–47.

[115] Naliboff BD, Berman S, Suyenobu B, Labus JS, Chang L, Stains J, Mandelkern MA, Mayer EA. Longitudinal change in perceptual and brain activation response to visceral stimuli in irritable bowel syndrome patients. Gastroenterology 2006;131:352–65.

[116] Naliboff BD, Derbyshire SWG, Munakata J, Berman S, Mandelkern M, Chang L, Mayer EA. Cerebral activation in irritable bowel syndrome patients and control subjects during rectosigmoid stimulation. Psychosom Med 2001;63:365–75.

[117] Naliboff BD, Munakata J, Fullerton S, Gracely RH, Kodner A, Harraf F, Mayer EA. Evidence for two distinct perceptual alterations in irritable bowel syndrome. Gut 1997;41:505–12.

[118] Nance DM, Sanders VM. Autonomic innervation and regulation of the immune system (1987–2007). Brain Behav Immun 2007;21:736–45.

[119] Nastaskin I, Mehdikhani E, Conklin J, Park S, Pimentel M. Studying the overlap between IBS and GERD: a systematic review of the literature. Dig Dis Sci 2006;51:2113–20.

[120] Neal KR, Hebden J, Spiller R. Prevalence of gastrointestinal symptoms six months after bacterial gastroenteritis and risk factors for development of the irritable bowel syndrome: postal survey of patients. BMJ 1997;314:779–82.

[121] Nyhlin H, Bang C, Elsborg L, Silvennoinen J, Holme I, Ruegg P, Jones J, Wagner A. A double-blind, placebo-controlled, randomized study to evaluate the efficacy, safety and tolerability of tegaserod in patients with irritable bowel syndrome. Scand J Gastroenterol 2004;39:119–26.

[122] Nyrop KA, Palsson OS, Levy RL, Korff MV, Feld AD, Turner MJ, Whitehead WE. Costs of health care for irritable bowel syndrome, chronic constipation, functional diarrhoea and functional abdominal pain. Aliment Pharmacol Ther 2007;26:237–48.

[123] O'Mahony L, McCarthy J, Kelly P, Hurley G, Luo F, Chen K, O'Sullivan GC, Kiely B, Collins JK, Shanahan F, Quigley EM. Lactobacillus and Bifidobacterium in irritable bowel syndrome: symptom responses and relationship to cytokine profiles. Gastroenterology 2005;128:541–51.

[124] O'Sullivan M, Clayton N, Breslin NP, Harman I, Bountra C, McLaren A, O'Morain CA. Increased mast cells in the irritable bowel syndrome. Neurogastroenterol Motil 2000;12:449–57.

[125] Pare P, Gray J, Lam S, Balshaw R, Khorasheh S, Barbeau M, Kelly S, McBurney CR. Health-related quality of life, work productivity, and health care resource utilization of subjects with irritable bowel syndrome: baseline results from LOGIC (Longitudinal Outcomes Study of Gastrointestinal Symptoms in Canada), a naturalistic study. Clin Ther 2006;28:1726–35.

[126] Park MI, Camilleri M. Is there a role of food allergy in irritable bowel syndrome and functional dyspepsia? A systematic review. Neurogastroenterol Motil 2006;18:595–607.

[127] Pimentel M, Park S, Mirocha J, Kane SV, Kong Y. The effect of a nonabsorbed oral antibiotic (rifaximin) on the symptoms of the irritable bowel syndrome: a randomized trial. Ann Intern Med 2006;145:557–63.

[128] Posserud I, Agerforz P, Ekman R, Bjornsson ES, Abrahamsson H, Simren M. Altered visceral perceptual and neuroendocrine response in patients with irritable bowel syndrome during mental stress. Gut 2004;53:1102–8.

[129] Poynard T, Regimbeau C, Benhamou Y. Meta-analysis of smooth muscle relaxants in the treatment of irritable bowel syndrome. Aliment Pharmacol Ther 2001;15:355–61.

[130] Prior A, Sorial E, Sun WM, Read NW. Irritable bowel syndrome: differences between patients who show rectal sensitivity and those who do not. Eur J Gastroenterol Hepatol 1993;5:343–9.

[131] Quartero AO, Meineche-Schmidt V, Muris J, Rubin G, de Wit N. Bulking agents, antispasmodic and antidepressant medication for the treatment of irritable bowel syndrome. Cochrane Database Syst Rev 2005;CD003460.

[132] Quigley EM, Flourie B. Probiotics and irritable bowel syndrome: a rationale for their use and an assessment of the evidence to date. Neurogastroenterol Motil 2007;19:166–72.

[133] Rainville P, Duncan GH, Price DD, Carrier B, Bushnell MC. Pain affect encoded in human anterior cingulate but not somatosensory cortex. Science 1997;277:968–71.

[134] Rapps N, van Oudenhove L, Enck P, Aziz Q. Brain imaging of visceral functions in healthy volunteers and IBS patients. J Psychosom Res 2008;64:599–604.

[135] Reilly MC, Bracco A, Ricci JF, Santoro J, Stevens T. The validity and accuracy of the Work Productivity and Activity Impairment questionnaire--irritable bowel syndrome version (WPAI:IBS). Aliment Pharmacol Ther 2004;20:459–67.

[136] Riedl A, Schmidtmann M, Stengel A, Goebel M, Wisser AS, Klapp BF, Monnikes H. Somatic comorbidities of irritable bowel syndrome: a systematic analysis. J Psychosom Res 2008;64:573–82.

[137] Ringel Y, Drossman DA, Leserman JL, Suyenobu BY, Wilber K, Lin W, Whitehead WE, Naliboff BD, Berman S, Mayer EA. Effect of abuse history on pain reports and brain responses to aversive visceral stimulation: an FMRI study. Gastroenterology 2008;134:396–404.

[138] Sagami Y, Shimada Y, Tayama J, Nomura T, Satake M, Endo Y, Shoji T, Karahashi K, Hongo M, Fukudo S. Effect of a corticotropin releasing hormone receptor antagonist on colonic sensory and motor function in patients with irritable bowel syndrome. Gut 2004;53:958–64.

[139] Saito YA, Schoenfeld P, Locke GR, 3rd. The epidemiology of irritable bowel syndrome in North America: a systematic review. Am J Gastroenterol 2002;97:1910–5.

[140] Sandler RS. Epidemiology of irritable bowel syndrome in the United States. Gastroenterology 1990;99:409–15.

[141] Sandler RS, Drossman DA, Nathan HP, McKee DC. Symptom complaints and health care seeking behavior in subjects with bowel dysfunction. Gastroenterology 1984;87:314–8.

[142] Sandler RS, Everhart JE, Donowitz M, Adams E, Cronin K, Goodman C, Gemmen E, Shah S, Avdic A, Rubin R. The burden of selected digestive diseases in the United States. Gastroenterology 2002;122:1500–11.

[143] Schmulson M, Lee OY, Chang L, Naliboff B, Mayer EA. Symptom differences in moderate to severe IBS patients based on predominant bowel habit. Am J Gastroenterol 1999;94:2929–35.

[144] Sharara AI, Aoun E, Abdul-Baki H, Mounzer R, Sidani S, Elhajj I. A randomized double-blind placebo-controlled trial of rifaximin in patients with abdominal bloating and flatulence. Am J Gastroenterol 2006;101 326–33.

[145] Shiotani A, Miyanishi T, Takahashi T. Sex differences in irritable bowel syndrome in Japanese university students. J Gastroenterol 2006;41:562–8.

[146] Simren M, Abrahamsson H, Svedlund J, Bjornsson ES. Quality of life in patients with irritable bowel syndrome seen in referral centers versus primary care: the impact of gender and predominant bowel pattern. Scand J Gastroenterol 2001;36:545–52.

[147] Simren M, Agerforz P, Bjornsson ES, Abrahamsson H. Nutrient-dependent enhancement of rectal sensitivity in irritable bowel syndrome (IBS). Neurogastroenterol Motil 2007;19:20–9.

[148] Simren M, Mansson A, Langkilde AM, Svedlund J, Abrahamsson H, Bengtsson U, Bjornsson ES. Food-related gastrointestinal symptoms in the irritable bowel syndrome. Digestion 2001;63:108–15.

[149] Smith RC, Greenbaum DS, Vancouver JB, Henry RC, Reinhart MA, Greenbaum RB, Dean HA, Mayle JE. Psychosocial factors are associated with health care seeking rather than diagnosis in irritable bowel syndrome. Gastroenterology 1990;98:293–301.

[150] Sperber AD, Atzmon Y, Neumann L, Weisberg I, Shalit Y, Abu-Shakrah M, Fich A, Buskila D. Fibromyalgia in the irritable bowel syndrome: studies of prevalence and clinical implications. Am J Gastroenterol 1999;94:3541–6.

[151] Sperber AD, Carmel S, Atzmon Y, Weisberg I, Shalit Y, Neumann L, Fich A, Friger M, Buskila D. Use of the Functional Bowel Disorder Severity Index (FBDSI) in a study of patients with the irritable bowel syndrome and fibromyalgia. Am J Gastroenterol 2000;95:995–8.

[152] Spiegel BM HL, Lucak SL, Mayer EA, Naliboff BD, Bolus RE, Estralian E, Chey WD, Lembo A, Karsan HA, Tillisch K, Dulai GS, Strickland A, Chang L. Predictor of work productivity in irritable bowel syndrome (IBS): Results from the PROOF Cohort. Gastroenterology 2008;134:A28.

[153] Spiegel BM, Strickland A, Naliboff BD, Mayer EA, Chang L. Predictors of patient-assessed illness severity in irritable bowel syndrome. Am J Gastroenterol 2008;103:1–8.

[154] Spiegel BMR, Gralnek IM, Mayer EA, Bolus R, Chang L, Dulai GS, Naliboff B. Clinical determinants of health-related quality of life in irritable bowel syndrome. Gastroenterology 2003;124: A398.

[155] Spiller R, Aziz Q, Creed F, Emmanuel A, Houghton L, Hungin P, Jones R, Kumar D, Rubin G, Trudgill N, Whorwell P. Guidelines for the management of irritable bowel syndrome. Gut 2007;56:1770–98.

[156] Sternberg EM. Neuroendocrine factors in susceptibility to inflammatory disease: focus on the hypothalamic-pituitary-adrenal axis. Horm Res 1995;43:159–61.

[157] Stewart M, Brown JB, Donner A, McWhinney IR, Oates J, Weston WW, Jordan J. The impact of patient-centered care on outcomes. J Fam Pract 2000;49:796–804.

[158] Tabas G, Beaves M, Wang J, Friday P, Mardini H, Arnold G. Paroxetine to treat irritable bowel syndrome not responding to high-fiber diet: a double-blind, placebo-controlled trial. Am J Gastroenterol 2004;99:914–20.

[159] Tack J, Broekaert D, Fischler B, Oudenhove LV, Gevers AM, Janssens J. A controlled cross-over study of the selective serotonin reuptake inhibitor citalopram in irritable bowel syndrome. Gut 2006;55:1095–103.

[160] Tack J, Talley NJ, Camilleri M, Holtmann G, Hu P, Malagelada JR, Stanghellini V. Functional gastroduodenal disorders. Gastroenterology 2006;130:1466–79.

[161] Talley NJ, Dennis EH, Schettler-Duncan VA, Lacy BE, Olden KW, Crowell MD. Overlapping upper and lower gastrointestinal symptoms in irritable bowel syndrome patients with constipation or diarrhea. Am J Gastroenterol 2003;98:2454–9.

[162] Talley NJ, Gabriel SE, Harmsen WS, Zinsmeister AR, Evans RW. Medical costs in community subjects with irritable bowel syndrome. Gastroenterology 1995;109:1736–41.

[163] Talley NJ, Zinsmeister AR, Melton III LJ. Irritable bowel syndrome in a community: symptom subgroups, risk factors, and health care utilization. Am J Epidemiol 1995;142:76–83.

[164] Tillisch K, Mayer EA, Labus JS, Stains J, Chang L, Naliboff BD. Sex-specific alterations in autonomic function among patients with irritable bowel syndrome. Gut 2005;54:1396–401.

[165] Trimble KC, Farouk R, Pryde A, Douglas S, Heading RC. Heightened visceral sensation in functional gastrointestinal disease is not site-specific. Evidence for a generalized disorder of gut sensitivity. Dig Dis Sci 1995;40:1607–13.

[166] Vahedi H, Merat S, Rashidioon A, Ghoddoosi A, Malekzadeh R. The effects of fluoxetine in patients with pain and constipation-predominant irritable bowel syndrome: a double-blind randomized-controlled study. Aliment Pharmacol Ther 2005;22 381–5.

[167] van der Horst HE, van Dulmen AM, Schellevis FG, van Eijk JT, Fennis JF, Bleijenberg G. Do patients with irritable bowel syndrome in primary care really differ from outpatients with irritable bowel syndrome? Gut 1997;41:669–74.

[168] Vassallo M, Camilleri M, Phillips SF, Brown ML, Chapman NJ, Thomforde GM. Transit through the proximal colon influences stool weight in the irritable bowel syndrome. Gastroenterology 1992;102:102–8.

[169] Vege SS, Locke GR, 3rd, Weaver AL, Farmer SA, Melton LJ 3rd, Talley NJ. Functional gastrointestinal disorders among people with sleep disturbances: a population-based study. Mayo Clin Proc 2004;79:1501–6.

[170] Verne GN, Himes NC, Robinson ME, Gopinath KS, Briggs RW, Crosson B, Price DD. Central representation of visceral and cutaneous hypersensitivity in the irritable bowel syndrome. Pain 2003;103:99–110.

[171] Videlock EJ, Chang L. Irritable bowel syndrome: current approach to symptoms, evaluation, and treatment. Gastroenterol Clin North Am 2007;36:665–85.

[172] Viramontes BE, Camilleri M, McKinzie S, Pardi DS, Burton D, Thomforde GM. Gender-related differences in slowing colonic transit by a 5-HT3 antagonist in subjects with diarrhea-predominant irritable bowel syndrome. Am J Gastroenterol 2001;96:2671–9.

[173] Whitehead WE, Cheskin LJ, Heller BR, Robinson JC, Crowell MD, Benjamin C, Schuster MM. Evidence for exacerbation of irritable bowel syndrome during menses. Gastroenterology 1990;98:1485–9.

[174] Whitehead WE, Holtkotter B, Enck P, Hoelzl R, Holmes KD, Anthony J, Shabsin HS, Schuster MM. Tolerance for rectosigmoid distention in irritable bowel syndrome. Gastroenterology 1990;98:1187–92.

[175] Whitehead WE, Palsson O, Jones KR. Systemic review of the comorbidity of irritable bowel syndrome with other disorders: What are the causes and implications? Gastroenterology 2002;122:1140–56.

[176] Whorwell PJ, McCallum M, Creed FH, Roberts CT. Non-colonic features of irritable bowel syndrome. Gut 1986;27:37–40.

[177] Wilder-Smith CH, Schindler D, Lovblad K, Redmond SM, Nirkko A. Brain functional magnetic resonance imaging of rectal pain and activation of endogenous inhibitory mechanisms in irritable bowel syndrome patient subgroups and healthy controls. Gut 2004;53:1595–601.

[178] Wilson S, Maddison T, Roberts L, Greenfield S, Singh S, Group BIR. Systematic review: The effectiveness of hypnotherapy in the management of irritable bowel syndrome. Aliment Pharmacol Ther 2006;24:769–80.

[179] Zar S, Benson MJ, Kumar D. Rectal afferent hypersensitivity and compliance in irritable bowel syndrome: Differences between diarrhoea-predominant and constipation-predominant subgroups. Eur J Gastroenterol Hepatol 2006;18:151–8.

[180] Zuo XL, Li YQ, Li WJ, Guo YT, Lu XF, Li JM, Desmond PV. Alterations of food antigen-specific serum immunoglobulins G and E antibodies in patients with irritable bowel syndrome and functional dyspepsia. Clin Exp Allergy 2007;37:823–30.

Correspondence to: Lin Chang, MD, Center for Neurobiology of Stress, David Geffen School of Medicine at UCLA, 11301 Wilshire Boulevard, Building 115, Room 215, Los Angeles, CA 90073, USA. Tel: 1-310-312-9276; email: linchang@mednet.ucla.edu.

Sensitive Heart: A Chronic Cardiac Pain Syndrome

Stuart D. Rosen[a,b] and Paolo G. Camici[a]

[a]National Heart and Lung Institute, Imperial College, London, United Kingdom;
[b]Department of Cardiology, Ealing Hospital, Middlesex, United Kingdom

Angina Pectoris and Ischemic Heart Disease

An association between chest pain and cardiac pathology has been recognized for at least two and a half centuries. Traditionally, the first detailed description of angina pectoris is considered to be that of Heberden [32]. About half a century later, a discrepancy between the extent of anatomical coronary artery disease and patients' symptoms was noted by John Warren in the very first issue of the *New England Journal of Medicine* [90]. Warren noted the poor correlation between the symptoms described by his patients and the extent of "ossification" of the coronary arteries that he found when, in the fullness of time, he performed their post mortem examinations. Later in the 19th century, the anatomy of the neural pathways were elucidated by, among others, François-Franck [23], who drew particular attention to the role of the sympathetic nerves. The early 20th century saw the establishment of the link between angina and reversible myocardial ischemia, initially suggested by Keefer and Resnik in 1928 [39]. The overall historical development of understanding of the mechanisms through which coronary artery disease (CAD) contributes to myocardial ischemia and angina has been reviewed by Bing [4].

Painful Myocardial Ischemia

In the patient with CAD, a critical stenosis of an epicardial artery sharply reduces coronary flow reserve (CFR, the ratio of maximal to resting myocardial blood flow) in the myocardial territory subtended by the stenosed vessel. Under these circumstances, oxygen supply cannot increase adequately to satisfy the increased myocardial demand, and aerobic metabolism can no longer be sustained downstream [85]. The well-known ischemic cascade proceeds, as shown in Fig. 1, and ultimately regional contractile function is compromised.

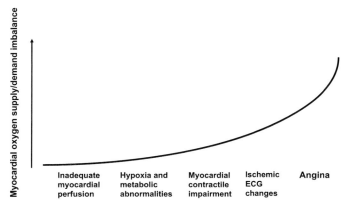

Fig. 1. Ischemic cascade leading to angina.

Tissue-Level Chemical Effects

At the tissue level, ischemia has a number of consequences. These include: (1) a buildup of adenosine from the breakdown of adenosine triphosphate (ATP), as well as the products of anaerobic metabolism, in particular hydrogen ions; (2) altered function of ionic transport mechanisms, increasing intracellular calcium loading and allowing leakage of intracellular potassium ions; and (3) changed local mechanical forces, most acutely in the border zone between ischemic and nonischemic myocardium [56]. All these factors combine to stimulate undifferentiated nerve endings within the myocardium (there are no known specific no-ciceptive nerve endings in the myocardium) and generate an increase in afferent nerve traffic [48].

Neural Pathways from the Heart to the Brain

Once the undifferentiated nerve endings in the heart have been sub-jected to an adequate stimulus, the afferent nerve traffic evoked by myocardial ischemia is carried by the cardiac sympathetic and vagal nerve fibers. These pathways, as determined from animal studies, have been reviewed in detail elsewhere [16,51,80]. The main methods used in these studies have been recording with microelectrodes in very specific brainstem and cortical sites to register the effect of discrete pe-ripheral stimuli; in addition, retrograde neuronal transport techniques have also been employed, using agents such as horseradish peroxidase. More recently, Albutaihi and colleagues have used elegant histological techniques to demonstrate significantly elevated neuronal *c-fos* synthe-sis in brain regions activated by capsaicin-induced cardiac pain in a rat model [1].

In broad terms, the sympathetic afferent fibers travel predomi-nantly via the dorsal columns to the ventral posterior lateral (VPL) thalamus. Neurons in the VPL also receive visceral afferent inputs via the spinothalamic tracts. Vagal fibers mainly connect to the nucleus of the solitary tract and thence to the parabrachial nucleus (in the pons) and to the parvocellular region ventral to the ventral posterior thala-mus. Beyond the thalamus, cardiopulmonary inputs have been shown to activate neurons in the ventral and caudal (agranular) zone of the insular cortex. This zone is also connected to medial prefrontal cortical regions and to the contralateral agranular insular cortex. Altogether, the physiological and anatomical evidence is consistent with the idea that the insula is involved in monitoring common visceral sensations and in modifying and integrating autonomic responses. In addition, there are projections to the ventrolateral orbital cortex and to the primary somatosensory cortex. The parabrachial nuclei also have efferent con-nections to the hypothalamus and amygdala. A simplified schema is presented in Fig. 2.

In Vivo Studies of the Role of the Central Nervous System in Cardiac Pain Perception

As noted above, the pathways described have largely been established from invasive animal experiments. To explore the role of the higher centers of the brain in vivo, we adopted an interdisciplinary approach employing positron emission tomography (PET). The latter is a powerful technique for the assessment of regional brain function. The parameter quantified by the PET method is regional cerebral blood

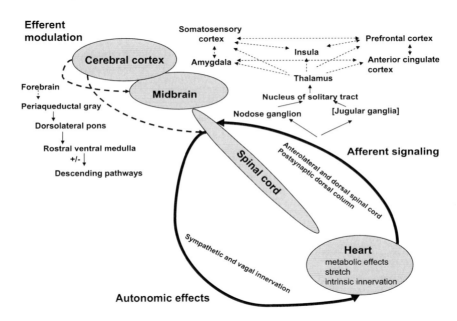

Fig. 2. Schematic of afferent and efferent pathways involved in the perception of chest pain.

flow (rCBF). In most circumstances, rCBF is a highly reliable index of cerebral glucose consumption, which rises regionally when a given cerebral territory is activated [26,49,64]. Glucose consumption is, in turn, coupled with Na/K-dependent ATPase and therefore with neuronal firing rates [25]. Measurements of rCBF have largely been confined to neurological studies to investigate, for example, brain responses to various motor tasks or to auditory or visual stimuli [24]. Applying this approach to the investigation of the cardiovascular system, we reported a study using PET with ^{15}O-labeled water to define the functional central nervous pathways activated by dobutamine-induced angina pectoris [69].

Compared to the resting state, angina was associated with increased rCBF in the hypothalamus and periaqueductal gray, bilaterally in the thalamus and lateral prefrontal cortex, and in the left inferior anterocaudal cingulate cortex. In contrast, rCBF was reduced bilaterally in the mid-rostrocaudal cingulate cortex and fusiform gyrus and in the right posterior cingulate and left parietal cortices. Several minutes after cessation of the dobutamine infusion, when the patients were no longer experiencing angina and the electrocardiographic changes had resolved, thalamic, but not cortical, activation could be demonstrated. We proposed that the central structures activated constituted the pathways for perception of anginal pain. An important finding was the persistence of thalamic activation after the cessation of the signs and symptoms of myocardial ischemia. This finding prompted us to propose that gating [52] of painful signals might occur at the thalamic level.

"Silent" Myocardial Ischemia

During the 20th century, the relationship between pain and ischemia was found to be more complex than might have been thought. It was observed that myocardial ischemia and infarction could occur in the absence of pain, either when infarction was discovered incidentally on a patient's electrocardiogram (ECG) or when myocardial ischemia could be assumed retrospectively after post mortem demonstration of significant CAD. The invention by Holter of a reliable tape-recording device that allowed ambulatory ECG monitoring brought about the discovery that episodes of painless ST segment depression were common and reflected reversible "silent" myocardial ischemia [19]. Indeed, up to 70% of episodes of myocardial ischemia in patients with CAD may be asymptomatic. In the case of acute myocardial infarction, the incidence of painless events has been estimated at 30% [3,38].

From the clinical perspective, insofar as ischemia-related chest pain can be considered an early warning system alerting one to myocardial injury, silent ischemia can be viewed as a failure of that system. The importance of this failure lies in its association with a poor prognosis after an episode of unstable angina or myocardial infarction [30,84]. Silent ischemia has also been assumed in cases of sudden death without any prior presentation of coronary disease. Silent ischemia has been found during exercise in cardiac arrest survivors and in patients with life-threatening arrhythmias [34].

Mildness of the ischemic episode, diabetes-related autonomic neuropathy, enhanced activity of the central nervous opioid system, and attentional factors have all been offered as reasons for the occurrence of silent ischemia [21]. However, the fact that silent ischemia often coexists with painful ischemia in the same patient precludes any simple explanation related to the particular characteristics of an individual patient [33].

We used the PET-based method described above to test whether the silence of painless myocardial ischemia is due to abnormal central nervous handling of afferent messages from the heart [70]. We examined rCBF changes during myocardial ischemia compared to baseline conditions and to placebo. During myocardial ischemia in patients known to experience angina, rCBF increased in the left thalamus, and bilaterally in the prefrontal, basal frontal, and ventral cingulate cortices. In a group of age- and sex-matched nondiabetic patients, who were experiencing silent myocardial ischemia (proven by stress echo), both thalami were shown to be activated, but cortical activation was limited to the right frontal region. A formal comparison of the two groups revealed significant differences for activation of the basal frontal cortex, ventral cingulate cortex, and left temporal pole (Fig. 3). In both groups, thalamic rCBF remained elevated after the symptoms and signs of ischemia had ceased.

In both angina and silent ischemia, bilateral activation of the thalamus was shown, so we felt that peripheral nerve dysfunction could not offer a complete explanation for silent ischemia. Frontal cortical activation appeared to be necessary for the sensation of pain. We suggested that abnormal central processing of afferent pain messages from the heart might have an etiologic role in silent myocardial ischemia, and gating at the thalamic level seemed a plausible explanation (Fig. 4). If our study achieved

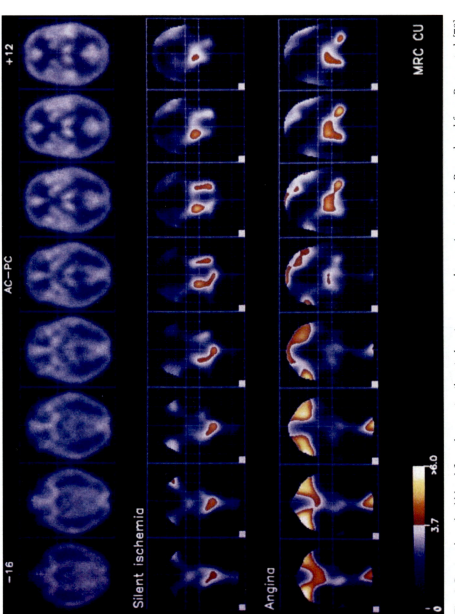

Fig. 3. Regional cerebral blood flow changes in silent ischemia compared to angina pectoris. Reproduced from Rosen et al. [70], with permission.

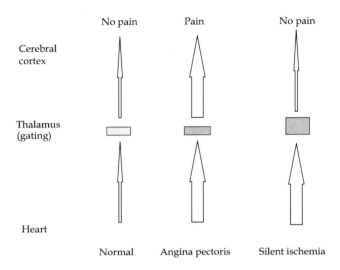

Fig. 4. Schematic of thalamic level gating in silent ischemia.

nothing else, it moved the focus of attention of research on cardiac pain to the brain and away from the heart.

Lessons from Recent Studies in Somatic Pain: The "Tools" with Which to Explore Functional Cardiac Pain

As evident from the rest of this book, pain research is a rapidly growing area, with a burgeoning literature. Several developments in the field have great relevance to the notion of a chronic cardiac pain syndrome. They will now be briefly reviewed. On a practical, clinical level, it is clear that chronic pain syndromes are very prevalent (affecting approximately 20% of the general population) and that the response to treatment is modest (rarely better than 40% in any treatment trial).

The Pain Matrix

An important concept that has emerged is that of the "pain matrix" [6,31,52,82]. In this view, rather than the conceptualization of a localized and specific "pain center," a more accurate notion is that of a looser network of different brain regions that—among several other functions—subserve the perception of pain. However, they interact in complex ways, so that pain not only is registered, but can also be modulated. The spectrum of modulation is extremely broad and can range from the complete blocking out of conscious pain sensations to feelings of extreme pain with little or even no peripheral stimulation.

Pain Modulation and Central Sensitization

Mood, cognitive set, context, and structural and neurochemical factors have all been shown to contribute to the modulation of pain perception. Depression [73] and anxiety [61] increase perceived pain, and there are now also hard data on the impact of expectation and anticipation [91], as well as belief and empathy [78]. The role of attention and distraction has been explored by Critchley et al. [18], focusing on interoception, and by Dunckley et al. with regard to attention [20]. Direct stimulation of brain regions has also been shown to generate pain in the absence of remote disease [28,57]. Lenz has also demonstrated that cardiac pain can be generated in this way [44].

Antinociception: The GABAergic System

An important role for γ-aminobutyric acid (GABA) receptor antagonists in the modulation of secondary hyperalgesia—a useful model of central sensitization—been reported by Iannetti and colleagues [35]. Electrical modulation of these pathways can also be achieved, particularly using spinal cord stimulation [53], and combinations of these treatments may be of value [89].

Neurophysiological Insights

When multichannel EEG is used to measure responses to painful peripheral stimuli, the resulting negative and positive potentials (the peak early latency components N1 and P1 and later latencies N2 and P2) permit researchers to discriminate regions involved in primary registration of a painful stimulus from other areas likely to mediate pain modulation or other processing. The ability of the central nervous system to habituate to repeated stimuli can thereby also be quantified [37].

The Sensitive Heart: Cardiac Syndrome X as a Chronic Central Pain Syndrome

A Reverse Disparity between Pain and Ischemia: Cardiac Syndrome X and "Minor Coronary Artery Disease"

With the advent of coronary arteriography in the early 1960s, the syndrome of anginal pain with a normal coronary arteriogram first became recognized. Indeed, early reports suggested that about 30% of all patients undergoing coronary arteriography for a chest pain syndrome had a normal coronary arteriogram [60,63], although contemporary data may put the figure lower.

In 1967, Kemp et al. [41] reported on 50 patients who lacked "significant" CAD and separated them into three groups according to the predictability of exertional chest pain and the similarity of the chest pain to angina pectoris due to "coronary insufficiency." Of the 50 patients, 34% had overt diabetes or abnormal glucose tolerance. In 4 out of 26 patients tested, lactate production (a metabolic marker of myocardial ischemia) was found during isoproterenol stress. Five additional patients with ischemic-like changes on the exercise ECG did not, however, show evidence of lactate production during stress.

The same year, Likoff et al. [45] described a series of 15 patients, all female, nondiabetic and normotensive, with normal coronary arteriograms, who had resting ECG abnormalities that were exacerbated by exercise. Nine of these patients were reported to have typical features of angina pectoris. Eight of the 15 patients were assessed in terms of cardiac output, oxygen consumption, and pulmonary artery pressures; all of these parameters remained normal during exercise despite the ECG changes.

Arbogast and Bourassa [2] investigated patients with angina pectoris and coronary arteriograms that were "normal or near-normal" (Group X) and patients with typical CAD (Group C). They noted that despite ischemic-like ECG changes with exercise, left ventricular function during atrial pacing remained normal or was even enhanced in the Group

X patients compared to the Group C patients, even though they detected lactate production in 5 of the 10 Group X patients during atrial pacing. In an editorial in the same issue, commenting upon Arbogast and Bourassa's paper, Kemp [40] noted that patients with chest pain and normal coronary arteriograms were a heterogeneous group and used the term "syndrome X" to convey the uncertainty over pathophysiology that has characterized this disorder up to the present day.

The substantial interest that this condition attracts is due to two main reasons. The first is clinical. Does the patient have heart disease? Can the condition be effectively treated? Is the patient's life expectancy shortened? The second reason relates to the pathophysiology of this condition. Is the chest pain in patients with syndrome X of ischemic origin? And, if the pain is due to myocardial ischemia, what are the mechanisms?

Since these early descriptions, a large number of studies have been performed in patients with angina and a "normal" coronary arteriogram. It must be noted, however, that as exemplified by the papers discussed above, inclusion and exclusion criteria in the vast majority of these studies have not been especially strict. In particular, the category of "normal coronary arteriogram" has been a broad one, often including cases of CAD ranging from minimal disease to coronary stenoses up to 50% of luminal diameter. Therefore, the patients described in such studies are clinically heterogeneous, and possible causes of their chest pain are numerous.

The Question of Definition

Clinically, a much more homogeneous set of patients is defined if the following criteria of selection are applied: greater than 0.1 mV rectilinear or downsloping ST segment depression on the exercise ECG; absence of left bundle branch block either on the resting or exercise ECG; the absence of even minimal irregularities on the arteriogram; and no evidence of diabetes mellitus, arterial hypertension, valve disease (including mitral valve prolapse), epicardial arterial spasm, or cardiomyopathy. This definition removes several potential confounding factors from a constructive discussion of pathophysiology. With these criteria, the incidence of the disorder is probably of the order of 1–3% of all patients presenting to the cardiologist with a chest pain syndrome [9,12].

These exclusion criteria are also essential because, more recently, it has become clear that abnormalities in the function and structure of the coronary microcirculation, which may be severe enough to contribute to myocardial ischemia, occur in many of the above conditions. Most commonly, myocardial ischemia is demonstrated in patients with CAD in whom CFR is reduced in parallel with the severity of coronary stenoses [56]. However, a reduced CFR can also be demonstrated in patients with angiographically normal epicardial arteries, and in this circumstance, it suggests coronary microvascular dysfunction (CMD). CMD has been demonstrated in patients who are at higher risk of developing CAD; it is thought to represent the functional counterpart of traditional coronary risk factors. CMD can also occur in patients with primary (e.g., hypertrophic) or secondary (e.g., hypertensive) cardiomyopathies and is most commonly due to adverse remodeling of intramural arterioles (for a detailed review of CMD see Camici and Crea [8]). Originally, the term "syndrome X" was coined to stress the uncertainty over the pathophysiology of chest pain. Therefore, this term should not be used in patients, such as those with risk factors for CAD or cardiomyopathies, in whom myocardial ischemia due to CMD is known to occur.

Evidence for Abnormal Pain Perception in Syndrome X

Although earlier papers sought to account for the features of syndrome X in terms of myocardial ischemia due to microvascular dysfunction, more recent studies of myocardial blood flow and ventricular function have considerably undermined this pathophysiological hypothesis. It has not been possible—despite numerous efforts—to demonstrate either ischemia of any significance or the reduction in regional contractility that the latter would bring about. This issue has been reviewed elsewhere [68]. Conversely, the case for abnormal visceral pain perception being a crucial etiological component of syndrome X is becoming well established. The many strands of evidence pointing in this direction are reviewed below.

Comparisons of Threshold for Cardiac Pain between Syndrome X Patients during Pharmacological Stress

Sylvén and colleagues, working to elucidate the mechanisms of chest pain perception, explored the role of adenosine in the generation of chest pain in normal volunteers, patients with CAD, and patients with angina and normal coronary arteries [42]. The latter group were shown to have a lower threshold for adenosine-induced chest pain administered as an intravenous (i.v.) bolus, as shown by a lower minimum dose of adenosine required for the provocation of pain and a lower maximal tolerable dose of adenosine.

Subsequently, the same group of investigators studied the effect of epinephrine infusion in eight syndrome X patients [22] in three experiments: (1) epinephrine was administered i.v. in incremental fashion, and hemodynamic responses and a rating of chest pain were recorded; (2) epinephrine was administered on two occasions, with a further infusion of placebo or the nonspecific α-adrenergic antagonist phentolamine given according to a randomized, crossover protocol; and (3) the epinephrine infusion was repeated with simultaneous echocardiography to assess left ventricular function. The findings of the study were that the patients' typical pain was reproduced in most cases, in the absence of ST segment changes on the ECG, with little hemodynamic difference from baseline and with no evidence at all of left ventricular wall motion abnormality. Phentolamine had no effect upon the development of chest pain. It was concluded that syndrome X might be "a sympathetic maintained pain of neurogenic origin due to dysregulation in the complex cardiac nervous system."

Studies to Assess the Relationships among Myocardial Blood Flow, Chest Pain, and Electrocardiogram Changes

Using PET, Camici et al. [9] assessed myocardial blood flow and coronary vasodilator reserve using ^{13}N-labeled ammonia in a large group of syndrome X patients (n = 45) with a history of chest pain and a normal coronary arteriogram, with or without ischemic-like changes in the stress ECG. No normal controls were studied. The data indicated that myocardial blood flow (MBF) values following dipyridamole were widely dispersed, and analysis of the frequency of distribution suggested that a subgroup of patients could be identified with a lower CFR. However, the authors found no correspondence between the flow data and ECG changes on exercise. Increased adrenergic activity was hypothesized in these patients, and it was suggested that limitation of the MBF response to dipyridamole, observed in some syndrome X patients, might be due to α_1-mediated coronary vasoconstriction. A preliminary open study [10] was then performed to measure the effect of the α_1 antagonist doxazosin in the subgroup of patients with CFR at the lower end of the range. Doxazosin was indeed shown to increase MBF following dipyridamole. However, in 7 out of 10 patients, dipyridamole-induced chest pain persisted despite a significant improvement of CFR. Furthermore, a subsequent study by Lorenzoni et al. showed that doxazosin was also able to induce a significant increase in resting and hyperemic MBF in normal volunteers [46].

In 1994, we followed Camici's 1992 study with a series of 29 syndrome X patients (tightly defined and all with ischemic-like ECG changes during exercise stress) and 20 matched true normal controls [72]. Our principal findings were that MBF values at rest and after dipyridamole were comparable in patients and controls. In addition, as in Camici et al's study [9], no relationships were demonstrable amongst MBF, chest pain, and ECG changes under stress. It is the combination of the above MBF data, as well as the failure of careful studies to demonstrate release of lactate [11] or H^+ [65] by syndrome X patients during stress, as well as the preservation (or even enhancement) of left ventricular function during stress [55,58], that have, in our opinion, significantly undermined the case for myocardial ischemia having much pathophysiological relevance in syndrome X.

Studies of Direct Cardiac Stimulation

Shapiro et al. [76] in 1988 reported a study of seven patients with syndrome X; four patients with chest pain, normal coronary arteries, and a negative exercise test; seven patients with CAD; and nine patients with mitral valve disease. Six out of seven syndrome X patients and all four patients with chest pain, normal coronary arteries, and a negative exercise test experienced pain when a catheter was rapidly turned, advanced, or retracted between the right atrium and the superior vena cava. All the coronary disease and mitral valve disease patients were insensitive to this maneuver.

A larger study by Cannon et al. [14] investigated 36 patients with chest pain and angiographically normal coronary arteries, 33 symptomatic patients with hypertrophic cardiomyopathy, and 33 patients with

CAD. Cardiac sensitivity was assessed in terms of awareness of, or pain provoked by, pacing, first from the right atrium and then from the right ventricular apex, at a rate 5 beats faster than the patient's basal heart rate. Another feature noted was whether patients experienced pain during the first injection of contrast medium into the left coronary artery. In the same study, cutaneous sensitivity was also measured in terms of a subjective scaling of a thermal pain stimulus. A subset of patients ($n = 14$) underwent investigation of esophageal sensitivity to balloon distension and/or instillation of hydrochloric acid.

Of the 36 patients with chest pain and angiographically normal coronary arteries, 29 experienced their typical chest pain during catheter manipulation, pacing, or contrast injection, compared to 15/33 hypertrophic cardiomyopathy patients, 2/33 CAD patients, and 1/10 patients with valve disease. Paradoxically, the cutaneous pain threshold was *higher* in the patients with chest pain and angiographically normal coronary arteries. No relationship was demonstrable between cardiac sensitivity and cutaneous thermal sensitivity.

In 1994, Chauhan and colleagues [17] reported a similar study of 36 syndrome X patients; 36 patients with normal coronaries, mitral valve disease, and CAD; and 36 cardiac transplant patients with normal coronaries. The stimulus was rapid rotation and movement of a Gensini catheter first in the right atrium and then in the right ventricle. Pain provoked by contrast injection was also assessed. In the same patients, coronary blood flow velocity was also measured at rest and after intracoronary papaverine.

The intracardiac stimulation produced typical chest pain in 34/36 syndrome X patients, but in only 5 patients with mitral valve disease and normal coronaries, 7 patients with mitral valve and coronary disease, and no patients with coronary disease alone. An important observation was that there were no significant changes in coronary flow velocity during chest pain in the syndrome X patients (regardless of whether there was any blunting of CFR).

Pasceri and colleagues [59] raised the question of whether patients with syndrome X have a genuinely increased perception of pain or just a greater tendency to complain. They explored this issue using the model of right atrial and ventricular pacing, 5–10 beats faster than the patient's basal heart rate, at varying stimulus intensities. True and false pacing protocols were employed. Their principal finding was that syndrome X patients had both increased perception of pain and a greater tendency to complain.

Comparison of Threshold for Somatic Pain between Syndrome X Patients during Peripheral Stimulation

In 1987, Turiel et al. [83] investigated the pain threshold to forearm ischemia and to electrical skin stimulation in women with syndrome X and in others with CAD and found a lower threshold in the latter group. However, the threshold for cutaneous pain in response to multiple thermal stimuli was greater in a study by Cannon et al. [13], and sensitivity to both thermal and electrical stimuli was found to be normal by Frøbert and colleagues [27]. The issue may find a potential explanation in terms of (1) the distinction of the pain pathways involved and (2) dissociation of the central opioid response to somatic versus visceral stimuli [36].

Abnormal Central Nervous Processing in Cardiac Syndrome X Demonstrated by Neurophysiological Measurements

Valeriani et al. [86] employed neurophysiological measurement techniques to measure laser-evoked potentials—cortical electrical responses to laser-evoked peripheral pain stimuli—in patients with chronic CAD and other patients with cardiac syndrome X. While the former demonstrated a gradual decrease in N2/P2 amplitude with sequences of stimuli, indicating habituation to the stimulus, this decrease was noticeably absent in the syndrome X group.

Effects of Spinal Cord Stimulation in Syndrome X Patients

After spinal cord stimulation was shown to be of benefit in patients with chronic CAD and intractable angina pectoris, the technique was applied with good effect by Lanza and colleagues to patients with syndrome X [43,74]. Long-term treatment is also effective [75]. In addition, by combining the technique of laser-evoked potential measurement with the therapeutic use of spinal cord stimulation in syndrome X patients, Sestito et al. [74] were able to show that this approach could restore the ability of the central nervous system of these patients to habituate to the painful stimulus.

Therapeutic Intervention with Psychotropic Drugs

When the dominant pathophysiological hypothesis of chest pain was that of myocardial ischemia, several anti-ischemic agents were used to treat syndrome X patients, including nitrates, beta-blockers, and calcium antagonists. More recently, from the advocates of other pathophysiological hypotheses, such as those relating to estrogen deficiency or to inappropriate adenosine release, have come recommendations that syndrome X patients be treated with hormone replacement therapy or aminophylline, respectively. Overall, however, the results of all of these agents have been less than satisfactory.

A different approach has been adopted by Cannon and colleagues [13]. In a large-scale study, 60 patients with chest pain and normal coronary arteries were investigated with the following tests: exercise ECG; technetium blood pool scan; right ventricular pacing 5 beats/minute faster than the patient's resting heart rate; adenosine infusion into the right coronary artery; balloon inflation in the esophagus, acid instillation into the esophagus, and assessment of esophageal motility; and a diagnostic interview by a psychiatric nurse. Subjects then embarked upon a randomized, double-blind, placebo-controlled trial of clonidine, imipramine, or placebo, preceded by a single-blind placebo phase for all participants. Patients had been referred because of recurrent chest pain, and 57/60 had previously been given anti-ischemic therapy that had failed to control their symptoms.

Of the 60 patients studied by Cannon and colleagues, 13 had a positive exercise test, 22 (of 54 tested) had abnormal esophageal motility (mainly distal high-amplitude peristalsis), 38 had at least one psychiatric disorder, and 52 had their characteristic pain provoked by right ventricular pacing or intracoronary adenosine. Imipramine therapy led to a 52% reduction in episodes of chest pain (which was statistically significant at $P = 0.03$), whereas clonidine produced a 39% reduction (statistically nonsignificant) compared to the baseline placebo phase. Of interest is that the response to imipramine was independent of the results of the cardiac, esophageal, and psychiatric testing at baseline. Also, the results for the subset of patients who could strictly be diagnosed with syndrome X (i.e., those with a positive exercise test) were entirely comparable to those of the wider patient group. The authors suggested that imipramine exerted its effects in the patients with chest pain and normal coronaries through a visceral analgesic action, similar to its effects when used in other chronic pain syndromes.

Psychological Aspects of Cardiac Syndrome X

Psychological aspects of cardiac syndrome X have been reviewed extensively elsewhere [66], but they can be summarized in terms of syndrome X patients having, compared to patients with CAD, greater anxiety, a tendency to seek reassurance, more stressful life events, and more neuroticism. Unfortunately, their psychological morbidity is substantial and enduring.

Evidence for Abnormal Sympathetic Nervous System Activation in Patients with Syndrome X

It might reasonably be expected that abnormal processing of signals from the heart might have consequences in terms of altered activity of the sympathetic nervous system. Data to support an increase in sympathetic activity include hemodynamic observations and indirect metabolic evidence [11], as well as heart rate variability data; the latter studies have been reviewed, and they broadly suggest an alteration in sympathovagal balance in syndrome X patients [67].

Functional Neuroimaging in Cardiac Syndrome X

As indicated above, we have pioneered the technique of using PET with ^{15}O-labeled water to explore the central neural correlates of chest pain in patients with CAD. An obvious next step was to apply this technique to the study of patients with cardiac syndrome X.

In this study [71], we found that syndrome X patients and normal controls have comparable rCBF responses to dobutamine stress, with activations in the hypothalamus, thalami, right frontal cortex, and anterior temporal poles, associated with the sensation of a fast or powerful heartbeat. However, in the syndrome X patients, but not in the controls, the dobutamine stress additionally generated severe chest pain. This pain

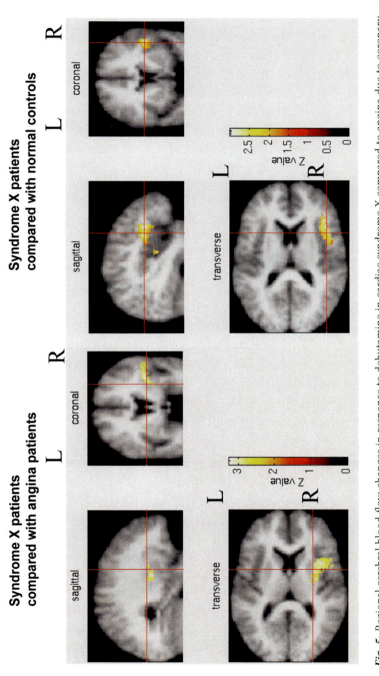

Fig. 5. Regional cerebral blood flow changes in response to dobutamine in cardiac syndrome X compared to angina due to coronary artery disease. Reproduced from Rosen et al. [71], with permission.

was associated with increased activity in the right anterior insula at the junction with the frontal operculum. Conversely, there was greater activity in the left insula and right cingulate cortex in controls. A comparison with our earlier published data from patients with angina due to CAD also showed greater right anterior insular activity in the syndrome X patients during the high-dose dobutamine infusion (Fig. 5). Therefore, we suggested that right insula activation has a significant role in the perception of chest pain in syndrome X. Moreover, the complete absence of echocardiographic evidence of left ventricular dysfunction during the chest pain in the syndrome X patients maintained the argument against the presence of myocardial ischemia.

Symptomatic Responses of Our Patient Groups to Dobutamine Infusion

All three of the groups we studied (syndrome X patients, CAD patients, and controls) received an equivalent dose of dobutamine, and the drug had comparable hemodynamic effects. Symptomatically, each group responded as expected: the normal subjects experienced a more powerful heart beat, but no frank pain; the syndrome X patients, despite the absence of echocardiographic evidence of left ventricular dysfunction, developed chest pain that persisted for many minutes after discontinuation of the dobutamine; and the CAD patients developed chest pain associated with ischemia, as demonstrated by the regional wall motion abnormality on their stress ECGs, which resolved on cessation of the dobutamine.

Differences between the Syndrome X Findings and Our Earlier Data in CAD Patients

Besides the obvious difference of the presence or absence of myocardial ischemia, functional differences of neural systems other than those associated with pain may explain some of the discrepancies between our recent study and our previous work in CAD patients. For example, abnormal laterality of cerebral activations has certainly been demonstrated in CAD patients, during mental arithmetic stress [79].

In our earlier reports of central neural correlates of painful and silent myocardial ischemia in patients with CAD, we suggested that the thalamus may exert a "gating" or filtering role in limiting the further afferent transmission of signals from the heart to the cerebral cortex. We might therefore have expected that in our recent study (if, indeed, in syndrome X the gate or filter was less effective), thalamic activation would be greater in syndrome X patients than in patients with CAD during high-dose dobutamine; indeed, for the right thalamus, this expectation was justified. However, the finding that both the syndrome X patients and the normal controls had substantial and equivalent increases in rCBF in the thalamus obviously refutes such a simple schema. In contrast, the findings of our recent study support the hypothesis that the chest pain in syndrome X involves modulation of cardiac afferent signals by altered cerebral cortical activity (Fig. 6).

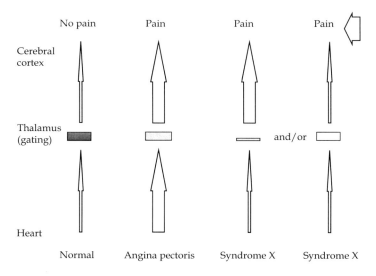

Fig. 6. Schematic of thalamic level gating in cardiac syndrome X, with or without cortical modification.

The Pain Matrix in the Patient with Cardiac Syndrome X

A consideration of the pain matrix outlined above shows that numerous routes of investigation and methodologies have identified elements whose dysfunction could contribute to a chronic pain syndrome. In this section, we have reviewed studies that point to abnormalities of pain perception in patients with syndrome X. It can readily be seen that there are probably several points in the matrix where abnormal modulation of afferent signals from the heart could lead to the establishment and maintenance of a chronic cardiac pain syndrome, even without any noteworthy innate cardiac dysfunction (Fig. 7).

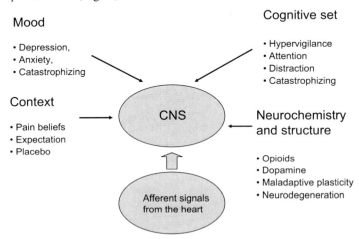

Fig. 7. Central modulation of afferent signals in cardiac syndrome X (after Tracey and Mantyh [81]).

The studies of thresholds for peripheral sensitivity do not establish a clear peripheral abnormality in the cardiac syndrome X patients, but it is likely that from the level of the spinal cord and upward, neural handling is abnormal [71]. However, the weight of evidence favors abnormal function even higher in the neuraxis, especially the functional imaging data and the therapeutic effect of imipramine. Failure of modulation might also relate to the psychological anomalies described (Fig. 7).

Applying these perspectives to our neuroimaging study, we observed that in response to dobutamine, the sensation experienced was different in the normal controls compared to the syndrome X patients. The former were aware of a rapid heart rate, a percept normally associated with exertion, excitement, or anxiety/fear. The dissociation between the perception of a fast heart rate and the appropriate trigger may have initially induced a transient emotional response in the normal subjects—unease or anxiety. However, it would be reasonable to suppose that the emotional

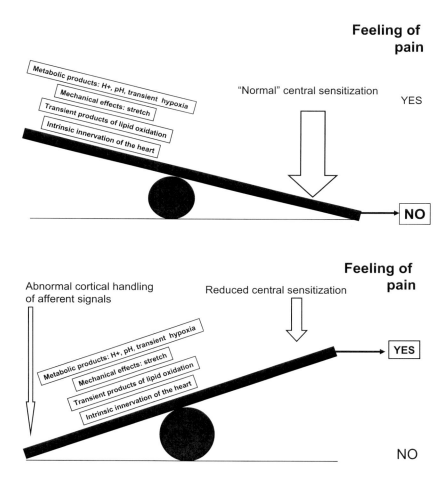

Fig. 8. Normal versus abnormal central sensitization in the generation of the pain percept in cardiac syndrome X.

response decayed as the subjects rapidly habituated to the sensation and related the heart rate response to the infusion. (Note the excessive anxiety reported above for syndrome X patients and the evidence of abnormal habituation.)

The syndrome X patients felt substantial pain after receiving dobutamine. Since pain is usually a signal that the sufferer is experiencing tissue injury, the pain percept is likely to be associated with an emotional response—fear and anxiety—to which the subject will only habituate slowly, if at all. Despite the rCBF changes observed in these syndrome X patients, the normal ECG findings indicated that (as far as we could tell) no myocardial damage was associated with the pharmacological stress. Overall, this finding suggests that the afferent signals in response to the dobutamine infusion in syndrome X patients were inappropriately encoded, generating the conscious experience of pain despite the absence of tissue injury. We propose that the differences in the cortical activations in response to high-dose dobutamine reflect the difference between sensory percepts in each group.

Normal controls have greater activation in the left insular and right anterior cingulate cortex, whereas greater activity in the right insular cortex differentiated syndrome X patients from normal controls. Furthermore, this regional difference was also present in the comparison of syndrome X patients with CAD patients, in whom pain is appropriately associated with tissue injury. We would therefore deduce that the right insular activation is specific for a perception of myocardial pain without ischemic injury and that this activation is the cortical expression of the abnormal percept.

Neuroanatomical Considerations and Functional Significance

The general involvement of the anterior cingulate and frontal cortex in the perception of cardiac pain is consistent with known neuroanatomy [54,87,88]. Yet the significance of the insular and prefrontal activation during chest pain in syndrome X invites further consideration. Luria and Simernitskaya [47] many years ago proposed a relatively more important role for the right hemisphere in the perception of visceral changes and suggested that feedback loop activity involving this region may be critical for emotional experience. Subsequent physiological and anatomical data have also pointed to the insula being involved in monitoring common visceral sensations and in modifying and integrating autonomic responses. The issue of abnormal interoception alluded to above may also be relevant in this context. Brooks and Tracey have recently written an elegant summary of current thinking on the unique role of the insula in pain perception [7].

Finally, this neurophysiological view of the etiology of chest pain in syndrome X might also account for one outstanding puzzling clinical feature in syndrome, namely the ST depression on the ECG during exercise stress. Thus, besides the more obvious common causes of a false-positive exercise ECG [50], such as overactivity of the sympathetic nervous system, abnormal transmembrane potassium flux [5,62], and hyperventilation [29], an efferent neural action upon the ECG during chest pain in syndrome X patients might also contribute to the ECG's "ischemic-like" appearance.

Chronic Functional Pain Aspects of Patients with Coronary Artery Disease

The above discussion has centered upon cardiac syndrome X as a model of a functional visceral pain syndrome, but many of the issues raised could be readily applied to the patient with minor CAD and "disproportionate" cardiac pain [77]. Clearly, these patients' disease needs to be managed optimally, but the disparity between their symptomatic status and objective measures of heart disease may find an explanation in the matters explored above.

Conclusion

Patients can be defined in whom—in simple terms—there is a "sensitive heart" [15,62]. A radically different, subtler, and more neurophysiologically aware approach might offer hope for a real improvement in the clinical status of these patients. Use of the pain matrix model should bring a focus on pain modulatory pathways and activities as the basis of future directions of treatment, and research should include exploration of factors modulating the experience of pain; routes may be psychological, neurophysiological, or pharmacological.

References

[1] Albutaihi IAM, deJongste MJL, ter Horst GJ. An integrated study of heart pain and behavior in freely moving rats (using fos as a marker for neuronal activation). Neurosignals 2004;13:207–26.
[2] Arbogast R, Bourassa MG. Myocardial function during atrial pacing in patients with angina pectoris and normal coronary arteriograms. Comparison with patients having significant coronary artery disease. Am J Cardiol 1973;32:257–63.
[3] Babey AM. Painless acute infarction of the heart. N Engl J Med 1939;220:410–2.
[4] Bing RJ. Coronary circulation and cardiac metabolism. In: Fishman AP, Richards DW, editors. Circulation of the blood: men and ideas. New York: Oxford University Press; 1964. p. 199–264.

[5]   Bøtker HE, Sonne HS, Frøbert O, Andreasen F. Enhanced exercise-induced hyperkalaemia in patients with syndrome X. J Am Coll Cardiol 1999;33:1056–61.
[6]   Brooks J, Tracey I. From nociception to pain perception: imaging the spinal and supraspinal pathways. J Anat 2005;207:19–33.
[7]   Brooks JCW, Tracey I. The insula: a multidimensional integration site for pain. Pain 2007;128:1–2.
[8]   Camici PG, Crea F. Coronary microvascular dysfunction. New Engl J Med 2007;356:830–40.
[9]   Camici PG, Gistri R, Lorenzoni R, Sorace O, Michelassi C, Bongiorni MG, Salvadori PA, L'Abbate A. Coronary reserve and exercise ECG in patients with chest pain and normal coronary angiograms. Circulation 1992;86:179–86.
[10] Camici PG, Marraccini P, Gistri R, Salvadori PA, Sorace O, L'Abbate A. Adrenergically mediated coronary vasoconstriction in patients with syndrome X. Cardiovasc Drugs Ther 1994;8:221–6.
[11] Camici PG, Marraccini P, Lorenzoni R, Buzzigoli G, Pecori N, Perissinotto A, Ferrannini E, L'Abbate A, Marzilli M. Coronary hemodynamics and myocardial metabolism in patients with syndrome X: response to pacing stress. J Am Coll Cardiol 1991;17:1461–70.
[12] Cannon RO, Camici PG, Epstein SE. Pathophysiological dilemma of syndrome X. Circulation 1992;85:883–92.
[13] Cannon RO, Quyyumi AA, Mincemoyer R, Stine AM, Gracely RH, Smith WB, Geraci MF, Black BC, Uhde TW, Waclawiw MA, et al. Imipramine in patients with chest pain despite normal coronary angiograms. N Engl J Med 1994;330:1411–7.
[14] Cannon RO, Quyyumi AA, Schenke WH, Fananapazir L, Tucker EE, Gaughan AM, Gracely RH, Cattau EL, Epstein SE. Abnormal cardiac sensitivity in patients with chest pain and normal coronary arteries. J Am Coll Cardiol 1990;16:1359–66.
[15] Cannon RO. The sensitive heart. A syndrome of abnormal cardiac pain perception. JAMA 1995;273:883–7.
[16] Cechetto DF. Supraspinal mechanisms of visceral representation. In: Gebhart GF, editor. Visceral pain. Progress in pain research and management, Vol. 5. Seattle: IASP Press; 1995. p. 261–90.
[17] Chauhan A, Mullins PA, Thuraisingham SI, Taylor G, Petch MC, Schofield PM. Abnormal cardiac pain perception in syndrome X. J Am Coll Cardiol 1994;24:329–35.
[18] Critchley HD, Wiens S, Rotshtein P, Ohman A, Dolan RJ. Neural systems supporting interoceptive awareness. Nature Neurosci 2004;7:189–95.
[19] Deanfield JE, Maseri A, Selwyn AP, Ribeiro P, Chierchia S, Krikler S, Morgan M. Myocardial ischaemia during daily life in patients with stable angina: its relation to symptoms and heart rate changes. Lancet 1983;2:753–8.
[20] Dunckley P, Aziz Q, Wise RG, Brooks J, Tracey I, Chang L. Attentional modulation of visceral and somatic pain. Neurogastroenterol Motil 2007;19:569–77.
[21] Epstein SE, Quyyumi AA, Bonow RO. Current concepts, myocardial ischaemia: silent or symptomatic. N Engl J Med 1988;318:1038–43.
[22] Eriksson B, Svedenhag J, Martinsson A, Sylvén C. Effect of epinephrine infusion on chest pain in syndrome X in the absence of signs of myocardial ischaemia Am J Cardiol 1995;75:241–5.
[23] François-Franck CA. Signification physiologique de la résection du sympathetique dans la maladie de Basedow, l'épilepsie, l'idiotie et le glaucome. Bull Acad Med Paris 1899;41:565–74.
[24] Friston KJ, Frackowiak RSJ. Imaging functional anatomy. In: Lassen NA, Ingvar DH, Raichle ME, Friberg L, editors. Brain work and mental activity. Alfred Benzon Symposium, Vol. 31. Copenhagen: Munksgaard; 1991. p. 267–79.
[25] Friston KJ, Frith CD, Liddle PF, Frackowiak RSJ. Comparing functional (PET) images: assessment of significant change. J Cereb Blood Flow Metab 1991;11:690–9.
[26] Friston KJ, Frith CD, Liddle PF, Lammertsma AA, Dolan RD, Frackowiak RSJ. The relationship between local and global changes in PET scans. J Cereb Blood Flow Metab 1990;10:458–66.
[27] Frøbert O, Arendt-Nielsen L, Bak P, Funch-Jensen P, Bagger JP. Pain perception and brain evoked potentials in patients with angina despite normal coronary angiograms. Heart 1996;75:436–41.
[28] Frot M, Mauguiere F. Dual representation of pain in the operculo-insular cortex in humans. Brain 2003;126:438–50.
[29] Gardin JM, Isner JM, Ronan JA, Fox SM. Pseudoischemic "false positive" ST-segment changes induced by hyperventilation in patients with mitral valve prolapse. Am J Cardiol 1980;45:952–8.

[30] Gottlieb SO, Weisfeldt ML, Ouyang P, Mellits ED, Gerstenblith G. Silent ischaemia as a marker for early unfavorable outcome in patients with unstable angina. N Engl J Med 1986;314:1214–9.

[31] Head H, Holmes G. Sensory disturbances from cerebral lesions. Brain Res 1911;34:102–254.

[32] Heberden W. Some account of a disorder of the breast. Med Trans Roy Coll Phys London 1772;2:59–67.

[33] Hofkamp SE, Henrikson CA, Wegener ST. An interactive model of pain and myocardial ischaemia. Psychosom Med 2007;69:632–39.

[34] Hong RA, Bhandari AK, McKay CR, Au PK, Rahimtoola SH. Life threatening ventricular tachycardia and fibrillation induced by painless myocardial ischaemia during exercise testing. JAMA 1987;257:1937–40.

[35] Ianetti GD, Zambreanu L, Wise RG, Buchanan TJ, Huggins JP, Smart TS, Vennart W, Tracey I. Pharmacological modulation of pain-related brain activity during normal and central sensitization states in humans. Proc Natl Acad Sci USA 2005;102:18195–200.

[36] Jarmukli N, Ahn J, Iranmanesh A, Russell D. Effect of raised plasma beta endorphin concentrations on peripheral pain and angina thresholds in patients with stable angina. Heart 1999;82:204–9.

[37] Kakigi R, Inui K, Tamura Y. Electrophysiological studies on human pain perception. Clin Neurophysiol 2005;116:743–63.

[38] Kannel WB, Abbott RD. Incidence and prognosis of unrecognised myocardial infarction: an update on the Framingham study. N Engl J Med 1984;311:1144–7.

[39] Keefer CS, Resnik WH. Angina pectoris: a syndrome caused by anoxemia of the myocardium. Arch Intern Med 1928;41:769–807.

[40] Kemp HG. The anginal syndrome associated with normal coronary arteriograms: report of a six year experience. Am J Med 1973;54:735–42.

[41] Kemp HG, Elliott WC, Gorlin R. The anginal syndrome with normal coronary arteriography. Trans Assoc Am Physicians 1967;80:59–70.

[42] Lagerqvist B, Sylvén C, Waldenstrom A. Lower threshold for adenosine induced chest pain in patients with angina and normal coronary arteries. Br Heart J 1992;68:282–5.

[43] Lanza GA, Sestito A, Sgueglia GA, Infusino F, Papacci F, Visocchi M, Ierardi C, Meglio M, Bellocci F, Crea F. Effect of spinal cord stimulation on spontaneous and stress-induced angina and 'ischaemia-like' ST-segment depression in patients with cardiac syndrome X. Eur Heart J 2005;26:983–9.

[44] Lenz FA, Dougherty PM, Traill TA. Thalamic mechanisms of chest pain in the absence of cardiac pathology. Heart 1996;75:429–30.

[45] Likoff W, Segal BI, Kasparian H. Paradox of normal selective coronary arteriograms in patients considered to have unmistakeable coronary heart disease. N Engl J Med 1967;276:1063–6.

[46] Lorenzoni R, Rosen SD, Camici PG. Effect of alpha 1-adrenoceptor blockade on resting and hyperemic myocardial blood flow in normal humans. Am J Physiol 1996;271:H1302–6.

[47] Luria AR, Simernitskaya EG. Interhemispheric relations and the functions of the minor hemisphere. Neuropsychologia 1977; 15:175–8.

[48] Malliani A. The conceptualisation of cardiac pain as a non-specific and unreliable alarm system. In: Gebhart GF, editor. Visceral pain. Progress in pain research and management, Vol. 5. Seattle: IASP Press; 1995. p. 63–74.

[49] Mata M, Fink DJ, Gainer H, Smith CB, Davidsen L, Savaki H, Schwartz WJ, Sokoloff L. Activity-dependent energy metabolism in rat posterior pituitary primarily reflects sodium pump activity. J Neurochem 1980;34:213–5.

[50] McHenry PL. The false positive ST segment response to stress testing: limitations of a technology. Am Coll Cardiol Current J Rev 1993;3:68–70.

[51] Meller ST, Gebhart GF. Visceral pain: a review of experimental studies. Neuroscience 1992;48:501–24.

[52] Melzack R, Wall P. Pain mechanisms: a new theory. Science 1965;150:971–99.

[53] Myerson BA, Linderoth B. Mechanisms of spinal cord stimulation in neuropathic pain. Neurol Res 2000;22:285–92.

[54] Neafsey EJ, Terreberry RR, Hurley KM, Ruit KG, Frysztak RJ. Anterior cingulate cortex in rodents: connections, visceral control functions and implications for emotion. In: Vogt BA, Gabriel M, editors. Neurobiology of cingulate cortex and limbic thalamus: a comprehensive handbook. Boston: Birkhäuser; 1993. p. 206–23.

[55] Nihoyannopoulos P, Kaski JC, Crake T, Maseri A. Absence of myocardial dysfunction during pacing stress in patients with syndrome X. J Am Coll Cardiol 1991;18:1463–70.
[56] Opie LH. The heart. Physiology and metabolism. New York: Raven Press; 1991. p. 52–66.
[57] Ostrowsky K, Magnin M, Ryvlin P, Isnard J, Guenot M, Mauguiere F. Representation of pain and somatic sensation in the human insula: a study of responses to direct electrical cortical stimulation. Cereb Cortex 2002;12:376–85.
[58] Panza JA, Laurienzo JM, Curiel RV, Unger EF, Quyyumi AA, Dilsizian V, Cannon RO 3rd. Investigation of the mechanism of chest pain in patients with angiographically normal coronary arteries using transesophageal dobutamine stress echocardiography. J Am Coll Cardiol 1997;29:293–301.
[59] Pasceri V, Lanza GA, Buffon A, Montenero AS, Crea F, Maseri A. Role of abnormal pain sensitivity and behavioural factors in determining chest pain in syndrome X. J Am Coll Cardiol 1998;31:62–6.
[60] Pepine CJ, Balaban RS, Bonow RO, Diamond GA, Johnson BD, Johnson PA, Mosca L, Nissen SE, Pohost GM; National Heart, Lung and Blood Institute; American College of Cardiology Foundation. Women's Ischemic Syndrome Evaluation: current status and future research directions: report of the National Heart, Lung and Blood Institute workshop: October 2–4, 2002: Section 1: diagnosis of stable ischemia and ischemic heart disease. Circulation 2004;109:44–6.
[61] Ploghaus A, Narain C, Beckmann CF, Clare S, Bantick S, Wise R, Matthews PM, Rawlins JN, Tracey I. Exacerbation of pain by anxiety is associated with activity in a hippocampal network. J Neurosci 2001;21:9896–903.
[62] Poole-Wilson PA. Potassium and the heart. Clin Endocrinol Metab 1984;13:249–68.
[63] Proudfit WL, Shirey EK, Sones FM. Selective cine coronary angiography. Correlation with clinical findings in 1000 patients. Circulation 1966;33:901–10.
[64] Raichle M. Circulatory and metabolic correlates of brain function in normal humans In: Mountcastle VB, Plum F, Geiger SR, editors. Handbook of physiology. Section 1: The nervous system. Vol. V. Higher functions of the brain. Bethesda: American Physiological Society; 1987. p. 643–74.
[65] Rosano GM, Kaski JC, Arie S, Pereira WI, Horta P, Collins P, Pileggi F, Poole-Wilson PA. Failure to demonstrate myocardial ischaemia in patients with angina and normal coronary arteries. Evaluation by continuous coronary sinus pH monitoring and lactate metabolism. Eur Heart J 1996;17:1175–80.
[66] Rosen SD. Hearts and minds: psychological factors and the chest pain of cardiac syndrome X. Eur Heart J 2004;25:1672–4.
[67] Rosen SD. The pathophysiology of cardiac syndrome X: a tale of paradigm shifts. Cardiovasc Res 2001;52:174–7.
[68] Rosen SD, Camici PG. Insights into the pathophysiology of syndrome X obtained using positron emission tomography (PET). In: Kaski JC, editor. Chest pain with normal coronary angiograms: pathogenesis, diagnosis and management. Dordrecht: Kluwer; 1999. p. 69–80.
[69] Rosen SD, Paulesu E, Frith CD, Jones T, Davies GJ, Frackowiak RSJ, Camici PG. Central neural correlates of angina pectoris as a model of visceral pain. Lancet 1994;344:147–50.
[70] Rosen SD, Paulesu E, Nihoyannopoulos P, Tousoulis D, Frackowiak RSJ, Frith CD, Jones T, Camici PG. Silent ischaemia as a central problem: regional brain activation compared in silent and painful myocardial ischaemia. Ann Intern Med 1996;124:939–49.
[71] Rosen SD, Paulesu E, Wise RJS, Camici PG. Central neural contribution to the perception of chest pain in cardiac syndrome X. Heart 2002;87:513–9.
[72] Rosen SD, Uren NG, Kaski J-C, Tousoulis D, Davies GJ, Camici PG. Coronary vasodilator reserve, pain perception and gender in patients with syndrome X. Circulation 1994;90:50–60.
[73] Schweinhardt P, Kalk N, Wartolowska K, Chessell I, Wordsworth P, Tracey I. Investigation into the neural correlates of emotional augmentation of clinical pain. Neuroimage 2008;40:759–66.
[74] Sestito A, Lanza GA, La Pera D, de Armas L, Sgueglia GA, Infusino F, Miliucci R, Tonali PA, Crea F, Valeriani M. Spinal cord stimulation normalizes abnormal cortical pain processing in patients with cardiac syndrome X. Pain 2008;139:82–9.
[75] Sgueglia GA, Sestito A, Spinelli A, Cioni B, Infusino F, Papacci F, Bellocci F, Meglio M, Crea F, Lanza GA. Long-term follow-up of patients with cardiac syndrome X treated by spinal cord stimulation. Heart 2007;93:591–7.

[76] Shapiro LM, Crake T, Poole-Wilson PA. Is altered cardiac sensation responsible for chest pain in patients with normal coronary arteries? Clinical observation during cardiac catheterization. BMJ 1988;296:170–1.
[77] Sheps DS, Creed F, Clouse RE. Chest pain in patients with cardiac and noncardiac disease. Psychosom Med 2004;66:861–7.
[78] Singer T, Seymour B, O'Doherty J, Kaube H, Dolan RJ, Frith CD. Empathy for pain involves the affective but not sensory components of pain. Science 2004;303:1157–62.
[79] Soufer R, Bremner JD, Arrighi JA, Cohen I, Zaret BL, Burg MM, Goldman-Rakic P. Cerebral cortical hyperactivation in response to mental stress in patients with coronary artery disease. Proc Natl Acad Sci 1998;95:6454–9.
[80] Spyer KM. Central nervous control of the cardiovascular system. In: Bannister R, Mathias CJ, editors. Autonomic failure. A textbook of clinical disorders of the autonomic nervous system. Oxford: Oxford University Press; 1992. p. 54–77.
[81] Tracey I, Mantyh PW. The cerebral signature for pain perception and its modulation. Neuron 2007;55:377–91.
[82] Tracey I, Ploghaus A, Gati JS, Clare S, Smith S, Menon RS, Matthews P. Imaging attentional modulation of pain in the periaqueductal gray in humans. J Neurosci 2002;22:2748–52.
[83] Turiel M, Galassi AR, Glazier JJ, Kaski JC, Maseri A. Pain threshold and tolerance in women with syndrome X and women with stable angina pectoris. Am J Cardiol 1987;60:503–7.
[84] Tzivoni D, Gavish A, Zin D, Gottlieb S, Moriel M, Keren A, Banai S, Stern S. Prognostic significance of ischemic episodes in patients with previous myocardial infarction. Am J Cardiol 1988;62:661–4.
[85] Uren NG, Melin JA, De Bruyne B, Wijns W, Baudhuin T, Camici PG. Relation between myocardial blood flow and the severity of coronary artery stenosis. New Engl J Med 1994;330:1782–8.
[86] Valeriani M, Sestito A, Le Pera D, de Armas L, Infusino F, Maiese T, Sgueglia GA, Tonali PA, Crea F, Restuccia D, Lanza GA. Abnormal cortical processing in patients with cardiac syndrome X. Eur Heart J 2005;26:975–82.
[87] Van Hoesen GW, Morecraft RJ, Vogt BA. Connections of the monkey cingulate cortex. In: Vogt BA, Gabriel M, editors. Neurobiology of cingulate cortex and limbic thalamus: a comprehensive handbook. Boston: Birkhäuser; 1993. p. 249–84.
[88] Vogt BA, Pandya DN. Cingulate cortex of the rhesus monkey: II. cortical afferents. J Comp Neurol 1987;262:271–89.
[89] Wallin J, Cui J-G, Yakhnitsa V, Schechtmann G, Myerson BA, Linderoth B. Gabapentin and Pregabalin suppresses tactile allodynia and potentiate spinal cord stimulation in a model of neuropathy. Eur J Pain 2002;6:261–72.
[90] Warren J. Remarks on angina pectoris. N Engl J Med Surg 1812;1:1–11.
[91] Wiech K, Kalisch R, Weiskopf N, Pleger B, Stephan KE, Dolan RJ. Anterolateral prefrontal cortex mediates the analgesic effect of expected and perceived control over pain. J Neurosci 2006, 26:11501–9.

Correspondence to: Stuart D. Rosen, MA, MD, FRCP, Department of Cardiology, Ealing Hospital, Uxbridge Road, Middlesex UB1 3HW, United Kingdom. Email: stuart.rosen@imperial.ac.uk.

Painful Bladder Syndrome/Interstitial Cystitis

Lori Birder[a] and Christopher Chapple[b]

[a]Department of Medicine, University of Pittsburgh School of Medicine, Pittsburgh, Pennsylvania, USA;
[b]Department of Urology, Sheffield Teaching Hospitals NHS Trust, The Royal Hallamshire Hospital, Sheffield, United Kingdom

Terminology

Normal bladder sensation governs the storage and voiding of urine. It is now evident that lower urinary tract symptoms occurring in both sexes as a consequence of pathology are not specific to underlying disease processes, but may have a different etiopathology in both sexes [28]. Lower urinary tract symptoms encompass storage, voiding, and postmicturition symptoms.

The term "overactive bladder" was first adopted by the International Continence Society (ICS) in a 1988 report on standardization of terminology to describe a chronic condition defined urodynamically as "detrusor overactivity" and characterized by involuntary bladder contractions during the filling phase of the micturition cycle [1]. The ICS refined the definition of overactive bladder as a symptom syndrome to serve as a symptomatic diagnosis that includes urinary urgency, with or without urgency incontinence, usually accompanied by urinary frequency (>8 micturitions/24 hours) and nocturia [2]. The symptoms occur in the absence of pathology (e.g., urinary tract infection, urinary stones, or inflammatory conditions) or metabolic factors (e.g., diabetes mellitus) that would explain them. In these situations, all other pathology such as bacterial infection, malignancy, stones, and detrusor overactivity has been excluded.

However, symptoms such as urgency, suprapubic pressure, and pain do coexist in some patients and may overlap with the classical picture of overactive bladder, and there is currently no clear consensus as to how (or whether) to distinguish between overactive bladder and the syndrome known variously as painful bladder syndrome, bladder pain syndrome, or interstitial cystitis. (For reasons of conciseness, this chapter will use the term "painful bladder syndrome.") A hallmark of functional pain syndromes, such as painful bladder syndrome, is pain in the absence of demonstrable pathology of the viscera or associated nerves. There are no proven etiologies, and no effective treatments to eradicate the symptoms. This condition is characterized by suprapubic pain, associated with bladder filling; it can also be accompanied by a sudden strong urge to void, increased frequency of urination, and nocturia [4,40,44,76,77,88]. Various theories explaining the pathology of painful bladder syndrome include an altered bladder lining and possible contribution of a bacterial agent [11,35,36,64,89].

Clearly, the pain syndromes are heterogeneous and usually of unknown etiology, because they usually represent a diagnosis made after other pathologies have been excluded. Painful bladder syndrome is a rare chronic, debilitating inflammatory condition typified by storage symptoms (frequency and urgency related to bladder pain), with sterile urine and with little in the way of pathognomonic histological findings. The true prevalence of this condition is unknown, because any figures for prevalence depend on the definition used, and on the cultural and geographic area. Painful bladder syndrome is predominantly a disease of women, but it has been known to occur in men, albeit with significantly lower frequency. A recent reevaluation of chronic pelvic pain in men (called "prostatodynia" or "chronic abacterial prostatitis") suggests that it shares many of its features with painful bladder syndrome in women. Indeed, "painful bladder syndrome/interstitial cystitis" has recently become a collective term for a variety of bladder pain syndromes [48], which are most commonly described according to symptoms. Homma [48] has explored lower urinary tract symptomatology in some detail, looking at the relationship of syndromes that fall within the umbrella of urgency-frequency syndromes. He suggests that the definitions of urgency for overactive bladder (sudden onset and/or fear of leakage) and bladder hypersensitivity (a persistent urge because of pain) can be distinguished.

One of the greatest problems concerning painful bladder syndrome is the lack of a clear definition of the condition. The NIDDK (National Institute of Diabetes, Digestive and Kidney Diseases) devised criteria to enable comparison between research studies [105]. The ICS introduced the term "painful bladder syndrome," defined as "the complaint of suprapubic pain related to bladder filling, accompanied by other symptoms such as increased daytime and night-time frequency, in the absence of proven urinary infection or other obvious pathology." The ICS restricts the diagnosis to typical cystoscopic and histological features, without further specifying what they are [2]. Experts at an international consensus meeting in Monaco decided to refer to the disease as "painful bladder syndrome/interstitial cystitis" [44].

Demographics

Not surprisingly, the demographics of painful bladder syndrome and overactive bladder differ greatly. Numerous studies indicate that painful bladder syndrome occurs at a much lower prevalence [44] (1–2 million in the United States) than overactive bladder (33 million in the United States) [94]. Overactive bladder tends to be a disease associated with aging, whereas painful bladder syndrome cuts across all age spectrums [32,84]. In addition, painful bladder syndrome is often associated with demonstrable changes in the appearance of the bladder urothelium after cystodistension, whereas the same is not true for overactive bladder, which includes a significant percentage of cases with detrusor overactivity, but in the remainder there is no demonstrable urodynamic abnormality.

The Pathophysiology
of Painful Bladder Syndrome

Shared and Organ-Specific Factors

Recent studies suggest that painful bladder syndrome has several mechanisms in common with other functional pain syndromes [76]. For example, patients with painful bladder syndrome may also have a variety of comorbid symptoms and disorders, which can include irritable bowel syndrome (IBS), endometriosis, vulvodynia, fibromyalgia, rheumatoid arthritis, and even asthma. The etiology of these syndromes is incompletely understood, but several factors may play an important role, which can include changes in urothelial or epithelial sensor/barrier function, neurogenic inflammation, and even autoimmune involvement [47,101]. In addition, comorbidities of other pelvic pain syndromes may be due in part to cross-talk between nerves supplying the different pelvic viscera [70,87]. Mechanistic differences are certain to exist, but a number of these visceral (and somatic) disorders may also share common features, including reports of psychological or physical stressors as contributing factors in symptom exacerbation [23,29–31,33,37,67,71]. Studies in animals have documented that stress-sensitization is associated with induction of hyperalgesic states similar to many functional pain syndromes [62].

In addition, there is abundant evidence that functional pain syndromes, including painful bladder syndrome, are associated with alterations in the epithelial layer. For example, alterations in the bladder uroepithelium at both the molecular and structural levels have been cited in both patients and animals diagnosed with the disease. Changes in the urothelial barrier can permit water, as well as urea and other toxic substances, to pass into the underlying tissue (neural and/or muscle layers), resulting in symptoms of urgency, frequency, and pain during bladder filling and voiding. Changes in epithelial signaling/barrier function would not be unique to the urinary bladder. For example, airway epithelia in asthmatic patients, intestinal epithelia in patients with IBS and in chronic stress models, and keratinocytes in certain types of skin disease also exhibit a number of similar abnormalities and compromised repair processes [5,12,19]. Taken together, epithelial cells can respond to a number of challenges, including luminal factors, such as bacteria and their products, environmental pollutants, and mediators released from nerves or nearby inflammatory cells. Their response may result in altered expression or sensitivity of various receptor/channels as well as changes in release of mediators, which may impact function.

Properties of Normal Urothelium and Alterations in Disease

Urothelial Barrier Function

The urothelium, the epithelial lining of the urinary tract between the renal pelvis and urinary bladder, is composed of at least three cell layers [7,8,9,68]. These consist of a basal cell layer, an intermediate layer, and a superficial or apical layer composed of cells termed "umbrella" cells, which are interconnected by tight junctions [3,65,102]. The urothelium maintains a tight barrier to ion and solute flux, but a number of local factors (e.g., tissue pH, mechanical or chemical trauma, and bacterial infection) as well as conditions such as painful bladder syndrome can modulate its barrier function [9,75]. For example, some of the changes reported in painful bladder syndrome include alterations in synthesis of a number of cell adhesion and tight junction proteins. Similarly, there is also evidence of epithelial dysfunctions in cats diagnosed with a natural idiopathic cystitis, termed "feline interstitial cystitis" (which exhibits nearly all the characteristics of nonulcerative painful bladder syndrome in humans) [15,20,21,22,66].

Disruption of the integrity of the urothelial barrier may be mediated by hormonal or neural mechanisms (such as by substances released by surrounding nerves and other cell types within the bladder wall). For example, nitric oxide (NO) has been found to be elevated in patients with painful bladder syndrome, as well as in cats with feline interstitial cystitis [17,63]. Excessive NO levels in the urinary bladder can increase permeability to water and urea, in addition to producing ultrastructural changes in the apical layer. Although the pathological mechanism is unknown, these findings appear to be similar to those in other epithelia where excess production of NO has been linked to changes in epithelial integrity [42]. Disruption of epithelial integrity may also be linked to expression of substances such as antiproliferative factor (APF), which has been character-ized as a frizzled-8-related sialoglycopeptide and is detected in the urine of patients with painful bladder syndrome [26,59,60,106]. Abnormalities in urothelial growth and proliferation may also be linked to changes in expression of trophic factors such as heparin-binding epidermal growth factor-like growth factor (HB-EGF) [27,57].

More Than a Barrier: Sensor/Transducer Properties of Bladder Urothelium

Although the urinary bladder urothelium has classically been thought of as a passive barrier to ions and solutes, several novel properties have been recently attributed to urothelial cells [16]. Studies have revealed that the urothelium is involved in sensory mechanisms (the ability to express a number of sensor molecules or respond to thermal, mechanical, and chemical stimuli) and can release chemical mediators. Thus, urothelial cells exhibit a number of "neuronal-like" properties, including possessing receptors and ion channels similar to those in sensory neurons (nociceptors and mechanoreceptors). The sensitivity of many of these molecular targets are significantly altered in a number of bladder pathologies.

Various studies have shown that pathology often results in aug-mented release of transmitters, most notably adenosine triphosphate (ATP), from the urothelium [18]. This process can lead to painful sensa-tions by exciting purinergic receptors on sensory fibers. There is specu-lation that this type of noncholinergic mechanism could have a role in a number of bladder pathologies, including idiopathic detrusor instabil-ity and painful bladder syndrome. Studies have shown that in sensory neurons, ATP can potentiate the response of vanilloids (by lowering the threshold for protons, capsaicin, and heat) [99]. This novel mechanism represents a means by which large amounts of ATP released from dam-aged or sensitized cells, in response to injury or inflammation, may trigger the sensation of pain. These findings have clinical significance; they indi-cate that alterations to afferent nerves or epithelial cells in pelvic viscera might contribute to the sensory abnormalities observed in pelvic disor-ders such as painful bladder syndrome. In this regard, targeting urothelial release mechanisms may prove important in the treatment for a number of bladder dysfunctions. For example, studies demonstrate the therapeutic benefit of botulinum toxins (BoNTA) in the treatment of neurogenic and non-neurogenic detrusor overactivity as well as in painful bladder syndrome [69]. Although the effectiveness of BoNTA may be due to a block of transmitters released from bladder nerves, recent evidence suggests that BoNTA may also block release of mediators from non-neuronal cells (including the urothelium) [92].

What Is the Source of Pain in Painful Bladder Syndrome?

Chronic pain conditions such as painful bladder syndrome are associated with changes in the central nervous system (CNS) as well as the periphery [13]. While the etiology or source of pain is unknown, the relationship is likely to be complicated, involving abnormalities in the neuroaxis as well as changes in the target organ.

Urothelium and Primary Afferents

Painful bladder syndrome has often been described as a disease of the urothelium [41,81,83]. The urothelium is likely to play an important role by actively communicating with bladder nerves, urothelial cells, smooth muscle, or even cells of the immune and inflammatory systems [16]. The localization of afferent nerves next to the urothelium suggests that urothelial cells could be targets for transmitters released from bladder nerves or that chemicals released by urothelial cells could alter afferent nerve excitability in addition to influencing other cells. For example, urothelial-released mediators including prostaglandins, acetylcholine, ATP, and NO [15,43,50,85,95] may influence bladder afferent nerve activity, while release of a "urothelial derived inhibitory factor" [97] is thought to affect smooth muscle function. In addition, studies using a range of imaging techniques and cross-sections of the bladder have revealed that both chemical and physical stimulation can generate a series of calcium "waves" that propagate across the urothelial-suburothelial layers before invading the underlying smooth muscle [51,52]. For some types of cells, intercellular calcium "waves" may be a common way of translating extracellular stimuli into functional processes that can spread as a "wave" to nearby cells, ultimately leading to release of neuroactive mediators [14,54,91]. These and other findings support a significant role for the urothelium in "receiving and integrating" information from the periphery and relaying this information (via release of mediators) to other cell types, including the nervous system.

There is abundant evidence that changes in afferent nerves contribute to processing of nociceptive information from the periphery, thus contributing to pain symptoms in patients with painful bladder syndrome. In this regard, augmented release of mediators related to functional pain disorders has been linked to activation of both neurons and glial cells in the spinal cord. Recent findings support an important role for activation of spinal cord glial cells in both initiation and maintenance of persistent pain [24,25,45,56,72,79,90,103,104]. While most studies have focused on the role of glial cell activation in peripheral nerve injury, preliminary reports have revealed that glial cells may also become "activated" in functional pain syndromes such as painful bladder syndrome, IBS, and fibromyalgia [93,96]. Thus, it is not inconceivable that increases in afferent activity in painful bladder syndrome (increased pain and urgency) could lead to glial cell activation, which could then play an important role in the modulation of pain.

Central Pain Amplification

In addition to peripheral mechanisms, visceral hypersensitivity and pain may also involve the persistent activation of dorsal horn neurons, resulting in changes within the spinal cord (i.e., central sensitization) that can mediate pain long after resolution of inflammation or other pelvic insult [6]. Factors that influence the processing of afferent signals at the level of the brain also may play an important role. Recent advances in functional brain imaging—both positron emission topography (PET) and functional magnetic resonance imaging (fMRI)—have had a major impact on understanding CNS control of the bladder and other pelvic viscera in humans [39,100]. For example, functional imaging studies have revealed that chronic pain affects the brain's ability to process information that could affect brainstem and cortical areas involved in learning and memory or perceptual responses to contraction and filling of viscera. There is also evidence that alterations in a single visceral organ can result in changes in the neural circuits processing information from other regions. These and other findings support the potential for interactions between somatic-visceral convergent inputs in the brainstem, which may explain (in part) the occurrence of functional pain.

Diagnosis and Patient Evaluation

Painful bladder syndrome is a "symptom syndrome" in which a presumptive diagnosis is made after the exclusion of other pathology affecting the bladder and adjacent structures including malignancies; infections caused by bacteria, parasites, fungi, or viruses; inflammation induced by physical or chemical agents such as irradiation or chemotherapy; other conditions such as pelvic endometriosis; and functional disorders affecting the lower urinary tract. Recommendations for the standardization of patient evaluation have been published [46].

A general, thorough medical history should be taken with attention to:

- previous pelvic operations
- previous urinary tract infections
- bladder history/urological diseases
- location of pelvic pain (referred pain) and its relation to bladder filling and emptying
- characteristics of pain: onset, correlation with other events, and description of pain
- previous pelvic radiation treatment
- autoimmune diseases
- drug therapy such as chemotherapy, immunosuppressants, and anti-inflammatory drugs (e.g., tiaprofenic acid)

A general physical examination should be performed, including palpation of the lower abdomen for bladder fullness and tenderness, as well as assessment of possible musculoskeletal pathology. Women should receive a vaginal examination with pain mapping of the vulval region and vaginal palpation for tenderness of the bladder, urethra, and the levator and adductor muscles of the pelvic floor. In men, digital rectal examination should be performed with pain mapping of the scrotal-anal region and palpation for tenderness of the bladder, prostate, the levator and adductor muscles of the pelvic floor, and the scrotal contents.

Laboratory tests should include the following:
- urine dipstick to assess pH, leucocytes, nitrate levels
- urine culture, including special cultures for *Chlamydia trachomatis*, *Ureaplasma urealyticum*, *Mycoplasma genitalium*, *M. hominis*, *Corynebacterium urealyticum*, and *Candida* species
- optional investigations for vaginal *Ureaplasma* and *Chlamydia* infections in females and prostatitis in men
- if sterile pyuria, culture for *Mycobacterium tuberculosis*
- urine cytology, in risk groups
- serum prostate-specific antigen (PSA) level, where appropriate
    Urodynamics and ultrasound scanning should include:
- a postvoid residual urine volume by ultrasound scanning
- flowmetry in all males, and if maximum flow rate is less than 20 mL/s, a pressure-flow study

Clinical symptom scales such as the O'Leary-Sant Interstitial Cystitis Symptom Index [78], the University of Wisconsin Interstitial Cystitis Inventory [61], and the Pelvic Pain and Urgency/Frequency (PUF) scale [82] have been used in this context, but experts have concluded that none of them can be used for diagnosis and that they require further evaluation [55].

The role of urodynamics remains controversial, but attention to this aspect can be useful in diagnosing detrusor overactivity and intravesical obstruction in men [53]. Parsons [80] introduced the potassium test, but its usefulness as a diagnostic tool has been questioned. Cystoscopy and hydrodistension is an important diagnostic test. In 1914, Hunner published the classic description of painful bladder syndrome as a bladder ulcer with a corresponding cystoscopic appearance of patches of red mucosa exhibiting small vessels radiating to a central pale scar [49]. Since then, glomerulations and postdistension bleeding observed after hydrodistension to 70–80 cm of water for 1–3 minutes has been reported as the primary cystoscopic feature of painful bladder syndrome [74], along with a rise in pulse and blood pressure under a light general anesthetic. However, neither the presence nor severity of glomerulations correlates with any of the primary symptoms of painful bladder syndrome [98], although the presence of a Hunner's ulcer is significantly associated with bodily pain and urinary urgency [73]. Some workers find a Hunner's ulcer in 50% of their patients with painful bladder syndrome, while others hardly ever see it [10]. Pathology of the bladder wall in painful bladder syndrome is also controversial [86]. If bladder biopsies are taken, it is usually to exclude carcinoma in situ. Changes specific to painful bladder syndrome have not been clearly defined.

Diagnostic biomarkers would be a very helpful future tool in the diagnosis of painful bladder syndrome [58]. Antiproliferative factor (APF), HB-EGF, epidermal growth factor (EGF), insulin-like growth factor 1 (IGF1), and insulin-like growth factor binding protein 3 (IGFBP3) have been shown to be correlated to painful bladder syndrome. APF, HB-EGF, and EGF seem to be most useful in discriminating between patients with painful bladder syndrome and asymptomatic controls [38]. A study in men with painful bladder syndrome, chronic prostatitis/chronic pelvic pain syndrome, and controls found increased NO in the urine of patients with inflammation of the bladder [34].

Summary

The available evidence has revealed that functional pain syndromes such as painful bladder syndrome/interstitial cystitis are associated with increased sensitivity to both physical and chemical stimulation. In this regard, increased uroepithelial sensitivity could lead to changes in the activity of pelvic pathways and associated pain. Changes in epithelial signaling/barrier function would not be unique to the urinary bladder. For example, airway epithelial cells from asthmatics exhibit a number of abnormalities and compromised repair processes. Taken together, epithelial cells can respond to a number of challenges (including environmental pollutants and mediators released from nerves or nearby inflammatory cells), resulting in altered expression of receptors and channels and the release of mediators, all of which may influence function.

Evidence-based recommendations for treatment are difficult to make due to the lack of well-designed, prospective, controlled, randomized studies. Readers are directed to excellent reviews of this subject such as the report from an advisory committee at the International Consultation on Incontinence [44].

References

[1]   Abrams P, Blaivas JG, Stanton SL, Andersen JT. Standardisation of terminology of lower urinary tract function. Neurourol Urodyn 1988;7:403–27.

[2]   Abrams P, Cardozo L, Fall M, Griffiths D, Rosier P, Ulmsten U, van Kerrebroeck P, Victor A, Wein AJ. The standardisation of terminology of lower urinary tract function: report from the standardisation sub-committee of the international continence society. Am J Obstet Gynecol 2002;187:116–26.

[3]   Acharya P, Beckel JM, Ruiz WG, Wang E, Rojas R, Birder LA, Apodaca G. Distribution of the tight junction proteins ZPO-1, occludin, and claudin-4, -8, and -12 in bladder epithelium. Am J Physiol 2004;287:F305–18.

[4]   Alagiri M, Chottiner S, Ratner V, Slade D, Hanno PM. Interstitial cystitis: unexplained associations with other chronic disease and pain syndromes. Urology 1997;49:52–7.

[5]   Alt-Belgnaoui A, Bradesi S, Floramonti J, Theodorou V, Bueno L. Acute stress-induced hypersensitivity to colonic distension depends upon increase in paracellular permeability: role of myosin light chain kinase. Pain 2005;113:141–7.

[6]   Anand P, Aziz Q, Willert R, Van Oudenhove L. Peripheral and central mechanisms of visceral sensitization in man. Neurogastroenterol Motil 2007;19:29–46.

[7]   Apodaca G. Modulation of membrane traffic by mechanical stimuli. Am J Physiol 2002;282: F179–90.

[8]   Apodaca G. The uroepithelium: not just a passive barrier. Traffic 2004;5:117–28.

[9]   Apodaca G, Kiss S, Ruiz WG, Meyers S, Zeidel M, Birder LA. Disruption of bladder epithelium barrier function after spinal cord injury. Am J Physiol 2003;284:F966–76.

[10] Bade J, Ishizuka O, Yoshida M. Future research needs for the definition/diagnosis of interstitial cystitis. Int J Urol 2003;10:S31–4.

[11] Baranowski AP, Abrams P, Berger RE, Buffington CAT, Williams AC, Hanno PM, Loeser JD, Nickel JC, Wesselmann U. Urogenital pain: time to accept a new approach to phenotyping and, as a consequence, management. Eur Urol 2008;53:33–6.

[12] Barbara G. Mucosal barrier defects in irritable bowel syndrome: who left the door open? Am J Gastroenterol 2006;101:1295–8.

[13] Berkley KJ. A life of pelvic pain. Physiol Behav 2005;86:272–80.

[14] Berridge MJ, Bootman MD, Roderick HL. Calcium signaling: dynamics, homeostasis and remodeling. Nat Rev Mol Cell Biol 2003;4:517–29.

[15] Birder LA, Barrick SR, Roppolo JR, Kanai AJ, deGroat WC, Kiss S, Buffington CAT. Feline interstitial cystitis results in mechanical hypersensitivity and altered ATP release from bladder urothelium. Am J Physiol 2003;285:F423–9.

[16] Birder LA, de Groat WC. Mechanisms of disease: involvement of the urothelium in bladder dysfunction. Nat Clin Pract 2007;4:46–54.

[17] Birder LA, Wolf-Johnston AS, Buffington CAT, Roppolo JR, De Groat WC, Kanai AJ. Altered inducible nitric oxide synthase expression and nitric oxide production in the bladder of cats with feline interstitial cystitis. J Urol 2005;173:625–9.

[18] Bodin P, Burnstock G. Purinergic signalling: ATP release. Neurochem Res 2001;26:959–69.

[19] Bosse Y, Pare PD, Seow CY. Airway wall remodeling in asthma: from the epithelial layer to the adventitia. Curr Allergy Asthma Rep 2008;8:357–66.

[20] Buffington CAT. Comorbidity of interstitial cystitis with other unexplained clinical conditions. J Urol 2004;172:1242–8.

[21] Buffington CAT, Blaisdell JL, Binns. S.P. J, Woodworth BE. Decreased urine glycosaminoglycan excretion in cats with interstitial cystitis. J Urol 1996;155:1801–4.

[22] Buffington CAT, Chew DJ. Presence of mast cells in submucosa and detrusor of cats with idiopathic lower urinary tract disease. J Vet Intern Med 1993;7:126A.

[23] Bunnett NW. The stressed gut: contributions of intestinal stress peptides to inflammation and motility. Proc Natl Acad Sci USA 2005;102:7409–10.

[24] Burnstock G, De Ryck M. UCB Pharma research day: 25 October 2007. Glia-neuron interactions and purinergic receptors in neurological disorders. Purinergic Signal 2008;4:79–84.

[25] Cao H, Zhang YQ. Spinal glial activation contributes to pathological pain states. Neurosci Biobehav Rev 2008;32:972–83.

[26] Chai TC, Keay S. New theories in interstitial cystitis. Nat Clin Pract Urol 2004;1:85–9.

[27] Chai TC, Zhang CO, Shoenfelt JL, Johnston HW Jr, Warren JW, Keay S. Bladder stretch alters urinary heparin-binding epidermal growth factor and antiproliferative factor in patients with interstitial cystitis. J Urol 2000;163:1440–4.

[28] Chapple CR, Wein AJ, Abrams P, Dmochowski RR, Giuliano F, Kaplan SA, McVary KT, Roehrborn CG. Lower urinary tract symptoms revisited: a broader clinical perspective. Eur Urol 2008;54:563–9

[29] Chen E, Miller GE. Stress and inflammation in exacerbations of asthma. Brain Behav Immmun 2007;21:993–9.

[30] Clauw DJ, Chrousos GP. Chronic pain and fatigue syndromes: overlapping clinical and neuroendocrine features and potential pathogenic mechanisms. Neuroimmunomodulation 1997;4:134–53.

[31] Clauw DJ, Schmidt M, Radulovic R, Singer A, Katz P, Bresette J. The relationship between fibromyalgia and interstitial cystitis. J Psych Res 1997;31:125–31.

[32] Clemens JQ, Meenan RT, O'Keeffe Rosetti MC, Brown SO, Gao SY, Calhoun EA. Prevalence of interstitial cystitis symptoms in a managed care population. J Urol 2005;174:576–80.

[33] Clemens JQ, R.T. M, O'Keeffe Rosetti MC, T.A. K. Case-control study of medical comorbidities in women with interstitial cystitis. J Urol 2008;179:2222–5.

[34] Ehren I, Hosseini A, Lundberg JO, Wiklund NP. Nitric oxide: a useful gas in the detection of lower urinary tract inflammation. J Urol 1999;162:327–9.

[35] Erickson DR. Urine markers of interstitial cystitis. Urology 2001;57:15–21.

[36] Erickson DR, Belchis DA, Babbs DJ. Inflammatory cell types and clinical features of interstitial cystitis. J Urol 1997;158:790–3.

[37] Erickson DR, Morgan KC, Ordille S, Keay SK, Xie SX. Nonbladder related symptoms in patients with interstitial cystitis. J Urol 2001;166:557–62.

[38] Erickson DR, Xie SX, Bhavanandan VP, Wheeler MA, Hurst RE, Demers LM, Kushner L, Keay SK. A comparison of multiple urine markers for interstitial cystitis. J Urol 2002;167:2461–9.

[39] Fowler CJ, Griffiths D, de Groat WC. The neural control of micturition. Nat Rev Neurosci 2008;9:453–66.

[40] Gillenwater JY, Wein AJ. Summary of the national institute of arthritis, diabetes, and kidney diseases workshop on interstitial cystitis. J Urol 1998;140:205.

[41] Graham E, Chai TC. Dysfunction of bladder urothelium and bladder urothelial cells in interstitial cystitis. Curr Urol Rep 2006;7:440–6.

[42] Han X, Fink MP, Yang R, Delude RL. Increased iNOS activity is essential for intestinal epithelial tight junction dysfunction in endotoxemic mice. Shock 2004;21:261–70.

[43] Hanna-Mitchell AT, Beckel JM, Barbadora S, Kanai AJ, DeGroat WC, Birder LA. Non-neuronal acetylcholine and urinary bladder urothelium. Life Sci 2007;80:2298–302.

[44] Hanno PM, Baranowski A, Fall M, Gajewski J, Nordling J, Nyberg L, Ratner V, Rosamilia A, Ueda T. Painful bladder syndrome (including interstitial cystitis). In: Abrams P, Cardozo L, Khoury S, Wein A, editors. Incontinence: Proceedings from the Third International Consultation on Incontinence. Paris: Health Publication; 2005. p. 1455–520.

[45] Hansson E. Could chronic pain and spread of pain sensation by induced and maintained by glial activation. Acta Physiol 2006;187:321–7.

[46] Held PJ, Hanno PM, Wein AJ. Epidemiology of interstitial cystitis. In: Hanno PM, Staskin DR, Krane RJ, Wein AJ, editors. Interstitial cystitis. London: Springer-Verlag; 1990. p. 29–48.

[47] Henrix S. Neuroimmune communication in skin: far from peripheral. J Invest Derm 2008;128:260–1.

[48] Homma Y. Lower urinary tract symptomatology: its definition and confusion. Int J Urol 2007;1442–2042.

164 L. Birder and C. Chapple

[49] Hunner GL. A rare type of bladder ulcer in women: report of cases. Trans South Surg Gynecol Assoc 1914;27:247–92.
[50] Hurst RE, Moldwin RM, Mulholland SG. Bladder defense molecules, urothelial differentiation, urinary biomarkers, and interstitial cystitis. Urology 2007;69:17–23.
[51] Ikeda Y, Fry C, Hayashi F, Stolz D, Griffiths D, Kanai AJ. Role of gap junctions in spontaneous activity of the rat bladder. Am J Physiol 2007;293:F1018–25.
[52] Ikeda Y, Kanai AJ. Urotheliogenic modulation of intrinsic activity in spinal cord transected rat bladders: the role of mucosal muscarinic receptors. Am J Physiol 2008;295:F454–61
[53] Irwin PP, Takei M, Sugino Y. Summary of the urodynamics workshops on IC Kyoto, Japan. Int J Urol 2003;10:S19–23.
[54] Isakson BE, Evans WH, Boitano S. Intercellular Ca^{2+} signaling in alveolar epithelial cells through gap junctions and by extracellular ATP. Am J Physiol 2001;280:L221–8.
[55] Ito T, Tomoe H, Ueda T, Yoshimura N, Sant GR, Hanno P. Clinical symptoms scale for interstitial cystitis for diagnosis and for following the course of the disease. Int J Urol 2003;10:S24–6.
[56] Ji RR, Kawasaki Y, Zhuang ZY, Wen YR, Decosterd I. Possible role of spinal astrocytes in maintaining chronic pain sensitization: review of current evidence with focus on bFGF/JNK pathway. Neuron Glia Biol 2006;2:259–69.
[57] Keay S, Kleinberg M, Zhang CO, Hise MK, Warren JW. Bladder epithelial cells from patients with interstitial cystitis produce an inhibitor of heparin-binding epidermal growth factor-like growth factor production. J Urol 2000;164:2112–8.
[58] Keay S, Takeda M, Tamaki M, Hanno P. Current and future directions in diagnostic markers in interstitial cystitis. Int J Urol 2003;10:S27–30.
[59] Keay S, Zhang CO, Shoenfelt JL, Chai TC. Decreased in vitro proliferation of bladder epithelial cells from patients with interstitial cystitis. Urology 2003;61:1278–84.
[60] Keay SK, Szekely Z, Conrads TP, Veenstra TD, Barchi JJ Jr, Zhang CO, Koch KR, Michejda CJ. An antiproliferative factor from interstitial cystitis patients is a frizzled 8 protein-related sialoglyco-peptide. Proc Natl Acad Sci USA 2004;101:11803–8.
[61] Keller ML, McCarthy DO, Neider RS. Measurement of symptoms of interstitial cystitis: a pilot study. Urol Clin North Am 1994;21:67–71.
[62] Khasar SG, Burkham J, Dina OA, Brown AS, Bogen O, Alessandri-Haber N, Green PG, Reichling DB, Levine JD. Stress induces a switch of intracellular signaling in sensory neurons in a model of generalized pain. J Neurosci 2008;28:5721–30.
[63] Koskela LR, Thiel T, Ehren I, De Verdier PJ, Wiklund NP. Localization and expression of inducible nitric oxide synthase in biopsies from patients with interstitial cystitis. J Urol 2008;180:737–41.
[64] Koziol JA. Epidemiology of interstitial cystitis. Urol Clin North Am 1994;21:7–20.
[65] Lai-Cheong JE, Arita K, McGrath JA. Genetic diseases of junctions. J Invest Derm 2007;127:2713–25.
[66] Lavelle JP, Meyers SA, Ruiz WG, Buffington CAT, Zeidel ML, Apodaca G. Urothelial pathophysiological changes in feline interstitial cystitis: a human model. Am J Physiol 2000;278:F540–53.
[67] Leistad RB, Nilsen KB, Stovner LJ, Westgaard RH, Ro M, Sand T. Similarities in stress physiology among patients with chronic pain and headache disorders: evidence for a common pathophysiological mechanism? J Headache Pain 2008;9:165–75.
[68] Lewis SA. Everything you wanted to know about the bladder epithelium but were afraid to ask. Am J Physiol 2000;278:F867–74.
[69] Liu HT, Kuo HC. Intravesical botulinum toxin A injections plus hydrodistension can reduce nerve growth factor production and control bladder pain in interstitial cystitis. Urology 2007;70:463–8.
[70] Malykhina AP, Qin C, Greenwood-van Meerveld B, Foreman RD, Lupu F, Akbarali HI. Hyperexcitability of convergent colon and bladder dorsal root ganglion neurons after colonic inflammation: mechanism for pelvic organ cross-talk. Neurogastroenterol Motil 2006;18:936–48.
[71] Mayer EA, Fanselow MS. Dissecting the components of the central response to stress. Nat Neurosci 2003;6:1011–2.
[72] McMahon SB, Cafferty WBJ, Marchand F. Immune and glial cell factors as pain mediators and modulators. Experimen Neurol 2005;192:444–62.
[73] Messing E, Pauk D, Schaeffer A, Nieweglowski M, Nyberg LM Jr, Landis JR, Cook YL, Simon LJ. Associations among cystoscopic findings and symptoms and physical examination findings in women enrolled in the Interstitial Cystitis Data Base (ICDB) Study. Urology 1997;49:81–5.

[74] Messing EM. The diagnosis of interstitial cystitis. Urology 1987;29:4–7.
[75] Neuhaus J, Pfeiffer F, Wolburg H, Horn LC, Dorschner W. Alterations in connexin expression in the bladder of patients with urge symptoms. BJU Int 2005;96:670–6.
[76] Nickel JC. Interstitial cystitis: an elusive clinical target? J Urol 2003;170:816–7.
[77] Nipkow L, Chai TC. Interstitial cystitis: modern tools for an accurate diagnosis. Curr Urol Rep 2003;4:381–4.
[78] O'Leary MP, Sant GR. The interstitial cystitis symptom and problem indices: rationale, development, and application. In: Sant GR, editor. Interstitial cystitis. Philadelphia: Lippincott-Raven; 1997. p. 271–6.
[79] Obata H, Eisenach JC, Hussain H, Bynum T, Vincler M. Spinal glial activation contributes to postoperative mechanical hypersensitivity in the rat. J Pain 2006;7:816–22.
[80] Parsons CL. Potassium sensitivity test. Tech Urol 1996;2:171–3.
[81] Parsons CL. The role of the urinary epithelium in the pathogenesis of interstitial cystitis/prostatitis/urethritis. Urology 2007;69:9–16.
[82] Parsons CL, Dell J, Stanford EJ, Bullen M, Kahn BS, Waxell T, Koziol JA. Increased prevalence of interstitial cystitis: previously unrecognized urologic and gynecologic cases identified using a new symptom questionnaire and intravesical potassium sensitivity. Urology 2002;60:573–8.
[83] Parsons CL, Lilly JD, Stein P. Epithelial dysfunction in nonbacterial cystitis (interstitial cystitis). J Urol 1991;145:732–5.
[84] Payne CK, Joyce GF, Wise M, Clemens JQ. Interstitial cystitis and painful bladder syndrome. J Urol 2007;177:2042–9.
[85] Rastogi P, Rickard A, Dorokhov N, Klumpp DJ, McHowat J. Loss of prostaglandin E$_2$ release from immortalized urothelial cells obtained from interstitial cystitis patient bladders. Am J Physiol 2008;294:F1129–35.
[86] Rosamilia A, Igawa Y, Higashi S. Pathology of interstitial cystitis. Int J Urol 2003;10:S11–5.
[87] Rudick CN, Chen MC, Mongiu AK, Klumpp DJ. Organ cross talk modulates pelvic pain. Am J Physiol 2007;293:R1191–8.
[88] Sant GR. Interstitial cystitis. Curr Opin Obstet Gynecol 1997;9:332–6.
[89] Schilling J, Hultgren S, Lorenz R. Recent advances in the molecular basis of pathogen recognition and host responses in the urinary tract. Int Rev Immunol 2002;21:291–304.
[90] Scholz J, Woolf CJ. The neuropathic pain triad: neurons, immune cells and glia. Nat Neuroscience 2007;10:1361–8.
[91] Shabir S, Southgate J. Calcium signaling in wound-responsive normal human urothelial cell monolayers. Cell Calcium 2008;44:453–64.
[92] Smith CP, Gangitano DA, Munoz A, Salas NA, Boone TB, Aoki KR, Francis J, Somogyi GT. Botulinum toxin type A normalizes alterations in urothelial ATP and NO release induced by chronic spinal cord injury. Neurochem Int 2007;52:1068–75.
[93] Staud R. Fibromyalgia pain: do we know the score? Curr Opin Rheumatol 2004;16:157–63.
[94] Stewart W, Van Rooyen J, Cundiff G, Abrams P, Herzog A, Corey R, Hunt T, Wein AJ. Prevalence and burden of overactive bladder in the United States. World J Urol 2003;20:327–36.
[95] Sun YN, Chai TC. Augmented extracellular ATP signaling in bladder urothelial cells from patients with interstitial cystitis. Am J Physiol 2006;290:C27–34.
[96] Sun YN, Luo JY, Rao ZR, Lan L, Duan L. GFAP and Fos immunoreactivity in lumbo-sacral spinal cord and medulla oblongata after chronic colonic inflammation in rats. World J Gastroenterol 2005;11:4827–32.
[97] Templeman L, Chapple CR, Chess-Williams R. Urothelium derived inhibitory factor and cross-talk among receptors in the trigone of the bladder of the pig. J Urol 2002;167:742–5.
[98] Tomaszewski JE, Landis JR, Russack V, Williams TM, Wang LP, Hardy C, Brensinger C, Matthews YL, Abele ST, Kusek JW, et al. ICDS. Biopsy features are associated with primary symptoms in interstitial cystitis: results from the interstitial cystitis database study. Urology 2001;57:67–8.
[99] Tominaga M, Wada M, Masu M. Potentiation of capsaicin receptor activity by metabotropic ATP receptors as a possible mechanism for ATP-evoked pain and hyperalgesia. Proc Natl Acad Sci USA 2001;98:6951–6.
[100] Tracey I. Imaging pain. Br J Anaesth 2008;101:32–9.
[101] Van de Merwe J. Interstitial cystitis and systemic autoimmune diseases. Nat Clin Pract Urol 2007;4:8.

[102] Van Itallie CM, Anderson JM. Claudins and epithelial paracellular transport. Ann Rev Physiol 2006;68:403–29.

[103] Watkins LR, Maier SF. Beyond neurons: evidence that immune and glial cells contribute to pathological pain states. Physiol Rev 2002;82:981–1011.

[104] Watkins LR, Maier SF. Glia: A novel drug discovery target for clinical pain. Nat Rev Drug Discov 2003;2:973–85.

[105] Wein AJ, Hanno PM, Gillenwater JY. Interstitial cystitis: an introduction to the problem. In: Hanno PM, Staskin D, Krane RJ, Wein AJ, editors. Interstitial cystitis. London: Springer-Verlag; 1990. p. 3–15.

[106] Zhang CO, Wang JY, Koch KR, Keay S. Regulation of tight junction proteins and bladder epithelial paracellular permeability by an antiproliferative factor from patients with interstitial cystitis. J Urol 2005;174:2382–7.

Correspondence to: Lori Birder, PhD, Department of Medicine, University of Pittsburgh School of Medicine, A1207 Scaife Hall, Pittsburgh, PA 15261, USA. Email: lbirder@pitt.edu.

Part III

Common Comorbid Syndromes in Relation to Pain

Combat-Related Psychiatric Syndromes

J. Douglas Bremner

*Departments of Psychiatry and Radiology, Emory University
School of Medicine, Atlanta, Georgia, USA*

This chapter reviews the complex relationship between exposure to stress, post-traumatic stress disorder (PTSD), and the functional pain disorders, including irritable bowel syndrome (IBS), fibromyalgia, nonspecific low back pain, chronic pelvic pain, temporomandibular pain, and chronic chest pain or sensitive heart. A functional disorder is one that, after appropriate medical assessment, cannot be explained in terms of a conventionally defined medical disease based on biochemical or structural abnormalities [30,32,95]. The fact that the functional pain disorders are not typically responsive to conventional medical therapy but are nevertheless responsible for the consumption of a great deal of medical resources [89,90,95] indicates that a better understanding of their etiologies is an important priority for the medical field.

Several psychiatric disorders involving pain disorders that are characterized by medically unexplained symptoms are outlined in the *Diagnostic and Statistical Manual* [3]. Somatoform disorders are disorders where physical symptoms are not attributable to a known organic etiology and are not secondary to anxiety or depression. Somatization disorder involves at least eight physical symptoms in four bodily systems. Other terms include psychogenic disease, chronic multisymptom illness, affective spectrum disorders, and central sensitization syndromes, as well as functional pain disorders [6,21,22,53,54,95].

This chapter's focus is the relationship between the functional pain disorders and combat-related psychiatric disorders. However, studies in a range of PTSD populations are informative to the question of the role of stress, trauma, and PTSD in functional pain disorders. This literature shows that although stress exposure plays a role in the development of functional pain disorders in many patients, and that PTSD is specifically associated with fibromyalgia and other pain disorders, specific traumas such as childhood abuse or combat exposure are not necessarily required for the development of functional pain disorders [5,65,66,67]. The development of functional pain disorders is probably related to a complex interplay of environmental events (including specific traumas in childhood and adulthood, as well as variables such as parenting style), genetics, and an interplay between central nervous system (CNS) processing of information and neural control of the gut, heart, and other peripheral organs [68]. There is a high comorbidity of the functional pain disorders with each other and with stress-related psychiatric disorders such as PTSD, panic disorder, and depression, as well as with chronic fatigue syndrome and headache [82]. This comorbidity may represent a common etiology (e.g., stress, a common genetic factor, or common neural circuitry), or the fact that they are involved in each other's etiology (e.g., pain leads to depression, or depression is involved in maintenance of pain after minor injury).

Post-Traumatic Stress Disorder

Post-traumatic stress disorder (PTSD) is a disabling condition that is associated with exposure to a traumatic stressor, defined as a threat to life or one's integrity accompanied by intense fear, horror, or helplessness. PTSD is characterized by specific symptoms, including intrusive thoughts, hyperarousal, flashbacks, nightmares, sleep disturbance, changes in memory and concentration, and startle responses, which develop following exposure to extreme stress [78]. PTSD affects 8% of people at some time during their lives [59]. Twelve percent of returning Iraq veterans suffer from PTSD [52] and 15% of Vietnam combat veterans suffer from chronic PTSD [60]. Other psychiatric disorders that are increased following exposure to combat and other stressors include depression, alcohol and substance abuse, anxiety, and dissociative disorders [60]. PTSD patients have an increase in chronic pain [7], as well as increased somatization [8], poorer health [81], and increased utilization of health resources [99]. Although PTSD patients report more pain symptoms, they report lower experiences of pain in laboratory settings, associated with increased hippocampal and decreased amygdalar and medial prefrontal brain activation [40,41].

Dissociation and Somatization

Symptoms of dissociation include feeling like you are in a dream, distortions of bodily perception (depersonalization), gaps in memory (amnesia), and distortions of perception such as feeling like you are in a tunnel (derealization). Dissociative symptoms are more common in traumatized individuals, and they were once thought to represent a defense mechanism or adaptive response to trauma. However, research studies have clearly shown that dissociative responses are a marker for poor outcome in both combat veterans and civilians exposed to trauma [15,20,64].

In the field of psychiatry there has long been an interest in the relationship between trauma, dissociation, and somatization. This interest dates to the psychoanalytic conception of unconscious conflicts becoming "dissociated" from consciousness and emerging as bodily symptoms. Indeed, symptoms of dissociation can resemble symptoms of conversion disorder, such as "glove and stocking anesthesia," which, like depersonalization, can involve distortions of bodily perception. This similarity has led to use of the term "somatoform dissociation" [74]. However, dissociative symptoms such as feeling as if you are in a dream are perhaps better described as a trauma-induced splitting of consciousness along the lines of Pierre Janet, the contemporary of Sigmund Freud, rather than as the result of suppression of unconscious conflicts as described in psychoanalysis.

Studies have examined the relationship between somatization disorder, stress, and dissociation. Somatization disorder patients, when compared to medical patients, were shown to have increased symptoms of dissociative amnesia, but not depersonalization, derealization, or identity confusion or alteration [16]. Somatization patients were found to have more history of emotional and physical abuse (but not sexual abuse), more family conflict, and less family cohesion.

Irritable Bowel Syndrome

Irritable bowel syndrome (IBS) accounts for 20–50% of all consultations to gastroenterologists and is the most common gastrointestinal disease [48,70]. The syndrome is characterized by abdominal pain and discomfort and associated alterations in bowel habits. The absence of any detectable structural or biochemical abnormalities in IBS patients has led to psychosocial factors being increasingly invoked as part of the disease etiology [5,33,65,66,67]. Like other functional syndromes, IBS has been defined negatively as "symptoms not explained by structural or biochemical abnormalities," and the diagnosis has been determined by symptom criteria (e.g., a change in pain with bowel movement).

Patients with IBS more commonly report symptoms such as disturbed sleep and libido and reduced energy [36,37,53], as well as headaches, back pain, myalgias and dyspareunia, and urinary urgency and pain [1,22,37,71]. IBS patients, like patients with some of the other functional pain disorders described in this chapter (e.g., temporomandibular pain or fibromyalgia) are thought to have generalized alterations in the processing of viscerosensory information [65], with a tendency to selectively attend to negative information and a memory bias for negative events [43]. Alterations in processing of sensory information and changes in pathways to and from the CNS and the viscera, including alterations in brain areas responsible for the mediation of pain, such as the anterior cingulate cortex (ACC), may underlie the pathophysiology of IBS [65,72,87].

Studies have examined the relationship between stress and IBS. Exposure to a threat is associated with changes in bowel function in animals, including an increase in defecation and changes in colonic motility. These changes are thought to be modulated by corticotropin-releasing factor (CRF) and by autonomic (vagal, sacral parasympathetic) influences on the gut [87]. Stress exposure in human subjects has been correlated with functional bowel symptoms [97]. Studies have shown an increase in childhood sexual abuse trauma and exposure to general traumatic events in IBS patients [76,77,79,83]. Other studies have shown that parental style, specifically hostility and rejection from paternal figures, plays a greater role in the development of IBS than childhood sexual abuse [61]. Rates of PTSD in IBS patients have ranged from rates that are not much higher than in the general population (8%) [23] to elevations as high as 36% [56]. An increase in symptoms of anxiety and depression has been reported in IBS patients [63]. IBS patients did not have an increase in dissociative symptoms compared to medical patient controls [77]. One theory is that hyperarousal characterizes IBS, PTSD, and depression, representing a common thread in the etiology of these disorders and an explanation for their high comorbidity [58].

An increase in gastrointestinal symptoms has been reported in veterans of combat. In a study of Gulf War veterans, deployed versus non-deployed veterans had more abdominal symptoms of gas, bloating and cramps, as well as diarrhea [39]. Vietnam combat veterans with PTSD were found to have increased self-reported digestive disease [9]. These studies show that the stress of combat is associated with an increase in gastrointestinal complaints.

Fibromyalgia

Fibromyalgia, which affects about 5% of women and 2% of men [96], is associated with chronic widespread pain, diffuse tenderness, fatigue, and sleep disturbance; diagnostic criteria require at least 3 months of widespread pain and pain upon digital palpation at no fewer than 11 of 18 characteristic tender points [98]. The original view that fibromyalgia would be explained either by local pathology or psychocultural factors alone [26] has given way to an understanding of fibromyalgia having a complex and multifactorial etiology.

Although trauma and stress are associated with fibromyalgia, there is not good evidence that exposure to traumatic stress is a prerequisite for development of the disorder. Some studies, though, have associated sexual assault in adulthood with fibromyalgia [19,93]. Some studies in patients with fibromyalgia have found elevated rates of childhood physical abuse [93], while others have not [19]. Childhood sexual abuse has not been consistently associated with fibromyalgia.

Studies consistently show an increase in PTSD rates in patients with fibromyalgia, with about 50% of fibromyalgia patients affected [24,84]. Furthermore, the link between PTSD and fibromyalgia does not appear to be necessarily related to a common exposure such as childhood abuse. Fibromyalgia symptoms are also seen in at least a fifth of PTSD patients, and PTSD patients with fibromyalgia symptoms have worse quality of life and more psychological distress than PTSD patients without fibromyalgia [2,27]. Fibromyalgia patients also have increased rates of anxiety, depression, and somatization [42,88]. Vietnam veterans reported an increase in musculoskeletal complaints [9]. Veterans deployed to the Gulf War had an increase in self-reported fibromyalgia (19% vs. 10% of non-deployed veterans) [55].

Current models of fibromyalgia conceptualize the disorder as being related at least in part to alterations in brain regions involved in pain. The known relationship of stress and negative affect to pain have led to suggestions that various stimuli ranging from injury elsewhere in the body to emotional and cognitive inputs from higher neural centers, such as the ACC, are involved in the initiation or maintenance of fibromyalgia symptoms [44,45]. Recently it has been demonstrated that catastrophizing—focusing upon the most negative outcomes associated with pain—in patients with fibromyalgia is correlated with enhanced activation of the dorsal ACC [44]. Fibromyalgia patients, especially those with a history of early trauma, have also been shown to have a blunting of the cortisol diurnal rhythm similar to that seen in patients with PTSD [46,94].

Nonspecific Low Back Pain

Back pain is the second leading symptomatic reason for physician visits in the United States [62]. As with fibromyalgia and IBS, there is a lack of observable pathology to account for nonspecific low back pain, treatment is difficult, and the relationship with emotional factors is not well defined.

Studies have shown that subjects with nonspecific low back pain have similar levels of lower back pathology to normal controls [29,57]; fewer than 15% of persons with back pain can be assigned to a category of specific low back pain with identifiable cause and treatment [86]. This leaves a substantial proportion of people suffering back pain without reliable indicators of injury or a physiological or anatomical defect [47].

About half of patients with low back pain have PTSD [28]. Prisoners of war from Vietnam reported an increase in back problems compared to non-POW servicemen [73]. Although it has not yet been empirically assessed, it has been observed that many U.S. veterans returning from Iraq have comorbid back pain and PTSD. Many veterans returning from Iraq are exhibiting high rates of pain related to mechanical wear and tear injuries from carrying more equipment than in prior wars (e.g., bulletproof vests). Low back pain and PTSD can maintain each other, with lack of mobility leading to increased avoidance.

Chronic Pelvic Pain

Chronic pelvic pain is intermittent or continuous pain in the pelvic area that lasts at least 3 months. Chronic pelvic pain is associated with increased rates of somatization [35] and has been conceptualized as representing a somatic response to childhood sexual trauma. Although rates of childhood sexual trauma are increased in pelvic pain patients [35], exposure to childhood sexual trauma is not a necessary antecedent of the disorder [85]. However, studies have shown elevated rates of childhood physical and sexual abuse as well as rates of PTSD of about 50% [49,51]. Women with chronic pelvic pain also exhibit a pattern of hypocortisolism that is similar to PTSD [50].

Temporomandibular Joint Disorder

Temporomandibular joint disorder (TMJD) refers to pain in the jaw that can be caused by a number of factors, one of which is gnashing of teeth associated with stress [83]. About one-fourth of patients with orofacial pain suffer from PTSD [83].

Chest Pain and Sensitive Heart

Sensitive heart refers to chest pain in the absence of objective signs of coronary artery disease [5]. Although an increase in cardiovascular disease has been associated with PTSD, research has not focused on PTSD and sensitive heart syndrome. Prisoners of war released from Serbian detention camps were shown to have an increase in electrocardiographic abnormalities [25].

Integrative Model of Stress, PTSD, and Functional Pain Syndromes

Appreciation is growing for the role of psychosocial factors, specifically stress and/or emotional factors, in the development and maintenance of functional pain disorders [6,95]. Brain imaging studies show that pain processing in patients with functional pain is dependent upon brain regions including the thalamus, insula cortex, prefrontal cortex, primary and secondary somatosensory cortex, and ACC [18,29,30,41,72]. These brain areas overlap with those implicated in the neural circuitry of stress and PTSD [10,13,38].

Animal models of stress have been used in the study of stress-related psychiatric disorders, including PTSD [91]. Animals exposed to repeated stress from which they cannot escape develop specific fear-related behaviors that are associated with lasting changes in stress-related neurochemical systems. Behavioral changes related to stress include weight loss and decreases in food intake, in active behavior in novel environments, and in competitiveness and normal aggressiveness, as well as reduced grooming, play activity, responding for rewards, and self-stimulation of brain reward centers. They also display deficits in memory and attention, sleep disturbances, and increased defecation. These behaviors are similar to stress-related behaviors seen in patients with PTSD, and are relevant to functional pain disorders such as IBS [87]. Brain regions felt to play an important role in PTSD include the hippocampus, amygdala, and medial prefrontal cortex [10]. Cortisol and norepinephrine are two neurochemical systems that are critical in the stress response [38,92] which have also been implicated in disorders like IBS and fibromyalgia.

The hypothalamic-pituitary-adrenal (HPA) axis plays an important role in the stress response. Activation of the HPA axis releases catecholamines from nerves and the adrenal medulla and leads to the secretion of corticotropin-releasing factor (CRF) from the pituitary. Adrenocorticotropin (ACTH), in turn, mediates the release of cortisol from the adrenal cortex. Chronic stress or poor adaption to stress can maintain activation of the HPA axis. Continuous activation of the HPA axis can have negative effects including exhaustion of the system and damage to neural structures [10–14]. A vulnerable link in the regulation of the HPA axis is the hippocampus. Continuous circulation of cortisol [80] and CRF [17] leads to the destruction of hippocampal cells, further dysregulates the HPA axis, and leads to disturbances in cognition. Stress can directly interfere with hippocampal-based mechanisms of memory function, including long-term potentiation [31]; studies have also shown that stress is associated with an inhibition of neurogenesis (or the growth of new neurons) in the hippocampus [34]. Animal studies have also shown that stress is associated with a decrease in neuronal branching in the medial prefrontal cortex/ACC [75]. Magnetic resonance imaging has shown that stress-related disorders such as recurrent depressive illness and PTSD are associated with atrophy of the hippocampus as well as the ACC [11,14]. A failure of medial prefrontal/ACC activation with stressful cues or reminders of the traumatic event is the most replicated finding in PTSD [12]. Since the medial prefrontal cortex/ACC inhibits amygdala function, such findings have led to the hypothesis that a failure of medial prefrontal function underlies the failure of extinction in PTSD. The hippocampus is also involved in inhibition of central stress circuits, through inhibitory inputs to the hypothalamus, which reduces CRF release and therefore reduces HPA axis activation [10,80]. Stress-induced damage to the hippocampus could play a role in the decreased ability of the hippocampus to inhibit limbic circuits and stress circuits [10,80].

Increased levels of CRH or glucocorticoids also result in enhanced firing of midbrain serotonergic raphe neurons, which may play a role in stress-mediated analgesia. As stress becomes more chronic, it may lead to depletion of central serotonin, upregulation of the brainstem presynaptic 5-HT$_{1A}$ receptor, and glucocorticoid-induced downregulation of the postsynaptic hippocampal 5-HT$_{1A}$ receptor [69]. Such events could lead to symptoms of depression and anxiety. Depletion of central serotonin might also lead to an increase in ascending nociceptive transmission.

The functional pain disorders have not been shown to share all the neurobiological alterations found in stress-related psychiatric conditions like depression and PTSD. For example, reduced hippocampal volume has not been reported in patients with long-standing chronic pain [4]. Although early abuse is associated with functional pain disorders in some patients, in others the disorders stem from a single traumatic event in adulthood, such as a motor vehicle accident or sexual assault. For these patients, the source of continual stress is the disorder itself, which is mediated through their cognitions about pain, self, and their affective state [90]. Some have hypothesized that these physical traumas can lead to an increased general neuronal hypersensitization, leading to a generalized increased sensitivity, which manifests itself in different ways in different individuals—multiple sensitivity points in fibromyalgia, for example, or increased sensitivity to one's own bowel contractions in IBS [90]. Thus, it is likely that the experience of functional pain will involve disturbance in higher cortical centers that process both cognition and affective state. The plasticity of cingulate function and the involvement of the ACC in both pain processing and emotion suggest the cingulate cortex as a potential area of increased vulnerability for functional pain.

Conclusions

The high degree of comorbidity between stress-related psychiatric disorders, such as PTSD and depression, and functional pain disorders suggests a connection between these two domains. In many patients this comorbidity is probably related to a common link to stress. However, the fact that not all patients with functional pain disorders have a history of severe stress exposure such as childhood abuse, nor for that matter the diagnosis of PTSD or depression, suggests that such stressors are not essential for the development of chronic pain disorders. Common brain areas, including the prefrontal cortex, and brain chemical systems, such as norepinephrine and the HPA axis, have been implicated in the etiology of both PTSD and functional pain disorders. For some disorders, such as IBS, the role of fear and the stress response is easy to understand, given the known effects of the fear response on bowel motility. For other disorders, such as fibromyalgia, the connection with stress is not as obvious, and invocations of stress in the etiology of this disorder may be related to the absence of physical manifestations of pathology. The etiology of these disorders probably involves a complex interplay between CNS control of peripheral organs and relay of information back to the CNS, as well as the impact of affective disorders on processing of information, and environmental exposures including stress and trauma. Certain brain areas play a role, including the cingulate cortex, which is important in the affective and cognitive dimensions of pain experience that are amplified in functional pain patients as well as being implicated in PTSD. Future studies are indicated to better understand the interplay between stress, PTSD, and functional pain disorders, and to map out better methods of treating these disabling disorders.

References

[1]   Alagiri M, Chottiner S, Ratner V, Slade D, Hanno PM. Interstitial cystitis: unexplained associations with other chronic disease and pain syndromes. Urology 1997;49:52–7.
[2]   Amir M, Kaplan Z, Neumann L, Sharabani R, Shani N, Buskila D. Posttraumatic stress disorder, tenderness and fibromyalgia. J Psychosom Res 1997;42:607–13.
[3]   APA. DSM-IV-TR: Diagnostic and statistical manual of mental disorders. Washington, DC: American Psychiatric Press; 2000.
[4]   Apkarian AV, Sosa Y, Sonty S, Levy RM, Harden RN, Parrish TB, Gitelman DR. Chronic back pain is associated with decreased prefrontal and thalamic gray matter density. J Neurosci 2004;24:10410–5.
[5]   Ballenger JC, Davidson JRT, Lecrubier Y, Nutt DJ, Lydiard RB, Mayer EA. Consensus statement on depression, anxiety, and functional gastrointestinal disorders. J Clin Psychiatry 2001;62(Suppl 8):48–51.
[6]   Barsky AJ, Borus JF. Functional somatic syndromes. Ann Intern Med 1999;130:910–21.
[7]   Beckham JC, Crawford AL, Feldman ME, Kirby AC, Hertzberg MA, Davidson JR, Moore SD. Chronic posttraumatic stress disorder and chronic pain in Vietnam combat veterans. J Psychosom Res 1997;43:379–89.
[8]   Beckham JC, Moore SD, Feldman ME, Hertzberg MA, Kirby AC, Fairbank JA. Health status, somatization, and severity of posttraumatic stress disorder in Vietnam combat veterans with posttraumatic stress disorder. Am J Psychiatry 1998;155:1565–9.
[9]   Boscarino JA. Diseases among men 20 years after exposure to severe stress: implications for clinical research and medical care. Psychosom Med 1997;59:605–15.
[10] Bremner JD. Does stress damage the brain? Understanding trauma-related disorders from a mind-body perspective. New York: W.W. Norton; 2002.

[11] Bremner JD. Stress and brain atrophy. CNS Neurol Disord Drug Targets 2006;5:503–12.

[12] Bremner JD. Functional neuroimaging in posttraumatic stress disorder. Expert Rev Neurother 2007;7:393–405.

[13] Bremner JD, Elzinga B, Schmahl C, Vermetten E. Structural and functional plasticity of the human brain in posttraumatic stress disorder. Prog Brain Res 2008;167:171–86.

[14] Bremner JD, Randall P, Scott TM, Bronen RA, Seibyl JP, Southwick SM, Delaney RC, McCarthy G, Charney DS, Innis RB. MRI-based measurement of hippocampal volume in patients with combat-related posttraumatic stress disorder. Am J Psychiatry 1995;152:973–81.

[15] Bremner JD, Southwick SM, Brett E, Fontana A, Rosenheck A, Charney DS. Dissociation and posttraumatic stress disorder in Vietnam combat veterans. Am J Psychiatry 1992;149:328–32.

[16] Brown RJ, Schrag A, Trimble MR. Dissociation, childhood interpersonal trauma, and family functioning in patients with somatization disorder. Am J Psychiatry 2005;162:899–905.

[17] Brunson KL, Avishai-Eliner S, Hatalski CG, Baram TZ. Neurobiology of the stress response early in life: evolution of a concept and the role of corticotropin releasing hormone. Mol Psychiatry 2001;6:647–56.

[18] Change L, Berman S, Mayer EA, Suyenobu B, Derbyshire S, Naliboff B, Vogt BA, Fitzgerald L, Mandelkern MA. Brain responses to visceral and somatic stimuli in patients with irritable bowel syndrome with and without fibromyalgia. Am J Gastroenterol 2003;98:1354–61.

[19] Ciccone DS, Elliott DK, Chandler HK, Nayak S, Raphael KG. Sexual and physical abuse in women with fibromyalgia syndrome: a test of the trauma hypothesis. Clin J Pain 2005;21:378–86.

[20] Classen C, Koopman C, Hales R, Spiegel D. Acute stress disorder as a predictor of posttraumatic stress symptoms. Am J Psychiatry 1998;155:620–4.

[21] Clauw DJ, Chrousos GP. Chronic pain and fatigue syndromes: overlapping clinical and neuroendocrine features and potential pathogenic mechanisms. Neuroimmunomodulation 1997;4:134–53.

[22] Clauw DJ, Schmidt M, Radulovic D, Singer A, Katz P, Bresette J. The relationship between fibromyalgia and interstitial cystitis. J Psychiatr Res 1997;31:125–30.

[23] Cohen H, Jotkowitz A, Buskila D, Pelles-Avraham S, Kaplan Z, Neumann L, Sperber AD. Posttraumatic stress disorder and other co-morbidities in a sample population of patients with irritable bowel syndrome. Eur J Intern Med 2006;17:567–71.

[24] Cohen H, Neumann L, Haiman Y, Matar MA, Press J, Buskila D. Prevalence of post-traumatic stress disorder in fibromyalgia patients: overlapping syndromes or post-traumatic fibromyalgia syndrome? Semin Arthritis Rheum 2002;32:38–50.

[25] Corovic N, Durakovic A, Zavalic M, Zrinscak J. Electrocardiographic changes in ex-prisoners of war released from detention camps. Int J Legal Med 2000;113:197–200.

[26] Croft P. Testing for tenderness: What's the point? J Rheumatol 2000;27:2531–3.

[27] Culclasure TF, Enzenauer RJ, West SG. Post-traumatic stress disorder presenting as fibromyalgia. Am J Med 1993;94:548–9.

[28] DeCarvalho LT, Whealin JM. What pain specialists need to know about posttraumatic stress disorder in Operation Iraqi Freedom and Operation Enduring Freedom returnees. J Musculoskel Pain 2006;14:37–45.

[29] Derbyshire SWG, Jones AKP, Creed F, Starz T, Meltzer CC, Townsend DW, Peterson AM, Firestone L. Cerebral responses to noxious thermal stimulation in chronic low back pain patients and normal controls. Neuroimage 2002;16:158–68.

[30] Derbyshire SWG, Whalley MG, Stenger VA, Oakley DA. Cerebral activation during hypnotically induced and imagined pain. Neuroimage 2004;23:392–401.

[31] Diamond DM, Fleshner M, Ingersoll N, Rose GM. Psychological stress impairs spatial working memory: relevance to electrophysiological studies of hippocampal function. Behav Neurosci 1996;110:661–72.

[32] Drossman DA, Corazziari E, Talley NJ, Thompson WG, Whitehead WE. Rome II. The functional gastrointestinal disorders: diagnosis, pathophysiology and treatment, a multinational consensus. 2nd ed. McLean, VA: Degnon; 2000.

[33] Drossman DA, Creed FH, Olden KW, Svedlund J, Toner BB, Whitehead WE. Psychosocial aspects of the functional gastrointestinal disorders. Gut 1999;45:1125–30.

[34] Duman RS. Depression: a case of neuronal life and death? Biol Psychiatry 2004;56:140–5.

[35] Ehlert U, Heim C, Hellhammer DH. Chronic pelvic pain as a somatoform disorder. Psychother Psychosom 1999;68:87–94.

[36] Farrar JT, Young JP, LaMoreaux L, Werth JL, Poole RM. Clinical importance of changes in chronic pain intensity measured on an 11-point numerical pain rating scale. Pain 2001;94:149–58.

[37] Fass R, Fullerton S, Naliboff B, Hirsh T, Mayer EA. Sexual dysfunction in patients with irritable bowel syndrome and non-ulcer dyspepsia. Digestion 1998;59:79–85.

[38] Francati V, Vermetten E, Bremner JD. Functional neuroimaging studies in posttraumatic stress disorder: review of current methods and findings. Depress Anxiety 2007;24:202–18.

[39] Fukuda K, Nisenbaum R, Stewart G, Thompson WW, Robin L, Washko RM, Noah DL, Barrett DH, Randall B, Herwaldt BL, Mawle AC, Reeves WC. Chronic multisystem illness affecting Air Force veterans of the Gulf War. JAMA 1998;280:981–8.

[40] Geuze E, Vermetten E, Jochims A, Bohus M, Schmahl C, Westenberg H. Neuroimaging of pain perception in Dutch veterans with and without posttraumatic stress disorder: preliminary results. Ann NY Acad Sci 2006;1071:401–4.

[41] Geuze E, Westenberg HG, Jochims A, de Kloet CS, Bohus M, Vermetten E, Schmahl C. Altered pain processing in veterans with posttraumatic stress disorder. Arch Gen Psychiatry 2007;64:76–85.

[42] Goldenberg DL, Sandhu HS. Fibromyalgia and post-traumatic stress disorder: another piece in the biopsychosocial puzzle. Semin Arthritis Rheum 2002;32:1–2.

[43] Gomborone JE, Dewsnap PA, Libby GW, Farthing MJG. Selective affective biasing in recognition memory in the irritable bowel syndrome. Gut 1993;34:1230–4.

[44] Gracely RH, Geisser ME, Giesecke T, Grant MAB, Petzke F, Williams DA, Clauw DJ. Pain catastrophizing and neural responses to pain among persons with fibromyalgia. Brain 2004;127:835–43.

[45] Gracely RH, Petzke F, Wolf JM, Clauw DJ. Functional magnetic resonance imaging evidence of augmented pain processing in fibromyalgia. Arthritis Rheum 2002;46:1333–43.

[46] Griep EN, Boersma JW, Lentjes EGWM, Prins APA, van der Korst JK, de Kloet ER. Function of the hypothalamic-pituitary-adrenal axis in patients with fibromyalgia and low back pain. J Rheumatol 1998;25:1374–82.

[47] Hadler NM. The injured worker and the internist. Ann Intern Med 1994;120:163–4.

[48] Harvey RF, Salih SY, Read AE. Organic and functional disorders in 2000 gastroenterology outpatients. Lancet 2000;1:632–4.

[49] Heim C, Ehlert U, Hanker JP, Hellhammer DH. Abuse-related posttraumatic stress disorder and alterations of the hypothalamic-pituitary-adrenal axis in women with chronic pelvic pain. Psychosom Med 1998;60:309–18.

[50] Heim C, Ehlert U, Hellhammer DH. The potential role of hypocortisolism in the pathophysiology of stress-related bodily disorders. Psychoneuroendocrinology 2000;25:1–35.

[51] Heim C, Ehlert U, Rexhausen J, Hanker JP, Hellhammer DH. Psychoendocrinological observations in women with chronic pelvic pain. Ann N Y Acad Sci 1997;821:456–8.

[52] Hoge CW, Castro CA, Messer SC, McGurk D, Cotting DI, Koffman RL. Combat duty in Iraq and Afghanistan, mental health problems, and barriers to care. N Engl J Med 2004;351:13–22.

[53] Hudson JI, Goldenberg DL, Pope HGJ, Keck PEJ, Schlesinger L. Comorbidity of fibromyalgia with medical and psychiatric disorders. Am J Med 1992;92:363–7.

[54] Hudson JI, Pope HG. Fibromyalgia and psychopathology: is fibromyalgia a form of "affective spectrum disorder"? J Rheumatol 1989;Suppl:15–22.

[55] Iowa. Self-reported illness and health status among Gulf War veterans: a population-based study (Iowa Persian Gulf Study Group). JAMA 1997;277:238–45.

[56] Irwin C, Falsetti SA, Lydiard RB, Ballenger JC, Brock CD, Brener W. Comorbidity of posttraumatic stress disorder and irritable bowel syndrome. J Clin Psychiatry 1996;57:576–8.

[57] Jensen MC, Brant-Zawadzki MN, Obuchowski N, Modic MT, Malkasian D, Ross JS. Magnetic resonance imaging of the lumbar spine in people without back pain. N Engl J Med 1994;331:69–73.

[58] Kendall-Tackett KA. Physiological correlates of childhood abuse: chronic hyperarousal in PTSD, depression, and irritable bowel syndrome. Child Abuse Negl 2000;24:799–810.

[59] Kessler RC, Sonnega A, Bromet E, Hughes M, Nelson CB. Posttraumatic stress disorder in the national comorbidity survey. Arch Gen Psychiatry 1995;52:1048–60.

[60] Kulka RA, Schlenger WE, Fairbank JA, Hough RL, Jordan BK, Marmar CR, Weiss DS. Trauma and the Vietnam War generation: report of findings from the National Vietnam Veterans Readjustment Study. New York: Brunner/Mazel; 1990.

[61] Lackner JM, Gudleski GD, Blanchard EB. Beyond abuse: the association among parenting style, abdominal pain, and somatization in IBS patients. Behav Res Ther 2004;42:41-56.
[62] Lemrow N, Adams D, Coffey R, Farley D. The 50 most frequent diagnosis-related groups (DRGs), diagnoses, and procedures: statistics by hospital size and location. DHHS Publication No. (PHS) 90-3465. Hospital Studies Program Research Note 13.
[63] Lydiard RB. Irritable bowel syndrome, anxiety, and depression: what are the links? J Clin Psychiatry 2001;62(Suppl 8):38–45; discussion 6–7.
[64] Marmar CR, Weiss DS, Schlenger DS, Fairbank JA, Jordan BK, Kulka RA, Hough RL. Peritraumatic dissociation and posttraumatic stress in male Vietnam theater veterans. Am J Psychiatry 1994;151:902–7.
[65] Mayer EA, Collins SM. Evolving pathophysiologic models of functional gastrointestinal disorders. Gastroenterology 2002;122:2032–48.
[66] Mayer EA, Craske M, Naliboff BD. Depression, anxiety, and the gastrointestinal system. J Clin Psychiatry 2001;62(Suppl 8):28–36; discussion 7.
[67] Mayer EA, Naliboff BD, Chang L, Coutinho SV. Stress and the gastrointestinal tract V. Stress and irritable bowel syndrome. Am J Physiol Gastrointest Liver Physiol 2001;280:G519–G24.
[68] McLean SA, Clauw DJ, Abelson JL, Liberzon I. The development of persistent pain and psychological morbidity after motor vehicle collision: integrating the potential role of stress response systems into a biopsychosocial model. Psychosom Med 2005;67:783–90.
[69] Mendelson SD, McEwen BS. Autoradiographic analyses of the effects of restraint-induced stress on 5-HT1A, 5-HT1C, and 5-HT2 receptors in the dorsal hippocampus of male and female rats. Neuroendocrinology 1991;54:454–61.
[70] Mitchell CM, Drossman DA. Survey of the AGA membership relating to patients with functional gastrointestinal disorders. Gastroenterology 1987;92:1282–4.
[71] Monga AK, Marrero JM, Stanton SL, Lemieux MC, Maxwell JD. Is there an irritable bladder in the irritable bowel syndrome? Br J Obstest Gynaecol 1997;104:1409–12.
[72] Naliboff BD, Derbyshire SW, Munakata J, Berman S, Mandelkern M, Chang L, Mayer EA. Cerebral activation in patients with irritable bowel syndrome and control subjects during rectosigmoid stimulation. Psychosom Med 2001;63:365–75.
[73] Nice S, Garland CF, Hilton SM, Baggett JC, Mitchell RE. Long-term health outcomes and medical effects of torture among US Navy prisoners of war in Vietnam. JAMA 1996;276:375–81.
[74] Nijenhuis ER, van Dyck R, ter Kuile MM, Mourits MJ, Spinhoven P, van der Hart O. Evidence for associations among somatoform dissociation, psychological dissociation and reported trauma in patients with chronic pelvic pain. J Psychosom Obstet Gynaecol 2003;24:87–98.
[75] Radley JJ, Sisti HM, Hao J, Rocher AB, McCall T, Hof PR, McEwen BS, Morrison JH. Chronic behavioral stress induces apical dendritic reorganization in pyramidal neurons of the medial prefrontal cortex. Neuroscience 2004;125:1–6.
[76] Reilly J, Baker GA, Rhodes J, Salmon P. The association of sexual and physical abuse with somatization: characteristics of patients presenting with irritable bowel syndrome and non-epileptic attack disorder. Psychol Med 1999;29:399–406.
[77] Ross CA. Childhood sexual abuse and psychosomatic symptoms in irritable bowel syndrome. J Child Sex Abuse 2005;14:27–38.
[78] Saigh PA, Bremner JD. Posttraumatic stress disorder: a comprehensive text. Needham Heights, MA: Allyn & Bacon; 1999.
[79] Salmon P, Skaife K, Rhodes J. Abuse, dissociation, and somatization in irritable bowel syndrome: towards an explanatory model. J Behav Med 2003;26:1-18.
[80] Sapolsky RM. Why stress is bad for your brain. Science 1996;273:749–50.
[81] Schnurr PP, Spiro A. Combat exposure, posttraumatic stress disorder symptoms, and health behaviors as predictors of self-reported physical health in older veterans. J Nerv Ment Dis 1999;187:353–9.
[82] Schur EA, Afari N, Furberg H, Olarte M, Goldberg J, Sullivan PF, Buchwald D. Feeling bad in more ways than one: comorbidity patterns of medically unexplained and psychiatric conditions. J Gen Intern Med 2007;22:818–21.
[83] Sherman JJ, Carlson CR, Wilson JF, Okeson JP, McCubbin JA. Post-traumatic stress disorder among patients with orofacial pain. J Orofac Pain 2005;19:309–17.

[84] Sherman JJ, Turk DC, Okifuji A. Prevalence and impact of posttraumatic stress disorder-like symptoms on patients with fibromyalgia syndrome. Clin J Pain 2000;16:127–34.

[85] Spinhoven P, Roelofs K, Moene F, Kuyk J, Nijenhuis E, Hoogduin K, Van Dyck R. Trauma and dissociation in conversion disorder and chronic pelvic pain. Int J Psychiatry Med 2004;34:305–18.

[86] Spitzer WO, Leblanc FE, Dupuis M. Scientific approach to the assessment and management of activity-related spinal disorders. Report of the Quebec Task Force on Spinal Disorders. Spine 1987;12:7S.

[87] Stam R, Akkermans LM, Wiegant VM. Trauma and the gut: interactions between stressful experience and intestinal function. Gut 1997;40:704–9.

[88] Thieme K, Turk DC, Flor H. Comorbid depression and anxiety in fibromyalgia syndrome: relationship to somatic and psychosocial variables. Psychosom Med 2004;66:837–44.

[89] Turk DC. Cognitive-behavioral approach to the treatment of chronic pain patients. Reg Anesth Pain Med 2003;28:573–9.

[90] Turk DC, Rudy TE. Cognitive factors and persistent pain: a glimpse into Pandora's Box. Cogn Ther Res 1992;16:99–122.

[91] Vermetten E, Bremner JD. Circuits and systems in stress. I. Preclinical studies. Depress Anxiety 2002;15:126–47.

[92] Vermetten E, Bremner JD. Circuits and systems in stress. II. Applications to neurobiology and treatment of PTSD. Depress Anxiety 2002;16:14–38.

[93] Walker EA, Keegan D, Gardner G, Sullivan M, Bernstein D, Katon WJ. Psychosocial factors in fibromyalgia compared with rheumatoid arthritis: II. Sexual, physical, and emotional abuse and neglect. Psychosom Med 1997;59:572–7.

[94] Weissbecker I, Floyd A, Dedert E, Salmon P, Sephton S. Childhood trauma and diurnal cortisol disruption in fibromyalgia syndrome. Psychoneuroendocrinology 2006;31:312–24.

[95] Wessely S, Nimnuan C, Sharpe M. Functional somatic syndromes: one or many? Lancet 1999;354:936–9.

[96] White KP, Speechley M, Harth M, Ostbye T. The London Fibromyalgia Epidemiology Study: the prevalence of fibromyalgia syndrome in London, Ontario. J Rheumatol 1999;26:1570–6.

[97] Whitehead WE, Crowell MD, Robinson JC, Heller BR, Schuster MM. Effects of stressful life events on bowel symptoms: subjects with irritable bowel syndrome compared with subjects without bowel dysfunction. J Gastroenterol 1992;33:825–30.

[98] Wolfe F, Smythe HA, Yunus MB, et al. The American College of Rheumatology 1990 criteria for the classification of fibromyalgia. Report of the multicenter criteria committee. Arthritis Rheum 1990;33:160–72.

[99] Zatzick DF, Marmar CR, Weiss DS, Browner WS, Metzler TJ, Golding JM, Stewart A, Schlenger WE, Wells KB. Posttraumatic stress disorder and functioning and quality of life outcomes in a nationally representative sample of male Vietnam veterans. Am J Psychiatry 1997;154:1690–5.

Correspondence to: J. Douglas Bremner, MD, Departments of Psychiatry and Radiology, Emory University School of Medicine, Atlanta, GA 30322, USA. Tel: 1-404-712-9569; email: jdbremn@emory.edu.

Anxiety in Functional Pain Disorders

Bruce D. Naliboff[a,b] and Jamie L. Rhudy[c]

[a]*Center for Neurobiology of Stress, Department of Psychiatry and Biobehavioral Sciences, David Geffen School of Medicine at UCLA, Los Angeles, California, USA;* [b]*VA Greater Los Angeles Healthcare System, Los Angeles, California, USA;* [c]*Human Psychophysiology Laboratory and Department of Psychology, The University of Tulsa, Tulsa, Oklahoma, USA*

Overview

Affective processes can interact with nociception and pain at a variety of levels—pain generation, pain modulation, and pain response. These relationships are found with pain regardless of its source, but there has been a special focus on the role of affective processes in functional pain disorders. This emphasis is due not only to a lack of good peripheral biological models for generation of symptoms in these disorders but also to empirical findings of increased comorbidity of functional syndromes with psychiatric disorders such as anxiety and depression. Anxiety is the negative affect most often identified as being linked with functional disorders, and this chapter will review the theory and evidence regarding the role of anxiety in the development, persistence, and treatment of functional syndromes.

How we approach such issues as the role of anxiety in functional pain disorders has shifted considerably with the development of affective neuroscience as a predominant paradigm for studying emotion. It is important to recognize that negative affect can be studied from multiple points of view. Much of what we know about the phenomenology of negative affect, and specifically anxiety, comes from self-report data and behavioral observations collected in questionnaires, in clinical interviews, or during laboratory experiments. From these data we now recognize specific anxiety disorders, which are based on a cluster of persistent symptoms that lead to life interference (e.g., panic disorder and generalized anxiety disorder), as well as dimensional characteristics that are related to anxiety but are present to some extent in the entire population (e.g., trait anxiety, worry, and specific fears).

For the purposes of this chapter, we have taken a broad conceptualization of the anxiety construct. We believe that anxiety emanates from the activation of a highly evolved neural network of cortical, subcortical, and brainstem regions that promote survival through threat detection and avoidance, i.e., the aversive/defensive system [13,29,61,63]. Negative affective states are the phenomenological experiences that result from the activation of this network, and the feeling of anxiety is one label for these experiences.

It is important to identify and define a number of anxiety-related terms that have been used throughout the pain literature to provide the reader with a framework for understanding our review. *State anxiety* is a diffuse negative affect associated with arousal, apprehension, and hypervigilance that is directed at the potential for future harm. *Trait anxiety* is the general tendency to experience state anxiety, reflecting a stable, trait-like disposition [115]. Similarly, *neuroticism* is a stable personality trait associated with the propensity to experience negative affect [34]. *Stress* is a term that has several meanings; however, for the purposes of this chapter it will be used to refer to the negative emotional reaction associated with exposure to a real or imagined threat that is typically concomitant with fight-or-flight reactions [70]. *Worry* is used to refer to cognitive responses to real or imagined threat [43,78], and *catastrophizing* involves cognitive processes associated with magnification, rumination, and helplessness about negative events such as pain. *Fear avoidance* and related terms (e.g., *kinesiophobia*) refer to negative affect stemming from the negative consequences (e.g., pain) of movement and physical activity [107,127]. Therefore, many of these terms clearly have significant conceptual overlap in that they are psychological responses to threat.

Affective neuroscience has emphasized the importance of examining the central nervous system (CNS) or neurocognitive processes that generate phenomenological categories and dimensions. For example, somewhat separate circuits within the limbic system have now been identified that subserve anxiety and fear-like behaviors in both humans and other mammals [128].

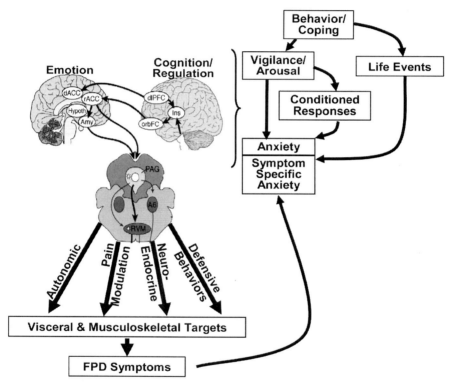

Fig. 1. Proposed model linking negative affect (e.g., anxiety) and functional pain disorders. Corticolimbic connections (dorsal lateral prefrontal cortex, dlPFC; insula, Ins; orbital frontal cortex, orbFC; rostral anterior cingulate cortex, rACC; dorsal anterior cingulate cortex, dACC; hypothalamus, Hypoth; amygdala, Amy) are believed to mediate the neurocognitive processes that lead to the evocation and regulation of emotional experience. Outputs from this corticolimbic network to regions of the brainstem (e.g., periaqueductal gray, PAG; rostral ventromedial medulla, RVM) are responsible for behaviors resulting from emotion, arousal, and defense, but also for descending modulation of nociception. These outputs influence visceral and musculoskeletal targets and symptoms of functional pain disorders (FPD). Further, functional pain symptoms provide feedback to the neurocognitive mechanisms that promote anxiety and negative affect. Adapted from Mayer and colleagues [74], with permission from Elsevier.

The focus on building-block neurocognitive processes that underlie both symptoms and behaviors associated with anxiety leads naturally to an examination of commonalities and interrelationships between processes involved in anxiety and those involved in pain modulation. Fig. 1 illustrates a proposed model of this relationship. Several key elements of this model are described as follows.

1) On a descriptive level, anxiety-related processes may influence the development and persistence of somatic symptoms via multiple interrelated pathways. These processes include increasing arousal and defensive responses to somatic information; altering interoceptive sensitivity, and particularly pain sensitivity, via descending modulatory pathways; increasing vigilance to somatic symptoms; and interfering with normal cognitive and behavioral strategies for coping with injury and illness.

2) Symptom-specific anxiety can be distinguished from more general anxiety in that the cues for triggering the negative affect are primarily related to the experience of symptoms and the contexts in which they occur.

3) At the level of neurocircuitry, these interacting processes are hypothesized to involve cortico-limbic-pontine interactions, with primary roles for the activity of the lateral prefrontal cortex interacting with limbic and paralimbic structures of the medial prefrontal cortex, anterior cingulate, and amygdala. Also involved are brainstem structures that mediate the various physiological and motor responses in response to stress.

4) Anxiety can also significantly influence functional syndromes at the level of behavior; for example, fear of movement may be a powerful incentive to rest, which in turn may lead to greater pain and fear.

Each of these processes will be discussed in more detail below.

Role of Anxiety in Development of Functional Pain Disorders

It is likely that the development of one or multiple functional pain disorders involves a summation of several vulnerabilities, of which some may be syndrome-specific and others are more common to functional pain disorders in general. It has been suggested that certain genetic predispositions and early life trauma may raise the probability of both functional pain disorders and anxiety-related conditions. Although a review of these literatures is beyond the scope of this chapter, it is relevant to note that there is some evidence that childhood abuse is most highly associated with panic disorder (as compared to other anxiety disorders or depression) [108]. In irritable bowel syndrome (IBS) it appears that vulnerability to anxiety (in the form of neuroticism) appears to be a primary pathway for translation of negative early experience into symptom generation [119] (see also Chapter 19 by Papp and Sobel; Chapter 5 by Chang and Drossman). Consistent with this conceptualization, a recent brain imaging study has shown that IBS patients with a history of abuse, compared to those without such a history, report more pain, greater mid-cingulate cortex activation (associated with affective experience of pain), and reduced activity of a region implicated in pain inhibition and arousal, the subgenual anterior cingulate cortex (ACC) [105].

The study of genetic vulnerability for functional pain disorders is in its infancy and is reviewed elsewhere in this volume (Chapter 19 by Papp and Sobel). So far, the results have shown intriguing relationships between genetic markers related to the serotonin and norepinephrine systems and the development and presentation of symptoms [23]. Many of these same markers have also been associated with anxiety and threat sensitivity [110]. Given the data suggesting a strong overlap of functional pain disorders with panic and generalized anxiety disorder (discussed below), it is interesting to note a recent report differentiating separate genetic vulnerabilities for panic versus generalized anxiety versus agoraphobia and other specific phobias [46]. It is likely that the relationships between genetic markers and both affective and pain symptoms are complex. For example, Diatchenko et al. [22] have recently reported a very strong association between haplotypes of the β_2 adrenergic receptor (ADRB2) and the development of temporomandibular joint disorder (TMD) (see also Chapter 3 by Maixner). Individuals who carried one haplotype coding for high expression and one coding for low expression of ADRB2 displayed the most positive psychological functioning and were about 10 times less likely to develop TMD than those without these haplotypes. However, of the anxiety measures used in this study, trait anxiety was negatively related to presence of one haplotype, current anxious mood was positively related to another, and several other measures were unrelated to the genetic markers. Overall, emerging but still preliminary data support the hypothesis that some of the common vulnerability between anxiety and functional pain disorders may be related both to overlapping genetic variables and to a history of trauma, and that these factors can be tied to specific CNS mechanisms of arousal and pain modulation.

Comorbidity of Anxiety and Functional Pain Disorders

A growing body of research demonstrates that functional somatic syndromes, including fibromyalgia syndrome (FM), irritable bowel syndrome (IBS), chronic fatigue syndrome (CFS), and chronic headache, are all associated with an increased prevalence of anxiety disorders as defined by the *Diagnostic and Statistical Manual* (DSM) criteria [1]. The data are not sufficient to pinpoint the degree of overlap with precision, but it appears that the combined rate of any anxiety disorder may be three or more times that of the general population and also greater than for clearly organic defined illnesses with similar symptom patterns such as gastrointestinal (GI) discomfort, pain, and fatigue. In clinic and especially tertiary care populations, the rates are even higher, with some findings of 60% or more of patients having a comorbid anxiety disorder. Examples of these studies are provided as follows.

Fibromyalgia syndrome. Epstein et al. [28] report a 17% rate of panic disorder, a 17% rate of simple phobia, and a 35% rate of any lifetime anxiety disorder in a clinic-based sample of FM patients. Arnold et al. [4] report a 28% rate for panic, a 21% rate for phobia, a 23% rate for post-traumatic stress disorder (PTSD), and a 60% rate for a lifetime diagnosis of anxiety. In agreement with these studies, a meta-analysis of five studies of FM also found panic disorder to be the most common of the comorbid anxiety diagnoses, with an odds ratio (OR) of 9.0 [4].

Irritable bowel syndrome. Kumano [56], in a large Japanese population study, found that panic disorder (OR = 3.58) and agoraphobia (OR = 1.96) were significantly more prevalent in subjects with IBS compared to those without. Several other authors have also reported increased rates of panic disorder and several other anxiety disorders as well as depression in IBS [66,129] in population studies, and an even greater prevalence of anxiety was found in GI clinic samples (30–60%) [64]. One study has also reported a high rate (36%) of PTSD in clinic patients with IBS [47]. A meta-analysis also found that anxiety, but not depressive symptoms, was associated with consulting for abdominal symptoms [45].

Chronic headache. In a large population study (*n* > 60,000), Zwart et al. [141] report significantly higher rates of anxiety disorders in individuals with both nonmigraine headaches (7.8%; OR = 2.7) and migraine headaches (9.2%; OR = 3.2). In another population study, Lake et al. [59] reported an increased prevalence of anxiety in subjects with recurrent headache as well as greater anxiety with more frequent headache. There was no greater risk for anxiety in subjects with infrequent headache.

Interstitial cystitis. While there is very little information about interstitial cystitis (IC), Wu et al. [136], studying a large population of patients in a health maintenance organization (HMO), reported significantly increased rates for depression (relative risk [RR] = 2.8) and even greater rates for anxiety (RR = 4.5) in patients diagnosed with IC. Talati et. al. [118] also report a genetically linked clustering of panic and social anxiety disorder with several medical syndromes including IC.

The only broad-based meta-analysis of anxiety and depression across functional syndromes [45] found that both anxiety and depression were consistency higher in the four disorders studied—IBS, FM, CFS, and functional dyspepsia. The effect sizes for the association of anxiety with these syndromes were of moderate magnitude but highly significant statistically when compared with healthy persons and control patients with medical disorders of known organic pathology. There were some differences in the relationships, however. For example, IBS had a stronger association with anxiety than did FM. Although there were insufficient data for most of the syndromes, the analysis of IBS also showed that consulting behavior and severity of somatization were significantly related to levels of anxiety.

Taken together, the studies to date indicate a substantially greater rate of lifetime anxiety disorders in patients with many of the functional disorders. However, it is not clear whether specific disorders in the anxiety spectrum are more closely associated with some or all of the syndromes. This type of analysis is complicated by extensive overlap among the anxiety disorders and by the focus of many studies on a limited set of disorders. The very limited data do, however, suggest that panic disorder and generalized anxiety disorder are the types of anxiety most consistently associated with IBS and FM. These findings may indicate a stronger overlap of mechanisms involved in these disorders with those of functional pain disorders.

Symptom-Specific Anxiety

Although the comorbidity studies described above point to increased general anxiety and other negative moods in patients with functional syndromes, growing evidence indicates that symptom-specific anxiety and fears may be even more relevant for understanding the relationship between negative affect and symptom development and persistence in these disorders. *Symptom-specific anxiety* can be defined as the cognitive, affective, and behavioral response stemming from fear of specific somatic (or visceral) sensations, symptoms, and the context in which these sensations and symptoms occur [5,58]. Examples of symptom-related contexts for a visceral sensation might include situations involving food and eating such as restaurants or parties or locations in which bathroom facilities are unknown. For a chronic pain condition, symptom-related contexts might include situations associated with movement or physical strain, such as a long stairway, an airport, or a long car ride. Symptom-specific anxiety includes hypervigilance to—and fear, worry, and avoidance of—relevant sensations and contexts. Symptom-specific anxiety may perpetuate symptoms through alterations in autonomic and pain facilitation, as well as through cognitive mechanisms [52,72]. Symptom-specific anxiety is thought to be associated with beliefs of poor symptom control and high illness impact and may, therefore, also be a critical element in the severe decrements in quality of life found in most functional syndrome patients [58].

Models of symptom-specific anxiety have been proposed for certain anxiety disorders [93,94] and more recently for chronic somatic pain [6,35] and functional GI disorders [58]. Anxiety sensitivity has been postulated as a constitutional predisposition characterized by hypersensitivity to anxiety-related somatic sensations (autonomic arousal) based upon beliefs that these sensations have harmful somatic, psychological, or social consequences [91,120]. Anxiety sensitivity can be distinguished from trait anxiety [92] in that it represents a specific tendency to respond fearfully to the interoceptive sensations of anxiety rather than the predisposition to respond anxiously to a wide range of stressors that characterizes trait anxiety. In a study of 8-year-old twins, Eley et al. [27] found a significant relationship between anxiety sensitivity and both panic symptoms and the ability to detect heartbeats (a measure of somatic vigilance). Genetic analysis suggested some common genetic vulnerability for these variables, although environmental influences appeared to be substantial.

Expansion of the anxiety sensitivity construct into multiple overlapping symptom-specific fears is partially an outgrowing of factor analytic research. For example, a recent factor analysis of a comprehensive measure of anxiety sensitivity revealed four specific somatic mechanisms or domains in addition to a single higher-order factor (general anxiety sensitivity trait) [120]. These domains corresponded to: (1) fear of respiratory symptoms, (2) fear of cardiovascular symptoms, (3) fear of cognitive dyscontrol, and (4) fear of GI symptoms. Overall, recent findings in the area of symptom-related anxiety support a common underlying vulnerability related to hypersensitivity to interoceptive information and threat, as well as specific content-related biases based on experience or other more specific vulnerabilities. In either case, clinical data suggest that symptom-specific anxiety is a powerful mediator of symptom severity, coping, and quality of life in patients with functional pain disorders.

Experimental Evidence for the Relationship between Negative Affect and Pain Processing

To understand the potential role of negative affect on functional pain, it is important to first characterize the experimental evidence in healthy

B.D. Naliboff and J.L. Rhudy

individuals. These data suggest that the relationship between negative affect and pain is nonmonotonic, such that the *intensity* of the emotional experience (typically assessed by level of arousal) determines the modulatory outcome (see Fig. 2) [99]. Specifically, negative emotions that are low to moderate in intensity (e.g., anxiety or apprehension) enhance pain, whereas very intense negative emotions (e.g., fear or panic) inhibit pain. Importantly, this effect is not simply due to arousal alone, because the relationship between positive affect intensity and pain is not nonmonotonic [99].

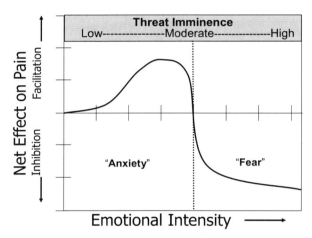

Fig. 2. Hypothesized relationship between negative affect and pain modulation in healthy persons. Negative affect with low to moderate intensity (arousal) enhances pain, whereas negative affect with high arousal inhibits pain. This figure also synthesizes ideas related to differences in emotional intensity and threat imminence. In particular, greater threat imminence (greater spatial or temporal proximity of a threatening stimulus or event) is associated with greater negative emotional intensity. Threat that is imminent and severe is likely to lead to intense negative affect (e.g., fear) that will inhibit pain processes. In contrast, threat that is less imminent (less proximal) will result in negative affect with less emotional intensity (e.g., anxiety). Therefore, threat that is not imminent and is less severe or unpredictable will lead to moderately intense negative affect that will facilitate pain processes. For persons with functional pain disorders, this relationship could be altered in several ways such that negative affect has a greater propensity to enhance pain (e.g., inhibitory processes are depleted, predictable threat enhances pain, and negative affect is generally exacerbated).

This nonmonotonic relationship of negative affect and pain is likely to have evolved as a means to promote survival during potential or immediate threat (conditions that would elicit negative affect). In situations associated with low to moderate threat (in which less intense negative affect would predominate), it is adaptive to promote environmental scanning, vigilance, and sensory intake as a means to improve threat detection [77,130]. In this situation, threat is more unpredictable, and hyperalgesia (enhanced pain) would be adaptive because it promotes detection of somatic threats and recuperation from tissue damage that might have been incurred during a time of high threat. However, when threat is present, imminent, and predictable (situations in which intense negative affect would predominate), pain and its associated reflexes and behaviors might interfere with active defense (fight-or-flight) [29,111]. In this latter situation, hypoalgesia (reduced pain) is adaptive.

Support for the relationship between negative affect and pain stems from research using various research methodologies. In preclinical studies, a large body of research has shown that acute and chronic stress leads to alterations in nociceptive sensitivity. Both analgesia and hyperalgesia have been demonstrated in studies of somatic pain, depending on the nature of the stress, the animal strain, and the behavioral indications of pain [54,67]. Studies of visceral sensitivity have shown long-lasting stress-induced hyperalgesia, suggesting potentially differential mechanisms for somatic and visceral pain modulation [12]. For example, Cornwall and Donderi [16] induced anxiety using a stressful interview or by providing a warning of an upcoming pressure pain test, compared to a no-anxiety condition. Findings suggested that both anxiety manipulations enhanced ratings of the pressure stimulus, with subjective stress showing a positive correlation with pain. In other studies, anxiety has been induced by verbal threat of electric shock and was found to reduce heat pain thresholds (causing hyperalgesia) [42,97]. Similar hyperalgesic effects occurred when instructions were given to generate anxiety about the same shock that was used to test pain [131]. Dougher and colleagues used emotionally charged statements to evoke negative affect, but also manipulated the focus of the emotion. They had participants read statements that produced general anxiety (e.g., walking down a dark alley), pain-specific anxiety (e.g., slamming a finger in a car door), or pain-task-specific anxiety (e.g., describing a device that produces extremely painful sensations) and found that only pain-specific anxiety reliably enhanced pain.

Evidence has shown that the repetitive application of a noxious stimulus leads to successively larger pain responses (temporal summation), an effect believed to be related to central sensitization. Robinson and colleagues [106] demonstrated that state anxiety during testing was positively correlated with temporal summation, suggesting that anxiety may engage mechanisms to enhance CNS pain processing. This effect was replicated by Granot and colleagues [38], and research by Edwards and colleagues [26] suggests that pain catastrophizing may have a similar facilitatory effect.

Ploghaus and colleagues [86] presented a neutral cue prior to the onset of a constant-intensity stimulus. However, in some trials the cue was followed by a stimulus of greater intensity. Thus, the cue came to elicit anxiety about the potential stronger stimulus. These authors found hyperalgesia to the constant-intensity stimulus, an effect that correlated with activation in the hippocampal formation as measured by functional magnetic resonance imaging.

As noted in the study by Ploghaus and colleagues, when a neutral cue (a conditioned stimulus) is paired with an aversive stimulus (an unconditioned stimulus), the conditioned stimulus comes to elicit negative affect—a procedure referred to as *fear conditioning*. In a variant of the fear conditioning paradigm, Williams and Rhudy [135] paired an unconditioned stimulus (a mild shock) with a conditioned stimulus consisting of a facial expression of fear. Later, the fear expression was presented to induce moderately intense negative affect (anticipatory anxiety) during pain testing. The investigators found that the fear expression reduced pain thresholds (causing hyperalgesia), despite the fact that fear expression had no influence on pain before being paired with shock.

Studies discussed thus far evoked negative affect by the presentation, or anticipation of, a *painful* stimulus; however, others have used nonpainful stimuli. Rhudy and Meagher [98] presented startling noise bursts to evoke negative affect. When the noises elicited negative affect and low arousal, *hyperalgesia* was produced, but when the noises elicited negative affect with high arousal, *hypoalgesia* ensued. Zelman and colleagues [139] had participants read emotionally charged statements unrelated to pain to produce sadness and found that negative affect reduced cold pressor tolerance (i.e., caused hyperalgesia). Other studies have used mental imagery, although rarely to induce negative emotions. Using personal negative imagery, Smith and Wolpin [113] found that cold pressor pain tolerance was decreased and that the effect was correlated with the vividness of the imagery. In three studies, Rainville and colleagues [90] used hypnotic suggestion to induce negative affect (anger, fear, sadness) and found that changes in negative affect were associated with changes in pain unpleasantness and pain-related heart rate responses.

In an innovative study, Villemure and colleagues [126] examined the influence of computer-delivered pleasant and unpleasant odors and found that, relative to pleasant odors, unpleasant odors increased negative mood and anxiety and enhanced pain unpleasantness. Further, odor-evoked mood was correlated with pain unpleasantness ratings. Unfortunately, this study did not include a neutral control condition to determine whether pleasant odors decreased, or unpleasant odors increased, pain unpleasantness. Indeed, when others included a control condition, evidence was mixed. One study found that pleasant odors reduced pain [89], whereas another found that unpleasant odors enhanced pain [69].

A problem with any experiment that manipulates emotion is the difficulty in standardizing the procedures so that emotion can be reliably manipulated across participants, laboratories, and studies. A recent technological advancement in this area was the development of the International Affective Picture System (IAPS) [60]. The IAPS is a normed set of emotionally charged visual stimuli that evoke reliable subjective and psychophysiological emotional responses in healthy participants [14] and engage corticolimbic systems [32,39,84]. Research has shown that unpleasant images from the IAPS (e.g., mutilated bodies, attack scenes, snakes, and spiders) reliably enhance pain threshold, pain tolerance, and pain ratings of noxious stimuli [21,76,80,137].

More recently, researchers have used the IAPS to determine whether physiological correlates of pain are modulated in the same manner as the subjective experience. This issue is important, given that the relationship between negative affect and pain could be due, at least in part, to experimental demands or report bias without any changes in nociceptive processing. In a series of studies, Rhudy and colleagues [102–104] assessed the influence of threatening images from the IAPS on the nociceptive flexion reflex (NFR). The NFR is a spinal reflex that promotes withdrawal from a noxious stimulus; it is dependent on the activation of Aδ-fiber nociceptors [109]. The threshold for eliciting the reflex correlates significantly with pain threshold, and the magnitude of the reflex covaries with subjective pain [109,112]. Thus, researchers have used the NFR as a physiological correlate of spinal nociception. Rhudy et al. [102–104] found that threatening images facilitated pain and increased the NFR, suggesting that emotion enhances nociceptive processing by activating descending brain-to-spinal cord circuitry. Given that pictures do not represent an immediate threat, the variation in emotional intensity elicited by pictures only elicits negative affect with low to moderate arousal (see Fig. 2). None-theless, the degree of nociceptive facilitation appeared to depend on the amount of arousal the pictures elicited, with greater facilitation resulting from greater emotional intensity [104].

It is also interesting to note that the ability of negative affect to engage descending facilitatory processes may depend on the predict-ability of the noxious stimulus. Rhudy and colleagues [103] manipulated whether the noxious shocks presented during emotional picture-viewing were predictable: half of participants received a cue (a light) just before each shock was delivered (predictable), whereas the other half received no cue (unpredictable). In both groups, unpleasant pictures facilitated pain report. However, the NFR was not modulated by unpleasant pictures when the noxious shock was predictable. This finding suggests that descending modulation was disengaged at the same time that supraspinal modulatory mechanisms that alter pain report remained intact.

In other studies, IAPS stimuli were found to modulate additional physiological responses to noxious stimuli, such as skin conductance re-sponse [96,104], heart rate acceleration [96,104], and eye blink magnitude [134]. Moreover, Kenntner-Mabialia and Pauli [51] demonstrated that pain-evoked somatosensory potentials were enhanced by unpleasant pic-tures. Taken together, studies of negative affect of low to moderate inten-sity suggest that hyperalgesia is observed and that this effect can involve descending circuits that modulate ascending nociception at spinal levels, especially when the noxious stimulus is unpredictable (and thus more anxiety provoking).

Relatively few studies have examined the influence of *intense* negative emotions on pain, primarily due to the difficulty of doing so in an ethical and safe manner. Nonetheless, a few well-controlled studies have been successful. Pitman and colleagues [85] exposed war veterans suffering from PTSD and a control group to a combat-related video. The video elicited highly arousing negative affect and hypoalgesia in the PTSD group, an effect that was opioid mediated. Janssen and Arntz [48] presented live spiders to arachnophobics to elicit intense negative affect. In this study, the manipulation also resulted in an opioid-mediated hypoalgesia, although it is unclear whether phobic stimuli reliably elicit hypoalgesia [c.f. 49].

Negative affect-induced hypoalgesia is not limited to clinical samples, however. For example, Janssen and Arntz [50] have shown that a parachute jump can induce an opioid-mediated hypoalgesia. Rhudy and Meagher [95,97,100,101] have shown that an intense, negative affect-producing shock results in elevated heat pain thresholds, and Willer [133] has shown that a neutral stimulus previously paired with a very intense shock of 70 mA inhibits spinal nociception (as assessed from the NFR).

To summarize, the influence of negative affect on pain can be facilitatory or inhibitory. While this complexity led to some initial confusion in the literature, it appears the direction of modulation is dependent on the intensity of the negative emotion that is elicited [99]. Negative affect of low to moderate intensity that stems from unpredictable, future threat (e.g., anxiety) results in hyperalgesia. In contrast, intense negative affect that stems from a present, immediate, predictable threat (e.g., fear) results in hypoalgesia.

Experimental Evidence for the Relationship between Negative Affect and Pain in Functional Pain Disorders

Numerous correlational studies have identified a relationship between negative affect and functional pain disorders [19,41,43,58,116,124]. However, there are relatively few experimental studies. Emotion-induction paradigms, combined with well-controlled experimental pain procedures, have the capacity to provide significant insight into pathophysiological mechanisms of chronic pain syndromes [25,81,104]. Sensitization or dysregulation of threat detection circuitry may lead to a lower threshold to experience negative emotions, more prolonged negative emotions, or exacerbated levels of negative emotions in patients with functional pain syndromes [73]. These mechanisms may result in a greater propensity toward negative affect-induced hyperalgesia. In addition, these patients may have depleted resources for engaging pain inhibitory mechanisms [62,114,132]. Thus, intense, highly arousing negative emotions may not elicit hypoalgesia, as noted in healthy individuals. If any or all of these circumstances are true, the net result would be enhanced pain sensitivity in these populations.

Evidence suggests that negative emotions and stress can exacer-bate clinical pain. Davis and colleagues [18] studied experimentally induced negative affect on clinical pain in persons with FM or osteoarthritis. Half of the participants were first primed using sad imagery, while the other half were not. All participants were then asked to recall a stressful inter-personal conflict. Results suggested that FM patients who were primed reported enhanced pain during the stress recall manipulation. This en-hanced pain also persisted during a subsequent recovery period, but only in the primed FM group. Gannon and colleagues [31] exposed headache patients and controls to a stressful mental arithmetic task. Over 68% of participants who suffered from frequent migraine or tension headaches developed a headache during this stressful procedure. However, only 25% of participants with infrequent headaches developed a headache. Mon-toya and colleagues [81] used pleasant and unpleasant pictures from the IAPS to manipulate affect in patients with FM or musculoskeletal pain without fibromyalgia. They found that unpleasant pictures enhanced FM pain relative to pleasant pictures and a no-picture baseline condition. This effect was not noted in the musculoskeletal pain group.

A few studies have experimentally induced emotion and pain in patients with functional pain disorders. Bach and colleagues [7] induced stress through anticipation of a public speaking task in IBS patients and controls before the participants were exposed to rectal distension. These authors found an abnormal physiological stress response in patients (in-creased heart rate reactivity), but the stress manipulation did not alter discomfort thresholds to distension for either group. Posserud and colleagues [88] tested pain and discomfort thresholds from rectal distension in IBS patients and controls after mental stress (induced by the Stroop test and mental arithmetic). Their results also suggested abnormal stress responses in IBS patients (greater subjective stress, higher corticotropin-releasing hormone and adrenocorticotropic hormone [ACTH] levels, and lower epinephrine and norepinephrine levels). Discomfort thresholds decreased in controls during and after stress, but only after stress in patients. Distension pain thresholds decreased (i.e., hyperalgesia occurred) in patients after stress. However, it is important to note that no controls experienced pain from the distension in this study; therefore, it is difficult to interpret these data. Dickhaus and colleagues [24] exposed IBS patients and controls to noise stress (conflicting music) or relaxing sounds (ocean waves) and examined the effect on pain due to rectal distension. Results suggested that IBS patients had slightly stronger negative emotional responses to the stressor, although there were no group differences in stress-related neuroendocrine responses (norepinephrine, ACTH, cortisol, and prolactin levels). Nonetheless, noise stress enhanced distension-related pain relative to relaxing noise only in IBS patients.

To date, only one study has examined the effects of picture-evoked emotions on experimental pain in persons with functional pain disorders. Arnold and colleagues [2] presented pain-related, unpleasant, neutral, and pleasant IAPS pictures to participants with FM, back pain, and somatoform disorder, and healthy controls. During picture-viewing, they tested pressure pain applied to the finger. They found that all groups showed a similar pattern of modulation, with unpleasant and pain-related pictures enhancing pain relative to neutral pictures. Pain-related pictures showed the greatest facilitatory effects.

In a recent imaging study, Berman and colleagues [9] examined the effect of a cue that predicted the onset of rectal distension in IBS patients and controls. Although the study design did not allow the authors to examine the influence of the cue on distension-related pain, it did provide a means of examining brain activation patterns associated with pain and pain expectation. Results suggested that the cue elicited greater negative affect (stress, anxiety, and anger) in patients. Moreover, the cue deactivated brain regions associated with nociceptive modulation (insula, ACC, amygdala, and dorsal brainstem) in controls to a greater extent than in patients (especially the insula and brainstem). Interestingly, anticipatory decreases in the brainstem were correlated with self-reported negative affect, suggesting that emotion may influence the activation of these regions involved with descending modulation.

To summarize, there appears to be a linkage between enhanced negative affect and functional pain disorders. However, there is a relative paucity of experimental studies examining the relationship between negative affect and enhanced pain in these populations. Nonetheless, there is some suggestion that emotion and stress reactivity may be dysregulated in some persons with functional pain disorders and that this dysregulation could contribute to enhanced pain. Clearly, additional well-controlled experimental research is needed.

Neurobiology of Anxiety and Functional Pain Disorders

Studies of the neurobiology of pain have identified structures and networks that may be important for the altered attention, affective response, and pain modulation seen in functional pain disorders. Although many of these aspects are discussed elsewhere in this volume, we will briefly review several that may directly play a role in the interplay of negative affect and functional pain symptoms. These involve corticolimbic interactions as well as brainstem areas involved in pain modulation, autonomic regulation, and peripheral manifestations of the defensive response (see Fig. 1).

A variety of corticocortical and corticolimbic interactions have been identified as playing a role in the response to both emotional and painful stimuli. Differential activation of subregions of the cingulate gyrus can be elicited by a wide variety of experimental stimuli, including somatic and visceral pain and emotional stimuli [11,37,74]. Areas of the dorsal cingulate cortex, especially an area toward the middle of the cingulate cortex, together with the insular cortex and the thalamus, respond to a wide range of painful and nonpainful, interoceptive, and exteroceptive stimuli and inform the brain about the homeostatic state of the organism. This group of structures has recently been labeled the "homeostatic afferent processing network" [74]. The most rostral aspect of the dorsal cingulate (subgenual ACC) and the adjacent medial prefrontal cortex have been implicated in negative feedback regulation of the amygdala and in arousal [68,87]. The same brain regions, which are rich in μ-opioid receptors, have also been implicated in the regulation of endogenous pain inhibition circuits [140]. Thus, the subgenual ACC/medial prefrontal cortex play important roles in the regulation both of emotional arousal and of pain perception [122].

It is therefore likely that altered activity in these same networks may be involved in the altered CNS responses associated with both chronic anxiety and functional pain disorders. A common finding across a variety of functional pain populations is an increased response in the mid-cingulate cortex to painful stimulation when compared to controls without pain disorders and in some cases when compared to patients with similar symptoms but with a clear peripheral organic cause [16,33,37,71,125]. In FM, activation in the dorsal ACC has been associated with greater cata-strophizing [36]. Of perhaps even more relevance for the overlap of anxi-ety and pain mechanisms is the finding of altered relationships between cognitive control areas of the lateral prefrontal cortex and limbic struc-tures such as the medial prefrontal cortex and amygdala in both anxiety and functional pain disorders [8,71]. Thus, it may be that a commonality across affective and functional pain disorders is primarily rooted in inef-fective neurocognitive control, leading to increased or sustained arousal responses, especially when the individual is confronted with a salient affective stimulus.

The primary circuit by which supraspinal centers can alter afferent nociception involves the periaqueductal gray (PAG), and its projections to the rostral ventromedial medulla (RVM) and dorsolateral pons/tegmentum [30,33]. This circuit has been implicated in both descending inhibition and facilitation of nociception [30,121]. The PAG-RVM circuit receives input from higher brain centers including the hypothalamus, cortex (e.g., anterior cingulate), and amygdala [30,40,79], and it is through these ex-tensive connections that cognitive, affective, and autonomic factors are believed to modulate nociception [30]. For example, ACC projections to the PAG-RVM are implicated in reductions in pain due to placebo

[10] and distraction [123]. Additionally, the amygdala is known to play an important role in fear and anxiety [20] and in conditioned fear reactions [44,53], and animal research has suggested that connections between the amygdala and PAG-RVM are involved in affective modulation of nociception [17,44,53,75]. Interestingly, evidence suggests that if the amygdala were to become sensitized, this condition could promote the initiation and/or maintenance of chronic pain in the absence of a peripheral organic cause [82].

Clinical Implications of Anxiety in Functional Pain Disorders

Assessment

The discussion above suggests several important areas of assessment related to anxiety that should be part of routine care for patients with functional pain disorders. These areas include general anxiety symptoms, symptom-specific anxiety, and history of trauma. Although these topics can be assessed relatively well during a clinical history, there are several advantages to using a validated self-report instrument. First, accurate assessment of anxiety requires an active questioning process regarding specific symptoms and their impact, which may be difficult in very brief primary care visits. Second, scales provide a better measure of the relative severity of the anxiety based on both general and functional pain norms. Fortunately, well-validated and brief instruments are available for these anxiety constructs. For anxiety symptoms, the Hospital Anxiety and Depression scales were specifically designed for use in a general medical context; this instrument is brief, with 11 items for the anxiety scale. Scales for symptom-specific anxiety in musculoskeletal pain and FM include the Tampa Scale for Kinesiophobia and the Fear-Avoidance Beliefs Questionnaire [117]. The Visceral Sensitivity Index is the only scale developed and validated specifically for anxiety related to visceral pain [57]. The Anxiety Sensitivity Index, although more targeted at panic symptoms, has been widely used in multiple pain disorders including headache [83]. Diagnosis of anxiety disorders is made using the DSM-IV categories and typically is beyond the scope of a general medical visit. However, familiarity with the most important disorders that may affect patient care, including panic disorder, generalized anxiety disorder, and PTSD, would be worthwhile for practitioners treating functional pain disorders [1].

Treatment

Many of the most widely used treatments for functional pain disorders act on overlapping mechanisms involved in pain and negative affect or anxiety. They include psychopharmacological treatments using antidepressants, anticonvulsants, and anti-anxiety medications; psychological therapies including cognitive behavioral therapy; and lifestyle interventions such as exercise programs. Most of these treatments have shown some efficacy, especially for global improvement measures; and these data are reviewed in the "Treatment" section of this volume. An important question relevant to the topic of this chapter regards whether improvements in mood and improvements in functional pain symptoms change in parallel, are independent, or if positive change in one results in secondary changes in the other. To date there has been little direct study of these questions. However, some recent research has shown that symptomatic improvements from both pharmacological and psychological therapies do not depend on changes in mood (e.g., [3,55]). Also, while several of the primary hypothesized methods of action of both psychological and pharmacological treatment involve anxiety-related mechanisms [65], there is good evidence that the presence of anxiety or depression is not a prerequisite for the efficacy of either type of treatment and that symptoms can be improved without working through major changes in general mood.

Future Research Directions

More well-controlled experimental research is needed that examines the relationship between negative affect and pain processing in patients with functional pain disorders. If true, the hypothesis that there is a non-monotonic relationship between negative affect and pain modulation has a number of important implications. First, it is important to consider individual differences in emotional responsiveness to different stimuli and stressors. When the effects of a stressor or emotionally-charged stimulus are examined, some patients may react with hyperalgesia whereas others will respond with hypoalgesia. If so, there would be a zero net influence on pain at the group level. This consideration leads to a second suggestion—that measures should be taken to assess the physiological and subjective indices of emotion. Individual differences in emotional reactivity may determine how pain is modulated. Third, measures that assess the degree and quality of emotional intensity should be used. In particular, differences in arousal (affective intensity) may help determine the degree of threat experienced by the individual (anxiety versus fear), but also the direction of negative affect-induced pain modulation (hyperalgesia versus hypoalgesia). Fourth, it is important to keep in mind that the predictability of the noxious event may affect the mechanisms by which negative affect modulates pain. As noted by Rhudy and colleagues [103], descending facilitation of spinal nociception can be disengaged when the noxious stimulus is predictable. This finding has important implications for clinical treatments that address the sense of unpredictability and lack of control experienced by patients with functional pain disorders. And finally, although we have focused specifically on the role of negative affective states, it is important to simultaneously examine the role of positive affect. For example, deficits in positive affect may be associated with symptom exacerbation during periods of stress and negative emotion [138].

It is also important to use experimental designs that provide a means of disentangling the direction of the negative emotion-pain relationship. One suggestion is to experimentally manipulate emotion using within-subject designs. However, this issue can also be addressed in treatment studies by making sure to assess various forms of negative affect and functional pain symptoms longitudinally. Another issue involves more careful study of the relationship between symptom-specific fear or anxiety and more general anxiety. While these two constructs may share primary mechanisms, symptom-specific fear or anxiety is likely to be the negative affect that is more influential in clinical situations, but it is often overlooked as a predictor and outcome measure in studies. Finally, more use of functional brain imaging and other measures of CNS activity (such as startle responses, brain electrical responses, and nociceptive reflexes) as both biomarkers and mechanistic tools will be extremely useful to test the neurocognitive mechanisms that underlie the relationship between negative affect and functional pain disorders.

Acknowledgments

Supported in part by NIH grants NR007768, P50 DK64539, VA Medical Research, University of Tulsa Summer Faculty Fellowships, and a grant from the Oklahoma Center for the Advancement of Science and Technology (HR06-177S).

References

[1]   American Psychiatric Association. Diagnostic and statistical manual for the mental disorders (DSM-IV). Washington, DC: American Psychiatric Association; 1994.
[2]   Arnold BS, Alpers GW, Suss H, Friedel E, Kosmutzky G, Geier A, Pauli P. Affective pain modulation in fibromyalgia, somatoform pain disorder, back pain, and healthy controls. Eur J Pain 2008;12:329–38.
[3]   Arnold LM, Crofford LJ, Martin SA, Young JP, Sharma U. The effect of anxiety and depression on improvements in pain in a randomized, controlled trial of pregabalin for treatment of fibromyalgia. Pain Med 2007;8:633–8.
[4]   Arnold LM, Hudson JI, Keck PE, Auchenbach MB, Javaras KN, Hess EV. Comorbidity of fibromyalgia and psychiatric disorders. J Clin Psychiatry 2006;67:1219–25.
[5]   Asmundson GJ. Commentary: Anxiety, sensitivity and the pain experience. Eur J Pain 2001;5:23–5.
[6]   Asmundson GJ, Norton PJ, Norton GR. Beyond pain: The role of fear and avoidance in chronicity. Clin Psychol Rev 1999;19:97–119.
[7]   Bach DR, Erdmann G, Schmidtmann M, Monnikes H. Emotional stress reactivity in irritable bowel syndrome. Eur J Gastroenterol Hepatol 2006;18:629–36.
[8]   Berman SM, Naliboff BD, Suyenobu B, Labus JS, Stains J, Ohning G, Kilpatrick L, Bueller JA, Ruby K, Jarcho J, Mayer EA. Reduced brainstem inhibition during anticipated pelvic visceral pain correlates with enhanced brain response to the visceral stimulus in women with irritable bowel syndrome. J Neurosci 2008;28:349–59.
[9]   Berman SM, Naliboff BD, Suyenobu B, Labus JS, Stains J, Ohning G, Kilpatrick L, Bueller JA, Ruby K, Jarcho J, Mayer EA. Reduced brainstem inhibition during anticipated pelvic visceral pain correlates with enhanced brain response to the visceral stimulus in women with irritable bowel syndrome. J Neurosci 2008;28:349–59.
[10] Bingel U, Lorenz J, Schoell E, Weiller C, Buchel C. Mechanisms of placebo analgesia: rACC recruitment of a subcortical antinociceptive network. Pain 2006;120:8–15.
[11] Bishop S, Duncan J, Brett M, Lawrence AD. Prefrontal cortical function and anxiety: controlling attention to threat-related stimuli. Nat Neurosci 2004;7:184–8.
[12] Bradesi S, Schwetz I, Ennes HS, Lamy CM, Ohning G, Fanselow M, Pothoulakis C, McRoberts JA, Mayer EA. Repeated exposure to water avoidance stress in rats: A new model for sustained visceral hyperalgesia. Am J Physiol Gastrointest Liver Physiol 2005;289:G42–G53.
[13] Bradley MM, Codispoti M, Cuthbert BN, Lang PJ. Emotion and motivation I: Defensive and appetitive reactions in picture processing. Emotion 2001;1:276–98.
[14] Center for the Study of Emotion and Attention (CSEA). The International Affective Picture System: Digitized photographs. Gainesville: The University of Florida. Available at: http://csea.phhp.ufl.edu/index.html.

[15] Chang L, Berman S, Mayer EA, Suyenobu B, Derbyshire S, Naliboff B, Vogt B, FitzGerald L, Mandelkern MA. Brain responses to visceral and somatic stimuli in patients with irritable bowel syndrome with and without fibromyalgia. Am J Gastroenterol 2003;98:1354–61.

[16] Cornwall A, Donderi DC. The effect of experimentally induced anxiety on the experience of pressure pain. Pain 1988;35:105–13.

[17] Crown ED, King TE, Meagher MW, Grau JW. Shock-induced hyperalgesia: III. Role of the bed nucleus of the stria terminalis and amygdaloid nuclei. Behav Neurosci 2000;114:561–73.

[18] Davis MC, Zautra AJ, Reich JW. Vulnerability to stress among women in chronic pain from fibromyalgia and osteoarthritis. Ann Behav Med 2001;23:215.

[19] De Benedittis G, Lorenzetti A. The role of stressful life events in the persistence of primary headache: major events vs. daily hassles. Pain 1992;51:35–42.

[20] De Oca BM, Fanselow MS. Amygdala and periaqueductal gray lesions only partially attenuate unconditional defensive responses in rats exposed to a cat. Integr Physiol Behav Sci 2004;39:318–33.

[21] de Wied M, Verbaten MN. Affective pictures processing, attention, and pain tolerance. Pain 2001;90:163–72.

[22] Diatchenko L, Anderson AD, Slade GD, Fillingim RB, Shabalina SA, Higgins TJ, Sama S, Belfer I, Goldman D, Max MB, Weir BS, Maixner W. Three major haplotypes of the beta2 adrenergic receptor define psychological profile, blood pressure, and the risk for development of a common musculoskeletal pain disorder. Am J Med Genet B Neuropsychiatr Genet 2006;141:449–62.

[23] Diatchenko L, Nackley AG, Slade GD, Fillingim RB, Maixner W. Idiopathic pain disorders: pathways of vulnerability. Pain 2006;123:226–30.

[24] Dickhaus B, Mayer EA, Firooz N, Stains J, Conde F, Olivas TI, Fass R, Chang L, Mayer M, Naliboff BD. Irritable bowel syndrome patients show enhanced modulation of visceral perception by auditory stress. Am J Gastroenterol 2003;98:135–43.

[25] Edwards RR, Sarlani E, Wesselmann U, Fillingim RB. Quantitative assessment of experimental pain perception: multiple domains of clinical relevance. Pain 2005;114:315–9.

[26] Edwards RR, Smith MT, Stonerock G, Haythornthwaite JA. Pain-related catastrophizing in healthy women is associated with greater temporal summation of and reduced habituation to thermal pain. Clin J Pain 2006;22:730–7.

[27] Eley TC, Gregory AM, Clark DM, Ehlers A. Feeling anxious: a twin study of panic/somatic ratings, anxiety sensitivity and heartbeat perception in children. J Child Psychol Psychiatry 2007;48:1184–91.

[28] Epstein SA, Kay G, Clauw D, Heaton R, Klein D, Krupp L, Kuck J, Leslie V, Masur D, Wagner M, Waid R, Zisook S. Psychiatric disorders in patients with fibromyalgia. A multicenter investigation. Psychosomatics 1999;40:57–63.

[29] Fanselow MS. Neural organization of the defensive behavior system responsible for fear. Psychonom Bull Rev 1994;1:429–38.

[30] Fields HL, Basbaum AI. Central nervous system mechanisms of pain modulation. In: Wall PD, Melzack R, editors. Textbook of pain. Edinburgh: Churchill Livingston; 1999. pp 309–29.

[31] Gannon LR, Haynes SN, Cuevas J, Chavez R. Psychophysiological correlates of induced headaches. J Behav Med 1987;10:411–23.

[32] Garrett AS, Maddock RJ. Separating subjective emotion from the perception of emotion-inducing stimuli: an fMRI study. Neuroimage 2006;33:263.

[33] Giesecke T, Gracely RH, Grant MA, Nachemson A, Petzke F, Williams DA, Clauw DJ. Evidence of augmented central pain processing in idiopathic chronic low back pain. Arthritis Rheum 2004;50:613–23.

[34] Goubert L, Crombez G, Van Damme S. The role of neuroticism, pain catastrophizing and pain-related fear in vigilance to pain: a structural equations approach. Pain 2004;107:234–41.

[35] Goubert L, Crombez G, Van Damme S. The role of neuroticism, pain catastrophizing and pain-related fear in vigilance to pain: A structural equations approach. Pain 2004;107:234–41.

[36] Gracely RH, Geisser ME, Giesecke T, Grant MA, Petzke F, Williams DA, Clauw DJ. Pain catastrophizing and neural responses to pain among persons with fibromyalgia. Brain 2004;127:835–43.

[37] Gracely RH, Petzke F, Wolf JM, Clauw DJ. Functional magnetic resonance imaging evidence of augmented pain processing in fibromyalgia. Arthritis Rheum 2002;46:1333–43.

[38] Granot M, Granovsky Y, Sprecher E, Nir RR, Yarnitsky D. Contact heat-evoked temporal summation: tonic versus repetitive-phasic stimulation. Pain 2006;122:295–305.

[39] Grimm S, Schmidt CF, Bermpohl F, Heinzel A, Dahlem Y, Wyss M, Hell D, Boesiger P, Boeker H, Northoff G. Segregated neural representation of distinct emotion dimensions in the prefrontal cortex-an fMRI study. Neuroimage 2006;30:325.

[40] Hadjipavlou G, Dunckley P, Behrens TE, Tracey I. Determining anatomical connectivities between cortical and brainstem pain processing regions in humans: a diffusion tensor imaging study in healthy controls. Pain 2006;123:169–78.

[41] Harrigan JA, Kues JR, Ricks DF, Smith R. Moods that predict coming migraine headaches. Pain 1984;20:385–96.

[42] Haslam DR. The effect of threatened shock upon pain threshold. Psychonom Sci 1966;6:309–10.

[43] Hazlett-Stevens H, Craske MG, Mayer EA, Chang L, Naliboff BD. Prevalence of irritable bowel syndrome among university students: the roles of worry, neuroticism, anxiety sensitivity and visceral anxiety. J Psychosom Res 2003;55:501–5.

[44] Helmstetter FJ. The amygdala is essential for the expression of conditional hypoalgesia. Behav Neurosci 1992;106:518–28.

[45] Henningsen P, Zimmermann T, Sattel H. Medically unexplained physical symptoms, anxiety, and depression: a meta-analytic review. Psychosom Med 2003;65:528–33.

[46] Hettema JM, Prescott CA, Myers JM, Neale MC, Kendler KS. The structure of genetic and environmental risk factors for anxiety disorders in men and women. Arch Gen Psychiatry 2005;62:182–9.

[47] Irwin C, Falsetti SA, Lydiard RB, Ballenger JC, Brock CD, Brener W. Comorbidity of posttraumatic stress disorder and irritable bowel syndrome. J Clin Psychiatry 1996;57:576–8.

[48] Janssen SA, Arntz A. Anxiety and pain: attentional and endorphinergic influences. Pain 1996;66:145–50.

[49] Janssen SA, Arntz A. No evidence for opioid-mediated analgesia induced by phobic fear. Behav Res Ther 1997;35:823–30.

[50] Janssen SA, Arntz A. Real-life stress and opioid-mediated analgesia in novice parachute jumpers. J Psychophysiol 2001;15:106–13.

[51] Kenntner-Mabiala R, Pauli P. Affective modulation of brain potentials to painful and nonpainful stimuli. Psychophysiol 2005;42:559–67.

[52] Keogh E, Cochrane M. Anxiety sensitivity, cognitive biases, and the experience of pain. J Pain 2002;3:320–9.

[53] Kim JJ, Rison RA, Fanselow MS. Effects of amygdala, hippocampus, and periaqueductal gray lesions on short- and long-term contextual fear. Behav Neurosci 1993;107:1093–8.

[54] King CD, Devine DP, Vierck CJ, Mauderli A, Yezierski RP. Opioid modulation of reflex versus operant responses following stress in the rat. Neuroscience 2007;147:174–82.

[55] Kroenke K, Swindle R. Cognitive-behavioral therapy for somatization and symptom syndromes: a critical review of controlled clinical trials. Psychother Psychosom 2000;69:205–15.

[56] Kumano H, Kaiya H, Yoshiuchi K, Yamanaka G, Sasaki T, Kuboki T. Comorbidity of irritable bowel syndrome, panic disorder, and agoraphobia in a Japanese representative sample. Am J Gastroenterol 2004;99:370–6.

[57] Labus J, Bolus R, Chang L, Wiklund I, Naesdal J, Mayer E, Naliboff B. The visceral sensitivity index: development and validation of a gastrointestinal symptom-specific anxiety scale. Aliment Pharmacol Ther 2004;20:89–97.

[58] Labus JS, Mayer EA, Chang L, Bolus R, Naliboff BD. The central role of gastrointestinal-specific anxiety in irritable bowel syndrome: further validation of the visceral sensitivity index. Psychosom Med 2007;69:89–98.

[59] Lake AE, 3rd, Rains JC, Penzien DB, Lipchik GL. Headache and psychiatric comorbidity: historical context, clinical implications, and research relevance. Headache 2005;45:493–506.

[60] Lang PJ, Bradley MM, Cuthbert BN. International Affective Picture System (IAPS): Technical Manual and Affective Ratings. NIMH Center for the Study of Emotion and Attention; 2001.

[61] Lang PJ, Davis M. Emotion, motivation, and the brain: Reflex foundations in animal and human research. Prog Brain Res 2006;156:3–29.

[62] Lautenbacher S, Rollman GB. Possible deficiencies of pain modulation in fibromyalgia. Clin J Pain 1997;13:189.

[63] LeDoux JE. Emotion circuits in the brain. Annu Rev Neurosci 2000;23:155–84.
[64] Lydiard RB. Irritable bowel syndrome, anxiety, and depression: what are the links? J Clin Psychiatry 2001;62 Suppl 8:38–45; discussion 6–7.
[65] Lydiard RB. Psychopharmacology in the treatment of irritable bowel syndrome. Primary Psychiatry 2007;14:40–2, 45–9.
[66] Lydiard RB, Greenwald S, Weissman MM, Johnson J, Drossman DA, Ballenger JC. Panic disorder and gastrointestinal symptoms: findings from the NIMH Epidemiologic Catchment Area project. Am J Psychiatry 1994;151:64–70.
[67] Marek P, Yirmiya R, Liebeskind JC. Strain differences in the magnitude of swimming-induced analgesia in mice correlates with brain opiate receptor concentration. Brain Res 1988;447:188–90.
[68] Maren S, Quirk GJ. Neuronal signalling of fear memory. Nat Rev Neurosci 2004;5:844–52.
[69] Martin GN. The effect of exposure to odor on the perception of pain. Psychosom Med 2006;68:613–6.
[70] Martin PR, Lae L, Reece J. Stress as a trigger for headaches: relationship between exposure and sensitivity. Anxiety Stress Coping 2007;20:393–407.
[71] Mayer EA, Berman S, Suyenobu B, Labus J, Mandelkern MA, Naliboff BD, Chang L. Differences in brain responses to visceral pain between patients with irritable bowel syndrome and ulcerative colitis. Pain 2005;115:398–409.
[72] Mayer EA, Craske MG, Naliboff BD. Depression, anxiety and the gastrointestinal system. J Clin Psychiatry 2001;62:28–36.
[73] Mayer EA, Naliboff BD, Chang L. Basic pathophysiologic mechanisms in irritable bowel syndrome. Dig Dis 2001;19:212–8.
[74] Mayer EA, Naliboff BD, Craig AD. Neuroimaging of the brain-gut axis: from basic understanding to treatment of functional GI disorders. Gastroenterology 2006;131:1925–42.
[75] McLemore S, Crown ED, Meagher MW, Grau JW. Shock-induced hyperalgesia: II. Role of the dorsolateral periaqueductal gray. Behav Neurosci 1999;113:539–49.
[76] Meagher MW, Arnau RC, Rhudy JL. Pain and emotion: effects of affective picture modulation. Psychosom Med 2001;63:79–90.
[77] Meagher MW, Ferguson AR, Crown ED, McLemore S, King TE, Sieve AN, Grau JW. Shock-induced hyperalgesia: IV. Generality. J Exp Psychol Anim Behav Process 2001;27:219–38.
[78] Meyer TJ, Miller ML, Metzger RL, Borkovec TD. Development and validation of the Penn State Worry Questionnaire. Behav Res Ther 1990;28:487–95.
[79] Millan MJ. Descending control of pain. Prog Neurobiol 2002;66:355–474.
[80] Mini A, Rau H, Montoya P, Palomba D, Birbaumer N. Baroreceptor cortical effects, emotions and pain. Int J Psychophysiol 1995;19:67.
[81] Montoya P, Sitges C, Garcia-Herrera M, Izquierdo R, Truyols M, Blay N, Collado D. Abnormal affective modulation of somatosensory brain processing among patients with fibromyalgia. Psychosom Med 2005;67:957.
[82] Neugebauer V, Li W, Bird GC, Han JS. The amygdala and persistent pain. Neuroscientist 2004;10:221–34.
[83] Norton PJ, Asmundson GJ. Anxiety sensitivity, fear, and avoidance behavior in headache pain. Pain 2004;111:218–23.
[84] Pissiota A, Frans O, Michelgard A, Appel L, Langstrom B, Flaten MA, Fredrikson M. Amygdala and anterior cingulate cortex activation during affective startle modulation: a PET study of fear. Eur J Neurosci 2003;18:1325–31.
[85] Pitman RK, van der Kolk BA, Orr SP, Greenberg MS. Naloxone-reversible analgesic response to combat-related stimuli in posttraumatic stress disorder. A pilot study. Arch Gen Psychiatry 1990;47:541–4.
[86] Ploghaus A, Narain C, Beckmann CF, Clare S, Bantick S, Wise R, Matthews PM, Rawlins JN, Tracey I. Exacerbation of pain by anxiety is associated with activity in a hippocampal network. J Neurosci 2001;21:9896.
[87] Porro CA, Lui F, Facchin P, Maieron M, Baraldi P. Percept-related activity in the human somatosensory system: Functional magnetic resonance imaging studies. Magn Reson Imaging 2004;22:1539–48.
[88] Posserud I, Agerforz P, Ekman R, Björnsson ES, Abrahamsson H, Simrén M. Altered visceral perceptual and neuroendocrine response in patients with irritable bowel syndrome during mental stress. Gut 2004;53:1102–8.

[89] Prescott J, Wilkie J. Pain tolerance selectively increased by a sweet-smelling odor. Psychol Sci 2007;18:308–11.

[90] Rainville P, Bao QVH, Chretien P. Pain-related emotions modulate experimental pain perception and autonomic responses. Pain 2005;118:306–18.

[91] Reiss S. Expectancy model of fear, anxiety, and panic. Clin Psychol Rev 1991;11:141–53.

[92] Reiss S. Trait anxiety: It's not what you think it is. J Anxiety Disord 1997;11:201–14.

[93] Reiss S, McNally RJ, Reiss S, Bootzon RR. The expectancy model of fear. In: editor. Theoretical Issues in Behavior Therapy. New York: Academic Press; 1985. pp 107–21.

[94] Reiss S, Peterson RA, Gursky DM, McNally RJ. Anxiety sensitivity, anxiety frequency and the predictions of fearfulness. Behav Res Ther 1986;24:1–8.

[95] Rhudy JL, Grimes JS, Meagher MW. Fear-induced hypoalgesia in humans: effects on low intensity thermal stimulation and finger temperature. J Pain 2004;5:458–68.

[96] Rhudy JL, McCabe KM, Williams AE. Affective modulation of autonomic reactions to noxious stimulation. Int J Psychophysiol 2007;63:105–9.

[97] Rhudy JL, Meagher MW. Fear and anxiety: divergent effects on human pain thresholds. Pain 2000;84:65–75.

[98] Rhudy JL, Meagher MW. Noise stress and human pain thresholds: divergent effects in men and women. J Pain 2001;2:57–64.

[99] Rhudy JL, Meagher MW. The role of emotion in pain modulation. Curr Opin Psychiatry 2001;14:241–5.

[100] Rhudy JL, Meagher MW. Individual differences in the emotional reaction to shock determine whether hypoalgesia is observed. Pain Med 2003;4:244–56.

[101] Rhudy JL, Meagher MW. Negative affect: effects on an evaluative measure of human pain. Pain 2003;104:617–26.

[102] Rhudy JL, Williams AE, McCabe K, Nguyen MA, Rambo P. Affective modulation of nociception at spinal and supraspinal levels. Psychophysiology 2005;42:579–87.

[103] Rhudy JL, Williams AE, McCabe KM, Rambo PL, Russell JL. Emotional modulation of spinal nociception and pain: the impact of predictable noxious stimulation. Pain 2006;126:221–33.

[104] Rhudy JL, Williams AE, McCabe KM, Russell JL, Maynard LJ. Emotional control of nociceptive reactions (ECON): do affective valence and arousal play a role? Pain 2008;136:250–61.

[105] Ringel Y, Drossman DA, Leserman JL, Suyenobu BY, Wilber K, Lin W, Whitehead WE, Naliboff BD, Berman S, Mayer EA. Effect of abuse history on pain reports and brain responses to aversive visceral stimulation: an FMRI study. Gastroenterology 2008;134:396–404.

[106] Robinson ME, Wise EA, Gagnon C, Fillingim RB, Price DD. Influences of gender role and anxiety on sex differences in temporal summation of pain. J Pain 2004;5:77–82.

[107] Roelofs J, McCracken L, Peters ML, Crombez G, van Breukelen G, Vlaeyen JW. Psychometric evaluation of the Pain Anxiety Symptoms Scale (PASS) in chronic pain patients. J Behav Med 2004;27:167–83.

[108] Safren SA, Gershuny BS, Marzol P, Otto MW, Pollack MH. History of childhood abuse in panic disorder, social phobia, and generalized anxiety disorder. J Nerv Ment Dis 2002;190:453–6.

[109] Sandrini G, Serrao M, Rossi P, Romaniello A, Cruccu G, Willer JC. The lower limb flexion reflex in humans. Prog Neurobiol 2005;77:353–95.

[110] Sen S, Burmeister M, Ghosh D. Meta-analysis of the association between a serotonin transporter promotor polymorphism (5-HTTLPR) and anxiety-related personality traits. Am J Med Genet B Neuropsychiatr Genet 2004;127:85–9.

[111] Sieve AN, King TE, Ferguson AR, Grau JW, Meagher MW. Pain and negative affect: evidence the inverse benzodiazepine agonist DMCM inhibits pain and learning in rats. Psychopharmacology (Berl) 2001;153:180–90.

[112] Skljarevski V, Ramadan NM. The nociceptive flexion reflex in humans: review article. Pain 2002;96:3–8.

[113] Smith LD, Wolpin M. Emotive imagery and pain tolerance. In: Shorr JE, Robin P, Connella JA, Wolpin M, editors. Imagery: current perspectives. New York: Plenum Press; 1989. pp 159–73.

[114] Song GH, Venkatraman V, Ho KY, Chee MWL, Yeoh KG, Wilder-Smith CH. Cortical effects of anticipation and endogenous modulation of visceral pain assessed by functional brain MRI in irritable bowel syndrome patients and healthy controls. Pain 2006;126:79–90.

[115] Spielberger CD. State-Trait Anxiety Inventory. Palo-Alto, CA: Consulting Psychologists Press; 1983.
[116] Staud R, Price DD, Robinson ME, Vierck CJ, Jr. Body pain area and pain-related negative affect predict clinical pain intensity in patients with fibromyalgia. J Pain 2004;5:338–43.
[117] Swinkels-Meewisse EJ, Swinkels RA, Verbeek AL, Vlaeyen JW, Oostendorp RA. Psychometric properties of the Tampa Scale for kinesiophobia and the fear-avoidance beliefs questionnaire in acute low back pain. Man Ther 2003;8:29–36.
[118] Talati A, Ponniah K, Strug LJ, Hodge SE, Fyer AJ, Weissman MM. Panic disorder, social anxiety disorder, and a possible medical syndrome previously linked to chromosome 13. Biol Psychiatry 2008;63:594–601.
[119] Talley NJ, Boyce PM, Jones M. Is the association between irritable bowel syndrome and abuse explained by neuroticism? A population based study. Gut 1998;42:47–53.
[120] Taylor S, Cox BJ. Anxiety sensitivity: Multiple dimensions and hierarchic structure. Behav Res Ther 1998;36:37–51.
[121] Urban MO, Gebhart GF. Supraspinal contributions to hyperalgesia. Proc Natl Acad Sci USA 1999;96:7687–92.
[122] Valet M, Sprenger T, Boecker H, Willoch F, Rummeny E, Conrad B, Erhard P, Tolle TR. Distraction modulates connectivity of the cingulo-frontal cortex and the midbrain during pain: an fMRI analysis. Pain 2004;109:399–408.
[123] Valet M, Sprenger T, Boecker H, Willoch F, Rummeny E, Conrad B, Erhard P, Tolle TR. Distraction modulates connectivity of the cingulo-frontal cortex and the midbrain during pain-an fMRI analysis. Pain 2004;109:399–408.
[124] van Middendorp H, Lumley MA, Jacobs JWG, van Doornen LJP, Bijlsma JWJ, Geenen R. Emotions and emotional approach and avoidance strategies in fibromyalgia. J Psychosom Res 2008;64:159–67.
[125] Verne GN, Himes NC, Robinson ME, Gopinath KS, Briggs RW, Crosson B, Price DD. Central representation of visceral and cutaneous hypersensitivity in the irritable bowel syndrome. Pain 2003;103:99–110.
[126] Villemure C, Slotnick BM, Bushnell MC. Effects of odors on pain perception: deciphering the roles of emotion and attention. Pain 2003;106:101–8.
[127] Vlaeyen JW, Linton SJ. Fear-avoidance and its consequences in chronic musculoskeletal pain: a state of the art. Pain 2000;85:317–32.
[128] Walker DL, Toufexis DJ, Davis M. Role of the bed nucleus of the stria terminalis versus the amygdala in fear, stress, and anxiety. Eur J Pharmacol 2003;463:199–216.
[129] Walker EA, Katon WJ, Jemelka RP, Roy-Byrne PP. Comorbidity of gastrointestinal complaints, depression, and anxiety in the epidemiologic catchment area (ECA) study. Am J Med 1992;92:26S-30S.
[130] Walters ET. Injury related behavior and neural plasticity: an evolutionary perspective on sensitization, hyperalgesia, and analgesia. Int Rev Neurobiol 1994;36:325–426.
[131] Weisenberg M, Aviram O, Wolf Y, Raphaeli N. Relevant and irrelevant anxiety in the reaction to pain. Pain 1984;20:371–83.
[132] Wilder-Smith CH, Schindler D, Lovblad K, Redmond SM, Nirkko A. Brain functional magnetic resonance imaging of rectal pain and activation of endogenous inhibitory mechanisms in irritable bowel syndrome patient subgroups and healthy controls. Gut 2004;53:1595–601.
[133] Willer JC. Anticipation of pain-produced stress: Electrophysiological study in man. Physiol Behav 1980;25:49–51.
[134] Williams AE, Rhudy JL. Affective modulation of eyeblink reactions to noxious sural nerve stimulation: a supraspinal measure of nociceptive reactivity? Int J Psychophysiol 2007;66:255–65.
[135] Williams AE, Rhudy JL. The influence of conditioned fear on human pain thresholds: does preparedness play a role? J Pain 2007;8:598–606.
[136] Wu EQ, Birnbaum H, Mareva M, Parece A, Huang Z, Mallett D, Taitel H. Interstitial cystitis: cost, treatment and co-morbidities in an employed population. Pharmacoeconomics 2006;24:55–65.
[137] Wunsch A, Philippot P, Plaghki L. Affective associative learning modifies the sensory perception of nociceptive stimuli without participant's awareness. Pain 2003;102:27–38.
[138] Zautra AJ, Fasman R, Reich JW, Harakas P, Johnson LM, Olmsted ME, Davis MC. Fibromyalgia: evidence for deficits in positive affect regulation. Psychosom Med 2005;67:147.
[139] Zelman DC, Howland EW, Nichols SN, Cleeland CS. The effects of induced mood on laboratory pain. Pain 1991;46:105–11.

[140] Zubieta JK, Smith YR, Bueller JA, Xu Y, Kilbourn MR, Jewett DM, Meyer CR, Koeppe RA, Stohler CS. Regional mu opioid receptor regulation of sensory and affective dimensions of pain. Science 2001;293:311–5.
[141] Zwart JA, Dyb G, Hagen K, Odegard KJ, Dahl AA, Bovim G, Stovner LJ. Depression and anxiety disorders associated with headache frequency. The Nord-Trondelag Health Study. Eur J Neurol 2003;10:147–52.

Correspondence to: Bruce D. Naliboff, PhD, Center for Neurobiology of Stress, VA GLAHS, Building 115, Room 223, 11301 Wilshire Boulevard, Los Angeles, CA 90073, USA. Email: naliboff @ucla.edu.

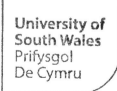

Chronic Pain and Depression

Alan F. Schatzberg

Department of Psychiatry and Behavioral Sciences, Stanford University School of Medicine, Stanford, California, USA

Chronic pain and depression are clearly linked, although the exact mechanisms are not entirely known. Epidemiological and clinical data both point to a clear relationship; however, the potentially bidirectional cause-versus-effect aspects have not been elucidated. The co-occurrence presents challenges to clinicians because patients with depression and pain are often more chronically depressed and more difficult to treat than depressives without pain. Optimal treatment strategies are not entirely clear. This chapter reviews key issues in the relationship between chronic pain and depression.

Prevalence

Most early studies on comorbidity were derived from clinical series, often in medical settings [21]. In patients with physical conditions and pain, depression rates range from 13% to 85% [4,44] and are higher than those seen in patients without pain. Conversely, similarly high rates of pain are observed in depressed patients in community-based medical settings. Generally, the estimated rates of comorbidity have been between 30% and 70%. For example, a recent study by Kroenke et al. [28] reported that in medical practices, 42% of depressed subjects had at least moderate pain.

These clinical sample data are somewhat intuitive; however, they leave a major question regarding whether such relationships are observed in the general community or merely reflect more severely ill clinical populations. To address this question, our group [34] analyzed data from a community-based sample of some 19,000 subjects studied in five European countries. The study assessed psychiatric syndromes, physical illnesses, sleep, and pain symptoms. Current major depression was observed in 4% of the sample. Of subjects who met current criteria for major depressive disorder, 43% had a chronic physical painful condition; this rate was over three times higher than the rate in subjects who did not meet criteria for major depression.

The diagnosis of depressive symptoms increased the risk of having a chronic pain condition. In subjects who had one depressive symptom, the rate of chronic physical pain was 26%. If two depressive symptoms were present, the percentage was 29%; in those with five depressive symptoms, it increased to 39%, and in those with eight or nine symptoms of major depression, it reached 62%.

The assessment process allowed for exploring the relative contribution of an organic major physical disorder versus functional pain to the likelihood of developing major depression. In subjects with one or more depressive symptoms, 28% reported chronic physical pain, and of these only a third (9% overall) had a medical condition that could account for the pain. Similarly, in those who met criteria for major depression, 43% had chronic physical pain, and of these again a third (14.5% overall) had a key medical disorder. Thus, the majority of patients with major depression and comorbid pain did not have a physical disorder that accounted for their pain. These data point to a relationship between chronic pain and depression that is not merely due to a comorbid medical disorder.

A recent Canadian epidemiological study reported that approximately a third of depressed subjects in the community had one of four common chronic pain disorders [32]. European groups have also explored major depression and anxiety disorders in relationship to chronic pain. In one study, 21,000 subjects were interviewed in six European countries. Chronic pain was reported in 29% of subjects without major depression. In those who met criteria for major depression, the prevalence was significantly higher, with 50% reporting chronic pain [9]. Similarly increased rates of comorbid pain were reported for anxiety disorders, with 29% of non-anxious subjects reporting pain in contrast to 45% of those who met criteria for an anxiety disorder [10]. Thus, both anxiety and depressive disorders are associated with increased risk for chronic pain.

Tsang et al. [44] assessed the prevalence of pain, depression, and anxiety in 18 countries in the World Mental Health Survey. A 12-month prevalence of chronic pain was reported in about 40% of subjects, with similar rates in both developing and developed countries. However, the vast majority of pain subjects did not appear to suffer from depression or anxiety.

The sequential relationship between pain and depression is not unidirectional. Either can precede the other. It is easy to posit that chronic pain is obviously stressful and understandably should lead to depression, but the number of studies that have confirmed that sequence is balanced by the number that have reported the converse—namely, that depression leads to a chronic pain syndrome. Moreover, the relationship between pain and depression in our community sample was independent of a major physical disorder, suggesting that pain was not a simple mediator or cause of depressive symptoms.

The bidirectional relationship could be explained by a common underlying biological factor that leads to both pain and depression. One notion has been that altered activity of both noradrenergic and serotonergic function peripherally and centrally could change pain perception and might point to possible targeted therapy. This hypothesis rests primarily on the observation that descending pathways from the brain into the spinal cord may be compromised both in depression and in chronic pain. These data are largely based on drug effects in animal models and require testing in humans. Alternatively, the comorbidity may reflect alterations in other systems, such as calcium or sodium ion channels, γ-aminobutyric acid, or glutamate.

Does Comorbidity Matter?

The comorbidity of depression and pain is of consequence. Several community samples have reported that it is associated with poorer social adjustment and higher rates of absenteeism. For example, a Canadian study of over 9 million individuals reported that subjects with pain who reported being absent from work were three times more likely to meet criteria for major depression than were those who did not miss work [31]. In a six-country European study, comorbid pain and depression—but not comorbid pain and anxiety—were associated with significantly increased work loss days [9]. A German study of 4,000 subjects in the community found that pain and depression were associated with poorer general functioning [5]. In a clinical sample of primary care patients in the Kaiser Permanente managed care system in the United States, comorbid pain and major depression were associated with a significantly greater clinical burden [2]. Thus, comorbidity of chronic pain with depression is associated with considerable medical and social morbidity, loss of productivity, and considerable direct and indirect financial costs.

Comorbidity of pain with depression is also associated with greater chronicity of depression. In our community-based study, the presence of one or more depressive symptoms with chronic pain was associated with longer duration of depressed mood than was observed in the pain-free comparator group [34]. Part of this chronicity may be due to patients not seeking help for their depression. In the large-scale multi-country European study, patients with comorbid major depression were less likely to seek help for their depression [9]. This reluctance was not observed for patients with comorbid anxiety and pain in that study [10]. Comorbid pain and depression appears to have greater social consequences than does the combination of anxiety and pain.

In two recent studies, we observed extremely high rates of chronic pain (about 80%) in recurrent major depression [1] or in refractory depression [37]. These data further indicate a relationship between chronicity or recurrence of depression and chronic pain.

Suicide

Chronic pain is associated with a threefold increase in risk for experiencing suicidal ideation [8,25,42] and a two- to eightfold increase in risk for committing suicide [30,35]. In a long-term study that followed farmers over 10 years, "successful suicides" were observed nine times more often in those with back pain than in pain-free controls [35]. In another study, Macfarlane and colleagues [30] reported a twofold increased risk in those with diffuse pain than in those without pain.

One obvious factor in this increased risk for suicide is comorbid major depression. For example, Treharne and colleagues in the United Kingdom reported suicidal ideation in 30% of patients with rheumatoid arthritis in comparison to 7% in controls [43]. In a U.S. community sample of young adults, Breslau noted an eightfold increase in risk for suicidal ideation in subjects with migraine with aura and coexisting major depression compared with subjects with migraine with aura alone and a 2.6-fold increase compared with subjects with major depression alone [8]. A study of 1,500 pain patients found that a catastrophizing cognitive style interacts with depression to result in increased suicidal ideation [18].

Pharmacological Treatment

Recent efforts to develop mixed norepinephrine-serotonin reuptake inhibitors have spurred considerable interest in the optimal treatment of comorbid major depression with chronic pain. Early trials reported that tricyclic antidepressants (TCAs), particularly those thought to have both serotonergic and noradrenergic effects, were effective in patients with depression and pain [23,45,46]. This observation has been particularly true for doxepin. However, although doxepin and other tertiary tricyclics (e.g., amitriptyline) were once thought to be both potently noradrenergic and serotonergic, after the development of selective serotonin reuptake blockers (SSRIs) it became clear that the serotonergic effects of the TCAs are modest at best. Instead, it is likely that the antihistaminic effects of the TCAs probably account for their usefulness in chronic pain. Often, the improvement in pain with TCA therapy was thought to reflect the improvement in depressive symptoms.

The development of the SSRIs was at one time looked upon as a potential major step forward in the treatment of patients with chronic pain because serotonin had been thought to play a key role in these patients' drug response. Indeed, a number of trials were conducted on SSRIs in chronic pain, but little was observed in regard to positive effects consistent with this theory. Indeed, TCAs are thought to be some three times as likely as SSRIs to provide relief, based on numbers needed to treat [39]. Bair et al. [3] reported that increasing pain ratings were associated with poorer responses to SSRIs.

This issue of relative efficacy has reemerged with the development of duloxetine, a combined norepinephrine-serotonin reuptake blocker without antihistaminic effects. In early trials of depressed patients, duloxetine appeared to be more effective than placebo in reducing pain as well as depression [11,12]. A subsequent study by Goldstein et al. [22] was positive, as was one by Perahia et al. [36]. None of these samples were enriched for pain, and subjects without pain at baseline were included in the analyses, suggesting that the results might be stronger if a sample of patients who had both pain and depression were studied. However, not all such duloxetine studies have been positive [13,27]. Paroxetine, an SSRI, has been explored at a relatively low dose as an SSRI comparator in several of these studies. It separated significantly from placebo in some studies [13,36], but not in all [22].

One meta-analysis argued that duloxetine was not significantly better than placebo in reducing pain symptoms in depression [41]. This study pointed out that trials with an enriched sample that included all patients with comorbid pain did show more favorable results. Indeed, two such studies have been reported. In the first (included in Spielmans' review), 141 patients who had major depression and had a Brief Pain Inventory score of at least 2 at baseline were randomized to receive duloxetine or placebo [6]. In this study, conducted in the United States, duloxetine separated significantly from placebo on most, but not all, pain measures. Scores on the Brief Pain Inventory showed that the drug was significantly superior over placebo on pooled measures, but it was not superior at the conclusion. On a visual analogue scale for pain, the drug did separate significantly from placebo. Interestingly, duloxetine was not statistically superior to placebo in reducing depression, in part due to high placebo responses. In this study, patients with one or more episodes of major depression were significantly more likely to respond. In a second, more recent study (not included in Spielmans' paper) conducted in five European countries, duloxetine did separate from placebo in reducing both pain and major depression in 337 comorbid patients. Reduction in average pain ratings on duloxetine separated from placebo as early as week 1 [7].

The recent Spielmans meta-analysis [41], which suggested that the drug may not have advantages over placebo in patients with comorbid pain and depression, is largely affected by the inclusion of the earlier trials that did not focus on homogeneously comorbid samples. Including these samples biases against finding differences between drug and placebo because nonpain patients cannot improve over a baseline pain score of or near zero. In another more recent review, Krebs et al. [27] reported that duloxetine was clearly superior to placebo but was not superior to paroxetine. This review did not include the Brecht et al. trial [7]. An intriguing question is whether patients who do not respond to an SSRI do better if crossed over to a mixed reuptake drug. In a recent trial [37], patients who failed to respond to an SSRI crossed over to one of two regimens with duloxetine. Both groups demonstrated high response rates for improvement in both pain and depression. All patients received duloxetine, so these data were not blinded.

The strong data on duloxetine in patients with diabetic neuropathic pain and fibromyalgia without comorbid depression also suggest anti-pain effects for the drug independent of antidepressant effects [38]. Further studies are needed to more fully understand the use and relative benefit of duloxetine in comorbid pain and depression.

The dual-acting agent venlafaxine and the newer agent desvenlafaxine have both been studied in comorbid pain and major depression. We have reported that venlafaxine and fluoxetine were both effective in reducing pain and depression in chronically depressed patients; the two agents were similar in effectiveness. In another study, desvenlafaxine at 100 mg per day appeared to be more effective than placebo in reducing both symptoms of depression and measures of pain [29]. The drug is also being studied in primary pain conditions.

The significance of pain in long-term treatment outcome has been examined prospectively in recent studies. As noted above, depression that is accompanied by pain tends to be associated with longer duration of depressive symptoms in community-based samples. In a treatment outcome study conducted at 60 community primary medical practices, pain at baseline and decrease in pain over time had significant effects on determining the likelihood of remission of the patients' depression [28]. In a recent prospective trial, patients were initially treated with open-label duloxetine at 60 mg per day for 12 weeks. Responders were then randomized to continuing on medication or crossing over to placebo. Baseline measures of pain were predictors of relapse; there was a treatment predictor interaction for pain at the randomization as well [20]. These data again point to a relationship between chronic pain and poorer outcome in depression.

Biology of Pain and Depression

Idiopathic pain disorders have been conceptualized to reflect an interaction between reaction to high psychological distress and increased pain sensitivity. These two dimensions may be affected by different biological systems. This overall approach has been nicely articulated in the recent literature by Diatchenko et al. [16]. A variety of systems that are commonly thought to underlie affect regulation and stress sensitivity have been hypothesized to play a role in heightened dysphoria and stress responses, whereas others appear to play a more pivotal role in pain transmission. Among the former are alterations in catecholamine and indoleamine functions. Indeed, clinical observations that newer antidepressants with combined noradrenergic and serotonergic (5-HT) reuptake blocking effects may have particular efficacy in comorbid pain and depression have led to increased interest in a possible unifying biology of the two disorders. Animal model and pharmacological studies point to noradrenergic and 5-HT descending pathways that inhibit pain transmission from the periphery to brain as well as a potential role for dual-acting agents in reducing pain in lower animals [26]. More recent studies on genetic polymorphisms have suggested that catecholamine alterations—particularly in epinephrine and norepinephrine—may play a greater role than do others involving 5-HT activity.

A number of studies on the functional significance of polymorphisms for one key catecholamine-degrading enzyme, catechol-O-methyltransferase (COMT), have yielded strong data that alterations in this enzyme have important effects on cognition, pain perception, and possibly mood. This enzyme degrades the catecholamines—dopamine, epinephrine, and norepinephrine—at the level of the synapse. Alterations in COMT activity have clinical significance in schizophrenia and depression [19] as well as in pain perception [33]. The effects of *COMT* alleles on risk of developing temporomandibular joint pain appear to be independent of the effect of psychological risk factors [40].

Low COMT activity in rats—produced by using an inhibitor—results in increased catecholamine levels and enhanced pain sensitivity. This hypersensitivity appears to be mediated via β_2 and/or β_3 receptors but not by β_1, α-adrenergic, or dopaminergic receptors [33]. Polymorphisms for *COMT* have been reported by the same group to account for a large percentage of the variance in pain sensitivity in humans [15,17]. Moreover, using haplotype analyses, the same group reported that β_2-receptor polymorphisms are associated with "stronger psychological traits" and a lower likelihood of developing a chronic pain condition [14]. Thus, these data suggest a preferential role for epinephrine or norepinephrine systems in pain. Zubieta et al. have also reported that a val/met allelic form of *COMT* was associated with changes in μ-opioid responses in humans [48].

Alterations of 5-HT transporter promoter have been implicated in risk for developing depression in the face of multiple untoward stressors—such as parental loss. Since the dual-acting antidepressants appear to be effective in patients with both depression and chronic pain, 5-HT transporter promoter variants would be an area worth exploring. Studies to date have been generally negative with regard to the transporter promoter affecting pain enhancement, but some data indicate an association with a 5-HT transporter intron allele and the risk for developing pain syndromes [24,47]. Further studies are needed to clarify the common underpinnings of comorbid pain and depression.

Acknowledgments

Dr. Schatzberg has consulted for Eli Lilly and Wyeth Pharmaceuticals.

References

[1]   Ahmed S, Schatzberg AF, Friedman ES, Rothschild AJ, Trivedi MH, Dunner DL, Gelenberg A, Ninan P, Shelton R, Zajecka JM. Prevalence and clinical correlates of pain in patients with recurrent major depressive disorder. Eur Neuropsychopharmacol 2007;17:S320–1.

[2]   Arnow BA, Hunkeler EM, Blasey CM, Lee J, Constantino MJ, Fireman B, Kraemer HC, Dea R, Robinson R, Hayward C. Comorbid depression, chronic pain, and disability in primary care. Psychosom Med 2006;68:262–8.

[3]   Bair MJ, Robinson RL, Eckert GJ, Stang PE, Croghan TW, Kroenke K. Impact of pain on depression treatment response in primary care. Psychosom Med 2004;66:17–22.

[4]   Bair MJ, Robinson RL, Katon W, Kroenke K. Depression and pain comorbidity: a literature review. Arch Intern Med 2003;163:2433–45.

[5]   Baune BT, Caniato RN, Garcia-Alcaraz MA, Berger K. Combined effects of major depression, pain and somatic disorders on general functioning in the general adult population. Pain 2008;138:310–7.

[6]   Brannan SK, Mallinckrodt CH, Brown EB, Wohlreich MM, Watkin JG, Schatzberg AF. Duloxetine 60 mg once-daily in the treatment of painful physical symptoms in patients with major depressive disorder. J Psychiatr Res 2005;39:43–53.

[7]   Brecht S, Courtecuisse C, Debieuvre C, Croenlein J, Desaiah D, Raskin J, Petit C, Demyttenaere K. Efficacy and safety of duloxetine 60 mg once daily in the treatment of pain in patients with major depressive disorder and at least moderate pain of unknown etiology: a randomized controlled trial. J Clin Psychiatry 2007;68:1707–16.

[8]   Breslau N. Migraine, suicidal ideation, and suicide attempts. Neurology 1992;42:392–5.

[9]   Demyttenaere K, Bonnewyn A, Bruffaerts R, Brugha T, De Graaf R, Alonso J. Comorbid painful physical symptoms and depression: prevalence, work loss, and help seeking. J Affect Disord 2006;92:185–93.

[10] Demyttenaere K, Bonnewyn A, Bruffaerts R, De Graaf R, Haro JM, Alonso J. Comorbid painful physical symptoms and anxiety: prevalence, work loss and help-seeking. J Affect Disord 2008;109:264–72.

[11] Detke MJ, Lu Y, Goldstein DJ, Hayes JR, Demitrack MA. Duloxetine, 60 mg once daily, for major depressive disorder: a randomized double-blind placebo-controlled trial. J Clin Psychiatry 2002;63:308–15.

[12] Detke MJ, Lu Y, Goldstein DJ, McNamara RK, Demitrack MA. Duloxetine 60 mg once daily dosing versus placebo in the acute treatment of major depression. J Psychiatr Res 2002; 36:383–90.

[13] Detke MJ, Wiltse CG, Mallinckrodt CH, McNamara RK, Demitrack MA, Bitter I. Duloxetine in the acute and long-term treatment of major depressive disorder: a placebo- and paroxetine-controlled trial. Eur Neuropsychopharmacol 2004;14:457–70.

[14] Diatchenko L, Anderson AD, Slade GD, Fillingim RB, Shabalina SA, Higgins TJ, Sama S, Belfer I, Goldman D, Max MB, Weir BS, Maixner W. Three major haplotypes of the beta$_2$ adrenergic receptor define psychological profile, blood pressure, and the risk for development of a common musculoskeletal pain disorder. Am J Med Genet B Neuropsychiatr Genet 2006; 141B:449–62.

[15] Diatchenko L, Nackley AG, Slade GD, Bhalang K, Belfer I, Max MB, Goldman D, Maixner W. Catechol-O-methyltransferase gene polymorphisms are associated with multiple pain-evoking stimuli. Pain 2006;125:216–24.

[16] Diatchenko L, Nackley AG, Slade GD, Fillingim RB, Maixner W. Idiopathic pain disorders: pathways of vulnerability. Pain 2006;123:226–30.

[17] Diatchenko L, Slade GD, Nackley AG, Bhalang K, Sigurdsson A, Belfer I, Goldman D, Xu K, Shabalina SA, Shagin D, Max MB, Makarov SS, Maixner W. Genetic basis for individual variations in pain perception and the development of a chronic pain condition. Hum Mol Genet 2005;14:135–43.

[18] Edwards RR, Smith MT, Kudel I, Haythornthwaite J. Pain-related catastrophizing as a risk factor for suicidal ideation in chronic pain. Pain 2006;126:272–9.

[19] Egan MF, Goldberg TE, Kolachana BS, Callicott JH, Mazzanti CM, Straub RE, Goldman D, Weinberger DR. Effect of COMT val108/158met genotype on frontal lobe function and risk for schizophrenia. Proc Natl Acad Sci USA 2001;98:6917–22.

[20] Fava M, Wiltse C, Walker D, Brecht S, Chen A, Perahia D. Predictors of relapse in a study of duloxetine treatment in patients with major depressive disorder. J Affect Disord 2008; Epub Jul 12.

[21] Garcia-Cebrian A, Gandhi P, Demyttenaere K, Peveler R. The association of depression and painful physical symptoms: a review of the European literature. Eur Psychiatry 2006;21:379–88.

[22] Goldstein DJ, Lu Y, Detke MJ, Wiltse C, Mallinckrodt C, Demitrack MA. Duloxetine in the treatment of depression: a double-blind placebo-controlled comparison with paroxetine. J Clin Psychopharmacol 2004;24:389–99.

[23] Hameroff SR, Weiss JL, Lerman JC, Cork RC, Watts KS, Crago BR, Neuman CP, Womble JR, Davis TP. Doxepin's effects on chronic pain and depression: a controlled study. J Clin Psychiatry 1984;45:47–53.

[24] Herken H, Erdal E, Mutlu N, Barlas O, Cataloluk O, Oz F, Guray E. Possible association of temporomandibular joint pain and dysfunction with a polymorphism in the serotonin transporter gene. Am J Orthod Dentofacial Orthop 2001;120:308–13.

[25] Hinkley BS, Jaremko ME. Effects of pain duration on psychosocial adjustment in orthopedic patients: the importance of early diagnosis and treatment of pain. J Pain Symptom Manage 1994;9:175–85.

[26] Iyengar S, Webster AA, Hemrick-Luecke SK, Xu JY, Simmons RM. Efficacy of duloxetine, a potent and balanced serotonin-norepinephrine reuptake inhibitor in persistent pain models in rats. J Pharmacol Exp Ther 2004;311:576–84.

[27] Krebs EE, Gaynes BN, Gartlehner G, Hansen RA, Thieda P, Morgan LC, DeVeaugh-Geiss A, Lohr KN. Treating the physical symptoms of depression with second-generation antidepressants: a systematic review and metaanalysis. Psychosomatics 2008;49:191–8.

[28] Kroenke K, Shen J, Oxman TE, Williams JW Jr, Dietrich AJ. Impact of pain on the outcomes of depression treatment: results from the RESPECT trial. Pain 2008;134:209–15.

[29] Liebowitz MR, Manley AL, Padmanabhan SK, Ganguly R, Tummala R, Tourian KA. Efficacy, safety, and tolerability of desvenlafaxine 50 mg/day and 100 mg/day in outpatients with major depressive disorder. Curr Med Res Opin 2008;24:1877–90.

[30] Macfarlane GJ, McBeth J, Silman AJ. Widespread body pain and mortality: prospective population-based study. BMJ 2001;323:1–5.

[31] Munce SE, Stansfeld SA, Blackmore ER, Stewart DE. The role of depression and chronic pain conditions in absenteeism: results from a national epidemiologic survey. J Occup Environ Med 2007;49:1206–11.

[32] Munce SE, Stewart DE. Gender differences in depression and chronic pain conditions in a national epidemiologic survey. Psychosomatics 2007;48:394–9.

[33] Nackley AG, Tan KS, Fecho K, Flood P, Diatchenko L, Maixner W. Catechol-O-methyltransferase inhibition increases pain sensitivity through activation of both beta$_2$- and beta$_3$-adrenergic receptors. Pain 2007;128:199–208.

[34] Ohayon MM, Schatzberg AF. Using chronic pain to predict depressive morbidity in the general population. Arch Gen Psychiatry 2003;60:39–47.

[35] Penttinen J. Back pain and risk of suicide among Finnish farmers. Am J Public Health 1995;85:1452–3.

[36] Perahia DG, Wang F, Mallinckrodt CH, Walker DJ, Detke MJ. Duloxetine in the treatment of major depressive disorder: a placebo- and paroxetine-controlled trial. Eur Psychiatry 2006;21:367–78.

[37] Perahia DG, Quail D, Desaiah D, Montejo AL, Schatzberg AF. Switching to duloxetine in selective serotonin reuptake inhibitor non- and partial-responders: effects on painful physical symptoms of depression. J Psychiatr Res 2008; Epub Aug 15.

[38] Russell IJ, Mease PJ, Smith TR, Kajdasz DK, Wohlreich MM, Detke MJ, Walker DJ, Chappell AS, Arnold LM. Efficacy and safety of duloxetine for treatment of fibromyalgia in patients with or without major depressive disorder: results from a 6-month, randomized, double-blind, placebo-controlled, fixed-dose trial. Pain 2008;136:432–44.

[39] Sindrup SH, Otto M, Finnerup NB, Jensen TS. Antidepressants in the treatment of neuropathic pain. Basic Clin Pharmacol Toxicol 2005;96:399–409.

[40] Slade GD, Diatchenko L, Bhalang K, Sigurdsson A, Fillingim RB, Belfer I, Max MB, Goldman D, Maixner W. Influence of psychological factors on risk of temporomandibular disorders. J Dent Res 2007;86:1120–5.

[41] Spielmans GI. Duloxetine does not relieve painful physical symptoms in depression: a meta-analysis. Psychother Psychosom 2008;77:12–6.

[42] Tang NK, Crane C. Suicidality in chronic pain: a review of the prevalence, risk factors and psychological links. Psychol Med 2006;36:575–86.

[43] Treharne G, Lyons AC, Kitas GD. Suicidal ideation in patients with rheumatoid arthritis. Research may help identify patients at high risk. BMJ 2000;321:18.

[44] Tsang A, Korff MV, Lee S, Alonso J, Karam E, Angermeyer MC, Borges GL, Bromet EJ, de Girolamo G, de Graaf R, et al. Common chronic pain conditions in developed and developing countries: gender and age differences and comorbidity with depression-anxiety disorders. J Pain 2008; Epub July 3.

[45] Ward NG, Bloom VL, Dworkin S, Fawcett J, Narasimhachari N, Friedel RO. Psychobiological markers in coexisting pain and depression: toward a unified theory. J Clin Psychiatry 1982; 43: 32-41.

[46] Ward N, Bokan JA, Phillips M, Benedetti C, Butler S, Spengler D. Antidepressants in concomitant chronic back pain and depression: doxepin and desipramine compared. J Clin Psychiatry 1984;45:54–9.

[47] Yilmaz M, Erdal ME, Herken H, Cataloluk O, Barlas O, Bayazit YA. Significance of serotonin transporter gene polymorphism in migraine. J Neurol Sci 2001;186:27–30.

[48] Zubieta JK, Heitzeg MM, Smith YR, Bueller JA, Xu K, Xu Y, Koeppe RA, Stohler CS, Goldman D. COMT val158met genotype affects mu-opioid neurotransmitter responses to a pain stressor. Science 2003;299:1240–3.

Correspondence to: Prof. Alan F. Schatzberg, MD, Department of Psychiatry and Behavioral Sciences, Stanford University School of Medicine, 401 Quarry Road, Third Floor, Stanford, CA 94305-5717, USA. Email: afschatz@stanford.edu.

Somatization and Pain Syndromes

Francis Creed

Psychiatry Research Group, School of Medicine, University of Manchester, Manchester, United Kingdom

This chapter aims to help the reader understand the relationship between somatization and the pain syndromes. I will commence with an explanation of the different ways in which the term "somatization" has been used. I will review the degree of overlap between somatization and the pain syndromes and then consider the meaning and the consequences of such an overlap. This review should enable clinicians to appreciate the importance of detecting somatization in their patients and help researchers realize why it is important to make independent assessments of somatization and pain.

Definitions of Somatization

Somatization is a common problem in patients with pain syndromes. Both somatization and functional syndromes share the attribute of bothersome symptoms without demonstrable pathology, and some authors have considered them to be synonymous. This chapter will demonstrate that this is not so.

Some of the confusion comes about because the term "somati-zation" has had different meanings at different times. An early definition of "somatization" was broad: a tendency to experience and communicate somatic distress and to attribute symptoms unexplained by pathological findings to physical illness and to seek medical help for them [58]. Another early definition considered somatization to be a kind of defense, in that individuals presented bodily symptoms instead of anxiety and depression. This idea could not be sustained when it became clear that those who report a large number of bodily symptoms also report many symptoms of anxiety and depression [39,46].

Primary care researchers operationalized the term "somatization," using four criteria: presentation of bodily symptoms to the doctor, a belief that the symptoms represent an underlying physical disease (somatic attri-bution), the presence of a psychiatric disorder (usually anxiety or depres-sion), and the considered judgment of an experienced clinician that treat-ment of the psychiatric disorder would lead to resolution of the symptoms [9]. This definition is too narrow, however, because somatization can oc-cur in the absence of another psychiatric disorder. The last condition—the considered opinion of a trained clinician—is not reliable because opinions vary so much in this respect [81].

Two major current usages of the term will be considered further in this chapter. First, somatization is considered as a rare psychiatric disor-der, "somatization disorder," in which a very large number of unexplained bodily symptoms is associated with the constructs of hypochondriasis and hysteria. Second, the term is applied simply to the reporting of numerous bodily symptoms, which is often associated with increased demand for health care and impairment of function [17,34].

Somatization Disorder

In the psychiatric diagnostic manuals, somatization disorder is defined in terms of bodily symptoms that are not fully explained by a general medical condition, by substance use, or by another mental disorder, and which are not intentionally produced (unlike factitious disorders). So-matization disorder is defined as: (a) a history of many such physical complaints beginning before 30 years of age that occur over a period of several years and result in treatment being sought or in significant impairment in social, occupational, or other important areas of functioning; and (b) the presence of all of the following at some time during the course of the disturbance: (i) four pain symptoms, (ii) two gastrointestinal tract symptoms, (iii) one sexual symptom, and (iv) one pseudoneurological symptom (e.g., weakness) [4]. This definition is a modified version of an earlier one, which required an even greater number of bodily symptoms.

There are two main problems with this definition of somatization disorder. First, the number of symptoms needed to reach the diagnostic criteria is so high that the disorder is made very rarely in primary care or population-based settings [15]. For this reason, researchers have used less stringent criteria, requiring only three to six medically unexplained symptoms [23,46,47,82]. Second, the diagnosis of somatization disorder includes only those symptoms that are "medically unexplained." When patients with a functional syndrome are interviewed, the researcher must make a decision regarding each symptom, and the prevalence varies greatly according to this decision [43].

Somatization as a Process

Somatization disorder probably represents the most extreme end of a continuum of number of bodily symptoms. There is a linear relationship between number of reported bodily symptoms and health status and health care use, without any clear cut-off point representing a "disorder" [8,14,41,50]. Therefore, somatization may be viewed as a normal process, but for most people the bodily symptoms are usually transient and have little impact on overall well-being. One of these symptoms may be troublesome at any one point in time in a quarter of the general population, but in a few a large number of bodily symptoms are troublesome and persist over time [36,52].

Somatization disorder can be assessed only by using a detailed interview to ascertain the number of bodily symptoms, each of which only counts toward a diagnosis of somatization disorder if it impairs function and the respondent has consulted a doctor, who has deemed it "unexplained" by a recognized medical illness or substance use. For example, the widely used Composite International Diagnostic Interview has questions about 46 bodily symptoms [96].

Alternatively, the number of bodily symptoms can be recorded on a self-report checklist of bodily symptoms. This type of instrument usually assesses whether each symptom causes some degree of discomfort or burden, but it cannot, of course, distinguish between medically explained and unexplained symptoms. There are numerous such questionnaires; an example is the PHQ-15 (Personal Health Questionnaire), which includes 15 symptoms [50]. Recent work using such questionnaires shows that total body symptom count, irrespective of whether each of the symptoms is medically explained or not, correlates strongly with functional impairment, health care use, and other psychiatric disorders [8,41,44,50].

In population-based samples there is a fairly consistent pattern, with the most commonly reported symptoms including fatigue, headaches, dizziness, abdominal pain, bloating, chest pain, and musculoskeletal pain [36,85]. Factor analytic or latent trait analyses have demonstrated clusters including fibromyalgia-like, irritable bowel-like, and chronic fatigue symptoms, but these are all largely attributable to one common higher-order factor explaining much of the variance—a general tendency to report bodily symptoms [20]. It is this general tendency that is referred to as somatization.

Somatization and Somatization Disorder in Pain Syndromes

There are very few studies of the prevalence of somatization disorder in patients with pain syndromes. In small samples of tertiary care patients with severe irritable bowel syndrome (IBS), it has been reported that 25% had somatization disorder diagnosed according to the *Diagnostic and Statistical Manual* (DSM-IV) [4] of the American Psychiatric Association [63,69]. As would be expected from the definition of somatization disorder, these patients had more gastrointestinal and other symptoms, more other psychiatric disorders, a greater number of physician contacts, and more medication changes and were less satisfied with their treatment compared to patients with severe IBS who did not have somatization disorder. They also missed more work days because of their illness. Somatization disorder has been recorded in approximately one-third of persons with IBS in a population-based study [45] and in 20% of clinic patients with low back pain compared to none in a healthy comparison group [61].

One of the difficulties with the diagnosis of somatization disorder in patients with a pain syndrome is the confusion caused by the pain symptoms that form part of the pain syndrome diagnosis but are also included in the diagnosis of somatization disorder.

There are numerous reports of individuals with a pain syndrome having a higher mean score on a questionnaire recording bodily symptoms than healthy comparison groups. For example, higher scores have been recorded for clinic patients and for people in population-based samples with functional gastrointestinal disorders [45,59,83,93], back pain, chronic widespread pain (fibromyalgia) [97], and temporomandibular joint disorder (TMD) [6,74]. Again, there is the difficulty that the score will be somewhat inflated, because the symptoms of the disorder may contribute several bodily symptoms to the overall score.

Causes of Somatization

Somatization (a large number of reported bodily symptoms) is associated with a number of risk factors. Predictors of persistent bodily symptoms include female gender, negative life events, a concurrent depressive disorder, a parental psychiatric disorder, and a predominance of pain as opposed to other bodily symptoms [24,52,53,57].

There is some evidence for a genetic factor in somatization [29], and rather stronger evidence for environmental factors, including childhood abuse, parental ill health/neuroticism, maternal somatization, and recent life stress [7,13,38,40,79]. A gene by environment interaction is likely [11]. Somatization is strongly correlated with neuroticism—the tendency to experience negative, distressing emotions [5,80]—and in severe forms, with personality disorder [26].

Somatization is very closely associated with anxiety or depressive disorders [55], and the time course of the two often correspond. There is some evidence that the painful condition precedes the anxiety or depression [25,56], but the reverse may also occur [57]. The peak onset appears to be during teenage years [42].

Somatization and the Pain Syndromes

The risk factors listed above for somatization are similar to risk factors for the pain syndromes. Furthermore, a number of studies have shown that somatization predicts the later onset of chronic widespread pain (fibromyalgia) [31,62], back pain [73], IBS [66], and TMD [54]. Interestingly many adults with TMD pain report that their pain started in adolescence.

Treatment studies suggest that psychological treatments that help the symptoms of a pain syndrome may help the additional bodily symptoms as well. Hypnotherapy, for example, leads to improvement in both the symptoms of IBS and all other bodily symptoms [92].

To some, this evidence implies that the pain syndromes are a form of somatization. This is a debated issue in relation to IBS [3,34,65,77,90], and fibromyalgia [84,95], and the counter-arguments will be reviewed here. A strong argument against the idea that the pain syndromes are a manifestation of somatization is the fact that many patients with pain syndromes do not have widespread symptoms relating to other bodily organs—i.e., they do not have the core feature of somatization—numerous bodily symptoms [34]. Thus, pain syndromes may be conceptualized as two types of disorder. In one type, the person has only a single organ-related set of symptoms, and in the other type the pain syndrome is accompanied by multiple bodily symptoms. What is not known is whether or not the same pathophysiology occurs in the two types of syndrome [3].

In population-based samples of people with disabling low back pain (interfering markedly with sleep and daily functioning), only 30% had a raised somatization score, and the remainder had one or no additional bodily symptoms other than the back pain [71]. In population-based samples of chronic widespread pain, orofacial pain, IBS, and chronic fatigue, between 26% and 36% had a raised somatization score [2]. In a primary-care-based sample of IBS patients, one-third had a raised somatization score [87].

The last study specifically aimed to test the "dual etiology" hypothesis, namely that IBS patients can be divided into those with evidence of excessive number of somatic symptoms—a "psychological etiology" group—and another group without such features in which the disease is presumed to have a biological etiology [87]. In that study, the group of patients with a high somatization score had significantly higher scores for neuroticism, mood disorder, and life events. They also had significantly greater impairment of function and were more likely to be off work for health reasons. The authors admitted that their simple split into "psychological" and "biological" etiologies may be an oversimplification and that an interaction between these two is likely to be important for many. However, they did reiterate the importance of the somatization subgroup with five to six different bodily symptoms outside of gastrointestinal tract [87].

A similar study of clinic patients with severe IBS found that half reported no, or only very few, bodily symptoms other than the gut symptoms of IBS [19]. These patients (the "IBS alone" group) might be described as having an organ-specific set of symptoms. A quarter reported four to seven additional bodily symptoms (moderate somatization), and a quarter reported a mean of eight bodily symptoms outside the gut (a high somatization score). The latter group, with numerous bodily symptoms, might be approaching the threshold for a diagnosis of somatization disorder if it could be shown that the additional symptoms were "medically unexplained."

There was a dose-response relationship between number of additional bodily symptoms and depressive disorder (Fig. 1a). Seventeen percent of those with IBS alone (with no or few additional bodily symptoms) had depressive disorder, compared to 33% and 49% of the groups with moderate and high somatization scores, respectively.

The group of patients with the highest somatization score (a mean of eight additional bodily symptoms) had a much greater proportion of individuals (52%) who were unemployed through ill health than the other groups (Fig. 1c). In this group, health status was greatly reduced, according to the physical component score on the Medical Outcomes Study 36-item Short-Form Health Survey (SF-36) (Fig. 1d). Patients in this group had also incurred much higher health costs than the other groups (mean = £2058,

SD= £329) compared to mean health care costs for the remaining three groups of between £976 and £1027 [19].

A rather similar study in the United States that compared health care costs and somatization score found a dose-response relationship between the two variables [83]. Patients with a somatization score two standard deviations above the mean had incurred health care costs over the previous year that were an average of US$2,481 more than those of patients with a mean somatization score.

In these studies it can be seen that between half to two-thirds of IBS patients did *not* report many bodily symptoms apart from the abdominal ones. Thus, it is not appropriate to equate their pain syndrome with somatization because they lacked the key feature of somatization—numerous bodily symptoms.

Two studies have used cluster analytic techniques to identify subgroups of patients with pain syndromes. Both studies identified a cluster that probably represented those with somatization. Among fibromyalgia

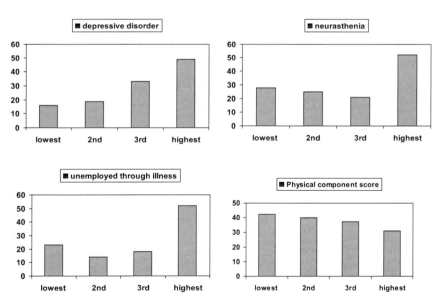

Fig. 1. Relationship between number of bodily symptoms, expressed as four quartiles, and (a) depressive disorder, (b) neurasthenia (chronic fatigue), (c) unemployment because of illness, and (d) the physical component score of the SF-36, in patients with irritable bowel syndrome. Data from Creed et al. [19].

patients one cluster, approximately one-third of the sample, had significantly elevated scores for anxiety, depression, and pain catastrophizing, with low scores for control over pain and marked tenderness on dolorimetry [23]. Somatization was not measured in this study.

In the study of IBS patients, mentioned above, there was a cluster with high scores for depression and other psychiatric diagnoses, a high frequency of sexual abuse, and a low threshold for pain on rectal distension, representing sensitivity to pain [32]. People in this cluster made frequent doctor visits and had the most marked impairment of health status. Further analysis of the data, for the purpose of this chapter, reveals that the somatization score was highest in this cluster at 1.35 (SD = 0.670), compared to another cluster with a low distension threshold but a lower burden of psychiatric disorders at 1.26 (SD = 0.82) and a third cluster of patients who did not have a low distension threshold (i.e., were not overly sensitive to distension of the rectum) (0.81; SD = 0.50; $P = 0.017$).

A considerable body of evidence supports the notion that people with a pain syndrome can be divided into one group, usually the majority, who appear to have an "organ-specific" set of symptoms, and another group whose pain syndrome is accompanied by numerous other bodily symptoms and who have, in a descriptive sense, somatization. The other symptoms are well recognized in IBS as "extra-intestinal" symptoms because of their location in different parts of the body.

Somatization and Multiple Pain Syndromes

There is considerable overlap among pain syndromes. For example, patients with one painful syndrome, such as chest pain, are likely to suffer concurrently other, similar syndromes such as IBS, TMD, and chronic fatigue syndrome [1,12,68,90]. This finding has been quoted as another piece of evidence that these syndromes share a common etiology [88]. There are alternative explanations, however.

One explanation argues that the overlap arises, in part, because the symptoms of one syndrome are also those of another; headache, for example, is a recognized symptom of several pain syndromes [67,88]. It is true also that the more bodily symptoms a patient reports, the more likely it is that multiple syndromes will be diagnosed, which leads to an overlap between somatization and functional bowel disorders [22,90].

The most likely explanation for the overlap of syndromes is the fact that somatization (and other psychiatric disorders) occur in a proportion of patients in each pain syndrome, and the shared risk factors reflect this fact, especially as the shared risk factors are also those for somatization: female predominance, a strong association with depression and anxiety, a history of childhood adversity, and exacerbation with stress.

In relation to patients with organ-specific pain syndromes, it has been pointed that there is very little overlap between the core symptoms of diarrhea (IBS), joint and muscular pains (fibromyalgia), and fatigue, and there is no pathophysiological mechanism that is common to such disparate symptoms [89]. Some preliminary work even suggests specificity in relationship to infection—*Campylobacter* gastroenteritis was a risk factor for IBS but not for chronic fatigue in one study [64], whereas infectious mononucleosis was a specific risk factor for chronic fatigue in another study [72].

In primary care or population-based samples, the overlap is somewhat less than in clinic studies [1,86]. In a primary care study, only 16% of IBS patients reported increased comorbidity with other conditions, and such comorbidity was greatest in those with a psychiatric disorder [91]. This finding is compatible with the notion that somatization accompanies IBS in some people and that this subgroup is responsible for the common risk factors across syndromes.

People who have two pain syndromes concurrently have higher somatization scores than those who only have one. Patients with both IBS and fibromyalgia have higher somatization scores than those with IBS alone [10]. Another study found that patients with both chronic pelvic pain and IBS differed from patients with chronic pelvic pain alone in terms of multiple pain sites, a higher somatization score, and a history of abuse [94]. The overlap between IBS and neurasthenia (chronic fatigue) occurs much more frequently in IBS patients who have high scores for somatization than in those with low scores (Fig. 1b) [19]. To some extent, this finding is predictable—the more symptoms that a person reports, the more likely he or she is to have multiple pain syndromes.

The Relationship between Somatization and the Pain Syndromes

At present the relationship between somatization and the pain syndromes is unclear. The evidence is inadequate to indicate which view of the relationship is correct, and it may prove to be more complex than currently considered [3]. We have seen that some speak of the "dual hypothesis" mentioned above, but such a neat dichotomy is rather unlikely. Others have distinguished between peripheral and central aspects of functional somatic syndromes or functional pain syndromes [35]. Peripheral aspects refer to muscular, endocrine, gastrointestinal, cardiac, and immunological changes, and central aspects may include central sensitization to pain and changes in cerebral blood flow. The distinction is apparent in the treatments offered: nonsteroidal anti-inflammatory drugs (NSAIDs), alosetron, and analgesics would be regarded as peripheral agents that are helpful in chronic widespread pain (fibromyalgia), IBS, and temporomandibular joint pain, respectively, whereas tricyclic antidepressants can be seen as central agents that may help patients with any of these conditions.

Present theories of etiology of the pain syndromes generally evoke some form of central sensitization in all patients, even those without pronounced psychological features. Further work is required that examines more fully the relationship between somatization and alterations of brain activations, because these alterations may be the result of disturbed central or peripheral mechanisms [76].

The mechanisms involved in somatization are, therefore, not clear. Few of the several potential mechanisms have been studied across different pain syndromes in a consistent fashion that would lead to firm conclusions. The mechanisms that have been studied may be conceptualized at different levels.

At the symptom level, many authors regard somatization as an amplification process, so that people with high somatization scores are those who experience and report normal bodily sensations as potential signs of disease [21,78,90]. These individuals would have a high neuroticism score on a personality inventory [78]. In relation to neuroticism, emotionally reactive individuals are more likely to perceive, overreact to, or complain about minor physical problems and sensations. Alternatively, they may over-report bodily symptoms on the basis of a negative reporting style, distorting retrospective accounts of daily experience [5].

In fibromyalgia patients, somatization is closely associated with an objective measure of sensitivity to pain and exertion. In one study, somatization mediated the effect of these measures on outcome [27]. Another study has shown that changes in cerebral blood flow in response to painful stimuli were associated with pain catastrophizing independently of depression [30]. The areas of the brain involved suggest that pain catastrophizing influences pain perception through its effect on affective and attentional responses to pain. This is probably one of several mechanisms underlying somatization [21,78].

With regard to pathophysiological mechanisms, some regard the disease-specific etiology and the generalized mechanisms related to somatization (e.g., the autonomic nervous system and brain-gut axis) as quite separate mechanisms; however, this observation appears to be based more on the presence or absence of a concurrent psychiatric disorder rather than on systematic studies of pathophysiology [77]. In IBS, peripheral mechanisms might include sensitization of peripheral processing of neuronal stimuli or, possibly, low-grade mucosal inflammation, whereas central nervous system mechanisms might include neuronal plasticity at the spinal cord level and attentional bias at the cortical level [65]. These peripheral and central events are invoked as distinct mechanisms in the two groups of patients [65].

Treatment of Somatization

A detailed description of the treatment of somatization is beyond the scope of this chapter. However, as stated above, somatization in patients with a pain syndrome is associated with marked impairment of daily function and increased health care use [8,41,50]. Increased morbidity has been clearly demonstrated in IBS in relation to somatization disorder [63,69] or lesser degrees of somatization [18,19,33,83]. A similar pattern is seen in other pain syndromes. Somatization also predicts a poor response to treatment [37,75].

Treatment must start, therefore, with an assessment of somatization and of the characteristics and severity of the pain syndrome. The severity of somatization can be assessed using one of the many scales that record the number of somatic symptoms [47,50,60]. If somatization is present, it will merit specific treatment in addition to the treatment offered for the pain syndrome. Assessment of the cause of the somatization may be simple or complex. The most frequent causes are also the simplest, namely concurrent depressive or anxiety disorders, which can be detected readily by the use of a few questions or the administration of a brief measure and treated by pharmacological or psychological means. If more complex personality and psychosocial factors are involved, referral to a psychiatrist or psychologist may be warranted.

Recent reviews of the treatment of somatization are quite optimistic regarding the use of both psychological methods and antidepressants [48,51,70]. It is interesting to note that improvement of somatization, whether by antidepressants or by cognitive behavioral treatment, is independent of any improvement in anxiety or depression, emphasizing that somatization is not the same as these psychological constructs [48,51,70].

Even quite severe forms of somatization appear to respond to psychological treatment or antidepressant treatment, with a marked reduction of health care use accompanying improvement in health status, even in the absence of marked improvement in somatic symptoms, as shown in our study in patients with severe IBS [19]. This response would support the notion that the dimension related to somatization, functional impairment, and health care seeking is somewhat separate from that related to IBS symptoms. In our study, improvement of somatization mediated the marked improvement that was observed in patients who reported a prior history of sexual abuse, emphasizing the close relationship between these variables [16]. As mentioned above, hypnotherapy is a successful treatment for somatization [92].

Conclusion

This chapter has focused on somatization as a process, rather than on the rare somatization disorder, and presented evidence that somatization is separate from, but coexists with, the functional pain syndromes. This point of view may or may not be correct, but it is intended to stimulate researchers to examine the pathophysiology of these disorders in patients with and without somatization separately to examine this possibility. In clinical practice, it is essential to detect somatization if it is present and treat it accordingly.

References

[1]   Aaron LA, Buchwald D. A review of the evidence for overlap among unexplained clinical conditions. Ann Intern Med 2001b;134:868–81.
[2]   Aggarwal VR, McBeth J, Zakrzewska JM, Lunt M, Macfarlane GJ, Aggarwal VR, McBeth J, Zakrzewska JM, Lunt M, Macfarlane GJ. The epidemiology of chronic syndromes that are frequently unexplained: do they have common associated factors? Int J Epidemiol 2006;35:468–76.
[3]   Alpers DH, Alpers DH. Multidimensionality of symptom complexes in irritable bowel syndrome and other functional gastrointestinal disorders. J Psychosom Res 2008;64:567–72.
[4]   American Psychiatric Association. Somatoform disorders. In: Diagnostic and statistical manual of mental disorders (DSM-IV). Washington, DC: American Psychiatric Association; 1994. p. 445–69.
[5]   Aronson KR, Barrett LF, Quigley K, Aronson KR, Barrett LF, Quigley K. Emotional reactivity and the overreport of somatic symptoms: somatic sensitivity or negative reporting style? J Psychosom Res 2006;60:521–30.
[6]   Baad-Hansen L, Leijon G, Svensson P, List T, Baad-Hansen L, Leijon G, Svensson P, List T. Comparison of clinical findings and psychosocial factors in patients with atypical odontalgia and temporomandibular disorders. J Orofac Pain 2008;22:7–14.
[7]   Barsky AJ, Borus JF. Functional somatic syndromes. Ann Intern Med 1999;130:910–21.
[8]   Barsky AJ, Orav EJ, Bates DW. Somatization increases medical utilization and costs independent of psychiatric and medical comorbidity. Arch Gen Psychiatry 2005;62:903–10.
[9]   Bridges KW, Goldberg DP. Somatic presentation of DSM III psychiatric disorders in primary care. J Psychosom Res 1985;29:563–9.
[10] Chang L, Mayer EA, Johnson T, FitzGerald LZ, Naliboff B. Differences in somatic perception in female patients with irritable bowel syndrome with and without fibromyalgia. Pain 2000;84:297–307.
[11] Cicchetti D, Rogosch FA, Sturge-Apple ML, Cicchetti D, Rogosch FA, Sturge-Apple ML. Interactions of child maltreatment and serotonin transporter and monoamine oxidase A polymorphisms: depressive symptomatology among adolescents from low socioeconomic status backgrounds. Dev Psychopathol 2007;19:1161–80.
[12] Ciccone DS, Natelson BH. Comorbid illness in women with chronic fatigue syndrome: a test of the single syndrome hypothesis. Psychosom Med 2003;65:268–75.
[13] Craig TK, Cox AD, Klein K, Craig TKJ, Cox AD, Klein K. Intergenerational transmission of somatization behaviour: a study of chronic somatizers and their children. Psychol Med 2002;32:805–16.
[14] Creed F. Can DSM-V facilitate productive research into the somatoform disorders? J Psychosom Res 2006;60:331–4.
[15] Creed F, Barsky A. A systematic review of the epidemiology of somatisation disorder and hypochondriasis. J Psychosom Res 2004;56:391–408.
[16] Creed F, Guthrie E, Ratcliffe J, Fernandes L, Rigby C, Tomenson B, Read N, Thompson DG. Reported sexual abuse predicts impaired functioning but a good response to psychological treatments in patients with severe irritable bowel syndrome. Psychosom Med 2005;67:490–9.

[17] Creed FH, Levy R, Bradley L, Drossman DA, Francisconi C, Naliboff BD, Olden KW. Psychosocial aspects of functional gastrointestinal disorders. In: Drossman DA, Corazziari E, Delvaux M, Spiller RC, Talley NJ, Thompson WG, Whitehead WE, editors. Rome III. The functional gastrointestinal disorders. McLean, VA: Degnon Associates; 2006. p. 295–368.

[18] Creed F, Ratcliffe J, Fernandez L, Tomenson B, Palmer S, Rigby C, Guthrie E, Read N, Thompson D. Health-related quality of life and health care costs in severe, refractory irritable bowel syndrome. Ann Intern Med 2001;134:860–8.

[19] Creed F, Tomenson B, Guthrie E, Ratcliffe J, Fernandes L, Read N, Palmer S TD. The relationship between somatisation and outcome in patients with severe irritable bowel syndrome. J Psychosom Res 2008;64:613–20.

[20] Deary IJ. A taxonomy of medically unexplained symptoms. J Psychosom Res 1999;47:51–9.

[21] Deary V, Chalder T, Sharpe M, Deary V, Chalder T, Sharpe M. The cognitive behavioural model of medically unexplained symptoms: a theoretical and empirical review. Clin Psychol Rev 2007;27:781–97.

[22] Enck P, Klosterhalfen S, Zipfel S, Martens U, Enck P, Klosterhalfen S, Zipfel S, Martens U. Irritable bowel syndrome: a single gastrointestinal disease or a general somatoform disorder? J Psychosom Res 2008;64:561–5.

[23] Escobar JI, Rubio-Stipec M, Canino G, Karno M. Somatic symptom index (SSI): a new and abridged somatization construct. Prevalence and epidemiological correlates in two large community samples. J Nerv Ment Dis 1989;177:140–6.

[24] Essau CA, Essau CA. Course and outcome of somatoform disorders in non-referred adolescents. Psychosomatics 2007;48:502–9.

[25] Frohlich C, Jacobi F, Wittchen HU, Frohlich C, Jacobi F, Wittchen HU. DSM-IV pain disorder in the general population. An exploration of the structure and threshold of medically unexplained pain symptoms. Eur Arch Psychiatry Clin Neurosci 2006;256:187–96.

[26] Garcia-Campayo J, Alda M, Sobradiel N, Olivan B, Pascual A, Garcia-Campayo J, Alda M, Sobradiel N, Olivan B, Pascual A. Personality disorders in somatization disorder patients: a controlled study in Spain. J Psychosom Res 2007;62:675–80.

[27] Geisser ME, Strader DC, Petzke F, Gracely RH, Clauw DJ, Williams DA, Geisser ME, Strader Donnell C, Petzke F, Gracely RH, et al. Comorbid somatic symptoms and functional status in patients with fibromyalgia and chronic fatigue syndrome: sensory amplification as a common mechanism. Psychosomatics 2008;49:235–42.

[28] Giesecke T, Williams DA, Harris RE, Cupps TR, Tian X, Tian TX, Gracely RH, Clauw DJ. Subgrouping of fibromyalgia patients on the basis of pressure-pain thresholds and psychological factors. Arthritis Rheum 2003;48:2916–22.

[29] Gillespie NA, Zhu G, Heath AC, Hickie IB, Martin NG. The genetic aetiology of somatic distress. Psychol Med 2000;30:1051–61.

[30] Gracely RH, Geisser ME, Giesecke T, Grant MA, Petzke F, Williams DA, Clauw DJ. Pain catastrophizing and neural responses to pain among persons with fibromyalgia. Brain 2004;127:835–43.

[31] Gupta A, Silman AJ, Ray D, Morriss R, Dickens C, Macfarlane GJ, Chiu YH, Nicholl B, McBeth J, Gupta A, et al. The role of psychosocial factors in predicting the onset of chronic widespread pain: results from a prospective population-based study. Rheumatology 2007;46:666–71.

[32] Guthrie E, Barlow J, Fernandes L, Ratcliffe J, Read N, Thompson DG, Tomenson B, Creed F; North of England IBS Research Group. Changes in tolerance to rectal distension correlate with changes in psychological state in patients with severe irritable bowel syndrome. Psychosom Med 2004;66:578–82.

[33] Halder SL, Locke GR, III, Talley NJ, Fett SL, Zinsmeister AR, Melton LJ III. Impact of functional gastrointestinal disorders on health-related quality of life: a population-based case-control study. Aliment Pharmacol Ther 2004;19:233–42.

[34] Henningsen P, Herzog W, Henningsen P, Herzog W. Irritable bowel syndrome and somatoform disorders. J Psychosom Res 2008;64:625–9.

[35] Henningsen P, Zipfel S, Herzog W, Henningsen P, Zipfel S, Herzog W. Management of functional somatic syndromes. Lancet 2007;369:946–55.

[36] Hiller W, Rief W, Brahler E, Hiller W, Rief W, Brahler E. Somatization in the population: from mild bodily misperceptions to disabling symptoms. Soc Psychiatry Psychiatr Epidemiol 2006;41:704–12.

[37] Holtmann G, Kutscher SU, Haag S, Langkafel M, Heuft G, Neufang-Hueber J, Goebell H, Senf W, Talley NJ. Clinical presentation and personality factors are predictors of the response to treatment in patients with functional dyspepsia; a randomized, double-blind placebo-controlled crossover study. Dig Dis Sci 2004;49:672–9.

[38] Hotopf M, Mayou R, Wadsworth M, Wessely S. Childhood risk factors for adults with medically unexplained symptoms: results from a national birth cohort study. Am J Psychiatry 1999;156:1796–800.

[39] Hotopf M, Wadsworth M, Wessely S, Hotopf M, Wadsworth M, Wessely S. Is "somatisation" a defense against the acknowledgment of psychiatric disorder? J Psychosom Res 2001;50:119–24.

[40] Hotopf M, Wilson-Jones C, Mayou R, Wadsworth M, Wessely S. Childhood predictors of adult medically unexplained hospitalisations. Results from a national birth cohort study. Br J Psychiatry 2000;176:273–80.

[41] Jackson J, Fiddler M, Kapur N, Wells A, Tomenson B, Creed F, Jackson J, Fiddler M, Kapur N, Wells A, Tomenson B, Creed F. Number of bodily symptoms predicts outcome more accurately than health anxiety in patients attending neurology, cardiology, and gastroenterology clinics. J Psychosom Res 2006;60:357–63.

[42] Jacobi F, Wittchen HU, Holting C, Hofler M, Pfister H, Muller N, Lieb R, Jacobi F, Wittchen HU, Holting C, et al. Prevalence, co-morbidity and correlates of mental disorders in the general population: results from the German Health Interview and Examination Survey (GHS). Psychol Med 2004;34:597–611.

[43] Johnson SK, DeLuca J, Natelson BH, Johnson SK, DeLuca J, Natelson BH. Assessing somatization disorder in the chronic fatigue syndrome. Psychosom Med 1996;58:50–7.

[44] Kisely S, Goldberg D, Simon G. A comparison between somatic symptoms with and without clear organic cause: results of an international study. Psychol Med 1997;27:1011–9.

[45] Koloski NA, Boyce PM, Talley NJ. Somatization an independent psychosocial risk factor for irritable bowel syndrome but not dyspepsia: a population-based study. Eur J Gastroenterol Hepatol 2006;18:1101–9.

[46] Kroenke K, Jackson JL, Chamberlin J, Kroenke K, Jackson JL, Chamberlin J. Depressive and anxiety disorders in patients presenting with physical complaints: clinical predictors and outcome. Am J Med 1997;103:339–47.

[47] Kroenke K, Kroenke K. Physical symptom disorder: a simpler diagnostic category for somatization-spectrum conditions. J Psychosom Res 2006;60:335–9.

[48] Kroenke K, Kroenke K. Efficacy of treatment for somatoform disorders: a review of randomized controlled trials. Psychosom Med 2007;69:881–8.

[49] Kroenke K, Spitzer RL, deGruy FV, III, Hahn SR, Linzer M, Williams JB, Brody D, Davies M. Multisomatoform disorder. An alternative to undifferentiated somatoform disorder for the somatizing patient in primary care. Arch Gen Psychiatry 1997;54:352–8.

[50] Kroenke K, Spitzer RL, Williams JB, Kroenke K, Spitzer RL, Williams JBW. The PHQ-15: validity of a new measure for evaluating the severity of somatic symptoms. Psychosom Med 2002;64:258–66.

[51] Kroenke K, Swindle R. Cognitive-behavioral therapy for somatization and symptom syndromes: a critical review of controlled clinical trials. Psychother Psychosom 2000;69:205–15.

[52] Leiknes KA, Finset A, Moum T, Sandanger I, Leiknes KA, Finset A, Moum T, Sandanger I. Course and predictors of medically unexplained pain symptoms in the general population. J Psychosom Res 2007;62:119–28.

[53] Leiknes KA, Finset A, Moum T et al. Overlap, comorbidity, and stability of somatoform disorders and the use of current versus lifetime criteria. Psychosomatics 2008;49:152–62.

[54] LeResche L, Mancl LA, Drangsholt MT, Huang G, Von Korff M, LeResche L, Mancl LA, Drangsholt MT, Huang G, Von Korff M. Predictors of onset of facial pain and temporomandibular disorders in early adolescence. Pain 2007;129:269–78.

[55] Lieb R, Meinlschmidt G, Araya R, Lieb R, Meinlschmidt G, Araya R. Epidemiology of the association between somatoform disorders and anxiety and depressive disorders: an update. Psychosom Med 2007;69:860–3.

[56] Lieb R, Pfister H, Mastaler M, Wittchen HU, Lieb R, Pfister H, Mastaler M, Wittchen HU. Somatoform syndromes and disorders in a representative population sample of adolescents and young adults: prevalence, comorbidity and impairments. Acta Psychiatr Scand 2000;101:194–208.

[57] Lieb R, Zimmermann P, Friis RH, Hofler M, Tholen S, Wittchen HU. The natural course of DSM-IV somatoform disorders and syndromes among adolescents and young adults: a prospective-longitudinal community study. Eur Psychiatry 2002;17:321–31.

[58] Lipowski ZJ. Somatization: the concept and its clinical application. Am J Psychiatry 1988;145:1358–1368.

[59] Locke GR III, Weaver AL, Melton LJ III, Talley NJ. Psychosocial factors are linked to functional gastrointestinal disorders: a population based nested case-control study. Am J Gastroenterol 2004;99:350–7.

[60] Lowe B, Spitzer RL, Williams JB, Mussell M, Schellberg D, Kroenke K, Lowe B, Spitzer RL, Williams JBW, Mussell M, et al. Depression, anxiety and somatization in primary care: syndrome overlap and functional impairment. Gen Hosp Psychiatry 2008;30:191–9.

[61] Manchikanti L, Pampati V, Beyer C, Damron K, Barnhill RC. Evaluation of the psychological status in chronic low back pain: comparison with general population. Pain Physician 2008;5:149–55.

[62] McBeth J, Macfarlane GJ, Benjamin S, Silman AJ. Features of somatization predict the onset of chronic widespread pain: results of a large population-based study. Arthritis Rheum 2001;44:940–6.

[63] Miller AR, North CS, Clouse RE, Wetzel RD, Spitznagel EL, Alpers DH. The association of irritable bowel syndrome and somatization disorder. Ann Clin Psychiatry 2001;13:25–30.

[64] Moss-Morris R, Spence M, Moss-Morris R, Spence M. To "lump" or to "split" the functional somatic syndromes: can infectious and emotional risk factors differentiate between the onset of chronic fatigue syndrome and irritable bowel syndrome? Psychosom Med 2006;68:463–9.

[65] Musial F, Hauser W, Langhorst J, Dobos G, Enck P, Musial F, Hauser W, Langhorst J, Dobos G, Enck P. Psychophysiology of visceral pain in IBS and health. J Psychosom Res 2008;64:589–97.

[66] Nicholl BI, Halder SL, Macfarlane GJ, Thompson DG, O'Brien S, Musleh M, McBeth J, Nicholl BI, Halder SL, Macfarlane GJ, et al. Psychosocial risk markers for new onset irritable bowel syndrome: results of a large prospective population-based study. Pain 2008;137:147–55.

[67] Nimnuan C, Hotopf M, Wessely S, Nimnuan C, Hotopf M, Wessely S. Medically unexplained symptoms: an epidemiological study in seven specialities. J Psychosom Res 2001;51:361–7.

[68] Nimnuan C, Rabe-Hesketh S, Wessely S, Hotopf M, Nimnuan C, Rabe-Hesketh S, Wessely S, Hotopf M. How many functional somatic syndromes? J Psychosom Res 2001;51:549–57.

[69] North CS, Downs D, Clouse RE, Alrakawi A, Dokucu ME, Cox J, Spitznagel EL, Alpers DH. The presentation of irritable bowel syndrome in the context of somatization disorder. Clin Gastroenterol Hepatol 2004;2:787–95.

[70] O'Malley PG, Jackson JL, Santoro J, Tomkins G, Balden E, Kroenke K. Antidepressant therapy for unexplained symptoms and symptom syndromes. J Fam Pract 1999;48:980–90.

[71] Palmer KT, Calnan M, Wainwright D, Poole J, O'Neill C, Winterbottom A, Watkins C, Coggon D, Palmer KT, Calnan M, et al. Disabling musculoskeletal pain and its relation to somatization: a community-based postal survey. Occup Med (Oxford) 2005;55:612–7.

[72] Petersen I, Thomas JM, Hamilton WT, White PD. Risk and predictors of fatigue after infectious mononucleosis in a large primary-care cohort. QJM 2006;99:49–55.

[73] Pincus T, Burton AK, Vogel S, Field AP, Pincus T, Burton AK, Vogel S, Field AP. A systematic review of psychological factors as predictors of chronicity/disability in prospective cohorts of low back pain. Spine 2002;27:E109–E120.

[74] Plesh O, Sinisi SE, Crawford PB, Gansky SA, Plesh O, Sinisi SE, Crawford PB, Gansky SA. Diagnoses based on the Research Diagnostic Criteria for Temporomandibular Disorders in a biracial population of young women. J Orofac Pain 2005;19:65–75.

[75] Porcelli P, De Carne M, Todarello O. Prediction of treatment outcome of patients with functional gastrointestinal disorders by the diagnostic criteria for psychosomatic research. Psychother Psychosom 2004;73:166–73.

[76] Rapps N, Van Oudenhove L, Enck P, Aziz Q, Rapps N, van Oudenhove L, Enck P, Aziz Q. Brain imaging of visceral functions in healthy volunteers and IBS patients. J Psychosom Res 2008;64:599–604.

[77] Riedl A, Schmidtmann M, Stengel A, Goebel M, Wisser AS, Klapp BF, Monnikes H, Riedl A, Schmidtmann M, Stengel A, Goebel M, Wisser AS, Klapp BF, Monnikes H. Somatic comorbidities of irritable bowel syndrome: a systematic analysis. J Psychosom Res 2008;64:573–82.

[78] Rief W, Broadbent E, Rief W, Broadbent E. Explaining medically unexplained symptoms-models and mechanisms. Clin Psychol Rev 2007;27:821–41.

[79] Roelofs K, Spinhoven P, Roelofs K, Spinhoven P. Trauma and medically unexplained symptoms towards an integration of cognitive and neurobiological accounts. Clin Psychol Rev 2007;27:798–820.

[80] Rosmalen JG, Neeleman J, Gans RO, de Jonge P, Rosmalen JGM, Neeleman J, Gans ROB, de Jonge P. The association between neuroticism and self-reported common somatic symptoms in a population cohort. J Psychosom Res 2007;62:305–11.

[81] Sharpe M, Mayou R, Walker J, Sharpe M, Mayou R, Walker J. Bodily symptoms: new approaches to classification. J Psychosom Res 2006;60:353–6.

[82] Smith RC, Gardiner JC, Lyles JS, Sirbu C, Dwamena FC, Hodges A, Collins C, Lein C, Given CW, Given B, et al. Exploration of DSM-IV criteria in primary care patients with medically unexplained symptoms. Psychosom Med 2005;67:123–9.

[83] Spiegel BM, Kanwal F, Naliboff B, Mayer E. The impact of somatization on the use of gastrointestinal health-care resources in patients with irritable bowel syndrome. Am J Gastroenterol 2005;100:2262–73.

[84] Staud R, Staud R. Somatization does not fit all fibromyalgia patients: comment on the article by Winfield. Arthritis Rheum 2002;46:564–5.

[85] van der Windt DA, Dunn KM, Spies-Dorgelo MN, Mallen CD, Blankenstein AH, Stalman WA, van der Windt DAWM, Dunn KM, Spies-Dorgelo MN, Mallen CD, et al. Impact of physical symptoms on perceived health in the community. J Psychosom Res 2008;64:265–74.

[86] Vandvik PO, Lydersen S, Farup PG, Vandvik PO, Lydersen S, Farup PG. Prevalence, comorbidity and impact of irritable bowel syndrome in Norway. Scand J Gastroenterol 2006;41:650–6.

[87] Vandvik PO, Wilhelmsen I, Ihlebaek C, Farup PG. Comorbidity of irritable bowel syndrome in general practice: a striking feature with clinical implications. Aliment Pharmacol Ther 2004;20:1195–1203.

[88] Wessely S, Nimnuan C, Sharpe M. Functional somatic syndromes: one or many? Lancet 1999;354:936–939.

[89] Wessely S, White PD, Wessely S, White PD. There is only one functional somatic syndrome. Br J Psychiatry 2004;185:95–96.

[90] Whitehead WE, Palsson O, Jones KR. Systematic review of the comorbidity of irritable bowel syndrome with other disorders: what are the causes and implications? Gastroenterology 2002;122:1140–1156.

[91] Whitehead WE, Palsson OS, Levy RR, Feld AD, Turner M, Von Korff M, Whitehead WE, Palsson OS, Levy RR, Feld AD, et al. Comorbidity in irritable bowel syndrome. Am J Gastroenterol 2007;102:2767–76.

[92] Whorwell PJ, Whorwell PJ. Hypnotherapy for irritable bowel syndrome: the response of colonic and noncolonic symptoms. J Psychosom Res 2008;64:621–3.

[93] Wilhelmsen I, Haug TT, Ursin H, Berstad A. Discriminant analysis of factors distinguishing patients with functional dyspepsia from patients with duodenal ulcer. Significance of somatization. Dig Dis Sci 1995;40:1105–11.

[94] Williams RE, Hartmann KE, Sandler RS, Miller WC, Steege JF, Williams RE, Hartmann KE, Sandler RS, Miller WC, Steege JF. Prevalence and characteristics of irritable bowel syndrome among women with chronic pelvic pain. Obstet Gynecol 2004;104:452–8.

[95] Winfield JB, Winfield JB. Does pain in fibromyalgia reflect somatization? Arthritis Rheum 2001;44:751–3.

[96] World Health Organization. Composite International Diagnostic Interview (CIDI). Geneva: World Health Organization Division of Mental Health; 1989.

[97] Yunus MB, Yunus MB. Central sensitivity syndromes: a new paradigm and group nosology for fibromyalgia and overlapping conditions, and the related issue of disease versus illness. Semin Arthritis Rheum 2008;37:339–52.

Correspondence to: Francis Creed, MD, FRCP, FRCPsych, FMedSci, Rawnsley Building, Manchester Royal Infirmary, Oxford Road, Manchester M13 9WL, United Kingdom. Email: francis.creed@manchester.ac.uk.

Chronic Fatigue Syndrome

Gudrun Lange[a,b] and Benjamin H. Natelson[c]

[a]Pain and Fatigue Study Center, New Jersey Medical School, Newark, New Jersey, USA; [b]War Related Illness and Injury Study Center, Department of Veterans Affairs New Jersey Health Care System, East Orange, New Jersey, USA; [c]Pain and Fatigue Study Center, Beth Israel Medical Center, Phillips Ambulatory Care Center, New York, New York, USA

Fatigue is a common condition afflicting many individuals worldwide. For many, fatigue is a temporary state following physical or mental exertion, is remedied by rest, and lasts for only a brief period of time. For some, however, fatigue persists longer and becomes chronic, either following a sudden onset, for instance after a bout of the flu, or after gradually building up over time. If the fatigue experienced by these individuals cannot be explained medically, some are eventually diagnosed with either prolonged fatigue (of 1 month's duration or more), idiopathic chronic fatigue (ICF), or chronic fatigue syndrome (CFS). To be diagnosed with ICF, an individual must have had persistent fatigue of new onset for at least 6 months. A diagnosis of CFS requires the same duration of fatigue, but the long-lived fatigue must be accompanied by a cluster of four or more of the following eight symptoms: cognitive difficulties; unrefreshing sleep; sore throat; tender lymph nodes; headaches of a new type, pattern, or severity; muscle pain; joint pain; and post-exertional malaise lasting for 24 hours or more. Over the years, several consensus case definitions have been used to diagnose the illness [7,24,26,47], but the one most commonly used in the United States is the "1994 case definition" [20] described above. The estimated prevalence of CFS in the United States using the 1994 case definition ranges from 0.24% [45] to 0.42% [27]. In the United States, CFS is most common in Latinos, next most in African Americans, and less common in whites [27,45]. The illness affects women more often than men [6,27,45], with women between the ages of 40 to 59 being most affected [27,45], but expression of the syndrome is generally not gender-specific [6,41,55]. Children and adolescents also suffer from CFS, although prevalence rates are significantly lower than in adults [8,18,29]. Gender distribution is similar to that of the adult sample.

Etiological Hypotheses

Chronic fatigue syndrome is a heterogeneous disease of unclear etiology as often reflected in the nomenclature used to define it, depending on the mechanism attributed putatively to its cause: myalgic encephalitis (ME), post-infectious fatigue, and chronic fatigue immune deficiency syndrome (CFIDS). A series of studies that has led to a hypothesis implicating infection as a possible cause for the illness has shown that about 9% of people, again women more often than men, have symptoms consistent with the diagnosis of CFS 6 months after sustaining severe viral infections [25,31]. However, efforts to find differences in viral burden between patients and controls have not succeeded [56]. Of interest are data from Glaser's group showing that animals reduce their activity when injected with an Epstein Barr viral antigen, i.e., a viral particle rather than the live virus [42]. This report may mean that aborted viral replication may still produce illness via release of toxic antigens.

Over the years, the immune system has been a prime candidate as a potential causal mechanism for CFS. The immunological hypothesis has to do with the well-known fact that humans feel sick when injected with pro-inflammatory cytokines. The idea is that viral infection produces immune dysregulation or onset of autoimmunity. Unfortunately, our own studies of cytokines in the blood have been negative [32]. However, in a study of spinal fluid, we did find increases in interleukin-10 (IL-10), an anti-inflammatory cytokine, in the subgroup of CFS patients reporting a sudden or flu-like illness onset [40]; the significance of this finding is unclear and bears replication. The most consistent immunological finding in CFS has been reduced natural killer cell count and function [39]. Recent work from the Miami group provides strong evidence that this finding is not an epiphenomenon of inactivity [48], but its significance in producing the syndrome remains unclear.

Early reports of laboratory abnormalities cited rates of up to 15% of patients with antinuclear antibodies [3]. These data led to the hypothesis that CFS could be an undiagnosed autoimmune disorder. In our clinic, we were impressed by the frequent CFS patient self-report of dry eyes and dry mouth and hypothesized that some might have had a mild form of Sjögren's disease, an autoimmune disease characterized by an inflammatory attack on lacrimal and salivary glands, among other glands, leading to dry eyes and mouth. To evaluate this hypothesis, we performed a case-control study with 25 patients and 18 healthy controls [50]. Fifty-two percent of the patients compared to none of the controls reported dry eyes and dry mouth. Of these 13 patients, 10 had abnormal rates of tear production, as assessed by Schirmer's test, compared to one control subject. Finally, and most impressively, 8 of these 10 CFS patients showed evidence of lymphoid infiltration of minor salivary glands following biopsy compared to none of the controls. This study indicates that up to a quarter of CFS patients have an undiagnosed autoimmune disorder consistent with primary Sjögren's disease.

The potential causal mechanism in which our group has been very interested is the possibility that CFS is a disorder of the central nervous system (CNS). Our first study was an outgrowth of an earlier study showing that individuals with CFS, like patients with multiple sclerosis (another illness in which fatigue is a major complaint), had objective evidence of cognitive dysfunction [17]. We evaluated several stratification strategies to determine which, if any, reduced the variability of the results. We found that stratifying according to the presence or absence of a comorbid psychiatric diagnosis was helpful. Specifically, we found that patients with a negative psychiatric history were the ones with the most cognitive dysfunction [16]. That result led us to use this stratification strategy a priori in our subsequent studies. The first of these was a blinded evaluation of brain magnetic resonance imaging (MRI) scans in CFS patients and healthy controls [34]. As was the case with our study of neuropsychological function, we found that individuals with CFS devoid of comorbid psychiatric disease were the ones with the highest number of MRI abnormalities—for the most part small T2 areas of uptake in frontal white matter. Importantly, in a subsequent study, we found that the patients with the MRI abnormalities had significantly poorer physical function than those without the abnormalities [12]; this result strongly suggested that the lesions were of functional significance.

Our inference from these data was that individuals with CFS devoid of psychiatric comorbidity had an occult encephalopathy producing their illness. We next turned to an examination of spinal fluid, comparing cell count and protein concentration to levels found in a group of healthy controls [40]. In contrast to the normal results for these variables in the 13 controls, 30% of 44 patients had either an elevated white cell count or elevated proteins, or both. Importantly, none of the patients with abnormal fluid had current depression, compared to nearly a quarter of those with normal fluids—again supporting the use of psychiatric comorbidity as an important stratifying variable. In a subsequent study using xenon computed tomography, we found reduced cerebral blood flow in all our patients compared to healthy controls [61]; however, the group without psychiatric comorbidity had the greatest reductions. Our new collaborator Dikoma Shungu has found a similar tendency showing increased cerebral ventricular lactate in CFS, in which patients with higher values had a lower rate of psychiatric comorbidity than those with normal lactate values [37A].

Finally, our most recent work has addressed the patient complaint of unrefreshing sleep and seeks to understand whether sleep disturbances could be causally related to CFS. We performed overnight polysomnography in individuals with CFS alone, in those with both CFS and fibromyalgia syndrome (FM), and in healthy controls [54]. One of the purposes of our study was to evaluate an earlier report of a high rate of sleep disturbed breathing in FM [23]. However, here we found similar results for those with CFS alone compared to those with CFS plus FM. Both groups had low rates of diagnosable sleep disorders. After excluding patients with specific sleep disorders, however, we found that individuals with CFS showed abnormalities in sleep structure. While we were not able to use psychiatric comorbidity to reduce variability in this study, we did find that patients who reported being sleepier after a night in the sleep laboratory were the ones with the most profound disturbances, characterized by poor sleep efficiency and sleep patterns consistent with broken sleep. In an experiment just completed, we asked patients and matched controls to remain awake all night and then determined the latency for them to fall asleep the next morning (unpublished data). The 13 controls fell asleep with latencies ranging from 0 to 540 seconds (median = 90 seconds), while the 15 patients fell asleep with latencies ranging from 0 to 3,240 seconds (median = 300 seconds; $P < 0.05$ for square-root-transformed data). Five of the 15 patients had sleep latencies longer than the longest of the controls (range 750 to 3,240 seconds; median 1,440 seconds). Thus, despite a night of sleep deprivation, one-third of the CFS patients had significant sleep delays indicative of a problem in falling asleep. We are currently investigating cytokine patterns to determine whether a shift from sleep-inducing to sleep-disrupting cytokines may be playing a role in the pathogenesis of CFS.

Similarities and Differences between Chronic Fatigue Syndrome and other Functional Syndromes

As discussed above, CFS is frequently comorbid with psychiatric illness, especially depression and anxiety, as well as with chronic pain disorders including FM, irritable bowel syndrome (IBS), and also multiple chemical sensitivity (MCS), a somatic response to exposure to odors with accompanying avoidant behavior [9]. Since many symptoms associated with these syndromes overlap with those defining CFS, some investigators have inferred that these conditions may be best referred to and managed as a single entity (i.e., the "one syndrome" hypothesis) and labeled "functional somatic syndromes" (FSS) [30,59]. This nomenclature is problematic in that the proponents of this view have not clearly defined what is meant by "functional." Does "functional" have its mid-20th century meaning of being due to psychogenic factors? Or does "functional" mean that organic pathology exists, but on an organizational or submicroscopic basis? Certainly, one reading of "functional" is that it is a manifestation of a psychiatric disorder called "somatization," in which distressed patients disregard emotional issues and focus instead on bodily sensations [2,58]. However, a diagnosis of somatization disorder allows for substantial variability in interpretation [28]. Using the symptoms constituting the 1994 case definition for CFS, rates of diagnosis of somatization disorder ranged from 97% to 0% when symptoms were coded either as psychiatric in cause or medical in cause, respectively. Since many physicians as well as patients view the diagnosis of somatization disorder as pejorative and judgmental, it was suggested that the term be replaced by "functional somatic syndromes" [46]. Relabeling somatization as a functional somatic syndrome does not seem to be a step forward in that it substitutes one vague label for another. Therefore, we prefer to describe such patients as having "medically unexplained symptoms." This name is not burdened with any preconceived notion of cause.

We agree with the London group [59] who suggest that it is unlikely that "improved understanding" of medically unexplained symptoms will result from statistical parsing of "symptoms and their occurrence." Yet it is surprising how little attention has been paid to looking for empirical differences among the syndromes. If all these medically unexplained health conditions reflect a unitary pathophysiological cause, then the mode of illness onset, symptoms, and comorbidity profile of each syndrome should be very similar to those of the next. Conversely, if differences exist in the pathophysiology causing the individual syndromes, then we should be able to find differences among the various syndromes on these variables.

In pursuing this line of reasoning, an important first research question is to ask whether the onset and comorbidity profile of CFS is similar in different patient groups with this diagnosis. To answer this question, we compared a civilian sample with sporadic onset of CFS to a sample of veterans who developed CFS after their return home from the Gulf War of 1990–91. As noted earlier, CFS in civilians is preponderantly a problem in women's health, but in veterans, related to the demographics of deployment to a war zone, it occurs more often in men than women [44].

To control for this gender-related discrepancy, we recently extended our earlier work to a sample restricted to male white patients (30 veterans with CFS and 84 non-veterans with CFS) [10]. Several differences in the comorbidity profiles emerged between groups. As one might expect, the rate of psychiatric comorbidity in veterans, specifically post-traumatic stress disorder (PTSD), was significantly higher than in civilians (27% vs. 3%). But more importantly, male veterans with CFS did not have comorbid FM, in contrast to male civilians with CFS (0% vs. 22%). Another difference between the groups was the rate of self-reported sudden or flu-like onset. More civilians than veterans reported a sudden, flu-like illness onset (43% vs. 10%), supporting the interpretation of different processes being responsible for illness onset between the groups. The differences provide strong support for the position that CFS in Gulf War veterans appears to have a pathophysiological basis that is different from that in civilians and argue against the one-syndrome hypothesis.

If CFS were a discrete syndrome, then we should also find differences in illness onset, physical functioning, and levels of symptom severity between patients with CFS only and those who have other medically unexplained illnesses such as FM and MCS [9]. To evaluate this issue, a consecutive series of 163 middle-aged women with CFS was assigned into groups of women with CFS only, those with CFS plus FM, those with CFS plus MCS, and those with CFS plus FM plus MCS. Thirty-eight percent of the sample had CFS only, while only 16% had all three diagnoses. Fibromyalgia was diagnosed in 43% and MCS in 35%. Patients with CFS alone had a significantly higher rate of sudden illness onset than those with CFS plus FM (47% vs. 25%); the rate of gradual onset increased once patients carried a diagnosis of FM. Physical function, as assessed with the Medical Outcomes Study 36-item Short-Form Health Survey (SF-36) [38], was in the severely disabled range across all groups when compared to other chronic illness groups. However, the CFS-only group functioned significantly better than groups of patients with comorbid FM, most likely due to inhibition of movement secondary to the presence of diffuse, four-quadrant pain central to a diagnosis of FM. Severity of general fatigue, as assessed by the Multi Fatigue Inventory (MFI) [51], was significantly greater in the group with CFS plus FM plus MCS compared to the

CFS-only group. The group with all three diagnoses also reported significantly more severe gland tenderness than any of the other groups. Muscle and joint pain was most severe in groups of patients with comorbid FM, as would be expected. Patient-reported severity of other core symptoms of CFS, including fever, sore throat, new-onset headache, muscle weakness, prolonged fatigue, unrefreshing sleep, and memory problems, did not differ across the four groups. In summary, the data suggest that while the CFS only group had less overall fatigue and enjoyed better physical function, most likely due to the absence of FM pain, the severity of core CFS symptoms was similar whether or not comorbid syndromes were present. This observation might argue for the one-syndrome hypothesis. However, the increased rate of sudden onset in the CFS-only group compared to a higher rate of gradual illness onset in patients who also have FM is consistent with the hypothesis that an infectious etiology is more common in CFS than in FM; obviously, it would be important to study a group with FM only to confirm this observation.

In a subset of women in the same study, we also assessed whether CFS patients had irritable bowel syndrome (IBS) as defined by the Rome III criteria (Ciccone and Natelson, unpublished data). (The Rome III criteria for IBS are shown in Table II of Chapter 5 by Chang and Drossman.) To determine whether rates of IBS in this subsample varied with presence or absence of other medically unexplained syndromes, we stratified the CFS only plus IBS patients into groups with and without coexisting FM and MCS. Table I shows the results of these previously unpublished data—a nonrandom distribution ($\chi^2 = 9.3$; $P < 0.05$).

Table I
Prevalence of irritable bowel syndrome in patients with
chronic fatigue syndrome (CFS) alone and in patients
with CFS and other comorbid syndromes
(FM, fibromyalgia; MCS, multiple chemical sensitivities)

	MCS Negative	MCS Positive
FM negative	4/26 or 15%	2/11 or 18%
FM positive	12/32 or 38%	10/18 or 56%

Source: Ciccone and Natelson, unpublished data.

Rates of IBS for the CFS-only group are at expected population rates (i.e., 15%) [5], but rates more than doubled in the face of comorbid FM (38%) and increased again when MCS was also present (56%). Given the small sample, we must consider these results preliminary, but nonetheless, they do suggest that the probability of having IBS increases in the face of having other medically unexplained syndromes. Looked at another way, the data suggest that CFS alone is a different illness from CFS plus FM plus MCS. The latter group seems to fit the model for "functional somatic syndromes" better than the former group.

Psychiatric comorbidity is another important factor when looking for differences and similarities across medically unexplained syndromes. The prevalence of having a lifetime concurrent psychiatric disorder, especially major depressive disorder (MDD), increased monotonically with the number of comorbid medically unexplained syndromes [9]. The rate of lifetime MDD in women with CFS plus FM plus MCS was more than double the rate in the CFS-only group (69% vs. 27%). This result is consonant with Wessely's earlier report of a linear relation between the number of CFS symptoms and psychiatric morbidity [57]. We found the same result when we looked at CFS plus IBS instead of MCS (Ciccone and Natelson, unpublished data). Rates of lifetime MDD for 31 women with CFS only were half of those for 22 women with CFS plus FM plus IBS (36% vs. 73%; $\chi^2 = 7.45$, $P = 0.05$). These data suggest a difference between patients with CFS only and others with multiple coexisting medically unexplained syndromes. Whether the greater prevalence of lifetime depression represents a response to an increased illness burden or an increased risk of having somatic symptoms related to the depressive diathesis is not known, but it remains an important question for future research.

Cognitive difficulties are characteristic in CFS [53] and have been associated with changes in brain structure [33,36] and function [35,49]. These complaints are also common in FM, but results of cognitive testing have varied with some showing deficits [43] and others not [52]. While the behavioral data suggest differences between CFS-only and CFS plus FM patient groups, available neuroimaging data provide evidence for some similarities. Neuroimaging studies of cognitive function found that FM patients had the same increased mental effort in response to cognitive tasks as occurred in CFS patients [22]. In an effort to deal with these discrepant results in FM and to directly compare cognitive function in CFS and FM, we challenged 20 patients with CFS only, 19 patients with CFS plus FM, and 26 healthy controls, all demographically similar, with a battery of cognitive tests designed to assess speed of information processing, performance variability, and efficiency [13]. One-way ANOVAs indicated that CFS-only patients displayed deficits in all three of these variables relative to healthy controls, while the CFS plus FM group performed similarly to controls. To our knowledge, no data exist comparing cognitive function in patients with CFS only, FM only, CFS plus FM, and healthy controls, either behaviorally or using neuroimaging. Thus, exploration of cognitive function remains an important area of future empirical research in medically unexplained syndromes.

Postexertional malaise is another core CFS symptom that, based on patient report, was similar in severity across CFS-only and "CFS plus" groups [9]; early studies suggested metabolic differences between CFS patients and controls [15]. To further evaluate this possibility, we asked individuals with CFS only, those with CFS plus FM, and healthy controls to perform a maximal exercise test by pedaling on a stationary bicycle as workload increased until they could pedal no longer [14]. Initial evaluation of the results indicated that CFS plus FM patients, but not CFS-only patients, had cardiorespiratory differences from controls. Specifically, the CFS plus FM group demonstrated lower ventilation, lower end-tidal CO_2, and higher ventilation to CO_2 production ratio (VE/VCO_2) compared to controls, and they had slower increases in heart rate compared to both CFS-only patients and controls. Peak oxygen consumption, ventilation, and workload were lower in the CFS plus FM group. However, when the two CFS groups were matched with one another and with healthy controls based on aerobic fitness, all these differences fell away. Thus, the differences we had originally found were related to small differences in baseline fitness or conditioning between groups. In summary, the two groups were physiologically similar, supporting the one-syndrome hypothesis.

However, a difference did emerge during subsequent submaximal exercise testing, during which participants cycled at 45% of their maximal oxygen uptake established in the previous study, a relatively easy task

(Cook and Natelson, unpublished data). Preliminary evaluation of the data revealed that, in the face of similar heart rates between groups, stroke volume (the amount of blood that is ejected from the left ventricle with each heartbeat) did not change for the CFS only group compared to controls but did increase significantly for the CFS plus FM group (see Fig. 1). This finding suggests more cardiac work at a constant workload for the latter group compared to those with CFS only. So here too, another pathophysiological difference emerges between patients with CFS only and those with CFS plus FM.

Finally, we looked at central serotonergic regulation in patients with CFS alone and others with CFS plus FM (Weaver and Natelson, unpublished data). Our reason for doing this study was that the available data

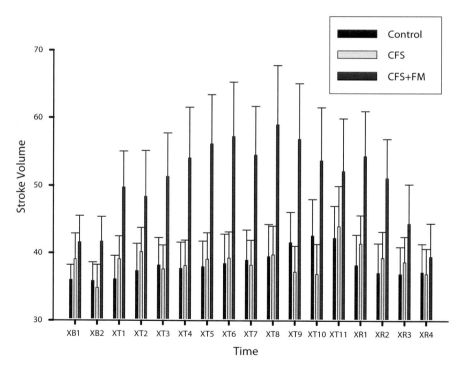

Fig. 1. Stroke volume for the three groups during baseline (XB1 and 2), during submaximal exercise at 45% VO$_2$max (XT1–11), and during recovery (XR1–4). Stroke volume changes little at this relatively easy task for controls and patients with chronic fatigue syndrome (CFS) alone, but it increases strikingly for patients with CFS plus fibromyalgia (FM).

suggested opposite effects of serotonin on fatigue and pain. When levels of brain serotonin (5-HT) are increased, either by exercise or administration of the 5-HT precursor tryptophan, fatigue follows [4,19]. Importantly, when levels are high, pain sensitivity is decreased and conversely, pain sensitivity increases when 5-HT levels are low [1,37,60]. These facts allowed us to hypothesize that brain serotonergic neurons would be upregulated in CFS and downregulated in FM. Finding such a result would be strong evidence against the one-syndrome hypothesis.

To evaluate brain serotonergic activity, we gave tryptophan intravenously to patients with CFS only and to others with CFS plus FM as well as to healthy controls over a 15-minute period (Weaver and Natelson, unpublished data). Serotonin is synthesized from the amino acid tryptophan via the enzyme tryptophan hydroxylase, which is not normally saturated with tryptophan. Thus, tryptophan loading increases serotonin synthesis in the brain in humans [21]. To reduce heterogeneity in the sample, we decided to study only women of reproductive age during the late follicular phase of their menstrual cycle (7 to 14 days after the first day of the subject's last menses) at the same time of day. All were medication free for at least 2 weeks prior to study, and we ascertained that none had current MDD because of the well-known effects of tryptophan in reducing plasma prolactin in patients with this diagnosis [11]. At least 30 minutes after venous catheterization, we drew an initial baseline sample and then another baseline sample, after which we began the 15-minute tryptophan infusion. Samples were drawn thereafter, and results can be seen in Fig. 2.

Baseline plasma prolactin concentrations did not differ among groups. Repeated-measures ANOVA showed a significant time effect, with prolactin increasing across all groups after tryptophan infusion ($P < 0.001$). A significant group effect was also seen ($P = 0.006$), with the responses of the CFS-only group being significantly greater than those of the CFS plus FM group and those of the healthy controls ($P < 0.05$ for both comparisons). The responses of the CFS plus FM group did not differ from those of healthy subjects.

This experiment showed that patients with CFS only have different serotonergic activity from those with CFS plus FM. As expected, those with CFS only showed upregulation, while those with CFS plus FM showed no difference from controls. Unfortunately, we did not have an FM-only group. Our hypothesis is that study of such a group would reveal a frank downregulated response. Nonetheless, the data reviewed above are important in supporting our working hypothesis that CFS and FM have different underlying pathophysiological processes.

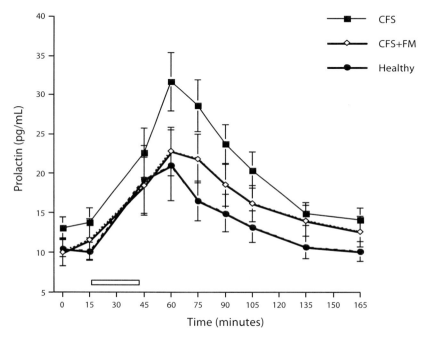

Fig. 2. Plasma prolactin response to exogenous tryptophan (infusion denoted by horizontal box along the horizontal axis) was significantly greater in chronic fatigue syndrome (CFS) patients than in patients with CFS plus fibromyalgia (FM) or healthy subjects. Patients with CFS plus FM did not differ from controls.

Conclusions

Using an empirical approach, we found substantial differences between veterans and civilians with CFS and between patients with CFS only and those with CFS plus FM or with other medically unexplained syndromes. Our ability to find such differences is strong evidence against the position that all these medically unexplained syndromes have a unitary cause. The data suggest that in patients with CFS, a different pathophysiological process may be responsible for symptoms than in those with CFS plus FM and multiple other medically unexplained syndromes. The take-home point from the research we have conducted to date is that differences can be found in empiric and biological data in subgroups of patients with medically unexplained illness. Rather than continue to focus on similarities among the syndromes, our work strongly supports the continued need for more empiric research focusing on uncovering differences.

Acknowledgments

Preparation of this chapter was supported in part by NIH grants AR053732 to G. Lange and AI54478 to B.H. Natelson. The authors thank their colleagues Drs. Donald Ciccone, Dane Cook, and Shelley Weaver for making available the unpublished data cited in this chapter.

References

[1]   Bakheit AM, Behan PO, Dinan TG, Gray CE, O'Keane V. Possible upregulation of hypothalamic 5-hydroxytryptamine receptors in patients with postviral fatigue syndrome. BMJ 1992;304:1010–2.
[2]   Barsky AJ, Borus JF. Functional somatic syndromes. Ann Intern Med 1999;130:910–21.
[3]   Bates DW, Buchwald D, Lee J, Kith P, Doolittle T, Rutherford C, Churchill WH, Schur PH, Wener M, Wybenga D, Winkelman J, Komaroff AL. Clinical laboratory test findings in patients with chronic fatigue syndrome. Arch Intern Med 1995;155:97–103.
[4]   Blomstrand E. Amino acids and central fatigue. Amino Acids 2001;20:25–34.
[5]   Boivin M. Socioeconomic impact of irritable bowel syndrome in Canada. Can J Gastroenterol 2001;15 Suppl B:8B–11B.
[6]   Buchwald D, Pearlman T, Kith P, Schmaling K. Gender differences in patients with chronic fatigue syndrome. J Gen Intern Med 1994;9:397–401.
[7]   Carruthers BM. Definitions and aetiology of myalgic encephalomyelitis: how the Canadian consensus clinical definition of myalgic encephalomyelitis works. J Clin Pathol 2007;60:117–9.
[8]   Chalder T, Goodman R, Wessely S, Hotopf M, Meltzer H. Epidemiology of chronic fatigue syndrome and self reported myalgic encephalomyelitis in 5–15 year olds: cross sectional study. BMJ 2003;327:654–5.
[9]   Ciccone DS, Natelson BH. Comorbid illness in women with chronic fatigue syndrome: a test of the single syndrome hypothesis. Psychosom Med 2003;65:268–75.
[10] Ciccone DS, Weissman L, Natelson BH. Chronic fatigue syndrome in male gulf war veterans and civilians: a further test of the single syndrome hypothesis. J Health Psychol 2008;13:529–36.
[11] Cleare AJ, Bearn J, Allain T, McGregor A, Wessely S, Murray RM, O'Keane V. Contrasting neuroendocrine responses in depression and chronic fatigue syndrome. J Affect Disord 1995;34:283–9.
[12] Cook DB, Lange G, DeLuca J, Natelson BH. Relationship of brain MRI abnormalities and physical functional status in CFS. Int J Neurosci 2001;107:1–6.
[13] Cook DB, Nagelkirk PR, Peckerman A, Poluri A, Mores J, Natelson BH. Exercise and cognitive performance in Chronic Fatigue Syndrome. Med Sci Sports Exerc 2005;37:1460–7.

[14] Cook DB, Nagelkirk PR, Poluri A, Mores J, Natelson BH. The influence of aerobic fitness and fibromyalgia on cardiorespiratory and perceptual responses to exercise in patients with chronic fatigue syndrome. Arthritis Rheum 2006;54:3351–62.

[15] De BP, Roeykens J, Reynders M, McGregor N, De MK. Exercise capacity in chronic fatigue syndrome. Arch Intern Med 2000;160:3270–7.

[16] DeLuca J, Johnson SK, Ellis SP, Natelson BH. Cognitive functioning is impaired in chronic fatigue syndrome patients devoid of psychiatric disease. J Neurol Neurosurg Psychiatry 1997;62:151–5.

[17] DeLuca J, Johnson SK, Natelson BH. Information processing efficiency in chronic fatigue syndrome and multiple sclerosis. Arch Neurol 1993;50:301–4.

[18] Farmer A, Fowler T, Scourfield J, Thapar A. Prevalence of chronic disabling fatigue in children and adolescents. Br J Psychiatry 2004;184:477–81.

[19] Fernstrom JD, Fernstrom MH. Exercise, serum free tryptophan, and central fatigue. J Nutr 2006;136:553S-9S.

[20] Fukuda K, Straus SE, Hickie I, Sharpe M, Dobbins JG, Komaroff AL. The chronic fatigue syndrome: a comprehensive approach to its definition and study. International Chronic Fatigue Syndrome Study Group. Ann Intern Med 1994;121:953–9.

[21] Gillman PK, Bartlett JR, Bridges PK, Hunt A, Patel AJ, Kantamaneni BD, Curzon G. Indolic substances in plasma, cerebrospinal fluid, and frontal cortex of human subjects infused with saline or tryptophan. J Neurochem 1981;37:410–7.

[22] Glass JM. Cognitive dysfunction in fibromyalgia and chronic fatigue syndrome: new trends and future directions. Curr Rheumatol Rep 2006;8:425–9.

[23] Gold AR, Dipalo F, Gold MS, Broderick J. Inspiratory airflow dynamics during sleep in women with fibromyalgia. Sleep 2004;27:459–66.

[24] Hairon N. NICE guidance on managing chronic fatigue syndrome/ME. Nurs Times 2007;103:21–2.

[25] Hickie I, Davenport T, Wakefield D, Vollmer-Conna U, Cameron B, Vernon SD, Reeves WC, Lloyd A. Post-infective and chronic fatigue syndromes precipitated by viral and non-viral pathogens: prospective cohort study. BMJ 2006;333:575.

[26] Holmes GP, Kaplan JE, Gantz NM, Komaroff AL, Schonberger LB, Straus SE, Jones JF, Dubois RE, Cunningham-Rundles C, Pahwa S. Chronic fatigue syndrome: a working case definition. Ann Intern Med 1988;108:387–9.

[27] Jason LA, Richman JA, Rademaker AW, Jordan KM, Plioplys AV, Taylor RR, McCready W, Huang CF, Plioplys S. A community-based study of chronic fatigue syndrome. Arch Intern Med 1999;159:2129–37.

[28] Johnson SK, DeLuca J, Natelson BH. Assessing somatization disorder in the chronic fatigue syndrome. Psychosom Med 1996;58:50–7.

[29] Jones JF, Nisenbaum R, Solomon L, Reyes M, Reeves WC. Chronic fatigue syndrome and other fatiguing illnesses in adolescents: a population-based study. J Adolesc Health 2004;35:34–40.

[30] Kanaan RA, Lepine JP, Wessely SC. The association or otherwise of the functional somatic syndromes. Psychosom Med 2007;69:855–9.

[31] Komaroff AL. Is human herpesvirus-6 a trigger for chronic fatigue syndrome? J Clin Virol 2006;37 Suppl 1:S39–S46.

[32] LaManca JJ, Sisto S, Ottenweller JE, Cook S, Peckerman A, Zhang Q, Denny TN, Gause WC, Natelson BH. Immunological response in chronic fatigue syndrome following a graded exercise test to exhaustion. J Clin Immunol 1999;19:135–42.

[33] Lange G, DeLuca J, Maldjian JA, Lee H, Tiersky LA, Natelson BH. Brain MRI abnormalities exist in a subset of patients with chronic fatigue syndrome. J Neurol Sci 1999;171:3–7.

[34] Lange G, DeLuca J, Maldjian JA, Lee HJ, Tiersky LA, Natelson BH. Brain MRI abnormalities exist in a subset of patients with chronic fatigue syndrome. J Neurol Sci 1999;171:3–7.

[35] Lange G, Steffener J, Bly BM, Christodoulou C, Liu W-C, DeLuca J, Natelson BH. Chronic fatigue syndrome affects verbal working memory: a BOLD fMRI study. Neuroimage 2005;26:513–24.

[36] Lange G, Wang S, DeLuca J, Natelson BH. Neuroimaging in chronic fatigue syndrome. Am J Med 1998;105:50S-3S.

[37] Lopez-Garcia JA. Serotonergic modulation of spinal sensory circuits. Curr Top Med Chem 2006;6:1987–96.

[37A] Mathew SJ, Mao X, Keegan KA, Levine SM, Smith EL, Heier LA, Otcheretko V, Coplan JD, Shungu DC. Ventricular cerebrospinal fluid lactate is increased in chronic fatigue syndrome compared with generalized anxiety disorder: an in vivo 3.0 T (1)H MRS imaging study. NMR Biomed 2008; Epub Oct 21.

[38] McHorney CA, Ware JE, Jr., Lu JFR. The MOS 36-item Short-Form Health Survey (SF-36): III. Tests of data quality, scaling assumptions, and reliability across diverse patient groups. Medical Care 1994;32:40–66.

[39] Natelson BH, Haghighi MH, Ponzio NM. Evidence for the presence of immune dysfunction in chronic fatigue syndrome. Clin Diagn Lab Immunol 2002;9:747–52.

[40] Natelson BH, Tseng C-L, Ottenweller JE. Spinal fluid abnormalities in patients with chronic fatigue syndrome. Clin Diagn Lab Immunol 2005;12:53–5.

[41] Natelson BH, Weaver SA, Tseng CL, Ottenweller JE. Spinal fluid abnormalities in patients with chronic fatigue syndrome. Clin Diagn Lab Immunol 2005;12:52–5.

[42] Padgett DA, Hotchkiss AK, Pyter LM, Nelson RJ, Yang E, Yeh PE, Litsky M, Williams M, Glaser R. Epstein-Barr virus-encoded dUTPase modulates immune function and induces sickness behavior in mice. J Med Virol 2004;74:442–8.

[43] Park DC, Glass JM, Minear M, Crofford LJ. Cognitive function in fibromyalgia patients. Arthritis Rheum 2001;44:2125–33.

[44] Pollet C, Natelson BH, Lange G, Tiersky L, DeLuca J, Policastro T, Desai P, Ottenweller JE, Korn L, Fiedler N, Kipen H. Medical evaluation of Persian Gulf veterans with fatigue and/or chemical sensitivity. J Med 1998;29:101–13.

[45] Reyes M, Nisenbaum R, Hoaglin DC, Unger ER, Emmons C, Randall B, Stewart JA, Abbey S, Jones JF, Gantz N, Minden S, Reeves WC. Prevalence and incidence of chronic fatigue syndrome in Wichita, Kansas. Arch Intern Med 2003;163:1530–6.

[46] Sharpe M, Mayou R. Somatoform disorders: a help or hindrance to good patient care? Br J Psychiatry 2004;184:465–7.

[47] Sharpe MC, Archard LC, Banatvala JE, Borysiewicz LK, Clare AW, David A, Edwards RH, Hawton KE, Lambert HP, Lane RJ. A report: chronic fatigue syndrome: guidelines for research. J R Soc Med 1991;84:118–21.

[48] Siegel SD, Antoni MH, Fletcher MA, Maher K, Segota MC, Klimas N. Impaired natural immunity, cognitive dysfunction, and physical symptoms in patients with chronic fatigue syndrome: preliminary evidence for a subgroup. J Psychosom Res 2006;60:559–66.

[49] Siessmeier T, Nix WA, Hardt J, Schreckenberger M, Egle UT, Bartenstein P. Observer independent analysis of cerebral glucose metabolism in patients with chronic fatigue syndrome. J Neurol Neurosurg Psychiatry 2003;74:922–8.

[50] Sirois DA, Natelson B. Clinicopathological findings consistent with primary Sjogren's syndrome in a subset of patients diagnosed with chronic fatigue syndrome: preliminary observations. J Rheumatol 2001;28:126–31.

[51] Smets EM, Garssen B, Bonke B, De Haes JC. The Multidimensional Fatigue Inventory (MFI) psychometric qualities of an instrument to assess fatigue. J Psychosom Res 1995;39:315–25.

[52] Suhr JA. Neuropsychological impairment in fibromyalgia: relation to depression, fatigue, and pain. J Psychosom Res 2003;55:321–9.

[53] Tiersky LA, Johnson SK, Lange G, Natelson BH, DeLuca J. Neuropsychology of chronic fatigue syndrome: a critical review. J Clin Exp Neuropsychol 1997;19:560–86.

[54] Togo F, Natelson BH, Cherniack NS, Fitzgibbons J, Garcon C, Rapoport DM. Sleep structure and sleepiness in chronic fatigue syndrome with or without coexisting fibromyalgia. Arthritis Res Ther 2008;10:R56.

[55] Tseng CL, Natelson BH. Few gender differences exist between women and men with chronic fatigue syndrome. J Clin Psychol Med Settings 2004;55–62.

[56] Wallace II HL, Natelson BH, Gause WC, Hay J. An evaluation of human herpesviruses in chronic fatigue syndrome. Clin Diagn Lab Immunol 1999;6:216–23.

[57] Wessely S, Chalder T, Hirsch S, Wallace P, Wright D. Psychological symptoms, somatic symptoms, and psychiatric disorder in chronic fatigue and chronic fatigue syndrome: a prospective study in the primary care setting. Am J Psychiatry 1996;153:1050–9.

[58] Wessely S, Nimnuan C, Sharpe M. Functional somatic syndromes: one or many? Lancet 1999;354:936–9.

[59] Wessely S, White PD. There is only one functional somatic syndrome. Br J Psychiatry 2004;185:95–6.

[60] Yoshimura M, Furue H. Mechanisms for the anti-nociceptive actions of the descending noradrenergic and serotonergic systems in the spinal cord. J Pharmacol Sci 2006;101:107–17.

[61] Yoshiuchi K, Farkas J, Natelson BH. Patients with chronic fatigue syndrome have reduced absolute cortical blood flow. Clin Physiol Funct Imaging 2006;26:83–6.

Correspondence to: Gudrun Lange, PhD, Department of Veterans Affairs New Jersey Health Care System, East Orange, 385 Tremont Avenue, East Orange, NJ 07018, USA. Email: gudrun.lange@va.gov.

Part IV

Neurobiological Mechanisms Contributing to Symptoms

Autonomic Nervous System Dysfunction

Wilfrid Jänig

Institute of Physiology, University of Kiel, Kiel, Germany

The Autonomic Nervous System Is a Motor System

Autonomic and endocrine homeostatic regulation is represented in the brain (in the hypothalamus, brainstem, and spinal cord) and under the control of the telencephalon. It is integrated on all central neural levels with the somatomotor and sensory representations of the body, leading to a tight coordination of autonomic and somatomotor regulation. The brain contains autonomic "sensorimotor programs" for the coordinated regulation of the internal environment of the body; it sends efferent commands to the peripheral target tissues through the autonomic and endocrine routes.

Autonomic regulation of body functions requires specific neural pathways in the periphery and a specific organization of neural circuits connected to these pathways in the central nervous system (CNS). Without these specific pathways and connections, it would be impossible to understand the precision with which the body makes rapid and slow adjustments during various behaviors. The effector cells of the autonomic nervous system are diverse, whereas those of the somatic efferent system are not. Thus, the autonomic nervous system is the major efferent component of the peripheral nervous system, surpassing the somatic efferent pathways in its size and diversity of function.

The model in Fig. 1 outlines the role of the autonomic nervous system in the generation of behavior. Behavior, defined as purposeful motor action of the body in the environment, is generated by coordinated activation of the three divisions of the motor system: the somatic, autonomic, and neuroendocrine motor systems [44,96,97,104]. The somatomotor system moves the body in the environment. The autonomic and neuroendocrine motor systems prepare and adjust the internal milieu, enabling the body to move. Both systems are also important in protecting the organism against real and potential short- and long-term injuries that threaten continuously from outside as well as from within the body.

The motoneuron pools of the somatomotor and autonomic nervous systems extend from the midbrain to the caudal end of the spinal cord, with gaps in the cervical and lower lumbar spinal cord for the autonomic system. The neuroendocrine motor neurons are located in the periventricular zone of the hypothalamus. The three divisions of the motor system are hierarchically organized in the spinal cord, brainstem, and hypothalamus, with the neuroendocrine motor system at the top of this hierarchy. The three divisions are integrated at each level of the hierarchy.

The activity of the motor system in generating behavior is dependent on three major classes of input: (1) the sensory systems, (2) the cortical system, and (3) the behavioral state system. The sensory systems monitor events in the body (*internal afferent* in Fig. 1) or in the environment (*external afferent* in Fig. 1). They are closely linked to the motor hierarchies, and at all levels of these hierarchies they generate reflex behaviors (*reflex* in Fig. 1). The cerebral hemispheres initiate and maintain behavior based on cognition and affective-emotional processes (*cortical* in Fig. 1). The behavioral state system consists of intrinsic neural systems that determine the state of the brain in which it generates motor behavior. The

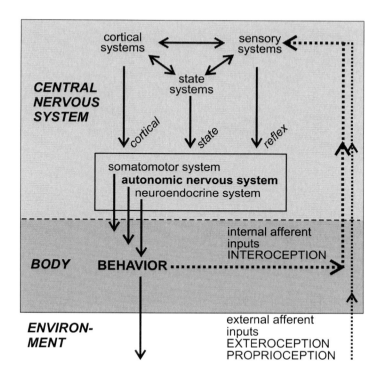

Fig. 1. Functional organization of the nervous system in relation to behavior. The brain controls behavior by way of the motor system, consisting of the somatomotor, autonomic (visceromotor), and neuroendocrine systems. The motor system is hierarchically organized in the spinal cord, brainstem, and hypothalamus. It receives three general types of input: (a) From the sensory systems monitoring processes in the body (small-diameter [Aδ and C] afferents) (interoception); in the environment, including the body surface (large-diameter afferents) (exteroception); or in skeletal muscles and joints (large-diameter afferents) (proprioception) to all levels of the motor system, generating reflex behavior (*reflex*). (b) From the cerebral hemispheres responsible for voluntary control of behavior, based on neural processes related to cognitive and affective-emotional processes (*cortical*). (c) From the behavioral system controlling attention, arousal, sleep/wakefulness, and circadian timing (*state*). The three general input systems communicate bidirectionally with each other (upper part of the figure). Modified from [96,97].

behavioral state system controls sleep and wakefulness, arousal, attention, vigilance, and circadian timing (*state* in Fig. 1).

This way of looking at the autonomic nervous system shows that the activity in the autonomic neurons is dependent on the intrinsic functional structure of the sensorimotor programs of the motor hierarchies and on the three global input systems (*sensory-reflex*, *cortical*, and *state*).

Any change in these peripheral and central input systems to the motor hierarchies is reflected in the activity of the autonomic pathways and therefore in autonomic regulation.

This chapter focuses on dysfunctions[1] of the autonomic nervous system. These dysfunctions can have a primarily peripheral origin (e.g., in autonomic neuropathy or pure autonomic failure) or a central origin (e.g., as a consequence of pathological stress, during essential hypertension, in orthostatic intolerance, in Parkinson's disease, in multiple systems atrophy, or after spinal cord injury or supraspinal injury) [2,74,85]. I will concentrate on central aspects of autonomic dysfunctions related to pain and hyperalgesia, including central malfunctioning following peripheral physical trauma, with or without an obvious nerve lesion (e.g., in patients with complex regional pain syndrome). Dysfunctional states of the autonomic nervous system that result from central lesions will not be covered.

The mechanisms of central autonomic dysfunctions are poorly understood. The subject is somewhat hypothetical because in most cases we are not able to locate the malfunctioning of the autonomic nervous system in the structures of the CNS. This problem has methodological reasons and is related to the fact that the anatomical, histochemical, and functional organization of the autonomic nervous system, both in the periphery and in the brain, has received insufficient research attention [44,56].

The Peripheral Parasympathetic and Sympathetic Systems Consist of Separate Pathways

The peripheral autonomic nervous system consists of the parasympathetic system, the sympathetic system, and the enteric nervous system [32,44,64]. The peripheral parasympathetic and sympathetic systems are composed of many pathways that transmit impulse activity from the spinal cord or brainstem to the effector cells. These pathways are separate

---

[1] The term *dysfunction* (abnormal function) is the opposite of *eufunction* (normal function). Both are old terms going back to the Greek concept of the functioning of the body in health and disease.

from each other and are functionally and anatomically distinct with respect to the effector cells. Thus, the impulses in the preganglionic neurons are transmitted in the autonomic ganglia within functionally defined pathways (and not between them), and the impulses in the postganglionic neurons are transmitted to many effector cells by specialized neuroeffector junctions. Each peripheral sympathetic or parasympathetic pathway is connected to distinct neural networks in the spinal cord, brainstem, and hypothalamus that generate the typical discharge patterns in the autonomic neurons. These central networks are responsible for the precise regulation of the target organs (cardiovascular regulation, thermoregulation, regulation of pelvic organs, regulation of the gastrointestinal tract, and so forth). They are responsible for the diverse types of homeostatic autonomic regulation and their coordination with somatomotor and neuroendocrine functions, and they are under powerful control by the cerebral hemispheres (Fig. 1).

The anatomical, histochemical, and functional organization of the autonomic nervous system, in the periphery and in the brain, has received insufficient attention in studies of the functioning of this system under pathobiological conditions. I emphasize three points: (1) The sympathetic nervous system is functionally as well differentiated as the parasympathetic nervous system. It does not react as a unitary system under normal physiological conditions, as originally conceived by Cannon [14]. (2) The terms *sympathetic* and *parasympathetic* are defined anatomically and not functionally. Thus, to use these terms functionally can be rather misleading. (3) The long-held view that the sympathetic and parasympathetic nervous systems always function antagonistically is also misleading. Both systems complement each other in their functions [44,56].

Autonomic Pathways and Small-Diameter Afferent Systems from the Body Tissues Form Feedback Systems

The definition of the terms *sympathetic* and *parasympathetic* does not include afferent neurons. About 85% of the axons in the vagus nerves and up to 50% of those in the (spinal) splanchnic nerves are afferent and are called vagal or spinal visceral afferents, respectively. They come from sensory receptors in the internal organs and have their cell bodies in the ganglia of the IXth and Xth nerves or in the dorsal root ganglia of the spinal segments corresponding to the autonomic outflow. To label thoracolumbar and sacral afferents "sympathetic" or "parasympathetic," respectively, is misleading. However, this statement does not contradict the idea that visceral afferents are integral components of most autonomic reflexes and processes of regulation [15,43,44,54,98]. In fact, visceral afferent neurons— together with the small-diameter (Aδ, C) afferent neurons that innervate almost all somatic tissues—monitor the mechanical, thermal, chemical, and metabolic state of the somatic and visceral body tissues. Thus, somatic afferent neurons with small-diameter fibers are also involved in homeostatic regulation and in regulation of body protection [20,23]. Their activation can lead to interoceptive body feelings that include pain, thermal sensations, sensual touch, itch, various visceral sensations, respiratory sensations, and sensations of deep somatic tissues (e.g., during exercise). Thus, these afferent neurons subserve interoception "as the sense of the physiological conditions of the body tissues." In primates, the physiological condition of the somatic and visceral body tissues seems to have a distinct representation in the posterior and basal part of the ventromedial thalamus and in the dorsal posterior insular cortex [20–23]. This concept of interoception extends that of Sherrington [89], who limited it to the viscera, in particular the gastrointestinal tract, which has a large inner surface area.

Brain and body are reciprocally "glued" together by the peripheral autonomic pathways and the small-diameter afferents that innervate all tissues and are involved in interoception. Furthermore, body and brain are welded together by neuroendocrine efferent systems, as well as by the hormonal and humoral feedback signals from the body tissues to the brain. Peripheral parasympathetic and sympathetic pathways and populations of small-diameter afferents form feedback loops between body tissues and brain.

The autonomic system regulates the visceral organs (the gastrointestinal tract, pelvic organs, kidneys, and airways), blood supply to body tissues via the cardiovascular system, body core temperature and other

functions. These neural functions and their failure can only be understood in the context of the reciprocal communication between brain and
body tissues. Afferent feedback informs the central representations of
the body domains at all times about the state of the tissues. This afferent
feedback reflects the effectiveness of the body's regulation by the autonomic systems, and the spatiotemporal pattern of the discharges in the
small-diameter afferents mirrors the patterns of discharge in the peripheral autonomic pathways. These feedback loops—consisting of peripheral
autonomic pathways, autonomic effector cells, and small-diameter afferents—connect the autonomic neural circuits in the brain that generate the
autonomic expression of emotions with the neural representations of the
body maps that are the basis for all bodily sensations. Thus, these feedback
loops ultimately give rise to or modulate emotional feelings (see Damasio
[25,26,27]). In view of the functional differentiation of the autonomic pathways and the central circuits connected with them [44], one would expect
that changes of activity in the autonomic pathways should be reflected by
changes in the activity patterns of the populations of small-diameter afferent neurons monitoring the mechanical, thermal, chemical, and metabolic
state of the tissues. These changes, in turn, would modulate the feeling
states of the organism, generated by patterns of activity in the representations of these body maps. This modulation of feeling states occurs
in the anterior insula, orbitofrontal cortex, prefrontal cortex, anterior cingulate cortex, and other cortical and subcortical centers [20–24].

The continuous process of activation of these cortical and subcortical centers in the generation of the different types of positive and negative
feeling states is the basis of what Sherrington [89] has called the *common
sensation*: "By common sensation is understood that sum of sensations
referred, not to external agents, but to the processes of the animal body.
Its 'object' is the body itself—the material 'me'. Sensations derived from the
body tissues and organs possess strong affective tone; while sensations of
special sense are relatively free from affective tone." Craig elaborated extensively on this aspect in his functional interpretation of the representation of various body sensations, related to the activation of small-diameter
afferents, which innervate all body tissues, including visceral organs, in
the basal and posterior part of the ventromedial nucleus of the thalamus

and in the posterior insula. Craig was the first to point out that, on the basis of functional morphological, neurophysiological, and imaging studies, these interoceptive body sensations are represented primarily in the posterior insula rather than in the primary and secondary somatosensory cortex [20].

Under normal physiological conditions, these systems are perfectly in balance, so that autonomic regulation and body feelings, both anchored in the state of the body tissues, adapt perfectly to one another, for example, during digestion, exercise, pelvic organ activity, and thermoregulatory challenge. This view does not conflict with the fact that the central circuits, generating somatomotor behavior and the autonomic adjustments of the body tissues, communicate directly with the (afferent) representations of the body domains (this communication could be the "as-if body loop" described by Damasio [25,26,27]). The important point to be emphasized is that the body loop is essential in this continuous afferent feedback for developing and maintaining the representations of the body domains in the brain. This feedback is a dynamic ongoing process that involves the efferent signals of the autonomic pathways.

In the following, I will argue that this active body loop, involving the autonomic pathways, is probably a very important component or a missing link in our understanding of the underlying pathobiological mechanisms of chronic pain disorders discussed in this volume and elsewhere [12,13,39,48,84,93] (Fig. 2). I am proposing that chronic pain syndromes are also characterized by changes in autonomic target cells that are dependent on changes in ongoing and reflex activity in neurons of the peripheral autonomic pathways. These autonomic changes are of central origin and appear to occur in parallel with changes in body perception (including pain, discomfort, fatigue, and feeling ill), endocrine changes, and changes expressed in the somatomotor system. It is generally assumed that centrally generated autonomic changes are adaptive responses to adjust visceral organs and somatic tissues that either follow or occur in parallel with the perceptual changes.

However, I hypothesize that changes in body perception are also the consequence of the autonomic changes generated by the brain. The connection between the efferent (autonomic) system and the afferent system occurs via the autonomic target cells in the body tissues. Alternatively, it occurs in the brain from the representations of autonomic functions to the afferent representation in the central body maps, or most likely in both ways. This first means of communication establishes autonomic-afferent (body) loops between the body and its central representations. Thus, activity in the efferent pathways shapes body perceptions by modulating the activity in afferent neurons with small-diameter axons via the autonomic target organs. The second means of communication occurs in the brain by communication between the representations of the autonomic motor systems and the central afferent body maps. This way of communication would correspond to the "as-if body loop" between the neural machinery of emotional expression and the neural machinery of body maps, as postulated by Damasio [25,26].

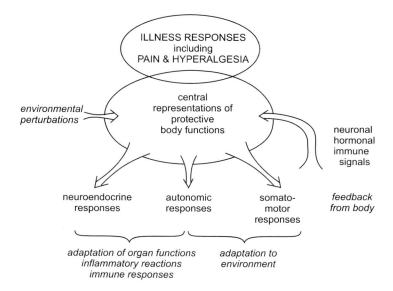

Fig. 2. Protective mechanisms of the body regulated by the brain: inputs, central representations, and outputs. Activation of the central circuits leads to neuroendocrine, autonomic, somatomotor, and illness responses (which include pain and hyperalgesia). The afferent feedback from the body tissues is neural and hormonal or mediated by cytokines from the immune system. The hypothetical central circuits in the spinal cord, brainstem, and hypothalamus are adapted by the telencephalon to the environmental situations and to the situations in the body. Modified after [52].

Normally, activity in the efferent (autonomic) outflow to the body tissues and in the afferent inflow from the body tissues to the brain is entirely in balance and perfectly adapted. However, in generalized functional chronic pain syndromes (often called *functional somatic syndromes* by specialists in psychosomatic medicine [10,39,105]), the sensory feedback from the body tissues has lost its precise temporal and spatial coordination with the central autonomic and somatic motor programs and with the sensory representations of the body within the brain. The resulting sensory-motor mismatch leads to the sensory-affective, somatomotor, autonomic motor, and endocrine abnormalities observed in these chronic pain syndromes.

Sympathetic Nervous System and Body Protection: A Concept

In addition to its "conventional" functions, the peripheral sympathetic nervous system also has functions that are conceptually best described in the context of regulation of protection of body tissues during the ongoing challenges that arise within the body or come from the environment. The organism's responses to these challenges involve the autonomic, neuroendocrine, and somatomotor systems, including the corresponding afferent feedbacks from the body tissues. These systems serve to adapt organ functions to changes in behavior and to behavioral responses to threatening environments, as discussed above (see Fig. 1). The organism's coordinated responses, which are represented in the brain (the brainstem, hypothalamus, limbic system, and neocortex), prepare the organism to generate the appropriate responses to the threatening events. The central representations receive neural afferent, hormonal, and humoral signals that continuously monitor the mechanical, thermal, metabolic, and chemical states of the tissues. Control of inflammation and hyperalgesia by the CNS is an integral component in this scenario and requires sympathetic systems that function in a differentiated way. During real or impending tissue damage, this integrated protective system is activated by the brain, leading to illness responses including pain, hyperalgesia, and other aversive sensations.

Regulation of pain and hyperalgesia are integral components of the fast defense system (fight or flight) and the slow (recuperative) defense system. *Fast defense*, organized by the hypothalamo-mesencephalic system, incorporates rapid analgesia (by active suppression of nociceptive impulse transmission to second-order neurons in the spinal or trigeminal dorsal horn, and probably by other supraspinal inhibitory processes as well). It calls for mobilization of energy, activation of various sympathetic channels (including the sympatho-adrenal system), and activation of the hypothalamo-pituitary adrenal (HPA) axis. It is accompanied by heightened vigilance and alertness, increased arterial blood pressure and heart rate, and vasodilation in the skeletal muscles of the extremities (to prepare for fighting or running away). It is accompanied by a non-opioid-mediated hypoalgesia. During *slow defense,* the organism switches to recuperation and healing of tissues. Slow defense is characterized by a state of quiescence and rest, with low blood pressure, bradycardia, and opioid-mediated hypoalgesia.

The neural representations of the integrative responses of the body during fast or slow defense are located in the periaqueductal gray (PAG) of the mesencephalon (Fig. 3) [4–6,59,60]:

• The neural representations of confrontational defense and flight (avoidance) are located in the dorsolateral and lateral columns of the PAG. These behavioral patterns can be activated from the medial prefrontal cortex (either directly or via the dorsal or ventromedial hypothalamus) or they can be generated reflexively from the body surface (skin) by stimulation of nociceptors via the spinal or trigeminal superficial dorsal horn (mainly lamina I neurons) and the lateral column of the PAG.

• The neural representation of quiescence (slow defense) is located in the ventrolateral column of the PAG. Quiescence can be generated from the orbital prefrontal cortex, either via direct projections to the ventrolateral PAG or via the lateral hypothalamus, or it can be generated reflexively by afferent nociceptive input from the deep somatic or visceral body domains (e.g., during chronic inflammation). It is probably also generated by vagal visceral afferent input via the solitary tract nucleus.

• The cortical signals and the afferent signals from the body always work together in the activation of these mesencephalic neural defense systems.

• The dorsolateral, lateral, and ventrolateral columns of the PAG have distinct reciprocal connections with the autonomic centers in the lower brainstem and in the hypothalamus that differentially regulate the activity in neurons of peripheral autonomic pathways.

• The neural systems in the PAG are integral nodal structures of the endogenous neural system. Via the ventromedial medulla (VMM) and the dorsolateral pontine tegmentum, they control nociceptive impulse transmission to the telencephalon in the spinal and trigeminal superficial dorsal horn, and possibly elsewhere. They are involved in the mechanisms underlying centrally generated antinociception and pronociception, and thus they are

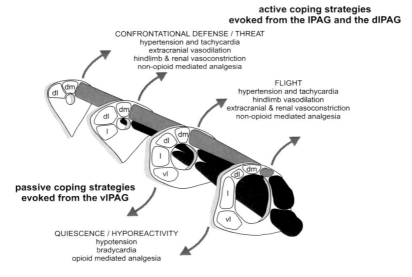

Fig. 3. Representation of defense behaviors in the dorsolateral, lateral, and ventrolateral periaqueductal gray (PAG). Schematic illustration of the dorsolateral (dl), lateral (l), and ventrolateral (vl) columns within the rostral, intermediate, and caudal PAG. The dorsomedial (dm) PAG column is also indicated. Stimulation of neuron populations in the dl-PAG, lPAG, and vlPAG by microinjections of the excitatory amino acid glutamate, which excites the cell bodies of neurons but not the axons, evokes distinct defense behaviors. Confrontational defense is elicited from the rostral portion of the dlPAG and lPAG; flight is elicited from the caudal part of the dlPAG and lPAG; and quiescence (cessation of spontaneous motor activity) is elicited from the vlPAG in the caudal portion of the PAG. These defense behaviors include typical autonomic cardiovascular reactions (changes in blood pressure, heart rate, and blood flow) and sensory changes (non-opioid or opioid-mediated analgesia). The representations of confrontational defense and flight are suggested to be the basis for active coping strategies produced by the cortex. The representation of quiescence is suggested to be the basis for passive coping strategies generated by the cortex. Modified from [5,6].

also implicated in hypoalgesia and hyperalgesia [30,38]. However, it should be emphasized that the main biological function of the PAG-VMM system is not the control of nociception and pain. This system has multiple roles in the regulation of behavior, which involves sensory, somatomotor, and autonomic systems. The modulation of nociception and pain is only part of these functions and must be seen in a wider behavioral context [71–73].

• The neural circuits in the PAG represent active and passive coping strategies that are activated by the cortex during ("psychological" or "physical") stress.

An important component of this protective neural system, promoting tissue repair and recuperation, is the bidirectional communication between the brain and the immune system. The brain is continuously influenced by signals from the immune system (via cytokines), and it modulates the reactivity of the immune system, mainly via the sympathoneural system and the hypothalamo-pituitary system. This bidirectional brain-immune system is probably of particular importance during slow defense. It furthers recuperation and tissue healing under normal biological conditions, although it appears to be switched on rather quickly. The defense systems organized in the brain are activated by peripheral signals from the immune system via afferent neurons (e.g., vagal afferent neurons and the solitary tract nucleus), or they are activated by cytokines via the circumventricular organs. The involvement of cytokines in the sensitization of nociceptors during inflammation, perhaps in part mediated by the terminals of sympathetic fibers [55,102], and the slow change in the sensitivity of nociceptors (linked to the activation of the sympatho-adrenal system), may also be components of the slow defense system [101,102].

It is unclear whether signaling from the brain to the immune system via the sympathetic nervous system occurs by a specific sympathetic channel that is anatomically and functionally different from sympathetic channels to other target cells, or whether it is a general functional characteristic of the peripheral sympathetic nervous system [1,11,40,66,67,88]. Based on various experimental observations, I favor the more likely hypothesis that the immune system is modulated by the brain by way of a functionally and anatomically distinct sympathetic pathway. However, this hypothesis has yet to be proven [44,51]. Therefore, I am skeptical whether

circulating catecholamines (epinephrine and norepinephrine) are as important in the brain's regulation of the immune system as the sympathetic

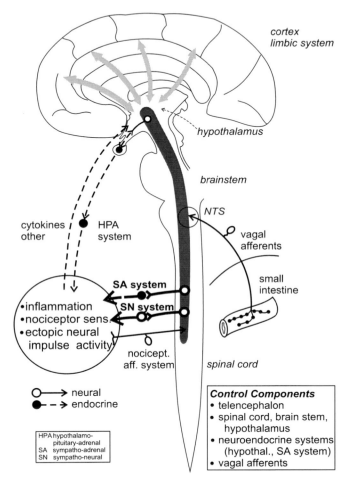

Fig. 4. The spinal cord, brainstem, and hypothalamus contain neural circuits that control
nociceptor sensitivity and inflammation in the periphery of the body via the sympatho-
adrenal (SA) system and the hypothalamo-pituitary-adrenal (HPA) system (shaded area).
Feedback information from the peripheral inflammatory process comes via nociceptive
primary afferent neurons and cytokines. The central circuits linked to the SA system and
the HPA system are modulated by activity in vagal afferents, probably those innervating
the small intestine (and here the gut-associated lymphoid tissue). The telencephalon controls the inflammation and sensitivity of nociceptors via the circuits in the spinal cord,
brainstem, and hypothalamus (see shaded double arrows). The sympatho-neural (SN)
system is also involved. Modified from [45].

innervation under physiological conditions [28,29]. Studies in monkeys have shown that chronic social stress enhances the sympathetic innervation of parenchymal areas of the lymph nodes containing T lymphocytes, but does not affect the innervation of blood vessels in lymph nodes [90,91]. These experiments support my hypothesis; again, however, they do not prove it.

The contexts in which the sympatho-neural system and the sympatho-adrenal system may be involved in generating protective body reactions—including nociception, pain, hyperalgesia, and inflammation—are listed in Table I and graphically expressed in Fig. 4. This complex

Table I
The sympathetic nervous system and body protection, inflammation, pain, and hyperalgesia

1. REACTIONS OF THE SYMPATHETIC NERVOUS SYSTEM IN NOCICEPTION AND PAIN

Protective spinal and supraspinal reflexes

Fight, flight, and quiescence, organized at the level of the periaqueductal gray

Sympathetically mediated changes in referred hyperalgesic zones during visceral and deep somatic pain

2. ROLE OF THE SYMPATHETIC NERVOUS SYSTEM IN THE GENERATION OF PAIN

Sympathetic-afferent coupling in the periphery

Coupling after a nerve lesion (norepinephrine, α-adrenoceptors)

Coupling via the micromilieu of the nociceptor and the vascular bed

Sensitization of nociceptors, mediated by sympathetic terminals independently of excitation and release of norepinephrine

Sensitization of nociceptors, initiated by cytokines or nerve growth factor and mediated by sympathetic terminals

The sympatho-adrenal system and nociceptor sensitization

3. THE SYMPATHETIC NERVOUS SYSTEM AND CENTRAL MECHANISMS

Control of inflammation and hyperalgesia by sympathetic and neuroendocrine mechanisms

Complex regional pain syndrome and the sympathetic nervous system

The immune system and the sympathetic nervous system

Rheumatic diseases and the sympathetic nervous system

Systemic chronic pain (e.g., fibromyalgia, irritable bowel syndrome) and the sympathetic nervous system

References: For point 1: [4–6,41,44]. For point 2: [34,42,43,46,52,53,55,58,61,62,77,78]. For point 3: [13,37,47–49,51,55,57,58,93–95,99].

subject has been extensively discussed elsewhere [45,55]. Four general aspects of this issue are distinguished (for references see Jänig [45] and Table I): (1) Reactions of the sympathetic nervous system during nociception and pain. These biological events include protective spinal and supraspinal reflexes, sympathetically mediated changes in referred hyperalgesic zones during deep somatic and visceral nociception and pain, and integrated autonomic reactions, as described in relation to Fig. 4. (2) Coupling (cross-talk) from sympathetic postganglionic neurons to afferent neurons under pathophysiological conditions, which generates pain (and perhaps other sensations). (3) The involvement of the sympathetic nervous system in inflammation, and the hyperalgesia associated with the inflammation. (4) Central mechanisms involving the sympathetic nervous system.

In the remaining part of this chapter I will argue (but not prove), by referring to experiments on animals and humans and to clinical observations, that activity in autonomic (efferent) systems — which, along with small-diameter afferent systems, form the body loop, via the somatic body tissues and the visceral organs — is an important aspect of our efforts to understand the mechanisms of chronic pain diseases (or functional somatic syndromes [39,105]). I will concentrate in this context on certain aspects of points 2 to 4 in Table I.

Pathophysiology of Sympathetic-Afferent Coupling: A Summary

As mentioned above, activity in sympathetic neurons that project to somatic and visceral body tissues and activity in afferent neurons with small-diameter fibers signaling the state of the body tissues to the brain occur under precisely adapted physiological conditions. There is no obvious sign for direct or indirect coupling between the efferent sympathetic systems and the afferent systems in the peripheral tissues leading to pain, discomfort, or other sensations maintained by the sympathetic outflow. This situation may change after trauma with or without nerve injury. In that case, activity in sympathetic neurons may lead to pain, known as sympathetically maintained pain (SMP). The concept is shown schematically in Fig. 5.

During inflammation or following nerve lesion, the efferent (noradrenergic) innervation of the affected tissue may feed back to the primary afferent neurons and activate them or enhance their activity. This process, in turn, would amplify the physiological impulse transmission in the spinal or trigeminal dorsal horn (causing sensitization of dorsal horn neurons) or would enhance the hyperexcitability of these neurons after nerve lesion [45].

Cross-talk from sympathetic postganglionic (noradrenergic) neurons may occur in several forms (for details, see [45]). Physiologically, the

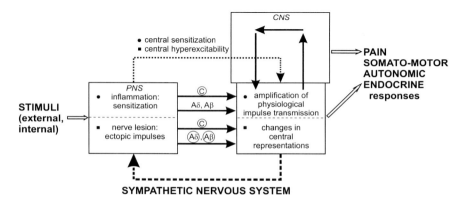

Fig. 5. Concept of generation of peripheral and central hyperexcitability during inflammatory pain and neuropathic pain involving the sympathetic nervous system. The pain is always associated with motor, autonomic, and endocrine responses. The upper dashed arrow indicates that the central changes are generated (and possibly maintained) (a) by persistent activation of nociceptors with unmyelinated (C) fibers (e.g., during chronic inflammation), called here "central sensitization," or (b) after trauma with nerve lesion by ectopic activity in myelinated (Aδ, Aβ) and C afferents and other changes in the lesioned afferent neurons, called here "central hyperexcitability." The lower dashed arrow indicates the efferent feedback via the sympathetic nervous system (including the sympatho-adrenal system). The transmission of nociceptive impulses is under multiple control of the brain (upper right). Primary afferent nociceptive neurons (in particular those with C fibers) are sensitized during inflammation. After nerve lesion, *all* lesioned primary afferent neurons (unmyelinated as well as myelinated ones) undergo biochemical, physiological, and morphological changes that become irreversible with time. These peripheral changes entail changes in the central representations (of the somatosensory system), which become irreversible if there is no regeneration of primary afferent neurons to their target tissue. The central functional changes, induced by persistent activity in afferent nociceptive neurons during chronic inflammation or by ectopic activity in afferent neurons after nerve lesion, are also reflected in the sympathetic efferent feedback system that may establish positive feedback loops to the primary afferent neurons. CNS, central nervous system; PNS, peripheral nervous system.

postganglionic neurons of the sympathoneural system are anatomically separate from the primary afferent neurons and do not communicate with them. Thus, excitation of the sympathetic neurons does not lead to activation of afferent neurons (except perhaps under rather artificial experimental conditions). However, under pathophysiological conditions, such as trauma with or without nerve lesion, this type of communication may occur. In that case, activity in sympathetic postganglionic neurons may activate or sensitize afferent nociceptive fibers and cause *sympathetically maintained pain*. This cross-talk between sympathetic postganglionic fibers and afferent neurons may be mediated by norepinephrine and α-adrenoceptors in the afferent neurons. It occurs in the peripheral tissues or even in the dorsal root ganglia (although I consider this latter type of coupling to be unlikely to represent an important peripheral mechanism underlying sympathetically maintained pain in patients [42,45]). The cross-talk may also occur indirectly via the vascular constriction generated by vasoconstrictor neurons and the ensuing changes in the affected tissue or by other changes involving the sympathetic postganglionic fibers (possibly inflammatory processes).

Postganglionic axons and afferent nociceptive fibers may also be coupled independently of excitation of sympathetic neurons and norepinephrine release. This type of coupling has been shown to occur in animal experiments studying mechanical hyperalgesic behavior elicited by intradermal injection of the inflammatory mediator bradykinin [61]. Surgical sympathectomy attenuates the bradykinin-induced mechanical hyperalgesic behavior, whereas decentralization of the sympathetic chain (transection of the preganglionic axons, leaving the postganglionic neurons intact) does not. We do not know whether this type of coupling is important in humans.

Behavioral experiments on rats show that part of the sensitizing effect of nerve growth factor on nociceptive afferents is mediated by sympathetic fibers, possibly via tyrosine kinase A (TrkA) receptors, release of norepinephrine, and β-adrenoceptors [76,106]. Furthermore, pharmacological experiments show that the sensitizing effect of the cytokine interleukin 8 (IL-8) also may be mediated by sympathetic terminals, release of norepinephrine, and β-adrenoceptors [82,107]. These sympathetically mediated effects on nociceptive afferent fibers must be confirmed and investigated in more detail by means of neurophysiological recording from afferent neurons [55].

A further category of coupling in which the sympatho-adrenal system is involved is the effect of epinephrine on the sensitivity of nociceptors. Epinephrine released by the adrenal medulla may sensitize nociceptors to mechanical stimulation. This sensitization develops after the nociceptive afferents are exposed to an increased concentrating of epinephrine in the blood plasma over several days. This type of sensitization has been demonstrated in a rat model of bradykinin-induced mechanical hyperalgesic behavior [61-63]. Such coupling between the sympatho-adrenal system and the peripheral nociceptive afferent neurons has only been shown to exist in behavioral experiments in rats. It remains to be shown whether it is relevant in physiological and pathophysiological conditions. Furthermore, it has to be verified in experiments using neurophysiological recordings from nociceptive and other afferent fibers.

Dysfunction of the Sympathetic Nervous System in Complex Regional Pain Syndrome Type I

Complex regional pain syndromes (CRPS) are painful disorders, typically affecting the limbs, that may develop as a consequence of trauma. Clinically, they are characterized by pain (spontaneous pain, hyperalgesia, and allodynia), active and passive movement disorders, including increased physiological tremor; abnormal regulation of blood flow and sweating; edema of the skin and subcutaneous tissues; and trophic changes in the skin, in appendages of the skin, and in subcutaneous tissues [7,8,37,47,48,57,92]. CRPS type I (previously called reflex sympathetic dystrophy) may develop after minor trauma (such as a bone fracture, sprain, bruises or skin lesions, or surgery) involving a small nerve lesion or no obvious nerve lesion in an extremity. In rare cases, CRPS-I may also develop after visceral trauma or after a lesion in the CNS (e.g., a stroke). An important feature of CRPS-I is that the severity and combination of clinical symptoms are *disproportionate* to the severity and type of trauma. The symptoms have a tendency to spread in the affected distal limb and are not confined to the innervation zone of an individual nerve. CRPS type II (previously called causalgia) develops after trauma with an obvious, usually extensive, nerve lesion [37,57,92].

On the basis of clinical observations, animal studies, and research in human patients, the hypothesis has been put forward that CRPS is a systemic disease involving the central and peripheral nervous systems (Fig. 6). Various traumas can trigger variable combinations of clinical phenomena in which the somatosensory system, the sympathetic nervous system, the somatomotor system, and peripheral (vascular and inflammatory) systems are involved. There is no correlation between the type of trauma and the pattern of clinical phenomenology [37,47,48]. The central changes are reflected in changes in somatic sensations (increased detection thresholds for mechanical, cold, warm, and heat stimuli [86,87]). There are also changes in motor performance and in neural regulation of sympathetic effector systems (involving the vasculature, sweat glands, and possibly inflammatory cells). The peripheral changes consist of inflammation involving blood vessels, inflammatory cells, and peptidergic afferent nerve fibers, as well as sympathetic-afferent coupling. The peripheral changes cannot be seen independently of the central changes; both interact with each other via afferent and efferent signals. In essence, the mechanisms that underlie CRPS cannot be reduced to only one mechanism (e.g., sympathetic-afferent coupling, an adrenoceptor disease, a peripheral inflammatory disease, or a psychogenic disease) [37,47,48].

Centrally generated activity in sympathetic neurons may be involved in various ways in the pathogenesis of CRPS-I, the main argument being that the peripheral changes are reversed or aggravated after intervention at the level of the peripheral sympathetic nervous system (sympathetic blocks or stimulation of the sympathetic nerves; Fig. 6). Several points that are relevant in the present context of dysfunction of the sympathetic nervous system, pain, and body protection need to be emphasized with regard to CRPS-I.

• In a subgroup of CRPS-I patients, pain or a component of pain obviously depends on activity in sympathetic neurons and is related to activation or sensitization of nociceptors by norepinephrine released by the

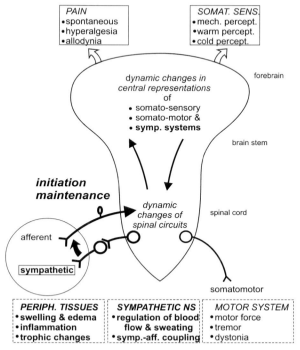

Fig. 6. Hypothetical development of complex regional pain syndrome (CRPS) as a disease of the central nervous system (CNS). Schematic diagram summarizing the sensory, autonomic, and somatomotor changes in CRPS-I patients. The figure symbolizes the CNS (forebrain, brainstem, and spinal cord). Changes occur in the central representations of the somatosensory, somatomotor, and sympathetic nervous system (which include spinal circuits) and are reflected in changes in the perception of painful and nonpainful stimuli, changes in cutaneous blood flow and sweating, and altered motor performance. These changes are triggered and possibly maintained by nociceptive afferent inputs from the somatic and visceral domains. It is unclear whether these central changes are reversible in chronic CRPS-I patients. The central changes also may affect the endogenous control system of nociceptive impulse transmission. Coupling between sympathetic neurons and afferent neurons in the periphery (see bold arrow) is one component of pain in CRPS-I patients with sympathetically maintained pain (SMP). However, it seems to be unimportant in CRPS-I patients without SMP. Modified from [47,48].

sympathetic fibers. This type of pain is sympathetically maintained pain. Either the nociceptors have expressed adrenoceptors, or the excitatory effect is generated indirectly, perhaps by way of changes in blood flow in the deep somatic tissues of an extremity [9]. Sympathetically maintained activity in nociceptive neurons may generate a state of central sensitization or hyperexcitability that is responsible for spontaneous pain (in particular in deep tissues), as well as for secondary evoked pain (mechanical and cold allodynia in the skin and deep mechanical allodynia and hyperalgesia).

• Many CRPS-I patients have distorted regulation of blood flow through the skin and abnormal sweating, although the peripheral vasoconstrictor and sudomotor pathways are intact [9,100,101]. This is a clear sign of central dysregulation of the sympathetic outflow to the skin and possibly to the deep somatic tissues as well.

• Swelling (edema) and inflammation may be generated by sympathetic and peptidergic afferent fibers interacting with each other at the arteriolar site of the vascular bed (influencing blood flow) and at the venular site (influencing plasma extravasation). Sympathetic fibers may influence inflammatory cells (macrophages and mast cells) by way of norepinephrine via adrenoceptors on the inflammatory cells [45,47,48].

• Trophic changes in the skin, appendages of the skin, and subcutaneous tissues (including the joints) are believed to depend, at least in part, on the sympathetic innervation. The nature of this neural influence on the tissue structure is unknown [37,48,57].

These observations in patients with CRPS-I (who have no nerve lesion and therefore by definition do not have neuropathic pain) suggest that altered activity in sympathetic neurons entails peripheral changes, which in turn may result in secondary activation or sensitization of primary afferent nociceptive and possibly also non-nociceptive neurons. The underlying mechanism of this activation and sensitization of nociceptive afferent neurons may involve short- and long-term processes, as discussed elsewhere [42,45]. Are the somatosensory, autonomic, and somatomotor changes observed in CRPS patients also a consequence of a disturbance in the body loop between the sympathetic outflow, target tissues, and small-diameter afferent neurons, leading to a central sensory-motor mismatch (see [65,75,80,81])? Sympathetic-afferent coupling, such as may occur after a major nerve lesion in patients with CRPS type II or in those with other types of pain following nerve lesion, is believed to be the mechanistic basis of sympathetically maintained pain in those patients (see Jänig [42,45]. Is CRPS a rather special pathophysiological case of a disturbed autonomic-afferent body loop?

An important observation, in CRPS-I patients with SMP (and possibly also in CRPS-II patients with SMP), is that pain relief following a conduction block of sympathetic neurons by a local anesthetic applied to the sympathetic chain mostly outlasts the conduction block by at least one order of magnitude (several days) (Fig. 7) [83]. The long-lasting pain-relieving effect of sympathetic blocks suggests that activity

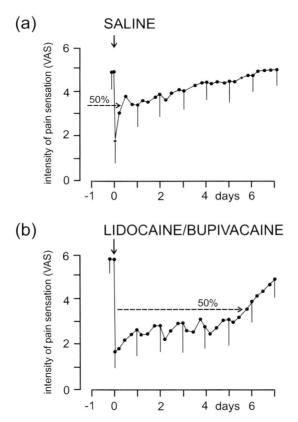

Fig. 7. Sympathetic blocks with a local anesthetic in patients with complex regional pain syndrome (CRPS) type I with sympathetically maintained pain (SMP) leads to a long-lasting significant reduction of pain. A local anesthetic (a) or saline (control) (b) was injected close to the corresponding paravertebral sympathetic ganglia in the same group of seven CRPS-I patients (stellate ganglion in four patients, lumbar ganglia in three patients) in a double-blind crossover study. Pain was measured repeatedly using a visual analogue scale (VAS) on the day of the injection and daily for 7 days after the injection. Both interventions produced pain relief (see 50% value of pain relief). However, the mean duration of the 50% pain relief after injection of the local anesthetic lasted for 6 days and was significantly longer than that following local injection of saline, which lasted for 6 hours (placebo block). The initial maximal peaks of relative analgesia were not statistically different. Means + SEM. Modified from [83].

in sympathetic neurons, which is of central origin, maintains a positive feedback circuit via the nociceptive and possibly non-nociceptive primary afferent neurons. This positive feedback circuit maintains a central state of hyperexcitability (e.g., of neurons in the spinal dorsal horn), via excitation of afferent neurons triggered by an intense noxious event. The persistent afferent activity needed to maintain such a state of central hyperexcitability is switched off during temporary block of conduction in the sympathetic chain lasting only a few hours. It cannot be immediately switched on again when the conduction block wears off and activity returns to the sympathetic postganglionic neurons (and sympathetically induced activity probably returns to afferent neurons). Afferent activity may need to occur over a long period to initiate and maintain the central state of hyperexcitability (via positive feedback). The mechanism underlying this important and interesting phenomenon needs to be studied experimentally in patients with SMP as well as in animal models that have yet to be designed.

Spinal Autonomic Systems and Visceral Pain

Visceral pain is dependent on the activation of spinal thoracolumbar or sacral visceral afferent neurons. With the exception of the proximal esophagus and proximal trachea, it does not rely on the activation of vagal afferent neurons innervating the viscera. However, vagal afferents are involved in the inhibitory, and possibly excitatory, control of impulse transmission from spinal visceral afferent neurons to neurons of the spinal dorsal horn [43,44]. Spinal visceral afferent neurons can be divided into low-threshold mechanosensitive, high-threshold mechanosensitive, and silent (mechanoinsensitive but chemosensitive) afferents. Some organs (such as the urinary bladder and hindgut) are innervated by all three types of afferents, and others (such as the gall bladder and ureter) are innervated only by high-threshold afferents. Visceral pain is believed to be generated by activation of high-threshold visceral and normally silent afferents, but the large group of low-threshold mechanosensitive afferents that are important for regulation of organs such as the pelvic organs, and for nonpainful sensations and non-nociceptive reflexes, most likely also contribute to visceral pain.

They faithfully encode in their activity non-noxious as well as noxious intraluminal pressures and are sensitized during inflammation ([35,36]; for review see [15–17,33]).

I hypothesize that spinal autonomic non-vasoconstrictor pathways to visceral organs are probably important in the generation of pain and other sensations in the visceral organs. The neurons of these autonomic pathways exhibit specific reflexes to physiological stimulation of afferent neurons innervating viscera and are integrated in the regulation of the visceral effector cells. Reflex activity in these spinal autonomic neurons may change when the spinal visceral afferent neurons are continuously active and sensitized or when normally silent visceral afferent neurons are recruited [17,33,79]. This process could lead to a sensitization of second-order neurons in the spinal dorsal horn, and by activation of spinal autonomic systems it might establish positive feedback loops between visceral afferent neurons, the spinal cord, spinal autonomic systems, and visceral effector organs. Furthermore, central supraspinal changes, via systems modulating spinal autonomic circuits and impulse transmission in the dorsal horn, could promote (or inhibit) these positive feedback loops between visceral organs and the spinal cord. Finally, changes in supraspinal centers occurring without any peripheral visceral trauma and without sensitization of spinal visceral afferents could establish positive feedback loops between visceral organs and the spinal cord and lead to visceral pain. Positive feedback loops between spinal autonomic systems, visceral organs, and visceral afferent neurons may turn out to be important mechanisms of cardiac pain without ischemia, noncardiac chest pain, pain in non-ulcer dyspepsia, pain in irritable bowel disease, and pain in other functional visceral diseases. These pain syndromes are described fully in the other chapters of this volume.

Cardiac Pain

Resting activity and physiological stimulation of spinal visceral afferents innervating the heart or the large blood vessels elicit no sensations under healthy conditions. This activity is integrated in the neural regulation of the heart (Fig. 8). During physical exercise, activity in spinal cardiac afferents enhances the synaptic activation by sympathetic premotor neurons

Cardiac Pain & Sympathetic Nervous System

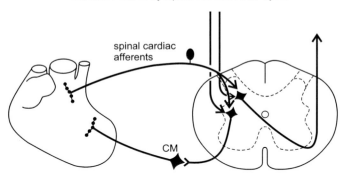

Fig. 8. Cardiac pain and the sympathetic innervation of the heart. A hypothetical positive feedback loop between spinal visceral cardiac afferent neurons and the sympathetic cardiomotor (CM) pathway(s) supplying the heart. Activation of this feedback loop enhances the activity of pacemaker cells and the inotropy of cardiac muscle cells. In physiological conditions, afferent feedback signals enhance the activity in descending sympathetic premotor neurons (located in the rostroventrolateral medulla and possibly the ventromedial medulla) in the adaptation of cardiac output during physical exercise. In pathophysiological conditions (such as coronary ischemia), sympathetic CM neurons and afferent feedback to sensitized dorsal horn neurons form a positive feedback loop that leads to cardiac pain. Activation of descending pathways could enhance or suppress this feedback loop. This feedback loop may also lead to cardiac pain without any peripheral pathological changes. Such pain may depend on the balance between the inhibitory and excitatory descending systems. The sympathetic pathway to the coronary arteries, which could also be involved in this scenario, is not shown. Modified from [50].

in the lower brain stem of spinal preganglionic (sympathetic) cardiomotor neurons (or of interneurons associated with them) that regulate the rate and contractility of the heart. In this way, cardiac output is adapted and maintained in relation to the level of exercise.

In pathophysiological conditions (e.g., atherosclerotic changes of the coronary arteries, resulting in ischemia), positive feedback coupling can have serious consequences. Cardiac spinal afferent neurons are excited and sensitized by ischemia, which leads to sensitization of neurons in the thoracic spinal dorsal horn, causing cardiac pain with referral to the dermatomes, myotomes, and sclerotomes that correspond to spinal segments T2 to T6 and possibly C2 to C4 [31]. Whether the cardiac spinal afferents that are excited by ischemia are the same as those that are

excited during exercise and increase of cardiac output, or whether a special group of cardiac afferents is excited that has a nociceptive function,
we do not know. The latter is tacitly assumed [3,19], but it may not be
the case (see [69,70]). Stimulation of the spinal cardiac afferent neurons
excites the sympathetic cardiomotor neurons via the cardio-cardiac spinal
reflex pathways. This activity, in turn, enhances the excitation of cardiac
afferents via greater contractility of ventricles and increased heart rate.
This idea of a positive feedback reflex loop, which adapts the work of the
heart under the physiological conditions of exercise and may have fatal
consequences under pathophysiological conditions, has been advanced by
Malliani and his coworkers and others [69,70].

Cardio-cardiac reflexes are under the control of supraspinal centers that are involved in regulation of cardiac output, perhaps via sympathetic cardiac premotor neurons in the rostroventrolateral medulla and
ventromedial medulla that synapse with the sympathetic preganglionic
cardiomotor neurons or with associated interneurons (not shown in Fig.
8). These reflexes also may be under the inhibitory or excitatory control
of impulse transmission from cardiac afferents to second-order neurons
in lamina I, lamina V, and deeper laminae of the dorsal horn, via supraspinal neurons located in the ventromedial medulla and the dorsolateral
pontine tegmentum [30,33,38]. Thus, it is possible that cardiac pain may
be generated without any pathophysiological changes in the coronary
arteries when transmission of ongoing activity in cardiac spinal afferents to second-order neurons is enhanced by descending control. By the
same token, it can be assumed that transmission of activity in spinal
cardiac afferents generated by ischemia in the heart due to coronary
occlusion is completely suppressed in the dorsal horn, resulting in the
absence of angina pain or pain during myocardial infarction [31]. The
neural mechanisms underlying the regulation of impulse transmission
from cardiac afferents to spinal second-order neurons and the regulation
of activity in sympathetic cardiomotor neurons by supraspinal centers
are not understood. Uncovering these mechanisms will teach us how
important the postulated positive feedback loop really is. We will learn
why patients may have cardiac pain without any peripheral pathological
changes in the coronary arteries and why humans, especially men, may

have no cardiac pain but clear-cut pathological changes of the coronary arteries with ischemia [18].

The Gastrointestinal Tract and Irritable Bowel Syndrome

Irritable bowel syndrome (IBS) is a functional disease of the gastrointestinal (GI) tract involving the brain ([12,13]; see Chapter 5 by Chang and Drossman). The mechanisms underlying the pain and motility changes seen in this disease are poorly understood. The pain cannot be reduced to a single peripheral mechanism, such as short- or long-term sensitization of spinal visceral afferent neurons innervating the GI tract, which could trigger central sensitization and activate spinal tract neurons projecting to the brainstem and/or thalamus. The motility changes also cannot be ascribed solely to the involvement of spinal neurons in the activation of parasympathetic and sympathetic neurons that regulate the motility or secretion of the GI tract. Functional, morphological, and biochemical markers, indicating inflammatory or other changes, in the GI tract, and in the visceral spinal primary afferent neurons that innervate the GI tract, appear to be absent. We do not know whether a pathological (inflammatory) process may have occurred in these patients that caused transient sensitization of spinal visceral afferents and triggered plastic changes in the spinal cord and elsewhere that were maintained for a long time after the peripheral inflammatory process had subsided.

Which hypothetical mechanism of IBS occurs first? (1) Changes in the spinal visceral afferent neurons, along with functional changes in the spinal dorsal horn (peripheral and central sensitization), and subsequent changes in the spinal (sacral and lumbar) autonomic systems. (2) Changes in the GI effector tissues of the spinal autonomic systems such as smooth musculature and the enteric nervous system. (3) Central supraspinal changes that influence the spinal circuits involved in regulating the GI tract and in controlling impulse transmission from spinal gastrointestinal afferent neurons to second-order neurons in the spinal cord.

The GI tract is innervated by several distinct classes of spinal autonomic pathways (sympathetic and parasympathetic) that are involved in regulating GI motility and secretions. These pathways are

Irritable Bowel Syndrome & Autonomic Nervous System

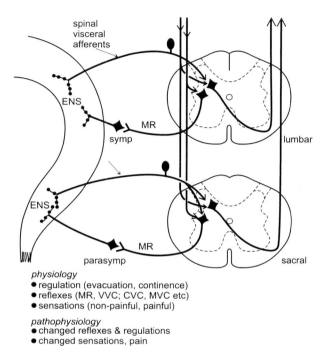

Fig. 9. Spinal visceral afferent neurons innervating the hindgut and spinal autonomic pathways supplying the hindgut form positive feedback loops that are controlled by descending supraspinal systems leading to pain: a hypothesis. Physiologically the spinal autonomic pathways are involved in evacuation and continence of the hindgut. These motility-regulating (MR) neurons include sacral parasympathetic and lumbar sympathetic pathways. The sacral visceral afferents are involved in regulation of evacuation and continence of the hindgut, in nonpainful as well painful sensations, and in various types of reflexes. These reflexes rely on MR neurons innervating other pelvic organs, and on other autonomic neurons such as muscle vasoconstrictor (MVC), visceral vasoconstrictor (VVC), and cutaneous vasoconstrictor (CVC) neurons. Activation of sacral visceral afferent neurons from the hindgut triggers coordinated activation of spinal autonomic systems and ascending systems leading to coordinated reactions of pelvic organs and the corresponding sensations. This coordinated neural spinal activity is under the control of descending systems. The lumbar visceral afferent neurons are also involved in reflexes, possibly in continence and in painful sensations as well as discomfort. It is hypothesized that under pathophysiological conditions visceral afferents and autonomic sacral outflow establish a positive feedback loop that enhances the activity in the visceral afferent neurons. This feedback loop may also occur without peripheral pathological changes and without sensitized visceral afferents innervating the hindgut, e.g., by changes of the balance of the descending supraspinal systems controlling the spinal circuits. ENS, enteric nervous system. Modified from [50].

collectively known as motility-regulating (MR) neurons. These spinal autonomic pathways are anatomically and functionally different from the visceral vasoconstrictor pathway innervating blood vessels of the GI tract (for references see [44]). The postganglionic neurons of the MR pathways either interfere with the enteric nervous system or innervate the nonvascular smooth muscle cells or secretory epithelia directly (Fig. 9). Blood flow through mucosa and submucosa is dependent on activity in post-ganglionic visceral vasoconstrictor fibers and locally on enteric neurons that induce vasodilation when activated. Most of these enteric neurons are secretomotor neurons.

I hypothesize that a "defect" occurs in IBS that is responsible for the pain and changed regulation of motility (and possibly secretion) of the GI tract. This possible defect involves the integration of spinal circuits, visceral afferents innervating the GI tract, and spinal autonomic non-vasoconstrictor pathways innervating the GI tract, and their control by supraspinal centers. These components may establish a positive feedback circuit in which the efferent spinal autonomic MR pathways are an important link (Fig. 9). This idea of a positive feedback circuit between the GI tract and spinal cord would be in accordance with the observation that supraspinal ("psychological" or pharmacological) interventions can attenuate, at least temporarily, the pain and increased or decreased motility of IBS.

Synopsis and Conclusions

Functional chronic pain syndromes are characterized by pain in deep somatic and visceral body tissues that has the tendency to generalize. The pain is correlated with changes involving the autonomic nervous system, the endocrine systems, and the somatomotor system. Their underlying mechanisms cannot be reduced to a peripheral process such as sensitized deep somatic or visceral nociceptors. Thus, pain and the correlated changes in the autonomic, endocrine, and somatic motor systems are the result of central dysregulation involving mechanisms in the spinal cord, brainstem, and forebrain. Are the centrally regulated autonomic changes, in particular those generated by the sympathetic nervous system, exaggerated adaptive responses of the body that occur in parallel to the pain, or are these autonomically mediated changes involved in the generation of pain in functional pain syndromes? Can activation of the autonomic outflow to the peripheral tissues stimulate the small-diameter afferents or enhance their activity in such a way that pain and associated changes are produced? In other words, are pain and changes in autonomic targets parallel events, or under certain conditions are they sequential events? Can this loop between efferent autonomic outflow to the tissues and afferent inflow from the tissues also occur in the brain between the central representations of the autonomic nervous systems and the central representations of the body tissues?

• The role of the sympathetic nervous system in the generation and maintenance of pain must be seen in the context of regulation of protection of body tissues orchestrated by the brain. This context includes fast defense and slow defense, leading to recuperation and healing, and it also involves the immune system.

• Dysfunction of the autonomic nervous system resulting in pain may occur in patients with SMP following trauma with or without nerve lesion (such as in patients with CRPS or neuropathic pain). The basis of SMP is suggested to be sympathetic-afferent coupling in the periphery of the body, which can occur in various systems, including the sympatho-neural system or the sympatho-adrenal system.

• Central dysfunction of the sympathetic nervous system, together with dysfunction of the somatosensory and somatomotor systems, is probably the basis of the development of CRPS. Thus, I suggest that CRPS is a disease of the CNS with several peripheral and central components. This concept may be applied to other chronic functional pain syndromes.

• Chronic visceral pain, such as GI pain in IBS, or cardiac pain, may also involve the spinal sympathetic or parasympathetic systems supplying the visceral organs. The spinal autonomic systems may amplify the afferent signals from the visceral organs without detectable pathology in the periphery of the organs. The primary cause of chronic visceral pain may be a central dysregulation that includes autonomic systems and visceral sensory systems.

Acknowledgment

Supported by the German Research Foundation, the Bundesministerium für Bildung und Forschung (BMBF) of Germany, and Pfizer.

References

[1] Ader A, editor. Psychoneuroendocrinology, Vols. 1 and 2. Amsterdam: Elsevier, 2007.
[2] Appenzeller O, editor. The autonomic nervous system. Part II: Dysfunctions. Handbook of Clinical Neurology, Vol. 75. Amsterdam: Elsevier, 2000.
[3] Baker DG, Coleridge HM, Coleridge JC, Nerdrum T. Search for a cardiac nociceptor: stimulation by bradykinin of sympathetic afferent nerve endings in the heart of the cat. J Physiol 1980;306:519–36.
[4] Bandler R, Keay KA, Floyd N, Price J. Central circuits mediating patterned autonomic activity during active vs. passive emotional coping. Brain Res Bull 2000;53:95–104.
[5] Bandler R, Price JL, Keay KA. Brain mediation of active and passive emotional coping. Prog Brain Res 2000;122:333–49.
[6] Bandler R, Shipley MT. Columnar organization in the midbrain periaqueductal gray: modules for emotional expression? Trends Neurosci 1994;17:379–89.
[7] Baron R. Complex regional pain syndromes. In: McMahon SB, Koltzenburg M, editors. Wall and Melzack's textbook of pain, 5th ed. Edinburgh: Elsevier Churchill Livingstone; 2006. p. 1011–27.
[8] Baron R. Complex regional pain syndromes. In: Bushnell MC, Basbaum, AI, editors. Pain. The Senses: A Comprehensive Reference, Vol. 5. San Diego: Academic Press; 2008. p. 909–18.
[9] Baron R, Schattschneider J, Binder A, Siebrecht D, Wasner G. Relation between sympathetic vasoconstrictor activity and pain and hyperalgesia in complex regional pain syndromes: a case-control study. Lancet 2002;359:1655–60.
[10] Barsky AJ, Borus JF. Functional somatic syndromes. Ann Intern Med 1999;130:910–21.
[11] Besedovsky HO, del Rey A. Immune-neuroendocrine interactions: facts and hypotheses. Endocr Rev 1995;17:64–102.
[12] Bradesi S, Mayer EA. Novel therapeutic approaches in IBS. Curr Opin Pharmacol 2007;7:598–604.
[13] Bradesi S, Mayer EA, Schwetz I. Irritable bowel syndrome. In: Bushnell MC, Basbaum, AI, editors. Pain. The Senses: A Comprehensive Reference, Vol. 5. San Diego: Academic Press; 2008. p. 571–8.
[14] Cannon WB. The wisdom of the body, 2nd ed. New York: Norton; 1939.
[15] Cervero F. Sensory innervation of the viscera: peripheral basis of visceral pain. Physiol Rev 1994;74:95–138.
[16] Cervero F. Visceral nociceptors. In: Belmonte C, Cervero F, editors. Neurobiology of nociceptors. Oxford: Oxford University Press; 1996. p. 220–40.
[17] Cervero F, Jänig W. Visceral nociceptors: a new world order? Trends Neurosci 1992;15:374–8.
[18] Cohn PF, Fox KM, Daly C. Silent myocardial ischemia. Circulation 2003;108:1263–77.
[19] Coleridge HM, Coleridge JC. Cardiovascular afferents involved in regulation of peripheral vessels. Annu Rev Physiol 1980;42:413–27.
[20] Craig AD. How do you feel? Interoception: the sense of the physiological condition of the body. Nat Rev Neurosci 2002;3:655–66.
[21] Craig AD. Interoception: the sense of the physiological condition of the body. Curr Opin Neurobiol 2003;13:500–5.
[22] Craig AD. A new view of pain as a homeostatic emotion. Trends Neurosci 2003;26:303–7.
[23] Craig AD. Pain mechanisms: labeled lines versus convergence in central processing. Annu Rev Neurosci 2003;26:1–30.
[24] Craig AD. Interoception and emotion. A neuroanatomical perspective. In: Lewis M, Haviland-Jones JM, Barrett Feldman L, editors. Handbook of emotions, 3rd ed. New York: Guilford Press; 2008. p. 272–88.

[25]   Damasio A. Descartes' error: emotion, reason, and the human brain. New York: Putman; 1994.
[26]   Damasio A. The feeling of what happens: body and emotions in the making of consciousness. New York: Harvest; 1999.
[27]   Damasio A. Looking for Spinoza: joy, sorrow, and the feeling brain. Orlando: Harvest; 2003.
[28]   Elenkov IJ, Wilder RL, Chrousos GP, Vizi ES. The sympathetic nerve: an integrative interface between two supersystems: the brain and the immune system. Pharmacol Rev 2000;52:595–638.
[29]   Elenkov IJ. Effects of catecholamines on the immune response. In: del Rey A, Chrousos GP, Besedovsky H, editors. The hypothalamus-pituitary-adrenal axis. NeuroImmune Biology, Vol. 7. Amsterdam: Elsevier; 2008. p. 189–206.
[30]   Fields HL, Basbaum AI, Heinricher MM. Central nervous system mechanisms of pain modulation. In: McMahon SB, Koltzenburg M, editors. Wall and Melzack's textbook of pain, 5th ed. Edinburgh: Elsevier Churchill Livingstone; 2006. p. 125–42.
[31]   Foreman RD. Mechanisms of cardiac pain. Annu Rev Physiol 1999;61:143–67.
[32]   Furness JB. The enteric nervous system. Oxford: Blackwell Science; 2006.
[33]   Gebhart GF, Bielefeldt TK. Visceral pain. In: Bushnell MC, Basbaum, AI, editors. Pain. The Senses: A Comprehensive Reference, Vol. 5. San Diego: Academic Press; 2008. p. 543–70.
[34]   Green PG, Jänig W, Levine JD. Sympathetic terminal: target for negative feedback neuroendocrine control of inflammatory response in the rat. J Neurosci 1997;17:3234–8.
[35]   Häbler HJ, Jänig W, Koltzenburg M. Myelinated primary afferents of the sacral spinal cord responding to slow filling and distension of the cat urinary bladder. J Physiol 1993;463:449-460.
[36]   Häbler HJ, Jänig W, Koltzenburg M. Receptive properties of myelinated primary afferents innervating the inflamed urinary bladder of the cat. J Neurophysiol 1993;69:395–405.
[37]   Harden RN, Baron R, Jänig W. Complex regional pain syndrome. Progress in Pain Research and Management, Vol. 22. Seattle: IASP Press; 2001.
[38]   Heinricher MM, Ingram SL. The brain stem and nociceptive modulation. In: Bushnell MC, Basbaum, AI, editors. Pain. The Senses: A Comprehensive Reference, Vol. 5. San Diego: Academic Press; 2008. p. 593–626.
[39]   Henningsen P, Zipfel S, Herzog W. Management of functional somatic syndromes. Lancet 2007;369:946–55.
[40]   Hori T, Katafuchi T, Take S, Shimizu N, Niijima A. The autonomic nervous system as a communication channel between the brain and the immune system. Neuroimmunomodulation 1995;2:203–15.
[41]   Jänig W. Spinal visceral afferents, sympathetic nervous system and referred pain. In: Vecchiet L, Albe-Fessard D, Lindblom U, Giamberardino MA, editors. New trends in referred pain and hyperalgesia. Pain Research and Clinical Management, Vol. 7. Amsterdam: Elsevier; 1993. p. 83–92.
[42]   Jänig W. Pain in the sympathetic nervous system: pathophysiological mechanisms. In: Mathias CJ, Bannister R, editors. Autonomic failure, 4th ed. New York: Oxford University Press; 2002. p. 99–108.
[43]   Jänig W. Vagal afferents and visceral pain. In: Undem B, Weinreich D, editors. Advances in vagal afferent neurobiology. Boca Raton: CRC Press; 2005. p. 465–93.
[44]   Jänig W. The integrative action of the autonomic nervous system: neurobiology of homeostasis. Cambridge: Cambridge University Press; 2006.
[45]   Jänig W. Autonomic nervous system and pain. In: Bushnell MC, Basbaum, AI, editors. Pain. The Senses: A Comprehensive Reference, Vol. 5. San Diego: Academic Press; 2008. p. 193–225.
[46]   Jänig W, Baron R. The role of the sympathetic nervous system in neuropathic pain: clinical observations and animal models. In: Hansson PT, Fields HL, Hill RG, Marchettini P, editors. Neuropathic pain: pathophysiology and treatment. Seattle: IASP Press; 2001. p. 125–49.
[47]   Jänig W, Baron R. Complex regional pain syndrome is a disease of the central nervous system. Clin Auton Res 2002;12:150–64.
[48]   Jänig W, Baron R. Complex regional pain syndrome: mystery explained? Lancet Neurol 2003;2:687–97.
[49]   Jänig W, Baron R. Experimental approach to CRPS. Pain 2004;108:3–7.
[50]   Jänig W, Häbler HJ. Visceral-autonomic integration. In: Gebhart GF, editor. Visceral pain. Progress in Pain Research and Management, Vol. 5. Seattle: IASP Press; 1995. p. 311–48.

[51] Jänig W, Häbler HJ. Specificity in the organization of the autonomic nervous system: a basis for precise neural regulation of homeostatic and protective body functions. Prog Brain Res 2000;122:351–67.

[52] Jänig W, Häbler HJ. Sympathetic nervous system: contribution to chronic pain. Prog Brain Res 2000;129:451–68.

[53] Jänig W, Koltzenburg M. What is the interaction between the sympathetic terminal and the primary afferent fiber? In: Basbaum AI, Besson J-M, editors. Towards a new pharmacotherapy of pain. Dahlem Workshop Reports. Chichester: John Wiley & Sons; 1991. p. 331–52.

[54] Jänig W, Koltzenburg M. Pain arising from the urogenital tract. In: Burnstock G, editor. The autonomic nervous system, Vol. 2. Chur: Harwood Academic; 1993. p. 523–76.

[55] Jänig W, Levine JD. Autonomic-neuroendocrine-immune responses in acute and chronic pain. In: McMahon SB, Koltzenburg M, editors. Wall and Melzack's textbook of pain, 5th ed. Edinburgh: Elsevier; 2006. p. 205–18.

[56] Jänig W, McLachlan EM. Neurobiology of the autonomic nervous system. In: Mathias CJ, Bannister R, editors. Autonomic failure, 4th ed. New York: Oxford University Press; 2002. p. 3–15.

[57] Jänig W, Stanton-Hicks M, editors. Reflex sympathetic dystrophy: a reappraisal. Seattle: IASP Press; 1996.

[58] Jänig W, Khasar SG, Levine JD, Miao FJP. The role of vagal visceral afferents in the control of nociception. Prog Brain Res 2000;122:273–87.

[59] Keay KA, Bandler R. Periaqueductal gray. In: Paxinos G, editor. The rat nervous system, 3rd ed. San Diego: Academic Press; 2004. p. 243–57.

[60] Keay K, Bandler R. Emotional and behavioral significance of the pain signal and the role of the midbrain periaqueductal gray (PAG). In: Bushnell MC, Basbaum, AI, editors. Pain. The Senses: A Comprehensive Reference, Vol. 5. San Diego: Academic Press; 2008. p. 627–34.

[61] Khasar SG, Miao FJP, Jänig W, Levine JD. Modulation of bradykinin-induced mechanical hyperalgesia in the rat skin by activity in the abdominal vagal afferents. Eur J Neurosci 1998;10:435–44.

[62] Khasar SG, Miao FJP, Jänig W, Levine JD. Vagotomy-induced enhancement of mechanical hyperalgesia in the rat is sympathoadrenal-mediated. J Neurosci 1998;18:3043–9.

[63] Khasar SG, Green PG, Miao FJ, Levine JD. Vagal modulation of nociception is mediated by adrenomedullary epinephrine in the rat. Eur J Neurosci 2003;17:909–15.

[64] Langley JN. The autonomic nervous system. Part I. Cambridge: W. Heffer; 1921.

[65] Lewis JS, Kersten P, McCabe CS, McPherson KM, Blake DR. Body perception disturbance: a contribution to pain in complex regional pain syndrome (CRPS). Pain 2007;133:111–9.

[66] Madden KS, Felten DL. Experimental basis for neural-immune interactions. Physiol Rev 1995;75:77–106.

[67] Madden KS, Sanders K, Felten DL. Catecholamine influences and sympathetic modulation of immune responsiveness. Rev Pharmacol Toxicol 1995;35:417–48.

[68] Maier SF, Watkins LR. Cytokines for psychologists: implications of bidirectional immune-to-brain communication for understanding behavior, mood, and cognition. Psychol Rev 1998;105:83–107.

[69] Malliani A. Cardiovascular sympathetic afferent fibers. Rev Physiol Biochem Pharmacol 1982;94:11–74.

[70] Malliani A, Lombardi F, Pagani M. Sensory innervation of the heart. Prog Brain Res 1986;67:39–48.

[71] Mason P. Contributions of the medullary raphe and ventromedial reticular region to pain modulation and other homeostatic functions. Annu Rev Neurosci 2001;24:737–77.

[72] Mason P. Ventromedial medulla: pain modulation and beyond. J Comp Neurol 2005;493:2–8.

[73] Mason P. Deconstructing endogenous pain modulations. J Neurophysiol 2005;94:1659–63.

[74] Mathias MC, Bannister R, editors. Autonomic failure, 5th ed. Oxford: Oxford University Press; in press.

[75] McCabe CS, Haigh RC, Halligan PW, Blake DR. Referred sensations in patients with complex regional pain syndrome type 1. Rheumatology (Oxford) 2003;42:1067–73.

[76] McMahon SB. NGF as a mediator of inflammatory pain. Philos Trans R Soc Lond B Biol Sci 1996;351:431–40.

[77] Miao FJP, Green PG, Coderre TJ, Jänig W, Levine JD. Sympathetic-dependence in bradykinin-induced synovial plasma extravasation is dose-related. Neurosci Lett 1996;205:165–8.

[78] Miao FJP, Jänig W, Levine JD. Role of sympathetic postganglionic neurons in synovial plasma extravasation induced by bradykinin. J Neurophysiol 1996;75:715–24.

[79] Michaelis M, Häbler HJ, Jänig W. Silent afferents: a separate class of primary afferents? Clin Exp Pharmacol Physiol 1996;23:99–105.

[80] Moseley GL. Graded motor imagery is effective for long-standing complex regional pain syndrome: a randomised controlled trial. Pain 2004;108:192–8.

[81] Moseley GL. Is successful rehabilitation of complex regional pain syndrome due to sustained attention to the affected limb? A randomised clinical trial. Pain 2005;114:54–61.

[82] Poole S, Woolf CJ. Cytokine-nerve growth factor interactions in inflammatory hyperalgesia. In: Watkins LR, Maier SF, editors. Cytokines and Pain. Basel: Birkhäuser Verlag; 1999. p. 89-132.

[83] Price DD, Long S, Wilsey B, Rafii A. Analysis of peak magnitude and duration of analgesia produced by local anesthetics injected into sympathetic ganglia of complex regional pain syndrome patients. Clin J Pain 1998;14:216–26.

[84] Prins JB, van der Meer JW, Bleijenberg G. Chronic fatigue syndrome. Lancet 2006;367:346–55.

[85] Robertson D, editor. Primer on the autonomic nervous system. Amsterdam: Elsevier; 2004.

[86] Rommel O, Gehling M, Dertwinkel R, Witscher K, Zenz M, Malin JP, Jänig W. Hemisensory impairment in patients with complex regional pain syndrome. Pain 1999;80:95–101.

[87] Rommel O, Malin JP, Zenz M, Jänig W. Quantitative sensory testing, neurophysiological and psychological examination in patients with complex regional pain syndrome and hemisensory deficits. Pain 2001;93:279–93.

[88] Schedlowski M, Tewes U, editors. Psychoneuroimmunology: an interdisciplinary introduction. New York: Kluwer Academic; 1999.

[89] Sherrington CS. Cutaneous sensation. In: Schäfer EA, editor. Textbook of physiology, Vol. 2. Edinburgh: Young J. Pentland; 1900. p. 920–1001.

[90] Sloan EK, Capitanio JP, Tarara RP, Mendoza SP, Mason WA, Cole SW. Social stress enhances sympathetic innervation of primate lymph nodes: mechanisms and implications for viral pathogenesis. J Neurosci 2007;27:8857–65.

[91] Sloan EK, Capitanio JP, Cole SW. Stress-induced remodeling of lymphoid innervation. Brain Behav Immun 2008;22:15–21.

[92] Stanton-Hicks M, Jänig W, Hassenbusch S, Haddox JD, Boas R, Wilson P. Reflex sympathetic dystrophy: changing concepts and taxonomy. Pain 1995;63:127–33.

[93] Staud R. Fibromyalgia. In: Bushnell MC, Basbaum, AI, editors. Pain. The Senses: A Comprehensive Reference, Vol. 5. San Diego: Academic Press; 2008. p. 775–82.

[94] Straub RH, Härle P. Sympathetic neurotransmitters in joint inflammation. Rheum Dis Clin North Am 2005;31:43–59.

[95] Straub RH, Baerwald CG, Wahle M, Jänig W. Autonomic dysfunction in rheumatic diseases. Rheum Dis Clin N Am 2005;31:61–75.

[96] Swanson LW. Cerebral hemisphere regulation of motivated behavior. Brain Res 2000;886:113–64.

[97] Swanson LW. The architecture of the nervous system. In: Squire LR, Bloom FE, McConnell SK, Roberts JL, Spitzer NC, Zigmond MJ, editors. Fundamental neuroscience, 2nd ed. San Diego: Academic Press; 2003. p. 15–45.

[98] Udem B, Weinreich D, editors. Advances in vagal afferent neurobiology. Boca Raton: CRC Press; 2005.

[99] Vierck CJ Jr. Mechanisms underlying development of spatially distributed chronic pain (fibromyalgia). Pain 2006;124:242–63.

[100] Wasner G, Heckmann K, Maier C, Baron R. Vascular abnormalities in acute reflex sympathetic dystrophy (CRPS I): complete inhibition of sympathetic nerve activity with recovery. Arch Neurol 1999;56:613–20.

[101] Wasner G, Schattschneider J, Heckmann K, Maier C, Baron R. Vascular abnormalities in reflex sympathetic dystrophy (CRPS I): mechanisms and diagnostic value. Brain 2001;124:587–99.

[102] Watkins LR, Maier SF, editors. Cytokines and pain. Basel: Birkhäuser Verlag; 1999.

[103] Watkins LR, Maier SF. The pain of being sick: implications of immune-to-brain communication for understanding pain. Annu Rev Psychol 2000;51:29–57.

[104] Watts AG, Swanson LW. Anatomy of motivational systems. In: Gallistel GR, editor. "Stevens" handbook of experimental psychology, 3rd ed. Vol. 3. New York: John Wiley; 2002. p. 563–631.
[105] Wessely S, Nimnuan C, Sharpe M. Functional somatic syndromes: one or many? Lancet 1999;354:936–9.
[106] Woolf CJ. Phenotypic modification of primary sensory neurons: the role of nerve growth factor in the production of persistent pain. Philos Trans R Soc Lond B Biol Sci 1996;351:441–8.
[107] Woolf CJ, Ma QP, Allchorne A, Poole S. Peripheral cell types contributing to the hyperalgesic action of nerve growth factor in inflammation. J Neurosci 1996;16:2716–23.

Correspondence to: Prof. Dr. Wilfrid Jänig, Physiologisches Institut, Christian-Albrechts-Universität zu Kiel, Olshausenstr. 40, 24098 Kiel, Germany. Tel: +431/8802036; fax: +431/8805256; email: w.janig@physiologie.uni-kiel.de.

HPA Axis and Sympathetic Influences on Pain and Fatigue in Fibromyalgia, Chronic Fatigue, and Overlapping Functional Pain Syndromes

Kathleen C. Light[a] and Charles J. Vierck[b]

[a]*Department of Anesthesiology, Health Sciences Center, University of Utah, Salt Lake City, Utah, USA;* [b]*Department of Neuroscience and McKnight Brain Institute, University of Florida College of Medicine, Gainesville, Florida, USA*

Pain and fatigue are the two symptoms most frequently reported by patients to their physicians. However, in overlapping multisymptom disorders [1,16,90], including fibromyalgia syndrome (FM), chronic fatigue syndrome (CFS), temporomandibular disorder (TMD) and irritable bowel syndrome (IBS), there is something exceptional about these symptoms—something that differs from acute cutaneous or postsurgical pain. The most notable characteristics of the pain and fatigue symptoms in these disorders is that they are chronic and very resistant even to treatments that are extremely effective in managing acute pain and fatigue such as opiates, stimulants, and sleep-inducing agents. Clearly, multiple physiological systems are dysregulated in patients with these disorders, affecting the processing of nociceptive input peripherally and the experience of pain centrally.

The first task of this chapter will be to discuss how nociceptive signals may be modulated as they are transmitted within the central nervous system (CNS). The second task will be to address how chronic pain develops and how it differs from acute pain, including ways in which acute pain sets the stage for development of chronic pain. Finally, we will turn our attention to the ways in which other systems contribute to the onset and maintenance of chronic pain and responses to treatment, specifically the body's primary stress systems, the hypothalamic-pituitary-adrenocortical (HPA) and the sympathetic-adrenomedullary (SAM) systems. We will also briefly address how immune function may be influenced by HPA and SAM dysregulation.

Investigating Nociceptive Transmission and Modulation at Early Stages of Processing

An enormous research effort has described details of connectivity between the spinal cord and brainstem and defined neurotransmitter relations between neurons at these sites [57]. These studies have been directed by an assumption that abnormal nociceptive processing can be controlled at early stages of synaptic processing [56], particularly by descending inhibition from the brainstem [6]. However, the relevance of these observations to mechanisms of chronic pain is unknown, because of the following procedural difficulties.

1) Most recordings or other characterizations of neurons in the dorsal horn are obtained from "interneurons" with unknown projections. The spinal recordings are obtained under anesthesia designed to eliminate pain, and the most common test for surgical anesthesia is obliteration of nociceptive flexion reflexes. Also, the dissection required for spinal recording generates nociceptive input. Therefore, most "normal" recordings used as comparisons with models of chronic pain are from neurons affected by extensive tissue injury, and relationships between neuronal discharge and any behavior indicative of nociceptive sensitivity cannot be determined in an anesthetized preparation.

2) The spinothalamic tract (STT) normally is a major pathway for nociceptive transmission to the cerebrum. However, the assumption that chronic pain can be understood by recording from STT cell bodies is suspect. Chronic central pain and hyperalgesia in humans can result from interruption of STT axons in the spinal cord [83,85,86] or the brainstem [62] or from lesions within thalamic terminations of the STT [40]. Thus,

pain transmission by routes other than the STT is important, as are adaptations of cerebral sites to disruption of the fastest, most direct route for passing of nociceptive signals to the cerebral cortex. A likely candidate for an alternate ascending pain pathway is the diffuse spinoreticulothalamo-cortical system [86], which has seldom been targeted by studies intended to reveal mechanisms of chronic pain.

3) The prevalent method for determining whether a manipulation affects pain has been to evaluate reflex responses. Reflex studies demand that any change in responsivity produced by an experimental manipulation results from actions on sensory processing in the dorsal horn. Obviously, changes in motoneuronal excitability could account for alterations of reflex responsivity, and controls for this possibility are not available. Similarly, stimulation of the brainstem inevitably generates both ascending and descending influences, but pain researchers have almost universally attended only to spinal effects of these manipulations. Ascending projections from the brainstem (e.g., serotonergic and noradrenergic projections) ramify extensively in the cerebrum [15,55]. Influences from the brainstem on cerebral sites involved in nociceptive transmission are not understood but are probably more relevant to chronic pain than descending control over reflexes.

Investigating Central Sensitization and Inhibition: Stress and Pain Modulation

Attempts to study mechanisms of chronic pain often have settled for examining nociceptive stimulation over minutes or hours. Long duration or repetitive nociceptive stimulation brings into play central mechanisms for amplification, prolongation, and spatial radiation of pain that contribute to, but are not sufficient to explain, most forms of chronic pain [96]. Therefore, tests of central sensitization can document the presence of pathology affecting pain transmission systems [84], but they do not identify the source or cause of chronically abnormal activity [82].

Understandably, pain researchers have thoroughly explored the possibility that pain can be inhibited. The prototypical inhibitory agents are opioid agonists. Extensive investigation of inhibitory control by opioids has been instructive but discouraging with regard to long-term therapy for chronic pain. Administration of opioid agonists is accompanied by a myriad of compensatory actions and reactions that impair opioid receptor activation and facilitate pain transmission [34,49,51,101]. Even when opiates are initially beneficial, problems can arise with long-term use [2]. Opioid inhibitory systems appear to be designed for short-term control of pain.

Psychological stress is thought to reduce pain sensitivity during acute emergencies, in part by activating opioidergic and adrenergic pathways, to aid fight or flight reactions to a perceived threat. Stress-induced analgesia is almost certainly present in the initial stages of a stressful event, when opioid release is maximal. However, investigations of stress effects on nociceptive processing have almost always involved post-stress evaluation. Nociceptive reflexes are attenuated after termination of a stressful experience (e.g., [14]). In contrast, operant testing reveals post-stress enhancement of escape responding to the same stimuli (stress-induced hyperalgesia [42]). The results of reflex testing have been misleading and have impeded recognition that stress does not inhibit pain over the long term but instead facilitates development of chronic pain and exacerbates it. Opioid release during stress is one component of an integrated reaction dominated by SAM arousal, which is intended to deal with an acute rather than a continuous threat. When stress is prolonged, it is not beneficial. Pain is distressing, and when it persists, excitatory effects on pain transmission predominate.

Investigating Mechanisms of Chronic Pain

Elucidating mechanistic bases for chronic pain conditions that afflict humans has proved to be a daunting challenge. Clinically relevant chronic pain goes on for months and years, not minutes or hours, and this time frame places extraordinary demands on mechanistic studies. Furthermore, a property of many forms of chronic pain is slow development in a subpopulation of individuals with apparently similar injuries. A delayed appearance of ongoing pain occurs following both peripheral and central injuries [62,73,83,85,86]. Characteristics of the pain depend upon the location and other features of a neural insult [38,70]. The painful sensations can change over time as the nervous system adjusts to nociceptive input and/or deafferentation [73]. These features of chronic pain dictate that we understand and learn to counteract long-term neural adaptations that occur gradually over time and endure, once established by an injury. This understanding is essential if we are to prevent development of chronic pain or cure it rather than attempting to partially manage it with inhibition. Chronic pain develops as abnormal sources of relentless activity overpower inhibitory influences. Either the original source of nociceptive input for each pain condition must be silenced (probably early on), or methods should be developed that attack the sources of abnormal activity that develop in reaction to an injury.

Tissue injury induces a variety of excitatory influences, both peripherally and at central locations that receive input from injured nociceptors. Inflammation is evident at peripheral sites of injury and at the central terminations of damaged afferents [102], resulting in hyperalgesia [87,97]. In addition, inflammation is a potent source of sympathetic activation, essentially producing a stress reaction [58]. Interruption of axons is a contributing factor in development of chronic pain, because deafferented central cells become spontaneously active [22]. In addition, constriction, demyelination, and inflammation of peripheral or central axons can result in abnormal activity in the affected nerve or pathway [78] and can trigger excitotoxic reactions of postsynaptic cells [91]. Similarly, direct insult to the CNS is accompanied by excitotoxic reactions of neurons in the vicinity of the infarct. For example, ischemia and associated neuronal discharge within spinal gray matter have been linked to spinal cord injury pain [85,92,99]. These consequences of peripheral or central neural injury are factors known to generate aberrant discharge within pain transmission systems, progressing gradually as potential sources of chronic pain.

Numerous forms of receptor up- and downregulation occur at the site of a neuronal insult and upstream from the trauma. Injuries to peripheral nerves provide abundant evidence for this plasticity. Partial nerve damage with formation of neuromas induces proliferation of noradrenergic receptors on nociceptive afferent terminals and ganglion cells that normally do not respond to noradrenergic agonists [65]. Excitatory influences of nerve injury result from this and numerous other forms of upregulation and phenotypic alteration of peripheral afferents [23]. Unfortunately, repeated application of receptor agonists or antagonists designed to counteract excitatory influences reliably produces compensatory receptor down- or upregulation that reduces therapeutic efficacy. This adaptation is the major challenge to be met with pain therapeutics.

A Model of Chronic Pain Involving Contributory Effects of Stress

The preceding discussion applies to any form of chronic pain resulting from neural trauma. Pain syndromes from injury to peripheral nerves or central pain pathways have been used as examples of how a generator of pain can become established by progressions of axonal injury and neuronal death, with attendant inflammatory reactions that generate abnormal spontaneous activity within pain transmission systems, elaborated by synaptic plasticity and receptor up-and downregulation. These reactions can far outlast apparent healing of the original injury [87], presenting the diagnostic nightmare of chronic pain. An additional category of chronic pain exemplifies the progressive development of excitatory influences, as outlined above, but it is not restricted to the innervation territory of damaged neurons. Instead, the chronic presence of a source of pain can result, over time, in the widespread pain and increased pain sensitivity that are characteristic of FM [82]. In the context in which an initial traumatic event or a chronic stressor is involved in the pathogenesis of chronic pain, we envision the following progression over time: (1) chronic activation of the body's stress systems, the HPA, and more importantly, the sympathetic or SAM system; (2) sympathetically mediated peripheral vasoconstriction (particularly in females); (3) eventual ischemia of deep tissues; and (4) sensitization of nociceptors consequent to receptor changes in the ischemic deep tissues, accounting for the widespread hypersensitivity that is characteristic of FM. We will next review evidence on how the body's primary stress systems, the HPA axis and the SAM systems, may be functionally altered in FM and related pain disorders.

Evidence of Complex Dysregulation of the HPA Axis in Fibromyalgia and Chronic Fatigue Syndrome

It was originally assumed that the HPA axis must be overactive in disorders such as FM, because patients report high levels of life stressors, and because chronic pain itself is a stressor. More recent evidence indicates that patients with FM can have lower or higher than normal cortisol levels, depending upon the time of day and the way in which cortisol was measured [50,53,77]. Urinary free-cortisol levels have been found to be low in FM patients in most studies (see [17]). In serum and saliva, due to the pulsatile release of cortisol and pronounced diurnal changes, cortisol levels are best studied by sampling throughout the day. Crofford et al. [21] found that half of 25 FM patients showed slowing in the diurnal decrease of serum cortisol over the waking hours of the day, resulting in elevated evening levels. Weissbecker et al. [88] found higher daytime cortisol responses only in FM women with a history of physical or sexual abuse: very low levels at awakening were followed by a marked rise and then a flattened decline later in the day. Many FM and CFS patients do report a history of childhood maltreatment and/or trauma, which are both known to be related to altered HPA activity [37,54].

In contrast to FM, patients with CFS have traditionally been labeled as having low levels of cortisol and adrenocorticotropin. As summarized by Cleare [17,18], about half of the studies using serum or salivary cortisol measures have supported this hypothesis, along with most studies using 24-hour urinary free cortisol. Many other studies have shown heightened negative glucocorticoid feedback to dexamethasone and similar challenges or diminished HPA responses to physical or psychological stressors [17]. The pattern of these findings, while not overwhelmingly consistent, was sufficient to stimulate two randomized controlled trials of hydrocortisone in CFS, but both yielded negative findings, with improvement seen in only about one-third of CFS patients treated [19,52]. In two other trials, hydrocortisone combined with fludrocortisone or galantamine, an acetylcholinesterase inhibitor that secondarily enhances cortisol secretion, also had no consistent benefit in CFS [8,9].

Cleare [18] summarized several prospective studies of cohorts at high risk for developing CFS and concluded that there are no HPA axis changes present during the early stages of CFS or FM. Thus, the mild hypocortisolism seen in later stages of CFS, the dysregulated diurnal cortisol pattern seen in some FM patients, and the heightened negative glucocorticoid feedback reported for both CFS and FM do not appear to be consistent initiating factors in these disorders. Instead, alterations in HPA responses in CFS and FM may be consequences of disordered sleep and breathing patterns, deconditioning, and excessive time spent lying down, and may be due to overlapping illnesses including depression and a history of maltreatment or trauma [32,37,43].

Evidence of Sympathetic Dysregulation in Fibromyalgia and Chronic Fatigue Syndrome

Several lines of evidence indicate that SAM activity is altered in patients with FM. Increased β_1-adrenergic activity and diminished parasympathetic tone are suggested by a number of studies of heart rate variability (HRV) in FM, documenting decreased HRV at rest while awake and during sleep [20,48,75]. Decreased HRV has also been reported in CFS, TMD, and IBS [10,13,66]. Vasoconstrictive and vasodilatory responses to cold, mental stress, and auditory stress are reduced in FM patients, suggesting an imbalance in β_2- vs. α-adrenergic activity in vascular smooth muscle that could manifest as impaired peripheral circulation [61,67,79]. This finding may explain the high frequency of Raynaud's syndrome and altered sensitivity to cold and heat in FM and CFS patients [25]. An imbalance in adrenergically mediated vascular responses with lower-body vasoconstriction and impaired venous return could also contribute to the hypotension and light-headedness during postural challenges and tilt-table tests seen in some patients with FM or CFS [30,68,98]. Evidence of downregulation of β-adrenergic and α-adrenergic receptors has been reported in FM and CFS patients, a marker of chronically enhanced adrenergic activity [47,76]. This chronic state may result in blunted or otherwise abnormal cardiac and vascular responses to stimuli such as postural challenge, mental stress, and exercise [31,61].

Several experts have hypothesized that a consequence of sympathetic dysregulation in FM is intramuscular hypoperfusion [39,46]. Recently, Katz and colleagues [39, p. 517] noted that FM patients describe their pain "in terms suggestive of the pain in muscles following extreme exertion and anaerobic metabolism." The muscle fatigue experienced by CFS and FM patients parallels that experienced by healthy subjects during exercise or the day after overexertion. Until recently, the peripheral processes involved in sensing this type of muscle fatigue and muscle pain were unknown. Animal model studies [35,36,44,60,72] have clarified that a complex of ion channel receptors on dorsal root ganglion cells (including the acid-sensing or ASIC, the purinergic 2 or P2X, and the capsaicin-responsive or TRPV1 receptors), working together, serve as the sensory mechanism detecting increased metabolic by-products of muscle exertion (adenosine triphosphate [ATP], lactate, and pH changes). There is also evidence that overworking the muscle or making the muscle ischemic may upregulate or otherwise sensitize these ion channel receptors [41,44,100]. Thus, if SNS and vasomotor dysregulation does lead to muscle hypoperfusion in FM and CFS, a secondary effect would be altered function of these receptors such that, even at resting levels of metabolites, enough of them are activated to be perceived as muscle fatigue and pain.

In support of the importance of sympathetic activity in FM, several randomized, placebo-controlled trials have indicated that duloxetine, which inhibits both norepinephrine reuptake and serotonin reuptake roughly equally, reduces fibromyalgia pain and stiffness, decreases tender points, and improves quality of life significantly in FM patients [3–5,11]. The benefits of duloxetine in these trials were not restricted to those FM patients with comorbid clinical depression and in fact were found to be independent of improvements in depression or anxiety symptoms. A similar combined reuptake inhibitor, venlafaxine, shows promise for reducing fatigue [26]. Since selective serotonin reuptake inhibitors (SSRIs) had previously been found to have only limited benefits in FM patients [94], this new study points to a critical contribution of norepinephrine reuptake inhibition in alleviating FM pain-related symptoms.

Pindolol, a drug that antagonizes both β_1 and β_2-adrenergic receptors as well as altering serotonin activity, was also shown in an uncontrolled open trial to decrease tender points and fibromyalgia impact, including pain [95]. Beta-receptor antagonists have also shown benefits in controlled studies. Propranolol, a β_1 and β_2 antagonist, was shown to reduce sensitivity to heat pain more than placebo in healthy young adults [12]. Likewise, in a randomized, placebo-controlled crossover study of 10 TMD and 10 FM patients, we found that on average the same subject's total pain score was reduced approximately 50% after propranolol vs. after placebo, and the number of body sites where pain was experienced was reduced by 30% [7]. Thus, chronically enhanced β-adrenergic activity may contribute to the onset or maintenance of FM and related disorders, and correction of dysregulated sympathetic function is linked to reduction in FM symptoms.

Dysregulation of Immune Responses Secondary to Beta-Adrenergic Activity

Elenkov and colleagues [27] have provided the most complete review of findings on how the SAM system serves as an integrative interface between the brain and the immune system, including the following three points. First, β-adrenergic activity inhibits pro-inflammatory thymus helper 1 (Th1) cell activity directly via specific β_2 receptors on these cells. Second, pro-inflammatory Th1 activity is inhibitory to anti-inflammatory Th2 cell activity; thus, by inhibiting Th1 activity, β-adrenergic activity should indirectly enhance Th2 activity. Third, although some circulating cytokines such as interleukin (IL)-6 have mixed pro- and anti-inflammatory effects, and others such as IL-8 are enhanced by stress and sympathetic activity and are primarily pro-inflammatory, the majority of pro-inflammatory cytokines are inhibited by stress and specifically by β-adrenergic activity, including interleukin (IL)-1β, IL-2, IL-12, and tumor necrosis factor (TNF-α), while the majority of anti-inflammatory cytokines (including IL-4, IL-10, and IL-13) are not. Thus, it would be expected that CFS and FM patients with excess SAM activity should show cytokine profiles where the balance between pro-inflammatory Th1 cytokines relative to anti-inflammatory Th2 cytokines is altered in favor of an anti-inflammatory predominance, as previously proposed by Patarca [63].

Recently, we reported cytokine findings from 19 FM and CFS patients and 17 healthy controls where blood was drawn before and four times after a 25-minute bout of moderate whole-body exercise [45]. We found that Th1/Th2 ratios were greatly reduced in CFS and FM patients vs. controls (ratios = 0.84 and 0.47 vs. 2.53, $P < 0.005$, based on weighted sums of IL-1β, IL-12, and TNF-α for Th1 and IL-10 and IL-13 for Th2). These observations are consistent with a number of prior reports on cytokine profiles in patients with FM and CFS [64,71,93]. We also found that β_1, β_2, and α_2 receptors on leukocytes were markedly increased for 48 hours after exercise in the CFS and FM groups, but not in controls. Finally, we found that specialized ion channel receptors on leukocytes (P2X4 and ASIC3 receptors), which are known to respond to combinations of ATP, pH, and lactate, were also increased in the CFS and FM patients but not in controls for 48 hours after exercise [45]. In animal models, P2X4 and ASIC3 receptors on dorsal root ganglion cells appear to be part of a specialized muscle fatigue and muscle pain sensory system [35,36,44,72,100].

Thus, patients with CFS and FM have three interactive systems that show dysregulation: (1) the SAM system, (2) the immune system, and (3) the ion channel-based sensory pathway that detects metabolites produced by muscle activity (presumed to be experienced at low levels as fatigue and at higher levels as both fatigue and pain). We suspect that these three components of dysregulation are linked, and that alterations in SAM function may lead both to the imbalance favoring anti-inflammatory over pro-inflammatory cytokine profile and to hypoperfusion of muscles. Thus, the normal, locally autoregulated vasodilatory response to muscle activity may be blunted in FM and CFS patients. In a vicious cycle, this dysregulation may limit the ability of the vasculature to remove muscle metabolites such as lactate, protons, and ATP, which may stimulate proliferation of the receptors sensing these metabolites, thereby further enhancing pain, which then further increases sympathetic activity. Physical activity may have the long-term benefit of increasing muscle perfusion by stimulating angiogenesis, but in the shorter term, CFS and FM patients may experience increased symptoms after exercise if they have upregulation of P2X4 and ASIC3 receptors. This finding may explain why carefully graded exercise regimens appear to be among the most effective interventions for reducing symptoms in CFS and FM [89].

More Insights on Treatment and Prevention

The ideal preventive approach for patients in whom chronic stress and an acute pain condition could lead to chronic widespread pain or FM would be to silence the source of chronic stress such as a localized pain condition. In the absence of procedures to eliminate pain localized to the distribution of neural trauma, attention could be directed to any portion of the nervous system involved in stress reactions to pain. Therapy might include behavioral or pharmacological procedures that reduce stress (e.g., by actions on limbic and hypothalamic structures). Behavioral and pharmacological methods of enhancing blood supply to deep tissues should alleviate muscular ischemia and attenuate nociceptor sensitization. Exercise, particularly if it incorporates whole-body aerobic exercise and resistance training, has already shown some effectiveness in normalizing the sympathetic dysregulation in FM [29]. Similarly, understanding the receptor changes responsible for nociceptor sensitization by ischemia of deep tissues should suggest ways to attenuate the sources of widespread FM pain and hypersensitivity.

Preventive approaches may in the near future be able to focus on individuals with known genetically based susceptibilities. Recent investigations have obtained initial evidence of an association between FM or CFS and gene pathways of interest based on the physiological information detailed above. These pathways include those involved in regulation of ion channel activity, cytokine-cytokine receptor interaction, neuroactive ligand-receptor interaction, adrenergic receptors, and synthesis of catechol-O-methyl transferase (COMT), an enzyme that metabolizes catecholamines [24,28,33,59,69,74,80]. Further, it is important to continue to address gene expression and factors that regulate such expression as well as more traditional genetic markers in FM and CFS [81].

Acknowledgments

Supported in part by National Institutes of Health grant R21 NS057821 to the first author.

References

[1]   Aaron LA, Burke MM, Buchwald D. Overlapping conditions among patients with chronic fatigue syndrome, fibromyalgia and temporomandibular disorder. Arch Intern Med 2000;160:221–7.

[2]   Angst MS, Clark JD. Opioid-induced hyperalgesia: a qualitative systematic review. Anesthesiology 2006;104:570–87.

[3]   Arnold LM, Lu Y, Crofford LJ, Wohlreich M, Detke MJ, Iyengar S, Goldstein DJ. A double-blind, multicenter trial comparing duloxetine with placebo in the treatment of fibromyalgia patients with or without major depressive disorder. Arthritis Rheum 2004;50:2974–84.

[4]   Arnold LM, Pritchett YL, D'Souza DN, Kajdasz DK, Iyengar S, Wernicke JF. Duloxetine for the treatment of fibromyalgia in women: pooled results from two randomized, placebo-controlled clinical trials. J Womens Health (Larchmt) 2007;16:1145–56.

[5]   Arnold LM, Rosen A, Pritchett YL, D'Souza DN, Goldstein DJ, Iyengar S, Wernicke JF. A randomized, double-blind, placebo-controlled trial of duloxetine in the treatment of women with fibromyalgia with or without major depressive disorder. Pain 2005;119:5–15.

[6]   Basbaum A, Fields H. Endogenous pain control mechanisms: review and hypothesis. Ann Neurol 1978;4:451–62.

[7]   Bhalang K, Light K, Maixner W. Effect of propranolol on TMD and fibromyalgia pain: preliminary findings. IADR/AADR/CADR 82nd General Session, Hawaii; 2004.

[8]   Blacker CV, Greenwood DT, Wesnes KA, Wilson R, Woodward C, Howe I, Ali T. Effect of galantamine hydrobromide in chronic fatigue syndrome: a randomized controlled trial. JAMA 2004;292:1195–1204.

[9]   Blockmans D, Persoons P, Van Houdenhove B, Lejeune M, Bobbaers H. Combination therapy with hydrocortisone and fludrocortisone does not improve symptoms in chronic fatigue syndrome: a randomized, placebo-controlled, double-blind, crossover study. Am J Med 2003;114:736–41.

[10] Boneva RS, Decker MJ, Maloney EM, Lin JM, Jones JF, Helgason HG, Heim CM, Rye DB, Reeves WC. Higher heart rate and reduced heart rate variability persist during sleep in chronic fatigue syndrome: a population-based study. Auton Neurosci 2007;137:94–101.

[11] Brecht S, Courtecuisse C, Debieuvre C, Croenlein J, Desaiah D, Raskin J, Petit C, Demyttenaere K. Efficacy and safety of duloxetine 60 mg once daily in the treatment of pain in patients with major depressive disorder and at least moderate pain of unknown etiology: a randomized controlled trial. J Clin Psychiatry 2007;68:1707–16.

[12] Bushnell MC, Schweinhardt P, Gramigni E, Baldini G, Clemente A, Carli F. The beta-blocker propranolol decreases pain perception in healthy volunteers. Soc Neurosci Abstracts 2007;826.9.

[13] Cain KC, Jarrett ME, Burr RL, Hertig VL, Heitkemper MM. Heart rate variability is related to pain severity and predominant bowel pattern in women with irritable bowel syndrome. Neurogastroenterol Motil 2007;19:110–8.

[14] Calcagnetti D, Holtzman S. Potentiation of morphine analgesia in rats given a single exposure of restraint stress immobilization. Pharmacol Biochem Behav 1992;37:193–9.

[15] Carstens E, Leah J, Lechner J, Zimmermann M. Demonstration of extensive brainstem projections to medial and lateral thalamus and hypothalamus in the rat. Neuroscience 1990;35:609–26.

[16] Chapman CR, Tuckett RP, Song CW. Pain and stress in a systems perspective: reciprocal neural, endocrine, and immune interactions. J Pain 2008;9:122–45.

[17] Cleare AJ. The neuroendocrinology of chronic fatigue syndrome. Endocr Rev 2003;24:236–52.

[18] Cleare AJ. The HPA axis and the genesis of chronic fatigue syndrome. Trends Endocrinol Metab 2004;15:55–9.

[19] Cleare AJ, Heap E, Malhi GS, Wessely S, O'Keane V, Miell J. Low-dose hydrocortisone in chronic fatigue syndrome: a randomised crossover trial. Lancet 1999;353:455–58.
[20] Cohen H, Neumann L, Shore M, Amir M, Cassuto Y, Buskila D. Autonomic dysfunction in patients with fibromyalgia: application of power spectral analysis of heart rate variability. Semin Arthritis Rheum 2000;29:217–27.
[21] Crofford LJ, Young EA, Engleberg NC, Korszun A, Brucksch CB, McClure LA, Brown MB, Demitrack MA. Basal circadian and pulsatile ACTH and cortisol secretion in patients with fibromyalgia and/or chronic fatigue syndrome. Brain Behav Immun 2004;18:314–25.
[22] Dalal A, Tata M, Allègre G, Gekiere F, Bons N, Albe-Fessard D. Spontaneous activity of rat dorsal horn cells in spinal segments of sciatic projection following transection of sciatic nerve or of corresponding dorsal roots. Neuroscience 1999;94:217–28.
[23] Devor M. Sodium channels and mechanisms of neuropathic pain. J Pain 2006;7:S3–S12.
[24] Diatchenko L. Slade GD, Nackley AG, Bhalang K, Sigurdsson A, Belfer A, Goldman D, Xu K, Shabalina SA, Shagin D, Max MB, Makarov SS, Maixner W. Genetic basis for individual variations in pain perception and the development of a chronic pain condition. Hum Mol Genet 2005;14:135–43.
[25] Dinerman H, Goldenberg DL, Felson DT. A prospective evaluation of 118 patients with the fibromyalgia syndrome: prevalence of Raynaud's syndrome, sicca symptoms, ANA, low complement, and Ig deposition at the dermal-epidermal junction. J Rheumatol 1986;13:368–73.
[26] Dhir A, Kulkarni SK. Venlafaxine reverses chronic fatigue-induced behavioral, biochemical and neurochemical alterations in mice. Pharmacol Biochem Behav 2008;89:563–71.
[27] Elenkov IJ, Wilder RL, Chrousos GP, Vizi ES. The sympathetic nerve: an integrative interface between two supersystems: the brain and the immune system. Pharmacol Rev 2000;52:595–638.
[28] Fang H, Xie Q, Boneva R, Fostel J, Perkins R, Tong W. Gene expression profile exploration of a large dataset on chronic fatigue syndrome. Pharmacogenomics 2006;7:429–40.
[29] Figueroa A, Kingsley JD, McMillan V, Panton LB. Resistance exercise training improves heart rate variability in women with fibromyalgia. Clin Physiol Funct Imaging 2008;28:49–54.
[30] Furlan R, Colombo S, Perego F, Atzeni F, Diana A, Barbic F, Porta A, Pace F, Malliani A, Sarzi-Puttini P. Abnormalities of cardiovascular neural control and reduced orthostatic tolerance in patients with primary fibromyalgia. J Rheumatol 2005;32:1787–93.
[31] Giske L, Vøllestad NK, Mengshoel AM, Jensen J, Knardahl S, Røe C. Attenuated adrenergic responses to exercise in women with fibromyalgia: a controlled study. Eur J Pain 2008;12:351–60.
[32] Gur A, Cevik R, Sarac AJ, Colpan L, Em S. Hypothalamic-pituitary-gonadal axis and cortisol in young women with primary fibromyalgia: the potential roles of depression, fatigue, and sleep disturbance in the occurrence of hypocortisolism. Ann Rheum Dis 2004;63:1504–6.
[33] Gursoy S, Erdal E, Herken H, Madenci E, Alasehirli B, Erdal N. Significance of catechol-O-methyltransferase gene polymorphism in fibromyalgia syndrome. Rheumatol Int 2003;23:104–7.
[34] Haller V, Bernstein M, Welch S. Chronic morphine treatment decreases the Ca_v 1.3 subunit of the L-type calcium channel. Eur J Pharmacol 2008;578:101–7.
[35] Hayes SG, Kindig AE, Kaufman MP. Blockade of acid sensing ion channels attenuates the exercise pressor reflex in cats. J Physiol 2007;581:1271–82.
[36] Hayes SG, McCord JL, Kaufman MP. Role played by P2X and P2Y receptors in evoking the muscle chemoreflex. J Appl Physiol 2008;104:538–41.
[37] Heim C, Wagner D, Maloney E, Papanicolaou DA, Solomon L, Jones JF, Unger ER, Reeves WC. Early adverse experience and risk for chronic fatigue syndrome: results from a population-based study. Arch Gen Psychiatry 2006;63:1258–66.
[38] Jensen T, Gottrup H, Sindrup S, Bach F. The clinical picture of neuropathic pain. Eur J Pharmacol 2001;429:1–11.
[39] Katz DL, Greene L, Ali A, Faridi Z. The pain of fibromyalgia syndrome is due to muscle hypoperfusion induced by regional vasomotor dysregulation. Med Hypoth 2007;69:517–25.
[40] Kim J, Greenspan J, Coghill R, Ohara S, Lenz F. Lesions limited to the human thalamic principal somatosensory nucleus (ventral caudal) are associated with loss of cold sensations and central pain. Neurobiol Dis 2007;27:4995–5005.
[41] Kindig AE, Hayes SG, Kaufman MP. Purinergic 2 receptor blockade prevents the responses of group IV afferents to post-contraction circulatory occlusion. J Physiol 2007;578:301–8.

[42] King C, Devine D, Vierck C, Mauderli A, Yezierski R. Opioid modulation of reflex versus operant responses following stress in the rat. Neuroscience 2007;147:174–82.

[43] Lasikiewicz N, Hendrickx H, Talbot D, Dye L. Exploration of basal diurnal salivary cortisol profiles in middle-aged adults: associations with sleep quality and metabolic parameters. Psychoneuroendocrinology 2008;33:143–51.

[44] Light AR, Hughen RW, Zhang J, Rainier J, Liu Z, Lee J. Dorsal root ganglion neurons innervating skeletal muscle respond to physiological combinations of protons, ATP and lactate mediated by ASIC, P2X and TRPV1. J Neurophysiol 2008;100:1184–201.

[45] Light KC, White A, Light AR. Post-exercise dysregulation of adrenergic and sensory receptors and altered cytokine profiles in patients with chronic fatigue/fibromyalgia. Presented at: Spring Brain Conference, Palm Springs, 13 March 2008.

[46] Maekawa K, Clark GT, Kuboki T. Intramuscular hypoperfusion, adrenergic receptors, and chronic muscle pain. J Pain 2002;3:251–60.

[47] Maekawa K, Twe C, Lotaif A, Chiappelli F, Clark GT. Function of beta-adrenergic receptors on mononuclear cells in female patients with fibromyalgia. J Rheumatol 2003;30:364–8.

[48] Martínez-Lavín M, Hermosillo AG, Rosas M, Soto ME. Circadian studies of autonomic nervous balance in patients with fibromyalgia: a heart rate variability analysis. Arthritis Rheum 1998;41:1966–71.

[49] Mayer D, Mao J, Holt J, Price D. Cellular mechanisms of neuropathic pain, morphine tolerance, and their interactions. Proc Natl Acad Sci USA 1999;96:7731–6.

[50] McBeth J, Chiu YH, Silman AJ, Ray D, Morriss R, Dickens C, Gupta A, Macfarlane GJ. Hypothalamic-pituitary-adrenal stress axis function and the relationship with chronic widespread pain and its antecedents. Arthritis Res Ther 2005;7:R992–R1000.

[51] McCleane G. The cholecystokinin antagonist proglumide enhances the analgesic effect of dihydrocodeine. Clin J Pain 2003;19:200–1.

[52] McKenzie R, O'Fallon A, Dale J, Demitrack M, Sharma G, Deloria M, Garcia-Borreguero D, Blackwelder W, Straus SE. Low-dose hydrocortisone for treatment of chronic fatigue syndrome: a randomized controlled trial. JAMA 1998;280:1061–6.

[53] McLean SA, Williams DA, Harris RE, Kop WJ, Groner KH, Ambrose K, Lyden AK, Gracely RH, Crofford LJ, Geisser ME, Sen A, Biswas P, Clauw DJ. Momentary relationship between cortisol secretion and symptoms in patients with fibromyalgia. Arthritis Rheum 2005;52:3660–9.

[54] Meewisse ML, Reitsma JB, de Vries GJ, Gersons BP, Olff M. Cortisol and post-traumatic stress disorder in adults: systematic review and meta-analysis. Br J Psychiatry 2007;191:387–92.

[55] Meller ST, Dennis BJ. Efferent projections of the periaqueductal gray in the rabbit. Neuroscience 1991;40:191–216.

[56] Melzack R, Wall PD. Pain mechanisms: a new theory. Science 1965;150:971–9.

[57] Millan M. Descending control of pain. Prog Neurobiol 2002;66:355–474.

[58] Molna P. Neurobiology of the stress response: contribution of the sympathetic nervous system to the neuroimmune axis in traumatic injury. Shock 2005;24:3–10.

[59] Nackley AG, Tan KS, Fecho K, Flood P, Diatchenko L, Maixner W. Catechol-O-methyltransferase inhibition increases pain sensitivity through activation of both β2- and β3-adrenergic receptors. Pain 2007;128:199–208.

[60] Naves IA, McCleskey EW. An acid-sensing ion channel that detects ischemic pain. Braz J Med Biol Res 2005;38:1561–9.

[61] Nilsen KB, Sand T, Westgaard RH, Stovner LJ, White LR, Bang Leistad R, Helde G, Rø M. Autonomic activation and pain in response to low-grade mental stress in fibromyalgia and shoulder/neck pain patients. Eur J Pain 2007;11:743–55.

[62] Pagni C. Central pain due to spinal cord and brain stem damage. In: Wall P, Melzack R, editors. Textbook of pain. New York: Churchill Livingstone; 1994. p. 481–96.

[63] Patarca R. Cytokines and chronic fatigue syndrome. Ann NY Acad Sci 2001;933:185–200.

[64] Patarca-Montero R, Antoni M, Fletcher MA, Klimas NG. Cytokine and other immunologic markers in chronic fatigue syndrome and their relation to neuropsychological factors. Appl Neuropsychol 2001;8:51–64.

[65] Perl E. Causalgia, pathological pain, and adrenergic receptors. Proc Natl Acad Sci USA 1999;96:7664–7.

[66] Perry F, Heller PH, Kamiya J, Levine JD. Altered autonomic function in patients with arthritic or with chronic orofacial pain. Pain 1989;39:77–84.

[67] Qiao ZG, Vaeroy H, Morkrid L. Electrodermal and microcirculatory activity in patients with fibromyalgia during baseline, acoustic stimulation and cold pressor tests. J Rheumatol 1991;18:1383–9.

[68] Raj SR, Brouillard D, Simpson CS, Hopman WM, Abdollah H. Dysautonomia among patients with fibromyalgia: a noninvasive assessment. J Rheumatol 2000;27:2660–5.

[69] Rakvag TT, Klepstad P, Baar C, Kvam TM, Dale O, Kaasa S, Krokan HE, Skorpen F. The Val-158Met polymorphism of the human catechol-O-methyltransferase (COMT) gene may influence morphine requirements in cancer pain patients. Pain 2005;116:73–8.

[70] Siddall P, Taylor D, McClelland J, Rutkowski S, Cousins M. Pain report and the relationship of pain to physical factors in the first 6 months following spinal cord injury. Pain 1999;81:187–97.

[71] Skowera A, Cleare A, Blair D, Bevis L, Wessely SC, Peakman M. High levels of type 2 cytokine-producing cells in chronic fatigue syndrome. Clin Exp Immunol 2004;135:294–302.

[72] Sluka KA, Radhakrishnan R, Benson CJ, Eshcol JO, Price MP, Babinski K, Audette KM, Yeomans DC, Wilson SP. ASIC3 in muscle mediates mechanical but not heat hyperalgesia associated with muscle inflammation. Pain 2007;129:102–12.

[73] Smith W, Bourne D, Squair J, Phillips D, Chamgers W. A retrospective cohort study of post mastectomy pain syndrome. Pain 1999;83:91–5.

[74] Snapir A, Koshkenvuo J, Toikka J, Orho-Melander M, Hinkka S, Saraster M, Hartiala J, Scheinin M. Effects of common polymorphisms in the alpha-1A-, alpha-2B-, beta-1- and beta-2-adreno-receptors on haemodynamic responses to adrenaline. Clin Sci 2003;104:509–20.

[75] Stein PK, Domitrovich PP, Ambrose K, Lyden A, Fine M, Gracely RH, Clauw DJ. Sex effects on heart rate variability in fibromyalgia and Gulf War illness. Arthritis Rheum 2004;51:700–8.

[76] Streeten DH. Role of impaired lower-limb venous innervation in the pathogenesis of the chronic fatigue syndrome. Am J Med Sci 2001;321:163–7.

[77] Tanriverdi F, Karaca Z, Unluhizarci K, Kelestimur F. The hypothalamo-pituitary-adrenal axis in chronic fatigue syndrome and fibromyalgia syndrome. Stress 2007;10:13–25.

[78] Ueda H. Peripheral mechanisms of neuropathic pain: involvement of lysophosphatidic acid receptor-mediated demyelination. Mol Pain 2008;4:11.

[79] Vaeroy H, Qiao ZG, Morkrid L, Forre O. Altered sympathetic nervous system response in patients with fibromyalgia. J Rheumatol 1989;16:1460–5.

[80] Vargas-Alarcón G, Fragoso JM, Cruz-Robles D, Vargas A, Vargas A, Lao-Villadóniga JI, García-Fructuoso F, Ramos-Kuri M, Hernández F, Springall R, et al. Catechol-O-methyltransferase gene haplotypes in Mexican and Spanish patients with fibromyalgia. Arthritis Res Ther 2007;9:R110.

[81] Vernon SD, Unger ER, Dimulescu IM, Rajeevan M, Reeves WC. Utility of the blood for gene expression profiling and biomarker discovery in chronic fatigue syndrome. Dis Markers 2002;18:193–9.

[82] Vierck CJ. Mechanisms underlying development of spatially distributed chronic pain (fibromyalgia). Pain 2006;124:242–63.

[83] Vierck CJ Jr, Greenspan JD, Ritz LA. Long term changes in purposive and reflexive responses to nociceptive stimulation in monkeys following anterolateral chordotomy. J Neuroscience 1990;10:2077–95.

[84] Vierck CJ, Hansson PT, Yezierski, RP. Clinical and pre-clinical pain assessment: are we measuring the same thing? Pain 2008;135:7–10.

[85] Vierck C Jr, Light A. Effects of combined hemotoxic and anterolateral spinal lesions on nociceptive sensitivity. Pain 1999;83:447–57.

[86] Vierck CJ Jr., Luck MM. Loss and recovery of reactivity to noxious stimuli in monkeys with primary spinothalamic chordotomies, followed by secondary and tertiary lesions of other cord sectors. Brain 1979;102:233–48.

[87] Vierck C, Yezierski R, Light A. Long-lasting hyperalgesia and sympathetic dysregulation after formalin injection into the rat hindpaw. Neuroscience 2008;153:501–6.

[88] Weissbecker I, Floyd A, Dedert E, Salmon P, Sephton S. Childhood trauma and diurnal cortisol disruption in fibromyalgia syndrome. Psychoneuroendocrinology 2006;31:312–24.

[89]   White PD, Sharpe MC, Chalder T, DeCesare JC, Walwyn R; PACE trial group. Protocol for the PACE trial: a randomised controlled trial of adaptive pacing, cognitive behaviour therapy, and graded exercise, as supplements to standardised specialist medical care versus standardised specialist medical care alone for patients with the chronic fatigue syndrome/myalgic encephalomyelitis or encephalopathy. BMC Neurol 2007;7:6.

[90]   Whitehead WE, Palsson O, Jones KR. Systematic review of the comorbidity of irritable bowel syndrome with other disorders: what are the causes and implications? Gastroenterology 2002;122:1140–56.

[91]   Whiteside G, Munglani R. Cell death in the superficial dorsal horn in a model of neuropathic pain. J Neurosci Res 2001;64:168–73.

[92]   Widerström-Noga E, Turk D. Types and effectiveness of treatments used by people with chronic pain associated with spinal cord injuries: influence of pain and psychosocial characteristics. Spinal Cord 2003;41:600–9.

[93]   Wolbeek M, van Doornen LJ, Kavelaars A, van de Putte EM, Schedlowski M, Heijnen CJ. Longitudinal analysis of pro- and anti-inflammatory cytokine production in severely fatigued adolescents. Brain Behav Immun 2007;21:1063–74.

[94]   Wolfe F, Cathey MA, Hawley DJ. A double-blind placebo controlled trial of fluoxetine in fibromyalgia. Scand J Rheumatol 1994;23:255–9.

[95]   Wood PB, Kablinger AS, Caldito GS. Open trial of pindolol in the treatment of fibromyalgia. Ann Pharmacother 2005;39:1812–6.

[96]   Woolf C. Dissecting out mechanisms responsible for peripheral neuropathic pain: implications for diagnosis and therapy. Life Sci 2004;74:2605–10.

[97]   Woolf C, Shortland P, Reynolds M, Ridings J, Doubell T, Coggeshall R. Reorganization of central terminals of myelinated primary afferents in the rat dorsal horn following peripheral axotomy. J Comp Neurol 1995;360:121–34.

[98]   Wyller VB, Saul JP, Walløe L, Thaulow E. Sympathetic cardiovascular control during orthostatic stress and isometric exercise in adolescent chronic fatigue syndrome. Eur J Appl Physiol 2008;102:623–32.

[99]   Yezierski R, Yu C-G, Mantyh P, Vierck C, Lappi D. Spinal neurons involved in the generation of at-level pain following spinal injury in the rat. Neurosci Lett 2004;361:232–6.

[100] Yokoyama T, Lisi TL, Moore SA, Sluka KA. Muscle fatigue increases the probability of developing hyperalgesia in mice. J Pain 2007;8:692–9.

[101] Yue X, Tumati S, Navratilova E, Strop D, St John P, Vanderah T, et al. Sustained morphine treatment augments basal CGRP release from cultured primary sensory neurons in a Raf-1 dependent manner. Eur J Pharmacol 2008;584:272–7.

[102] Zhang F-Y, Wan Y, Zhang Z-K, Light A, Fu K-Y. Peripheral formalin injection induces long-lasting increases in cyclooxygenase 1 expression by microglia in the spinal cord. J Pain 2007;8:110–7.

Correspondence to: Kathleen C. Light, PhD, Department of Anesthesiology, University of Utah, 3C444 SOM, 30 North 1900 East, Salt Lake City UT 84132-2304, USA. Tel: 1-801-581-6393; fax: 1-801-581-4367; email: kathleen.c.light@hsc.utah.edu.

15

Central Neuroglial Interactions in the Pathophysiology of Neuropathic Pain

Ji Zhang[a] and Yves De Koninck[a,b]

[a]The Alan Edwards Centre for Research on Pain, McGill University, Montreal, Quebec, Canada;
[b]Robert-Giffard Research Centre, Laval University, Quebec, Quebec, Canada

Pathogenesis of Neuropathic Pain

The pathogenesis of neuropathic pain is very complex, involving several structural, physiological, and pharmacological changes throughout the neuraxis (from peripheral nerves to the spinal cord and the brain). For decades, a neuron-centric view has predominated to explain the pathophysiology of chronic pain, but recent work has uncovered extensive neuroimmune interactions as substrates of neuropathic pain. Interactions between the immune and nervous systems occur at multiple levels, and different types of immune and glial cells and immune-derived substances are implicated at different stages of pathogenesis [55]. Injuries—not only to the central nervous system, but also to peripheral nerves—trigger an important central neuroinflammatory response that causes pain hypersensitivity. In this chapter, we will primarily focus on neuroimmune interactions at the spinal level in response to peripheral nerve injury, with the understanding that several of the interactions are likely to take place in supraspinal areas, particularly in central pain conditions.

Nerve Injury and Glial Activation

Within the central nervous system (CNS), microglia and astrocytes represent two highly reactive intraparenchymal cell populations. Microglia (resident macrophages in the CNS) are quiescent in normal conditions, fulfilling a constitutive surveillance function [17]. They become activated early in response to injury, infections, ischemia, brain tumors, or neurodegeneration. Activated microglia are characterized by a specific morphology, proliferation, increased expression of cell surface markers or receptors, and changes in functional activities, such as migration to areas of damage, phagocytosis, and the production and release of pro-inflammatory substances or cell-signaling mediators [16]. Astrocytes also respond to different types of insult, and this activation is characterized by morphological changes, increased production of intermediate filaments such as glial fibrillary acidic protein (GFAP), increased production of signaling molecules, and alterations in homeostatic activity [36].

Both microglial and astrocytic activations are multidimensional. There are many different activational states, with various components expressed with different time-courses and intensities that are dependent on the stimulus that triggers activation. Functional and morphological changes are not time-locked; one can be detected in the absence of the other [49].

Microglial Activation and Neuropathic Pain

Peripheral nerve injury can induce spinal microglial activation [10,15,76]. Under different conditions, activated microglia release known pronociceptive substances such as adenosine triphosphate (ATP), brain-derived neurotrophic factor (BDNF), pro-inflammatory cytokines, excitatory amino acids, nitric oxide, and prostaglandins [20,37]. These substances are likely to excite spinal nociceptive neurons, either directly or indirectly, and promote the release of other transmitters that can act on nociceptive neurons [37,74]. Consistent with these findings, several experimental approaches reversed spinal hypersensitivity in animal models of neuropathic pain, including (1) targeting microglial activation [40,48], (2) inhibiting cytokine synthesis or signaling [40,62–64], (3) blocking glial ATP-receptor signaling [38,69], and (4) blocking spinal BDNF signaling [12]. Thus, by releasing these factors, spinal cord microglia can be important players in pain hypersensitivity. Recent results have also revealed that nerve-injury-induced spinal microglial response can include not only activation of preexisting resident microglia, but also the proliferation of new microglia [13] and the recruitment of peripheral monocytes and macrophages [77]. Both resident and bone-marrow-derived microglia may be involved in the central component of sensitization to enhance neuronal excitability. The ability of blood-borne monocytes and macrophages to populate the CNS parenchyma has been observed in adult animals, especially in certain special pathological conditions [60]. Interestingly, either resident microglia or peripheral monocytes and macrophages (active at the site of peripheral injury and infiltrating into the spinal cord) appear sufficient to cause full development of tactile allodynia after nerve injury [77].

Astrocyte Activation and Neuropathic Pain

Compared to the ample evidence for microglial regulation of pain hypersensitivity, much less is known about the importance of astrocytes in chronic pain. A correlation between persistent activation of spinal astrocytes, often evidenced by increased expression of GFAP, and pain hypersensitivity has been observed in different animal models of chronic pain involving peripheral nerve injury [75], spinal cord injury [42], and bone cancer [35]. Compared with nerve-injury-induced microglial activation, astrocyte activation is characterized by a delayed, moderate, long-lasting GFAP upregulation for several months in models of persistent pain hypersensitivity [75]. Basic fibroblast growth factor, a primary "activator" of astrocytes, appears to be required for producing chronic pain [33].

Injured Neurons Talk to Their Surrounding Glial Cells to Trigger Glial Activation

Almost all reported animal models of nerve-injury-induced exaggerated pain appear to be associated with the activation of spinal microglia, and the site of microglial activation is restricted to the central projection of the injured afferents [5]. Thus, microglial activation is likely to be controlled by damaged or degenerating neurons. It is not the degeneration itself (e.g., the formation of cellular debris) that triggers microglial activation, because rhizotomy produces only a weak microglial reaction within the spinal cord gray matter [54]. Thus, activation of microglia must occur in response to a cell-to-cell signaling mechanism (Fig. 1). The factors that cause the spinal microglia to shift from a resting to an activated state remain an active subject of investigation. Many efforts have been devoted to identifying the molecules involved in neuron-to-microglia signaling in different injury conditions.

Extracellular ATP Mediates Interaction between Damaged Neurons and Their Surrounding Glial Cells

Adenosine triphosphate (ATP) is an important signaling molecule mediating interactions among various cell types in the CNS. Substantial release of ATP occurs after metabolic stress and injury [14], and high levels of ATP persist for hours after the insult [72]. Although astrocytes and endothelial cells are likely to release large amounts of ATP after an injury, the amount of ATP released by damaged or dead neurons appears to be significant [6,18]. Upon stimulation, ATP can be released from primary afferent terminals and axons of dorsal root ganglion (DRG) neurons [53,58],

Fig. 1. Summary of CNS neuroimmune interactions involved in the early phase of pathogenesis of neuropathic pain. Pain hypersensitivity is caused by a neuron-to-microglia-to-neuron signaling cascade that results in increased neuronal excitability in the spinal dorsal horn. See the text for a detailed description of the evidence implicating each of the signaling events depicted here. Briefly, following nerve injury, damaged sensory neurons upregulate the chemokine MCP-1. The latter is released within the spinal cord to cause microglial activation and chemotaxis of circulating monocytes via activation of the CCR2 receptor. Stimulated monocytes infiltrate the spinal cord parenchyma and differentiate into activated microglia. Activated microglia proliferate and release cathepsin S (CatS), which cleaves fractalkine tethered to the extracellular surface of neurons. Cleaved fractalkine acts on CX3CR1 receptors on microglia to amplify microglial activation. Activated microglia express de novo the P2X4 receptors, and when stimulated by endogenously released ATP, they release brain-derived neurotrophic factor (BDNF). In turn, BDNF acts on neuronal tyrosine kinase B (TrkB) receptors to down regulate the potassium chloride cotransporter KCC2 in dorsal horn neurons. The loss of KCC2 causes an accumulation of resting intracellular chloride concentration and a decrease in chloride extrusion capacity, which effectively impairs the efficacy of $GABA_A$- and glycine receptor-mediated transmission. This event leads to a loss of spinal inhibition (disinhibition) and thus increases the excitability of dorsal horn neurons, allowing crosstalk between non-nociceptive and nociceptive sensory channels. The result is the aberrant relay of innocuous input via normally nociceptive relay pathways to the brain.

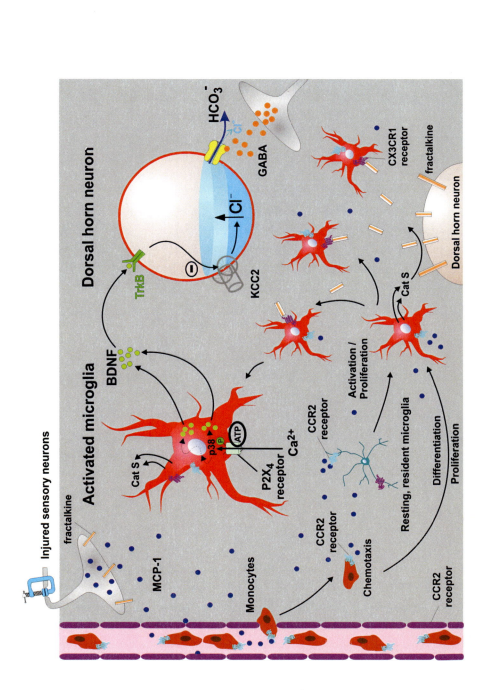

Injured sensory neurons

Activated microglia

Dorsal horn neuron

fractalkine

MCP-1

Monocytes

CCR2 receptor

Chemotaxis

CCR2 receptor

Cat S

p38

P

ATP

P2X₄ receptor

Ca²⁺

BDNF

TrkB

Cl⁻

KCC2

GABA

Cl⁻

HCO₃⁻

Resting, resident microglia

Differentiation
Proliferation

Activation/
Proliferation

Cat S

CX3CR1 receptor

fractalkine

Dorsal horn neuron

as well as from somatic cell bodies of DRG neurons [79]. Although precise data on the quantity and the time course of ATP release are still missing, it is reasonable to suggest that peripheral nerve injury can induce the release of ATP from primary afferent terminals in the spinal dorsal horn. ATP is thus likely to be involved in both sensory transmission and neuron-to-glia signaling [14]. There are two distinct classes of receptors for ATP: the P2X ionotropic ligand-gated ion channel receptors (P2X1–P2X7) and the P2Y metabotropic G-protein-coupled-receptors (P2Y1, 2, 4, 6, 11, 12, 13, and 14). Some of these receptors are expressed exclusively by glial cells. ATP, acting through purinergic receptors, can stimulate the release of various biologically active substances from microglia [26].

Following peripheral nerve injury, spinal microglia become activated, and P2X4 receptors are selectively induced in the activated microglia. In an animal model, P2X4 protein expression progressively increased in the days following nerve injury, in parallel with the development of tactile allodynia. Reducing the upregulation of P2X4 receptors in spinal microglia using an antisense oligodeoxynucleotide prevented the development of nerve-injury-induced mechanical allodynia [70]. These findings implied that P2X4 receptors in spinal microglia, activated by ATP, are necessary in the pain hypersensitivity associated with neuropathic pain.

Extracellular ATP has also been attributed a function as a chemoattractant. Microglial chemotaxis by ATP via P2Y12 receptors, originally detected by Honda et al. [23], has been confirmed in vivo in P2Y12 knockout mice [21]. A recent study demonstrated that P2Y12 mRNA and protein increased in the spinal cord following peripheral nerve injury; the P2Y12-expressing cells were exclusively microglia [31,68]. Both pharmacological blockades by intrathecal administration of P2Y12 antagonist and genetic modulation of P2Y12 expression (with antisense treatment) suppressed the development of pain behavior and the phosphorylation of p38 mitogen-activated protein kinase (MAPK) in spinal microglia in animals that had undergone nerve lesion. Therefore, activation of P2Y12 by released ATP stimulates the MAPK signaling pathway and plays a role in the pathogenesis of neuropathic pain.

However, blockade or knockdown of P2X4 receptors [70] nor of P2Y12 receptors [68] could not reverse the peripheral-nerve-injury-induced increase in immunoreactivity in OX-42 (a specific marker for microglia) in the spinal cord, indicating that other signaling mechanisms, upstream of ATP signaling, are necessary for microglial activation.

P2X7 is a ligand-gated cation channel, expressed predominantly by cells of immune origin. When activated, it can cause the release of biologically active inflammatory cytokines, including interleukin (IL)-1β. P2X7 receptors are expressed on DRG satellite cells [80]. A recent study revealed that electrical stimulation of DRG neurons elicits robust vesicular ATP release from their somata, which suggests that by activating P2X7 receptors on satellite cells, somatic ATP released from DRG neurons may underlie communication between neurons and satellite glial cells [79]. It has been demonstrated that P2X7 deletion or antagonism significantly inhibits neuropathic pain behaviors [8,38]. However, no data are available on the presence of P2X7 receptors in CNS glia; thus, the involvement of these receptors in the pathogenesis of neuropathic pain may occur primarily in the periphery.

Microglia–Neuron–Microglia Communication via Cathepsin S–Fractalkine–CX3CR1 Signaling

Fractalkine, also named CX3CL1, has been suggested to act as a neuron-to-glia signal. Fractalkine is the only chemokine that is expressed constitutively on neurons [3]. In the spinal cord dorsal horn, fractalkine is expressed on neurons and sensory terminals, whereas its receptor, CX3CR1, is expressed primarily on microglia [71]. In addition, fractalkine is unique among the typically promiscuous chemokines in that it binds only one known receptor, CX3CR1, and this receptor binds only fractalkine [27].

Fractalkine is also unique in that it is tethered to the extracellular surface of neurons and can be cleaved to form a diffusible signal [7]. Lysosomal cysteine protease cathepsin S (CatS), when expressed on activated spinal microglia, is responsible for the cleavage of neuronal transmembrane fractalkine into active soluble fractalkine [9]. After nerve injury, CatS-expressing activated microglia in the spinal cord dorsal horn innervated by damaged fibers release CatS, which then liberates soluble fractalkine from afferent terminals and surrounding spinal neurons. The released fractalkine feeds back onto microglia cells via the CX3CR1 receptors to activate the p38 MAPK pathway, and then it modulates the synthesis and release of other pronociceptive mediators.

Both exogenous or endogenous fractalkine and CatS have pronociceptive effects [4,41]. Inhibition of CatS enzymatic activity and neutralization of the CX3CR1 receptor successfully reversed the hypersensitivity in an animal model of neuropathic pain with nerve injury [9,41]. CatS-induced-hyperalgesia is lost in CX3CR1 null mice [9]. Thus, while neurons are the source of fractalkine signaling to CX3CR1 on microglia, the initiating signal appears to be microglial CatS. Activated microglia may be signaling to other microglia via the cleavage of fractalkine on neurons. The concurrent increase in CatS expression by microglia and fractalkine by neurons could serve as a mechanism of amplification and coincidence detection. Because it is activated microglia that appear to release CatS, expression of CatS is unlikely to be the initiating mechanism causing the activation of microglia. Another signaling mechanism must trigger microglial activation, followed by an amplification of microglial activation via the CatS-fractalkine-CX3CR1 signaling cascade.

Neuron–Microglia/Monocyte Communication via MCP-1–CCR2 Signaling

Monocyte chemoattractant protein-1 (MCP-1), a CC family chemokine (also called CCL2), which specifically attracts monocytes to sites of inflammation [32], has been attributed a key role in cell-to-cell communication. Absent in the normal CNS, MCP-1 was found to be induced in DRG sensory neurons by chronic constriction of the sciatic nerve [65,75]. The MCP-1 induced in DRG neurons is transported to the spinal dorsal horn [75] and is released in the dorsal horn in response to electrical stimulation of sensory nerves [66]. CCR2, the receptor for MCP-1, is expressed selectively on cells of monocyte/macrophage lineage in the periphery [51] and can be induced in spinal microglia by peripheral nerve injury [1]. Both temporally and spatially, MCP-1 induction in terminals of damaged sensory neurons is closely correlated with the subsequent surrounding spinal microglial activation [75]. Notably, this nerve-injury-induced spinal microglial activation was completely abolished in mice lacking CCR2 [77]. We recently demonstrated that local spinal injection of exogenous MCP-1 could induce microglial activation and that this activation is lost in CCR2 knockout mice [77]. Together, these results implicate MCP-1 as a trigger for microglial activation and point to a critical role of MCP-1/CCR2 signaling in neuron-to-microglia crosstalk.

Following peripheral nerve injury, in addition to activation of microglia resident to the spinal cord, blood-borne monocytes and macrophages have the ability to infiltrate the spinal cord, where they proliferate and differentiate into activated microglia [77]. MCP-1/CCR2 signaling is also involved in the crosstalk between neurons and monocytes/macrophages from the CNS to the periphery, given that neutralization of MCP-1 at the spinal level prevented monocyte/macrophage infiltration after nerve injury [77]. Thus, both resident microglial activation and monocyte/macrophage infiltration appear to be due to a signaling mechanism within the spinal cord. Other evidence implicates MCP-1/CCR2 in the recruitment of monocytes/macrophages and activated lymphocytes into the CNS in a variety of inflammatory, infective, and trauma-related conditions [25,29,50]. CCR2-positive monocytes were identified as direct circulating precursors of microglia responsible for CNS infiltration [39]. A potential role of MCP-1 in the chemotaxis from the periphery to the CNS involves altering the expression of tight junction-associated proteins in the brain and spinal cord microvascular endothelial cells, thereby increasing the permeability of the barrier between the blood and the brain or spinal cord [59,61].

Not only is MCP-1 a necessary mediator for spinal microglial activation, but its action is necessary for the development of mechanical allodynia. It has been demonstrated that mice lacking CCR2 have impairment of the nociceptive response typically associated with neuropathy [1,77]. We recently were able to selectively delete CNS versus peripheral CCR2 to determine the respective role of central and peripheral CCR2 signaling. Interestingly, although total CCR2 knockout mice did not develop mechanical allodynia, CCR2 expression either in resident microglia or in the periphery was sufficient for the development of full mechanical allodynia [77]. Thus, to effectively relieve nerve-injury-induced mechanical allodynia, it appears that both CNS resident microglia and blood-borne macrophages need to be targeted.

Activated Glial Cells Signal to Neurons to Alter Their Excitability

After being activated by neurons, glial cells signal back to neurons to alter their excitability. This glia-to-neuron signaling appears to contribute to both the establishment and maintenance of the enhanced excitability, within the peripheral and central nociceptive pathways, that underlies neuropathic pain.

Microglia Affect Neuronal Excitability by Altering Neuronal Chloride Homeostasis

We recently identified a novel mechanism by which spinal activated microglia signal to neurons to increase their excitability. This mechanism involves the release of BDNF from activated microglia in response to ATP stimulation [12]. Stimulation of P2X4 receptors by ATP appears to be necessary for BDNF release from microglia [12,70]. BDNF acting on its receptor, the tyrosine kinase B (TrkB) receptor, in adult neurons is known to downregulate the potassium chloride co-transporter KCC2 [52]. KCC2 is responsible for extrusion of chloride from the cells and thus helps maintain a low intracellular chloride concentration in normal conditions. The result of this BDNF-TrkB signaling is thus a decrease in chloride extrusion capacity of the cells, which effectively decreases the inhibitory power of γ-aminobutyric acid A ($GABA_A$) and glycine receptors. This disinhibition results from two phenomena: first, from a collapse in the transmembrane chloride gradient, resulting in a loss of hyperpolarizing $GABA_A$- and glycine-receptor-mediated currents [47]; and second, from the fact that neurons are no longer able to maintain hyperpolarizing anion currents upon repeated $GABA_A$- and glycine-mediated synaptic input [11]. In a subset of spinal neurons, after peripheral nerve injury, $GABA_A$/glycine currents are reversed to the extent that they can even cause excitation [12,47]. The net result is the routing of innocuous tactile sensory input to nociceptive-specific spinal lamina I output neurons and thus the relay of innocuous signals via a normally nociceptive ascending pathway to the brain [30]. Blockade of P2X4 receptors and of BDNF-TrkB signaling reverses tactile allodynia in animals with nerve injury and reverses the depolarizing shift in chloride gradient [12], indicating continuous P2X receptor activation and BDNF-TrkB signaling during the maintenance phase of hypersensitivity.

After peripheral inflammation, BDNF released from primary afferents appears to be responsible for spinal hypersensitivity [22,34,67,81]. This source of BDNF also causes downregulation of KCC2 [78]. In neuropathic pain conditions, however, the source of spinal BDNF appears to be principally glia, because selective deletion of BDNF from nociceptive afferents prevents the development of pain hypersensitivity caused by peripheral inflammatory agents but not that caused by nerve injury [81].

Other Glia-to-Neuron Signaling Mechanisms

A variety of other mediators are released by glia in pathophysiological conditions [37,55]. Several of these putative mediators can produce pain and hyperalgesia when given intrathecally. The best evidence exists for IL-1β, tumor necrosis factor-α (TNF-α), prostaglandin E_2 (PGE$_2$), and ATP. IL-1β and TNF-α are both capable of producing neuropathic symptoms in adult rats when delivered centrally [45,46]. Receptors for IL-1β and TNF-α are expressed on both spinal neurons and primary sensory neurons. They may be increased in some persistent pain states [44]. Activation of these receptors can lead to rapid changes in neuronal excitability [43] or long-term changes in gene expression that modulate the responsiveness of the neurons [73]. These inflammatory cytokines may also act indirectly, via the release of other mediators, such as PGE$_2$ or nitric oxide. Because these agents act directly on nociceptors and are known to play a role in peripheral sensitization [55], it is difficult to evaluate their relative contribution to central versus peripheral effects. Interestingly, in addition to its effect on sensory fibers, PGE$_2$ has been shown to cause disinhibition of spinal dorsal horn neurons via a selective action on the α_3 subunit of the glycine receptor [2,19]. However, although this mechanism appears to be an important component of central sensitization in response to peripheral inflammation, it does not appear to play a role in neuropathic pain [24].

Roles of Different Cellular Elements in the Induction and Maintenance of Chronic Pain

Nerve injury activates not only spinal microglia, but also spinal astrocytes. The activation of these cells is linked to their contribution to neuropathic pain. The scanning of the microenvironment by microglia to sense any disturbance may involve assistance from astrocytes [21]. Although the signals that trigger and sustain astrocyte activation are unknown, it is intriguing to speculate that the astrocyte response occurs secondary to microglial activation, probably through proinflammatory substances released by the activated microglia [55]. Astrocytes can also induce antioxidant gene expression in microglia [57].

Accumulating evidence shows that persistent changes in spinal astrocytes in different chronic pain conditions often outlast microglial changes [75,82]. Consistent with these findings, the activation of extracellular signal-regulated kinase (ERK) in the spinal cord started in activated microglia (2 days post-injury) and then shifted to reactive astrocytes (3 weeks post-injury) [83]. A recent study demonstrated that after nerve injury, matrix metalloproteinase (MMP)-9 was induced in DRG sensory neurons within hours and returned to baseline 3 days after injury, whereas MMP-2 was induced in DRG satellite cells and in spinal astrocytes at later times (from several days to weeks after injury). Although cellular distribution and temporal profile are different, both MMPs require a common molecular player, the cytokine IL-1β. MMP-9 induces neuropathic pain through IL-1β cleavage and microglial activation at early time points, whereas MMP-2 maintains neuropathic pain through IL-1β cleavage and astrocyte activation at later times [28]. Future research must determine the relative involvement of microglia versus that of astrocytes in the signaling at later time points in the pathogenesis of neuropathic pain (several months in rodents or years in humans).

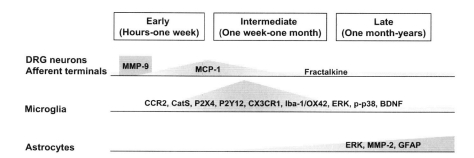

Fig. 2. Different cellular signaling elements are involved at different stages (induction and maintenance) of neuropathic pain. Shortly after nerve injury (within hours to a week), distressed sensory neurons and their central terminals release mediators such as matrix metalloproteinase-9 (MMP-9) and monocyte chemoattractant protein-1 (MCP-1) that trigger surrounding microglial activation. Within a week to a month, activated microglia, in turn, secrete other mediators such as brain-derived neurotrophic factor (BDNF) and adenosine triphosphate (ATP), produce and/or secrete enzymes such as cathepsin S (CatS), phosphorylated mitogen-activated protein kinase p38 (p-p38), and extracellular signal-regulated kinase (ERK), and upregulate chemokine and ion channel receptors (e.g., CCR2, P2X4, P2Y12, and CX3CR1) that amplify the immune response and modulate neuronal excitability. Molecules such as ERK, MMP-2, and glial fibrillary acidic protein (GFAP) are induced on activated astrocytes at a later stage, but they are sustained for a prolonged time and may thus be important for the maintenance phase. However, the relative involvement of microglia versus that of astrocytes in signaling at late time points of neuropathic pain remains to be determined.

Activation of different glial cells occurs along a complex temporal pattern; the contribution of each cell population to the modulation of nociceptive processing in pathological conditions follows a well-organized sequence of reciprocal communication between neurons and glia and among glial cells themselves (Fig. 2). Detailed understanding of each of the steps involved remains incomplete. More importantly, microglial activation can be caused by a wide variety of factors, each resulting in different response phenotype. The cascades of events leading to microglial activation in response to peripheral nerve injury are very distinct from the activation processes that follow spinal cord injury, multiple sclerosis, or brain ischemia, for example [56], and they are thus likely to underlie different pathophysiologies. How the mechanisms associated with nerve injury highlighted in this chapter relate to other pathologies remains to be determined. A more extensive dissection of the complex signaling mechanisms involved in neuroglial interactions in different conditions of injury to the nervous system will therefore be important for the development of disease-specific therapeutic treatments.

Conclusion

Neuropathic pain management is currently aimed only at reducing symptoms, generally by suppressing neuronal activity. The role of glial cells as pain mediators and modulators, as highlighted here, challenges conventional approaches in drug discovery. Targeting glial cells and modulating the central immune response to nerve injury will provide novel opportunities not only to relieve the symptoms of chronic pain, but possibly to reverse the pathology.

Acknowledgments

The authors acknowledge financial support from the Canadian Institute of Health Research (CIHR). J. Zhang is a CIHR New Investigator, and Y. De Koninck is a *Chercheur National* of the Fonds de la recherche en santé du Québec. We thank Mr. Sylvain Côté for expert assistance in the design of Fig. 1.

References

[1]   Abbadie C, Lindia JA, Cumiskey AM, Peterson LB, Mudgett JS, Bayne EK, DeMartino JA, MacIntyre DE, Forrest MJ. Impaired neuropathic pain responses in mice lacking the chemokine receptor CCR2. Proc Natl Acad Sci USA 2003;100:7947–52.
[2]   Ahmadi S, Lippross S, Neuhuber WL, Zeilhofer HU. PGE$_2$ selectively blocks inhibitory glycinergic neurotransmission onto rat superficial dorsal horn neurons. Nat Neurosci 2002;5:34–40.
[3]   Asensio VC, Campbell IL. Chemokines in the CNS: plurifunctional mediators in diverse states. Trends Neurosci 1999;22:504–12.
[4]   Barclay J, Clark AK, Ganju P, Gentry C, Patel S, Wotherspoon G, Buxton F, Song C, Ullah J, Winter J, Fox A, Bevan S, Malcangio M. Role of the cysteine protease cathepsin S in neuropathic hyperalgesia. Pain 2007;130:225–34.
[5]   Beggs S, Salter MW. Stereological and somatotopic analysis of the spinal microglial response to peripheral nerve injury. Brain Behav Immun 2007;21:624–33.
[6]   Burnstock G. Physiology and pathophysiology of purinergic neurotransmission. Physiol Rev 2007;87:659–797.
[7]   Chapman GA, Moores K, Harrison D, Campbell CA, Stewart BR, Strijbos PJ. Fractalkine cleavage from neuronal membranes represents an acute event in the inflammatory response to excitotoxic brain damage. J Neurosci 2000;20:RC87.

[8] Chessell IP, Hatcher JP, Bountra C, Michel AD, Hughes JP, Green P, Egerton J, Murfin M, Richardson J, Peck WL, et al. Disruption of the P2X7 purinoceptor gene abolishes chronic inflammatory and neuropathic pain. Pain 2005;114:386–96.

[9] Clark AK, Yip PK, Grist J, Gentry C, Staniland AA, Marchand F, Dehvari M, Wotherspoon G, Winter J, Ullah J, Bevan S, Malcangio M. Inhibition of spinal microglial cathepsin S for the reversal of neuropathic pain. Proc Natl Acad Sci USA 2007;104:10655–60.

[10] Colburn RW, Rickman AJ, DeLeo JA. The effect of site and type of nerve injury on spinal glial activation and neuropathic pain behavior. Exp Neurol 1999;157:289–304.

[11] Cordero-Erausquin M, Coull JA, Boudreau D, Rolland M, De Koninck Y. Differential maturation of GABA action and anion reversal potential in spinal lamina I neurons: impact of chloride extrusion capacity. J Neurosci 2005;25:9613–23.

[12] Coull JA, Beggs S, Boudreau D, Boivin D, Tsuda M, Inoue K, Gravel C, Salter MW, De Koninck Y. BDNF from microglia causes the shift in neuronal anion gradient underlying neuropathic pain. Nature 2005;438:1017–21.

[13] Echeverry S, Shi XQ, Zhang J. Characterization of cell proliferation in rat spinal cord following peripheral nerve injury and the relationship with neuropathic pain. Pain 2008;135:37–47.

[14] Fields RD, Stevens-Graham B. New insights into neuron-glia communication. Science 2002;298:556–62.

[15] Fu KY, Light AR, Matsushima GK, Maixner W. Microglial reactions after subcutaneous formalin injection into the rat hind paw. Brain Res 1999;825:59–67.

[16] Gehrmann J, Matsumoto Y, Kreutzberg GW. Microglia: intrinsic immuneffector cell of the brain. Brain Res Brain Res Rev 1995;20:269–87.

[17] Hanisch UK, Kettenmann H. Microglia: active sensor and versatile effector cells in the normal and pathologic brain. Nat Neurosci 2007;10:1387–94.

[18] Hansson E, Ronnback L. Glial neuronal signaling in the central nervous system. FASEB J 2003;17:341–8.

[19] Harvey RJ, Depner UB, Wassle H, Ahmadi S, Heindl C, Reinold H, Smart TG, Harvey K, Schutz B, Abo-Salem OM, et al. GlyR alpha3: an essential target for spinal PGE_2-mediated inflammatory pain sensitization. Science 2004;304:884–7.

[20] Hashizume H, DeLeo JA, Colburn RW, Weinstein JN. Spinal glial activation and cytokine expression after lumbar root injury in the rat. Spine 2000;25:1206–17.

[21] Haynes SE, Hollopeter G, Yang G, Kurpius D, Dailey ME, Gan WB, Julius D. The P2Y12 receptor regulates microglial activation by extracellular nucleotides. Nat Neurosci 2006;9:1512–9.

[22] Heppenstall PA, Lewin GR. BDNF but not NT-4 is required for normal flexion reflex plasticity and function. Proc Natl Acad Sci USA 2001;98:8107–12.

[23] Honda S, Sasaki Y, Ohsawa K, Imai Y, Nakamura Y, Inoue K, Kohsaka S. Extracellular ATP or ADP induce chemotaxis of cultured microglia through Gi/o-coupled P2Y receptors. J Neurosci 2001;21:1975–82.

[24] Hosl K, Reinold H, Harvey RJ, Muller U, Narumiya S, Zeilhofer HU. Spinal prostaglandin E receptors of the EP2 subtype and the glycine receptor alpha3 subunit, which mediate central inflammatory hyperalgesia, do not contribute to pain after peripheral nerve injury or formalin injection. Pain 2006;126:46–53.

[25] Huang DR, Wang J, Kivisakk P, Rollins BJ, Ransohoff RM. Absence of monocyte chemoattractant protein 1 in mice leads to decreased local macrophage recruitment and antigen-specific T helper cell type 1 immune response in experimental autoimmune encephalomyelitis. J Exp Med 2001;193:713–26.

[26] Inoue K, Koizumi S, Tsuda M. The role of nucleotides in the neuron-glia communication responsible for the brain functions. J Neurochem 2007;102:1447–58.

[27] Jung S, Aliberti J, Graemmel P, Sunshine MJ, Kreutzberg GW, Sher A, Littman DR. Analysis of fractalkine receptor CX_3CR1 function by targeted deletion and green fluorescent protein reporter gene insertion. Mol Cell Biol 2000;20:4106–14.

[28] Kawasaki Y, Xu ZZ, Wang X, Park JY, Zhuang ZY, Tan PH, Gao YJ, Roy K, Corfas G, Lo EH, Ji RR. Distinct roles of matrix metalloproteases in the early- and late-phase development of neuropathic pain. Nat Med 2008;14:331–6.

[29] Kelder W, McArthur JC, Nance-Sproson T, McClernon D, Griffin DE. Beta-chemokines MCP-1 and RANTES are selectively increased in cerebrospinal fluid of patients with human immunodeficiency virus-associated dementia. Ann Neurol 1998;44:831–5.

334   J. Zhang and Y. De Koninck

[30] Keller AF, Beggs S, Salter MW, De Koninck Y. Transformation of the output of spinal lamina I neu-
      rons after nerve injury and microglia stimulation underlying neuropathic pain. Mol Pain 2007;3:27.
[31] Kobayashi K, Yamanaka H, Fukuoka T, Dai Y, Obata K, Noguchi K. P2Y12 receptor upregu-
      lation in activated microglia is a gateway of p38 signaling and neuropathic pain. J Neurosci
      2008;28:2892–902.
[32] Leonard EJ, Skeel A, Yoshimura T. Biological aspects of monocyte chemoattractant protein-1
      (MCP-1). Adv Exp Med Biol 1991;305:57–64.
[33] Madiai F, Goettl VM, Hussain SR, Clairmont AR, Stephens RL Jr, Hackshaw KV. Anti-fibroblast
      growth factor-2 antibodies attenuate mechanical allodynia in a rat model of neuropathic pain. J
      Mol Neurosci 2005;27:315–24.
[34] Mannion RJ, Costigan M, Decosterd I, Amaya F, Ma QP, Holstege JC, Ji RR, Acheson A, Lind-
      say RM, Wilkinson GA, Woolf CJ. Neurotrophins: peripherally and centrally acting modula-
      tors of tactile stimulus-induced inflammatory pain hypersensitivity. Proc Natl Acad Sci USA
      1999;96:9385–90.
[35] Mantyh PW, Clohisy DR, Koltzenburg M, Hunt SP. Molecular mechanisms of cancer pain. Nat
      Rev Cancer 2002;2:201–9.
[36] Maragakis NJ, Rothstein JD. Mechanisms of disease: astrocytes in neurodegenerative disease.
      Nat Clin Pract Neurol 2006;2:679–89.
[37] Marchand F, Perretti M, McMahon SB. Role of the immune system in chronic pain. Nat Rev
      Neurosci 2005;6:521-32.
[38] McGaraughty S, Chu KL, Namovic MT, Donnelly-Roberts DL, Harris RR, Zhang XF, Shieh CC,
      Wismer CT, Zhu CZ, Gauvin DM, et al. P2X7-related modulation of pathological nociception in
      rats. Neuroscience 2007;146:1817–28.
[39] Mildner A, Schmidt H, Nitsche M, Merkler D, Hanisch UK, Mack M, Heikenwalder M, Bruck
      W, Priller J, Prinz M. Microglia in the adult brain arise from Ly-6ChiCCR2+ monocytes only
      under defined host conditions. Nat Neurosci 2007;10:1544–53.
[40] Milligan ED, Twining C, Chacur M, Biedenkapp J, O'Connor K, Poole S, Tracey K, Martin D,
      Maier SF, Watkins LR. Spinal glia and proinflammatory cytokines mediate mirror-image neuro-
      pathic pain in rats. J Neurosci 2003;23:1026–40.
[41] Milligan ED, Zapata V, Chacur M, Schoeniger D, Biedenkapp J, O'Connor KA, Verge GM, Chap-
      man G, Green P, Foster AC, et al. Evidence that exogenous and endogenous fractalkine can
      induce spinal nociceptive facilitation in rats. Eur J Neurosci 2004;20:2294–302.
[42] Nesic O, Lee J, Johnson KM, Ye Z, Xu GY, Unabia GC, Wood TG, McAdoo DJ, Westlund KN,
      Hulsebosch CE, Regino Perez-Polo J. Transcriptional profiling of spinal cord injury-induced cen-
      tral neuropathic pain. J Neurochem 2005;95:998–1014.
[43] Obreja O, Rathee PK, Lips KS, Distler C, Kress M. IL-1 beta potentiates heat-activated currents
      in rat sensory neurons: involvement of IL-1RI, tyrosine kinase, and protein kinase C. FASEB J
      2002;16:1497–1503.
[44] Ohtori S, Takahashi K, Moriya H, Myers RR. TNF-alpha and TNF-alpha receptor type 1 upregu-
      lation in glia and neurons after peripheral nerve injury: studies in murine DRG and spinal cord.
      Spine 2004;29:1082–8.
[45] Oka T, Oka K, Hosoi M, Aou S, Hori T. The opposing effects of interleukin-1 beta microinjected
      into the preoptic hypothalamus and the ventromedial hypothalamus on nociceptive behavior in
      rats. Brain Res 1995;700:271–8.
[46] Oka T, Wakugawa Y, Hosoi M, Oka K, Hori T. Intracerebroventricular injection of tumor
      necrosis factor-alpha induces thermal hyperalgesia in rats. Neuroimmunomodulation
      1996;3:135–40.
[47] Prescott SA, Sejnowski TJ, De Koninck Y. Reduction of anion reversal potential subverts the
      inhibitory control of firing rate in spinal lamina I neurons: towards a biophysical basis for neuro-
      pathic pain. Mol Pain 2006;2:32.
[48] Raghavendra V, Tanga F, DeLeo JA. Inhibition of microglial activation attenuates the devel-
      opment but not existing hypersensitivity in a rat model of neuropathy. J Pharmacol Exp Ther
      2003;306:624–30.
[49] Raivich G, Bohatschek M, Kloss CU, Werner A, Jones LL, Kreutzberg GW. Neuroglial activation
      repertoire in the injured brain: graded response, molecular mechanisms and cues to physiologi-
      cal function. Brain Res Brain Res Rev 1999;30:77–105.

[50] Rancan M, Otto VI, Hans VH, Gerlach I, Jork R, Trentz O, Kossmann T, Morganti-Kossmann MC. Upregulation of ICAM-1 and MCP-1 but not of MIP-2 and sensorimotor deficit in response to traumatic axonal injury in rats. J Neurosci Res 2001;63:438–46.
[51] Rebenko-Moll NM, Liu L, Cardona A, Ransohoff RM. Chemokines, mononuclear cells and the nervous system: heaven (or hell) is in the details. Curr Opin Immunol 2006;18:683–9.
[52] Rivera C, Li H, Thomas-Crusells J, Lahtinen H, Viitanen T, Nanobashvili A, Kokaia Z, Airaksinen MS, Voipio J, Kaila K, Saarma M. BDNF-induced TrkB activation down-regulates the K^+-Cl^- cotransporter KCC2 and impairs neuronal Cl- extrusion. J Cell Biol 2002;159:747–52.
[53] Salter MW, De Koninck Y, Henry JL. Physiological roles for adenosine and ATP in synaptic transmission in the spinal dorsal horn. Prog Neurobiol 1993;41:125–56.
[54] Scholz J, Abele A, Marian C, Haussler A, Herbert TA, Woolf CJ, Tegeder I. Low-dose methotrexate reduces peripheral nerve injury-evoked spinal microglial activation and neuropathic pain behavior in rats. Pain 2008;138:130–42.
[55] Scholz J, Woolf CJ. The neuropathic pain triad: neurons, immune cells and glia. Nat Neurosci 2007;10:1361–8.
[56] Schwartz M, Butovsky O, Bruck W, Hanisch UK. Microglial phenotype: is the commitment reversible? Trends Neurosci 2006;29:68–74.
[57] Shih AY, Fernandes HB, Choi FY, Kozoriz MG, Liu Y, Li P, Cowan CM, Klegeris A. Policing the police: astrocytes modulate microglial activation. J Neurosci 2006;26:3887–8.
[58] Soeda H, Tatsumi H, Katayama Y. Neurotransmitter release from growth cones of rat dorsal root ganglion neurons in culture. Neuroscience 1997;77:1187–99.
[59] Song L, Pachter JS. Monocyte chemoattractant protein-1 alters expression of tight junction-associated proteins in brain microvascular endothelial cells. Microvasc Res 2004;67:78–89.
[60] Soulet D, Rivest S. Bone-marrow-derived microglia: myth or reality? Curr Opin Pharmacol 2008; Epub May 16.
[61] Stamatovic SM, Keep RF, Kunkel SL, Andjelkovic AV. Potential role of MCP-1 in endothelial cell tight junction 'opening': signaling via Rho and Rho kinase. J Cell Sci 2003;116:4615–28.
[62] Sweitzer S, Martin D, DeLeo JA. Intrathecal interleukin-1 receptor antagonist in combination with soluble tumor necrosis factor receptor exhibits an anti-allodynic action in a rat model of neuropathic pain. Neuroscience 2001;103:529–39.
[63] Sweitzer SM, Medicherla S, Almirez R, Dugar S, Chakravarty S, Shumilla JA, Yeomans DC, Protter AA. Antinociceptive action of a p38alpha MAPK inhibitor, SD-282, in a diabetic neuropathy model. Pain 2004;109:409–19.
[64] Sweitzer SM, Schubert P, DeLeo JA. Propentofylline, a glial modulating agent, exhibits antiallodynic properties in a rat model of neuropathic pain. J Pharmacol Exp Ther 2001;297:1210–7.
[65] Tanaka T, Minami M, Nakagawa T, Satoh M. Enhanced production of monocyte chemoattractant protein-1 in the dorsal root ganglia in a rat model of neuropathic pain: possible involvement in the development of neuropathic pain. Neurosci Res 2004;48:463–9.
[66] Thacker MA, Clark AK, Bishop T, Grist J, Yip PK, Moon LD, Thompson SW, Marchand F, McMahon SB. CCL2 is a key mediator of microglia activation in neuropathic pain states. Eur J Pain 2008; Epub Jun 11.
[67] Thompson SW, Bennett DL, Kerr BJ, Bradbury EJ, McMahon SB. Brain-derived neurotrophic factor is an endogenous modulator of nociceptive responses in the spinal cord. Proc Natl Acad Sci USA 1999;96:7714–8.
[68] Tozaki-Saitoh H, Tsuda M, Miyata H, Ueda K, Kohsaka S, Inoue K. P2Y12 receptors in spinal microglia are required for neuropathic pain after peripheral nerve injury. J Neurosci 2008;28:4949–56.
[69] Tsuda M, Inoue K, Salter MW. Neuropathic pain and spinal microglia: a big problem from molecules in "small" glia. Trends Neurosci 2005;28:101–7.
[70] Tsuda M, Shigemoto-Mogami Y, Koizumi S, Mizokoshi A, Kohsaka S, Salter MW, Inoue K. P2X4 receptors induced in spinal microglia gate tactile allodynia after nerve injury. Nature 2003;424:778–83.
[71] Verge GM, Milligan ED, Maier SF, Watkins LR, Naeve GS, Foster AC. Fractalkine (CX3CL1) and fractalkine receptor (CX3CR1) distribution in spinal cord and dorsal root ganglia under basal and neuropathic pain conditions. Eur J Neurosci 2004;20:1150–60.
[72] Wang X, Arcuino G, Takano T, Lin J, Peng WG, Wan P, Li P, Xu Q, Liu QS, Goldman SA, Nedergaard M. P2X7 receptor inhibition improves recovery after spinal cord injury. Nat Med 2004;10:821–7.

[73] Watkins LR, Maier SF. Glia: a novel drug discovery target for clinical pain. Nat Rev Drug Discov 2003;2:973–85.
[74] Watkins LR, Milligan ED, Maier SF. Glial proinflammatory cytokines mediate exaggerated pain states: implications for clinical pain. Adv Exp Med Biol 2003;521:1–21.
[75] Zhang J, De Koninck Y. Spatial and temporal relationship between monocyte chemoattractant protein-1 expression and spinal glial activation following peripheral nerve injury. J Neurochem 2006;97:772–83.
[76] Zhang J, Hoffert C, Vu HK, Groblewski T, Ahmad S, O'Donnell D. Induction of CB2 receptor expression in the rat spinal cord of neuropathic but not inflammatory chronic pain models. Eur J Neurosci 2003;17:2750–4.
[77] Zhang J, Shi XQ, Echeverry S, Mogil JS, De Koninck Y, Rivest S. Expression of CCR2 in both resident and bone marrow-derived microglia plays a critical role in neuropathic pain. J Neurosci 2007;27:12396–406.
[78] Zhang W, Liu LY, Xu TL. Reduced potassium-chloride co-transporter expression in spinal cord dorsal horn neurons contributes to inflammatory pain hypersensitivity in rats. Neuroscience 2008;152:502–10.
[79] Zhang X, Chen Y, Wang C, Huang LY. Neuronal somatic ATP release triggers neuron-satellite glial cell communication in dorsal root ganglia. Proc Natl Acad Sci USA 2007;104:9864–9.
[80] Zhang XF, Han P, Faltynek CR, Jarvis MF, Shieh CC. Functional expression of P2X7 receptors in non-neuronal cells of rat dorsal root ganglia. Brain Res 2005;1052:63–70.
[81] Zhao J, Seereeram A, Nassar MA, Levato A, Pezet S, Hathaway G, Morenilla-Palao C, Stirling C, Fitzgerald M, McMahon SB, et al. Nociceptor-derived brain-derived neurotrophic factor regulates acute and inflammatory but not neuropathic pain. Mol Cell Neurosci 2006;31:539–48.
[82] Zhuang ZY, Gerner P, Woolf CJ, Ji RR. ERK is sequentially activated in neurons, microglia, and astrocytes by spinal nerve ligation and contributes to mechanical allodynia in this neuropathic pain model. Pain 2005;114:149–59.
[83] Zhuang ZY, Wen YR, Zhang DR, Borsello T, Bonny C, Strichartz GR, Decosterd I, Ji RR. A peptide c-Jun N-terminal kinase (JNK) inhibitor blocks mechanical allodynia after spinal nerve ligation: respective roles of JNK activation in primary sensory neurons and spinal astrocytes for neuropathic pain development and maintenance. J Neurosci 2006;26:3551–60.

Correspondence to: Ji Zhang, MD, PhD, 740 Dr. Penfield Avenue, Suite 3200C, Montreal, Quebec, Canada H3A 2B2. Tel: 1-514-398-7203; fax: 1-514-398-8900; email: ji.zhang@mcgill.ca.

16

Gut Microbiota and Abnormal Mucosal Neuroendocrine Immune Activation

Robin Spiller[a] and Fergus Shanahan[b]

[a]Nottingham Digestive Diseases Centre, Biomedical Research Unit, School of Medical and Surgical Sciences, Queen's Medical Centre, Nottingham, United Kingdom; [b]Alimentary Pharmabiotic Centre, University College, Cork, Ireland

Overview

The gastrointestinal (GI) tract's prime function is to digest and absorb nutrients, mostly in the small intestine. Absorption requires a large surface area, estimated at 400 m^2, and a short diffusion path, rendering the small intestine vulnerable to invasion by pathogenic organisms. A series of elaborate protection mechanisms—including salivary lysozyme, gastric acid, and bile—minimize the number of ingested bacteria reaching the small intestine. The remaining bacteria are controlled by mucosal immunocytes (macrophages, dendritic cells, and T and B lymphocytes) and by the mesenteric lymph nodes, which together comprise the largest single component of the immune system. Within the small-intestinal mucosa, Paneth cells, enteroendocrine cells, and mast cells also detect and react to bacterial products.

Despite these defenses, a commensal microbiota rapidly develops after birth, modulating the immune system, which exhibits a state of tolerance to resident microbiota. Within the colon, the bacterial population rises steeply from 10^7 proximally to 10^{13} distally. Here, fermentation of unabsorbed dietary residue, mainly nonstarch polysaccharides, contributes up to 10% of daily caloric intake, while bacteria themselves account for around 70% of stool weight. This chapter will examine each of these components of the gut and their interactions, focusing on examples of how disruption of this fine balance can contribute to painful GI disorders.

Gut Microbiota

The average human body contains around 10^{14} commensal organisms, whose combined genome contains more than 100 times the number of host genes. This diversity is reflected in the enormous variety of metabolic activities that the colonic microbiota are capable of performing [6]. Previous attempts at identifying colonic microbiota using standard culture techniques grossly underestimated the enormous diversity of commensal bacteria. However, the microbiota can now be assessed using culture-independent molecular phylogenetic approaches based on sequencing bacterial ribosomal RNA (16S rRNA) genes, or more recently, the entire metagenome. The human microbiota is individually distinctive and apparently stable over time [125], despite wide changes in dietary intake and attack by pathogenic viruses and bacteria.

Development of Gut Microbiota

The fetal gut is sterile, but the gut is rapidly colonized during vaginal birth by maternal vaginal and fecal organisms. Breastfed infants rapidly develop a microbiota dominated by 10^{11} colony-forming units (cfu)/mL *Bifidobacteria* spp. with 10^9 cfu/mL *Lactobacillus* spp. and 10^5 cfu/mL *Enterobacteriaceae* spp. Compared to breastfed infants, bottle-fed infants show a continuing dominance of *Enterobacteriaceae* spp., and at 1 month they have lower levels of *Lactobacillus* spp. and *Bifidobacteria* spp. [124]. The dominance of *Bifidobacteria* spp. appears to be related to their specific ability to metabolize human milk oligosaccharides [55]. Lower numbers of *Bifidobacteria* spp. are also found in infants born through cesarean section and infants treated with antibiotics [81].

Impact of Early Microbiota on the Immune System

This process of colonization has a profound effect on gut structure and immunology. Gnotobiotic animals have defective mucous layers [105], reduced numbers of goblet cells [50], and a marked impairment of Peyer's patches [84]. Exposure to certain bacteria specifically modulates the immune system. For example, *Bacteroides fragilis*, a ubiquitous Gram-negative anaerobe, has a capsular polysaccharide, which activates the immune system and corrects the Th2 imbalance characteristic of germ-free mice, normalizing the depleted lymphocyte zones in their spleens [65]. Oral tolerance, which is a key feature of the mucosal immune system, is defective in gnotobiotic animals, but this deficiency can be corrected by reconstituting their flora with *Bifidobacterium infantis* [104].

Impact of Infant Microbiota on Development of Allergic Disease

The "hygiene hypothesis" relates the rapid rise of atopy (a predisposition to develop allergies to environmental antigens) over the last two decades in Western Europe to a decrease in immune stimulation by infectious illness, which is associated with falling family size and rapid economic development. That this phenomenon might be mediated by changes in gut microbiota was supported by a study showing that atopic children had fewer *Lactobacillus* spp. and *Bacteroides* spp. but a higher proportion of coliforms [13]. Increases in *Clostridium* spp. and decreases in *Bifidobacterium* spp. at 3 weeks postpartum are also a feature of children who subsequently go on to develop atopy [48]. This idea has led to numerous attempts to prevent the development of atopy by altering the gut microbiota using probiotics. While treatment once the atopy has developed appears to be ineffective, according to numerous negative randomized controlled trials [15,34,37], one study that gave the probiotics before birth to the mother and subsequently to the child showed that the treatment was effective in reducing atopy when subjects were assessed at 4 years of age [49]. Interestingly, infants with older siblings who have a lower risk of subsequent atopy also have significantly higher numbers of *Bifidobacterium* spp. [81].

Effect of Disruption of Microbiota

The gut microbiota are most obviously disrupted iatrogenically by the ingestion of broad spectrum antibiotics, but acute infection with pathogenic agents is also a common cause of disruption. Both infections and antibiotics have marked effects on the gut mucosa and on the associated endocrine and immune systems.

Effect of Broad Spectrum Antibiotics

Broad spectrum antibiotics reduce bacterial counts dramatically and frequently induce diarrhea [12]. The diarrhea is due to a number of factors, including overgrowth of pathogens such as *C. difficile, Klebsiella oxytoca* [41], and *Candida albicans,* as well as loss of the normal "colonic salvage" function [86], whereby colonic bacteria ferment and allow absorption of otherwise undigestible dietary nonstarch polysaccharides, mostly of plant origin. This dysfunction is seen in the marked reduction in fecal short chain fatty acids [42], products that normally stimulate colonic sodium and water absorption.

Visceral Hypersensitivity Induced by Antibiotic Therapy

Human epidemiological studies have shown that patients with irritable bowel syndrome (IBS) consume more antibiotics than controls [70]. A subsequent prospective study showed that antibiotic therapy increased the risk of developing IBS threefold [64]. Antibiotic treatments are known to disturb the gut microbiota and change stool form and frequency, but how this effect would cause abdominal pain was less clear. However, recent animal studies have shown that broad spectrum antibiotics induce inflammatory changes in the gut, increase expression of the neuropeptide substance P, and cause increased abdominal contractions in response to colorectal distension [110]. These changes could be prevented by spent culture medium from *L. paracasei* cultures, suggesting that specific bacterial products normally control substance P expression and hence modulate visceral pain pathways.

Infectious Enteritis

Epidemiology

Recent community studies in the United Kingdom indicate that approximately 20% of the population have a bout of acute diarrhea once a year [119]. In most stool cultures, no infectious organism can be identified, but where an organism can be identified, the most common is a variant of *Escherichia coli* (including enterotoxigenic strains, enteroadherent strains, and *E. coli* 0157), followed by small round structured viruses (*Norovirus*), *Aeromonas, Campylobacter jejuni, Rotavirus, Yersinia,* and *Astrovirus,* in order of decreasing frequency.

Effects of Viral Gastroenteritis

Viral gastroenteritis is characterized in general by a short-lived diarrheal illness, which can be severe [97], with variable villus damage [72]. Despite the severe diarrhea, the lesions heal rapidly, and there is no increase in excretion of markers of inflammation found in the stool, such as calprotectin or the protein S100A12 [47]. A report of a foodborne *Norovirus* outbreak suggested a rapid recovery, and by 6 months the risk of persistent bowel symptoms was similar in exposed and nonexposed individuals [61], in contrast with the increased incidence of IBS after bacterial enteritis.

Effects of Bacterial Gastroenteritis

There are few human studies of acute bacterial gastroenteritis, but in general biopsies taken during the acute phase of *Shigellosis* [4] and *Campylobacter jejuni* infection show acute colitis [14]. Local cytokine responses in *Shigellosis* include significant increases in cells producing interleukin (IL)-1β, tumor necrosis factor (TNF)-α, IL-8, IL-10, IL-6, IL-4, γ-interferon, TNF-β, and transforming growth factor β. In one study, biopsies taken 30 days after the onset of the diarrhea continued to show upregulated local cytokine production, even though symptoms had subsided [87].

Studies of patients with *C. jejuni* enteritis have shown acute increases in CD3+ T lymphocytes, both in the lamina propria and within the epithelium. There is also an increase in CD68-staining macrophages and 5-hydroxytryptamine (5-HT)-positive enterochromaffin cells [100].

Postinfective Irritable Bowel Syndrome

Pathological Changes

A large study of 1,977 patients infected with *C. jejuni* identified 106 patients with previously normal bowel habit who had developed postinfective IBS 3 months after infection. When compared with 28 age- and sex-matched infected individuals who had recovered fully and 34 healthy volunteers, those with postinfective IBS had significantly elevated levels of both CD3+ T lymphocytes and 5-HT-containing enterochromaffin cells [28]. An earlier study had also shown that subjects with postinfective IBS had an increase in chronic inflammatory cells in a rectal biopsy 3 months after infection [40]; it also showed increased IL-1β mRNA both at onset and 3 months after infection [39]. Increased IL-1β mRNA was also reported after a *Shigella* outbreak in which 27 subjects with postinfective IBS underwent colonoscopy and were compared with 29 subjects with IBS with diarrhea but no history of infection and 12 controls [116]. In this study, the postinfective IBS group showed increased IL-1β mRNA in both the terminal ileum and the colon but increased mast cells only in the terminal ileum. This study was unique in that it also assessed innervation, measuring fibers staining for the pan-neuronal marker neuron-specific enolase (NSE) as well as for substance P, 5-HT, and calcitonin gene-related peptide (CGRP). Fibers staining for NSE and substance P were increased in both IBS groups. The authors also reported an increased number of mast cells in close proximity to nerve fibers in both IBS groups. These results are similar to findings by Barbara and colleagues, who reported that the proximity of nerve fibers to mast cells correlated well with the severity of abdominal pain [7].

Risk Factors

Earlier epidemiological studies indicated that the strongest risk factor for developing postinfective IBS was prolonged duration of the initial diarrhea. Those with diarrhea lasting more than 3 weeks had an 11.5-fold increased risk compared with those in whom the diarrhea lasted less than 1 week [74]. Another significant factor was female gender, with a threefold increased risk, while being over 60 years of age reduced the risk to 0.36 (95% CI = 0.1–0.09). Bacterial toxicity is important, given that patients infected with a toxin-producing *C. jejuni* strain had a 10.5-fold increased risk of persistent bowel dysfunction compared with those infected with a non-toxin-producing strain [106]. Subsequent studies have confirmed the impact of initial severity [67,116] and also of female gender [40]. There is no gender difference in inflammatory response or baseline mucosal histology [30]. A subsequent study found that the female gender effect was confounded by adverse psychological factors, and a multivariate analysis showed that gender was not an independent predictor of developing postinfective IBS, although depression was [28].

Increased Gut Permeability

C. jejuni enteritis produces a prolonged increase in small-bowel gut permeability [100], which was associated with developing postinfective IBS in the Walkerton outbreak, which involved infection with both *C. jejuni* and *E. coli* 0157 [62]. Abnormal gut permeability has also been reported in postinfective IBS many years after the initial infection as well as in IBS with diarrhea [27]. Possible mediators include the cytokines IL-4, interferon, and TNF-α [66,126], which appear to reduce the complexity of tight junctions, as revealed by electron microscopy and immunofluorescent staining [92].

Role of Serotonin in Gut Function

Role of 5-HT in the Gut

Ninety percent of the body's total serotonin (5-HT) is found in the enterochromaffin cells of the gut. Numbers of 5-HT-containing enteroendocrine or enterochromaffin cells are increased in several models of epithelial damage, including *Trichinella spiralis* [118] and *Trichuris muris* infection [114]. Recovery is mediated by CD4+ T cells and depends on the body's ability to mount a Th2-biased immune response, possibly via production of IL-13 [73]. Similar increases of enterochromaffin cells are seen after experimentally induced colitis in rodents [54]. Enterochromaffin cells are also increased in the inflamed duodenal mucosa of patients with celiac disease [21,96], in the colon of patients with ulcerative colitis [103], and in the rectum of individuals recovering from *C. jejuni* enteritis [28,100].

Evidence of Altered 5-HT Metabolism in Human Disease

Assessing 5-HT release in vivo is difficult because 5-HT has a very short half-life in plasma, since it is rapidly taken up by the serotonin transporter (SERT), which is ubiquitous in endothelial cells as well as in platelets. Levels of 5-HT in platelet-poor plasma are increased postprandially in individuals with IBS with diarrhea [5] or postinfective IBS [26], which could reflect impairment of SERT in either platelets or the gut, as some have reported [23]. However, other studies have not confirmed the depression of mucosal SERT in IBS [17]. SERT exhibits a promoter polymorphism, of which the short (S) form is associated with reduced production of SERT. Although some studies have suggested an increase in the S allele in IBS with diarrhea [122], a recent meta-analysis suggests that worldwide, there is no association [107]. There is a possibility of confounding influences in some studies because the S allele is associated with anxiety [68] and depression [46], which are both common in IBS.

Effect of Inflammatory Cytokines on Peripheral Gut Function

Role of Cytokines

Although cytokines are for the most part signaling molecules that coordinate the immune response, promoting T-cell proliferation and differentiation, they also act on peripheral nerves, forming part of the neuroimmune interaction. Early studies have observed that IL-1β, which is upregulated in many inflammatory conditions, inhibits release of acetylcholine [60] and norepinephrine [43] from the myenteric plexus. IL-1β also mediates the increase in substance P within the plexus seen in *Trichinella*-infected rats [44]. The overall impact of these presynaptic inhibitory effects is excitatory. Xia and colleagues found that IL-1β and IL-6 suppressed noradrenergic inhibitory postsynaptic potentials and increased the neuronal excitability of secretomotor neurons [121]. They hypothesized that removing the inhibitory sympathetic brake would allow overreaction of secretomotor nerves and contribute to the diarrheal symptoms of inflammatory bowel disease.

Cytokines also exert an important effect on the parasympathetic nervous system, particularly by acting on the vagal afferents to mediate some of the central behavioral effects of inflammation, including fever, anorexia, and a rise in plasma cortisol [59]. The interaction is not one way, however (Fig. 1), because the vagus also appears to exert an anti-inflammatory effect on the gut [36]. This cholinergic anti-inflammatory action appears to be mediated by the α_7 nicotinic acetylcholine receptor [115].

However, within the gut mucosa there is a system of checks and balances, and while acute inflammation increases the sensitivity of afferent nerves, chronic inflammation appears to decrease it. Recent studies have suggested that this effect could be mediated by increased

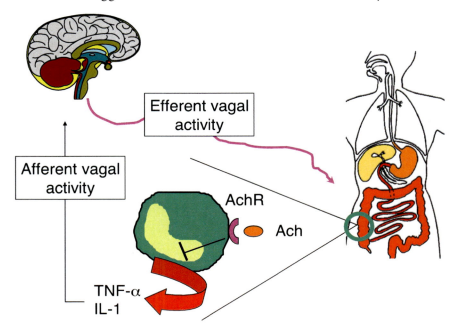

Fig. 1. Bidirectional interaction between vagus and immunocytes. The cytokines interleukin-1 (IL-1) and tumor necrosis factor alpha (TNF-α) signal via the vagus to the brainstem structures modifying behavior while vagus efferents exert an anti-inflammatory effect via acetylcholine receptors (AchR) on macrophages.

production by local T lymphocytes of inhibitory neurotransmitters such as the β-endorphins [112]. The key role of T lymphocytes is demonstrated in the visceral hypersensitivity characteristic of immune-deficient mice. This feature can be counteracted by the transfer of CD4 T lymphocytes, which increase local expression of β-endorphins and downregulate morphine receptors.

Evidence of Abnormal Cytokines in Human Disease

Overt inflammatory disease is often associated with increased cytokines, but even in functional disease in which the mucosa looks ostensibly normal, recent studies have found evidence of slightly elevated cytokine production, with increases in mRNA for IL-1β seen in postinfective IBS [39,116]. Circulating peripheral blood mononuclear cells include a substantial number of gut-homing lymphocytes, which also produce elevated quantities of cytokines [18,53]. Serum levels of IL-6 and IL-8 were also elevated in an IBS cohort in which persons with major psychiatric disorders had been excluded [25]. These elevations of IL-6 levels were correlated with the exaggerated release of both adrenocorticotropic hormone (ACTH) and cortisol following an infusion of corticotropin-releasing hormone. Plasma IL-8 and TNF-α levels were increased in subjects with bipolar affective disorders [78], and IL-6 and TNF-α were also reported to be elevated in depression [33]. Given the wide overlap of psychiatric disorders with functional GI diseases, the abnormal cytokines may very well reflect the psychiatric abnormalities.

Mast Cell Abnormalities and Stress

Evidence of Increased Mast Cell Numbers in Irritable Bowel Syndrome

Some investigators have reported increased mast cells in diarrhea-predominant IBS (IBS-D) in the terminal ileum [45] and caecum [80], whereas others have found no increase [20,29]. Although in postinfective IBS there was no change in the rectum [28,116], increased mast cells have been found in the terminal ileum in both postinfective IBS and IBS-D [116].

One group has also found increased mast cell numbers in constipation-predominant IBS (IBS-C) as well as IBS-D [7]. More recently, increased mast cell numbers have been reported in the duodenum and jejunum in IBS [38a].

Stress-Induced Changes in Colonic Function

Stress-related release of corticotropin-releasing factor (CRF) is a key mediator in stress-induced accelerated transit, increased colonocyte chloride secretion, and gut permeability [90]. Stress also aggravates chemically induced experimental colitis by decreasing colonic mucin secretion [82]. Chronic stress-induced barrier dysfunction allows bacterial adhesion and penetration into the enterocytes and beyond, which may account for the associated hyperplasia and activation of mast cells and the infiltration of neutrophil and mononuclear cells [98]. This increased bacterial translocation appears to occur most readily through the follicle-associated epithelium, where chronic stress can increase the passage of *E. coli* as much as 30-fold [109].

Stress and Mast Cell Activation

Acute stress in rats increases colonic histamine content and enhances visceral sensitivity, an effect that can be blocked by the mast cell stabilizer doxantrazole [38]. Similarly, acute stress induced by plunging the hand into ice-cold water stimulates the release of histamine and prostaglandins into the jejunum of healthy human volunteers [89]. Chronic stressors such as water avoidance for 1 hour per day for 5 days induces a marked increase in the number of mast cells in rats, which is associated with increased transcellular flux of horseradish peroxidase, an effect that is absent in mast-cell-deficient mice [91]. Recent human studies showing a correlation of fatigue and depression with mast cell numbers suggest that such a mechanism may also apply in patients with IBS [83].

How stress increases mast cell numbers is unclear, but CRF may play a role. Neonatal maternal deprivation in rats elevates corticosteroid levels and causes increased gut paracellular permeability, which can be mimicked by exogenous CRF, and this effect can be blocked by doxantrazole [9]. Studies in human biopsies show that human mast cells express CRF-1 and CRF-2 receptors and that CRF increases gut permeability, an effect that is mediated by mast cells and can be blocked by CRF antagonists and by lodoxamide, a mast cell stabilizer [113].

Most patients with functional GI diseases suffer from chronic rather than acute stress, and they often have a history of childhood abuse, which has led researchers to develop models of chronic stress such neonatal maternal deprivation, which generates neurotic behavior characteristic of chronic anxiety. Maternal deprivation sensitizes the gut to the effects of acute stress, which impairs barrier function and increases gut permeability; these effects can be reduced by a CRF antagonist [99]. The trophic changes of chronic stress may be mediated by nerve growth factor (NGF) because the increased mast cell density seen with maternal deprivation can be blocked by anti-NGF antibodies, a treatment that also prevents the increase in gut permeability and visceral hypersensitivity associated with this condition [8].

Activation of Mast Cells and Visceral Hypersensitivity

Mast cells contain a number of mediators, including histamine, tryptase, substance P, and prostaglandins, which are all potent sensitizers of afferent nerves. Activation of protease-activated receptor 2 (PAR-2) receptors by tryptase not only can mediate visceral hypersensitivity but also can stimulate intestinal secretion and increase gut permeability [111]. The importance of mast cells in visceral hypersensitivity is supported by the correlation between the severity of pain and the number of mast cells in close proximity to colonic nerves [7]. Increased proximity of mast cells to nerves is also seen in postinfective IBS [116] and in maternally deprived rats [10]. The rat study showed that the increased synaptogenesis at 4 weeks could be abolished by anti-NGF antibodies, a treatment that also blocked the increase in mast cell numbers [10].

Visceral Hypersensitivity and Stress-Induced Increased Gut Permeability

Stress-induced hypersensitivity to distension appears to be mediated by increased gut permeability because it can be blocked by

2,4,6-triaminopyrimidine, a drug that acts on tight junctions to prevent the increase in colonic permeability. This effect can also be blocked by an inhibitor of myosin light chain kinase (MLK), suggesting that stress increases colonic permeability by causing epithelial cell cytoskeletal contraction through MLK activation [1]. CRF stimulates mast cells to release NGF, which appears to contribute to the increase in gut permeability, because the effect is reduced by anti-NGF antibodies [9]. Given that these stress models involve inflammatory changes due to translocation of luminal bacteria into the lamina propria, an obvious next step was to modify the colonic bacteria to see whether that could modify the effect on permeability. Several studies have now been reported, suggesting that probiotic bacteria can counteract stress-induced gut permeability [2,31].

Mast Cell Activation in Irritable Bowel Syndrome: Implications for Treatment

Several uncontrolled studies had already suggested benefit of sodium cromoglycate, a mast cell stabilizer, in patients with IBS and food allergy [57,101]. Released mast cell tryptase can act in the mucosa or be secreted into the colonic lumen, where it can increase permeability. Fecal supernatants from patients with IBS-D, when instilled into the colon of mice, increased abdominal contractions in response to colorectal distension, an effect that could be blocked by protease inhibitors and did not occur with fecal supernatants from patients with IBS-C [35]. Chemical analysis showed increased levels of serine proteases in fecal supernatants from patients with IBS-D but not in those with IBS-C or an alternating bowel habit. It is unlikely that the source of these enzymes is the pancreas because the enzyme pancreatic elastase was not increased, nor were calprotectin or other markers of polymorphonuclear cell secretions. The visceral sensitizing effect appears to be specific to agents acting through PAR-2 receptors, since it was not seen in PAR-2 knockout mice [35]. Similar results were reported by another group, who showed that although mast cell numbers did not increase, tryptase mRNA as well as trypsin and tryptase protein levels did increase in both the rectum and ascending colon biopsies [19]. In this study, the authors also demonstrated somatic hyperalgesia induced by injecting the supernatants into the mouse paw, showing that the effect was not unique to visceral nerves.

Alteration of Mucosal Nerves

Mucosal inflammation with initial destruction is followed by restitution and repair in which mucosal nerves are prominently involved. Using a rat model of colitis experimentally induced by trinitrobenzene sulfonic acid, studied over an extended period, we have demonstrated an initial destruction of mucosal nerves followed by regrowth, resulting in a temporary excess of nerves followed by a remodeling in which the number of nerves returns toward normal, but the chemical coding appears to be changed. We noted increased expression of substance P, neurokinin A, vasoactive intestinal peptide, and galanin [95]. These changes are found not only in the mucosa, but also in the circular muscle layers. Mice infected with *Trichinella spiralis* show increased tachykinin expression in the mucosa as well as in the dorsal horn of the spinal column innervating the colon [24]. Recurring inflammation in humans due to ulcerative colitis is also associated with increases in tachykininergic neurons in rectal biopsies of those with the most severe disease [117] and in the myenteric plexus of resected colons of those who go on to colectomy [75].

Sensitization of nerves has been associated within an increase in expression of the transient receptor potential vanilloid 1 (TRPV1) receptor, a feature that is seen in inflammatory bowel disease [123], in the bladder of women with idiopathic sensory urgency [56], and in mucosal biopsies in esophagitis [63].

More recently, increased TRPV1 has also been demonstrated in patients with IBS [3], with the linear density of TRPV1 fibers correlating with the maximum severity of abdominal pain. Interestingly, there was an inverse relation with age, which may explain why the incidence of IBS declines in older persons. NGF also appears to be important in humans with rectal hypersensitivity, in whom the increase in TRPV1 was associated with an increase in nerve fibers expressing glial-derived neurotrophic factor (GDNF) and the receptor for NGF tyrosine kinase A [22].

Modulation of Gut Flora to Control Mucosal Neuroimmune Function

Probiotics are nonpathogenic bacteria, which when ingested by mouth can provide positive health benefits. These organisms are most typically *Lactobacilli* spp. or *Bifidobacteria* spp., which are common components of the infant gut. Animal studies have shown that such organisms can increase barrier function [58], stimulate mucous secretion [16], and exert anti-inflammatory effects [32,93]. Several probiotics also exert protective effects on tight junctions [71], including *E. coli* Nissle 1917, which has beneficial effects in preventing the relapse of inflammatory bowel disease [51]. Treatment with this probiotic enhanced the expression of zonula occludens-2 protein and prevented the upregulation of protein kinase C-zeta in T84 cells challenged with enteropathic *E. coli* [127]. A soluble protein from *L. rhamnosus* GG has also been shown to prevent hydrogen-peroxide-induced damage to the tight junction [94].

The anti-inflammatory effects may be mediated either by stimulating regulatory T lymphocytes or more directly by inhibiting TNF-α production [69]. *L. rhamnosus* increases the secretion of IL-10 by human peripheral blood mononuclear cells while decreasing secretion of TNF-α, IL-6, and interferon-γ in response to commensal microbiota [93]. One of the more successful probiotics, known as VSL#3, is a mixture containing 90×10^{10} cfu/mL *Lactobacillus* spp. (*casei, plantarum, acidophilus,* and *delbrueckii* ssp. *bulgaricus*) together with *Bifidobacterium* (*lungrum, breve,* and *infantis*) and one strain of *Streptococcus salivarians* ssp. *thermophilus*). This mixture was effective in preventing pouchitis in patients undergoing ileal pouch anal anastomosis for ulcerative colitis, where it was associated with a reduction in inflammation and in numbers of activated T cells [85].

Recently, novel probiotics have been designed to deliver specific compounds including IL-10 [102], nitric oxide [52], and trefoil factors [108], which may all have specific benefits in inflammatory disease.

Probiotics as a Treatment for Visceral Hypersensitivity

The nitric-oxide-secreting *Lactobacillus farciminis* has been shown to inhibit the visceral hypersensitivity and increased colonic permeability associated with partial restraint [2]. The authors also showed that *L. farciminis* prevented the increase in colonocyte MLK phosphorylation, which might mediate the permeability change.

A new chapter in the exploration of the interaction of the gut flora with the mucosa has opened with the recent demonstration that *L. acidophilus* reduces visceral hypersensitivity by inducing the expression of morphine and cannabinoid-2 (CB2) receptors in epithelial cells. When given by mouth for 15 days, probiotics increased the pain threshold, an effect similar to that seen with morphine. The analgesic effect was transitory, disappearing 3 days after oral dosing ceased [88]. Cannabinoid receptors are also important in feeding behavior and inflammation, so these studies offer potential new therapeutic options in modulation of gut-to-brain signaling.

Probiotics as Treatment for Pain in Irritable Bowel Syndrome

Pain or discomfort is one of the key symptoms in IBS, so the recent flurry of placebo-controlled trials of probiotics in IBS are of some relevance. Among the difficulties in evaluating these clinical trials is the wide variety of different probiotics used, as well as the fact that most trials were underpowered. One relatively consistent finding has been a reduction in flatulence seen with a number of different *Lactobacillus* spp. [11,76,77]. Whether probiotics specifically benefit pain is unclear because many studies have used unvalidated composite scores. One large, well-designed, randomized, double-blind, placebo-controlled trial did show a decrease in pain with *Bifidobacterium infantis* 1×10^8 cfu/day [120]. A previous smaller study with *B. infantis* 1×10^{10} cfu/day in 25 IBS patients also showed a reduction in pain and bloating, together with a normalization of the depressed IL-10/IL-12 ratio in peripheral blood mononuclear cells, suggesting a possible anti-inflammatory action [79].

Summary

The gut microbiota exist in a delicate equilibrium with the mucosa. Disturbances in the microbiota alter immune development and gut function. Acute infections leave long-lasting changes in the mucosa, including

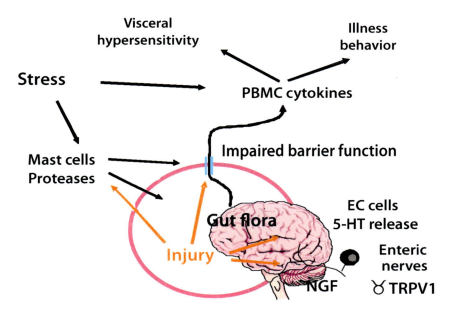

Fig. 2. Diagram showing how mucosal insult and stress interact to cause visceral hypersensitivity and illness behavior. EC = enterochromaffin, 5-HT = 5-hydroxytryptamine, NGF = nerve growth factor, PBMC = peripheral blood mononuclear cells, TRPV1 = transient receptor potential vanilloid 1.

increases in enterochromaffin cells, lymphocytes, and mast cells, which may lead to impaired barrier function and chronic immune activation (Fig. 2). Psychological stressors also modulate mast cells, whose activation increases gut permeability and sensitizes afferent nerves. Mucosal injury can also be followed by alterations in afferent nerve receptors, leading to visceral hypersensitivity.

References

[1]   Ait-Belgnaoui A, Bradesi S, Fioramonti J, Theodorou V, Bueno L. Acute stress-induced hypersensitivity to colonic distension depends upon increase in paracellular permeability: role of myosin light chain kinase. Pain 2005;113:141–7.

[2]   Ait-Belgnaoui A, Han W, Lamine F, Eutamene H, Fioramonti J, Bueno L, Theodorou V. *Lactobacillus farciminis* treatment suppresses stress induced visceral hypersensitivity: a possible action through interaction with epithelial cell cytoskeleton contraction. Gut 2006;55:1090–4.

[3]   Akbar A, Yiangou Y, Facer P, Walters JR, Anand P, Ghosh S. Increased capsaicin receptor TRPV1 expressing sensory fibres in irritable bowel syndrome and their correlation with abdominal pain. Gut 2008;57:923–9.

[4]   Anand BS, Malhotra V, Bhattacharya SK, Datta P, Datta D, Sen D, Bhattacharya MK, Mukherjee
      PP, Pal SC. Rectal histology in acute bacillary dysentery. Gastroenterology 1986;90:654–60.
[5]   Atkinson W, Lockhart S, Whorwell PJ, Keevil B, Houghton LA. Altered 5-hydroxytryptamine
      signaling in patients with constipation- and diarrhea-predominant irritable bowel syndrome.
      Gastroenterology 2006;130:34–43.
[6]   Backhed F, Ley RE, Sonnenburg JL, Peterson DA, Gordon JI. Host-bacterial mutualism in the
      human intestine. Science 2005;307:1915–20.
[7]   Barbara G, Stanghellini V, De Giorgio R, Cremon C, Cottrell GS, Santini D, Pasquinelli G, Mor-
      selli-Labate AM, Grady EF, Bunnett NW, et al. Activated mast cells in proximity to colonic nerves
      correlate with abdominal pain in irritable bowel syndrome. Gastroenterology 2004;126:693–702.
[8]   Barreau F, Cartier C, Ferrier L, Fioramonti J, Bueno L. Nerve growth factor mediates alterations
      of colonic sensitivity and mucosal barrier induced by neonatal stress in rats. Gastroenterology
      2004;127:524–34.
[9]   Barreau F, Cartier C, Leveque M, Ferrier L, Moriez R, Laroute V, Rosztoczy A, Fioramonti J, Bueno
      L. Pathways involved in gut mucosal barrier dysfunction induced in adult rats by maternal depriva-
      tion: corticotrophin-releasing factor and nerve growth factor interplay. J Physiol 2007;580:347–56.
[10] Barreau F, Salvador-Cartier C, Houdeau E, Bueno L, Fioramonti J. Long-term alterations of
      colonic nerve mast cell interactions induced by neonatal maternal deprivation in rats. Gut
      2008;57:582–90.
[11] Bausserman M, Michail S. The use of Lactobacillus GG in irritable bowel syndrome in children:
      a double-blind randomized control trial. J Pediatr 2005;147:197–201.
[12] Bergogne-Berezin E. Treatment and prevention of antibiotic associated diarrhea. Int J Antimi-
      crob Agents 2000;16:521–6.
[13] Bjorksten B, Naaber P, Sepp E, Mikelsaar M. The intestinal microflora in allergic Estonian and
      Swedish 2-year-old children. Clin Exp Allergy 1999;29:342–6.
[14] Blaser MJ. Epidemiologic and clinical features of Campylobacter jejuni infections. J Infect Dis
      1997;176(Suppl 2):S103–5.
[15] Brouwer ML, Wolt-Plompen SA, Dubois AE, van der Heide S, Jansen DF, Hoijer MA, Kauffman
      HF, Duiverman EJ. No effects of probiotics on atopic dermatitis in infancy: a randomized pla-
      cebo-controlled trial. Clin Exp Allergy 2006;36:899–906.
[16] Caballero-Franco C, Keller K, De Simone C, Chadee K. The VSL#3 probiotic formula induces
      mucin gene expression and secretion in colonic epithelial cells. Am J Physiol Gastrointest Liver
      Physiol 2007;292:G315–G322.
[17] Camilleri M, Andrews CN, Bharucha AE, Carlson PJ, Ferber I, Stephens D, Smyrk TC, Urrutia
      R, Aerssens J, Thielemans L, et al. Alterations in expression of p11 and SERT in mucosal biopsy
      specimens of patients with irritable bowel syndrome. Gastroenterology 2007;132:17–25.
[18] Campbell E, Richards M, Foley S, Hastings M, Whorwell P, Mahida Y, et al. Markers of inflam-
      mation in IBS: increased permeability and cytokine production in diarrhoea predominant sub-
      groups. Gastroenterology 130:A51.
[19] Cenac N, Andrews CN, Holzhausen M, Chapman K, Cottrell G, Andrade-Gordon P, Steinhoff
      M, Barbara G, Beck P, Bunnett NW, et al. Role for protease activity in visceral pain in irritable
      bowel syndrome. J Clin Invest 2007;117:636–47.
[20] Chadwick VS, Chen W, Shu D, Paulus B, Bethwaite P, Tie A, Wilson I. Activation of the mucosal
      immune system in irritable bowel syndrome. Gastroenterology 2002;122:1778–83.
[21] Challacombe DN, Dawkins PD, Baker P. Increased tissue concentrations of 5-hydroxytryptamine
      in the duodenal mucosa of patients with coeliac disease. Gut 1977;18:882–6.
[22] Chan CL, Facer P, Davis JB, Smith GD, Egerton J, Bountra C Williams NS, Anand P. Sensory
      fibres expressing capsaicin receptor TRPV1 in patients with rectal hypersensitivity and faecal
      urgency. Lancet 2003;361:385–91.
[23] Coates MD, Mahoney CR, Linden DR, Sampson JE, Chen J, Blaszyk H, Crowell MD, Sharkey
      KA, Gershon MD, Mawe GM, et al. Molecular defects in mucosal serotonin content and de-
      creased serotonin reuptake transporter in ulcerative colitis and irritable bowel syndrome. Gas-
      troenterology 2004;126:1657–64.
[24] De Giorgio R, Barbara G, Blennerhassett P, Wang L, Stanghellini V, Corinaldesi R, Collins SM,
      Tougas G. Intestinal inflammation and activation of sensory nerve pathways: a functional and
      morphological study in the nematode infected rat. Gut 2001;49:822–7.

[25] Dinan TG, Quigley EM, Ahmed SM, Scully P, O'Brien S, O'Mahony L, O'Mahony S, Shanahan F, Keeling PW. Hypothalamic-pituitary-gut axis dysregulation in irritable bowel syndrome: plasma cytokines as a potential biomarker? Gastroenterology 2006;130:304–11.

[26] Dunlop SP, Coleman NS, Blackshaw E, Perkins AC, Singh G, Marsden CA, Spiller RC. Abnormalities of 5-hydroxytryptamine metabolism in irritable bowel syndrome. Clin Gastroenterol Hepatol 2005;3:349–57.

[27] Dunlop SP, Hebden J, Campbell E, Naesdal J, Olbe L, Perkins AC, et al. Abnormal intestinal permeability in subgroups of diarrhea-predominant irritable bowel syndromes. Am J Gastroenterol 2006;101:1288–94.

[28] Dunlop SP, Jenkins D, Neal KR, Spiller RC. Relative importance of enterochromaffin cell hyperplasia, anxiety, and depression in postinfectious IBS. Gastroenterology 2003;125:1651–9.

[29] Dunlop SP, Jenkins D, Spiller RC. Distinctive clinical, psychological, and histological features of postinfective irritable bowel syndrome. Am J Gastroenterol 2003;98:1578–83.

[30] Dunlop SP, Jenkins D, Spiller RC. Age-related decline in rectal mucosal lymphocytes and mast cells. Eur J Gastroenterol Hepatol 2004;16:1011–5.

[31] Eutamene H, Lamine F, Chabo C, Theodorou V, Rochat F, Bergonzelli GE, Corthésy-Theulaz I, Fioramonti J, Bueno L. Synergy between *Lactobacillus paracasei* and its bacterial products to counteract stress-induced gut permeability and sensitivity increase in rats. J Nutr 2007;137:1901–7.

[32] Ezendam J, van Loveren H. Probiotics: immunomodulation and evaluation of safety and efficacy. Nutr Rev 2006;64:1–14.

[33] Fitzgerald P, O'Brien SM, Scully P, Rijkers K, Scott LV, Dinan TG. Cutaneous glucocorticoid receptor sensitivity and pro-inflammatory cytokine levels in antidepressant-resistant depression. Psychol Med 2006;36:37–43.

[34] Fölster-Holst R, Müller F, Schnopp N, Abeck D, Kreiselmaier I, Lenz T, von Rüden U, Schrezenmeir J, Christophers E, Weichenthal M. Prospective, randomized controlled trial on *Lactobacillus rhamnosus* in infants with moderate to severe atopic dermatitis. Br J Dermatol 2006;155:1256–61.

[35] Gecse K, Róka R, Ferrier L, Leveque M, Eutamene H, Cartier C, Ait-Belgnaoui A, Rosztóczy A, Izbéki F, Fioramonti J, et al. Increased faecal serine-protease activity in diarrhoeic IBS patients: a colonic lumenal factor impairing colonic permeability and sensitivity. Gut 2008;57:591–9.

[36] Ghia JE, Blennerhassett P, Kumar-Ondiveeran H, Verdu EF, Collins SM. The vagus nerve: a tonic inhibitory influence associated with inflammatory bowel disease in a murine model. Gastroenterology 2006;131:1122–30.

[37] Grüber C, Wendt M, Sulser C, Lau S, Kulig M, Wahn U, Werfel T, Niggemann B. Randomized, placebo-controlled trial of *Lactobacillus rhamnosus* GG as treatment of atopic dermatitis in infancy. Allergy 2007;62:1270–6.

[38] Gue M, Rio-Lacheze C, Eutamene H, Theodorou V, Fioramonti J, Bueno L. Stress-induced visceral hypersensitivity to rectal distension in rats: role of CRF and mast cells. Neurogastroenterol Motil 1997;9:271–9.

[38a] Guilarte M, Santos J, de Torres I, Alonso C, Vicario M, Ramos L, Martinez C, Casellas F, Saperas E, Malagelada JR. Diarrhoea-predominant IBS patients show mast cell activation and hyperplasia in the jejunum. Gut 2007;56:203–9.

[39] Gwee KA, Collins SM, Read NW, Rajnakova A, Deng Y, Graham JC, McKendrick MW, Moochhala SM. Increased rectal mucosal expression of interleukin 1beta in recently acquired post-infectious irritable bowel syndrome. Gut 2003;52:523–6.

[40] Gwee KA, Leong YL, Graham C, McKendrick MW, Collins SM, Walters SJ, Underwood JE, Read NW. The role of psychological and biological factors in postinfective gut dysfunction. Gut 1999;44:400–6.

[41] Högenauer C, Langner C, Beubler E, Lippe IT, Schicho R, Gorkiewicz G, Krause R, Gerstgrasser N, Krejs GJ, Hinterleitner TA. *Klebsiella oxytoca* as a causative organism of antibiotic-associated hemorrhagic colitis. N Engl J Med 2006;355:2418–26.

[42] Hove H, Tvede M, Mortensen PB. Antibiotic-associated diarrhoea, *Clostridium difficile*, and short-chain fatty acids. Scand J Gastroenterol 1996;31:688–93.

[43] Hurst S, Collins SM. Interleukin-1 beta modulation of norepinephrine release from rat myenteric nerves. Am J Physiol 1993;264:G30–5.

[44] Hurst SM, Stanisz AM, Sharkey KA, Collins SM. Interleukin 1 beta-induced increase in substance P in rat myenteric plexus. Gastroenterology 1993;105:1754–60.
[45] Hwang L, Leichter R, Okamoto A, Payan D, Collins SM, Bunnett NW. Downregulation of neutral endopeptidase (EC 3.4.24.11) in the inflamed rat intestine. Am J Physiol 1993;264:G735–43.
[46] Jarrett ME, Kohen R, Cain KC, Burr RL, Poppe A, Navaja GP, Heitkemper MM. Relationship of SERT polymorphisms to depressive and anxiety symptoms in irritable bowel syndrome. Biol Res Nurs 2007;9:161–9.
[47] Kaiser T, Langhorst J, Wittkowski H, Becker K, Friedrich AW, Rueffer A, Dobos GJ, Roth J, Foell D. Faecal S100A12 as a non-invasive marker distinguishing inflammatory bowel disease from irritable bowel syndrome. Gut 2007;56:1706–13.
[48] Kalliomaki M, Kirjavainen P, Eerola E, Kero P, Salminen S, Isolauri E. Distinct patterns of neonatal gut microflora in infants in whom atopy was and was not developing. J Allergy Clin Immunol 2001;107:129–34.
[49] Kalliomaki M, Salminen S, Poussa T, Arvilommi H, Isolauri E. Probiotics and prevention of atopic disease: 4-year follow-up of a randomised placebo-controlled trial. Lancet 2003;361:1869–71.
[50] Kandori H, Hirayama K, Takeda M, Doi K. Histochemical, lectin-histochemical and morphometrical characteristics of intestinal goblet cells of germfree and conventional mice. Exp Anim 1996;45:155–60.
[51] Kruis W, Schutz E, Fric P, Fixa B, Judmaier G, Stolte M. Double-blind comparison of an oral Escherichia coli preparation and mesalazine in maintaining remission of ulcerative colitis. Aliment Pharmacol Ther 1997;11:853–8.
[52] Lamine F, Fioramonti J, Bueno L, Nepveu F, Cauquil E, Lobysheva I, Eutamène H, Théodorou V. Nitric oxide released by *Lactobacillus farciminis* improves TNBS-induced colitis in rats. Scand J Gastroenterol 2004;39:37–45.
[53] Liebregts T, Adam B, Bredack C, Röth A, Heinzel S, Lester S, Downie-Doyle S, Smith E, Drew P, Talley NJ, Holtmann G. Immune activation in patients with irritable bowel syndrome. Gastroenterology 2007;132:913–20.
[54] Linden DR, Chen JX, Gershon MD, Sharkey KA, Mawe GM. Serotonin availability is increased in mucosa of guinea pigs with TNBS-induced colitis. Am J Physiol Gastrointest Liver Physiol 2003;285:G207–16.
[55] LoCascio RG, Ninonuevo MR, Freeman SL, Sela DA, Grimm R, Lebrilla CB, Mills DA, German JB. Glycoprofiling of bifidobacterial consumption of human milk oligosaccharides demonstrates strain specific, preferential consumption of small chain glycans secreted in early human lactation. J Agric Food Chem 2007;55:8914–9.
[56] Lowe EM, Anand P, Terenghi G, Williams-Chestnut RE, Sinicropi DV, Osborne JL. Increased nerve growth factor levels in the urinary bladder of women with idiopathic sensory urgency and interstitial cystitis. Br J Urol 1997;79:572–7.
[57] Lunardi C, Bambara LM, Biasi D, Cortina P, Peroli P, Nicolis F, Favari F, Pacor ML. Double-blind cross-over trial of oral sodium cromoglycate in patients with irritable bowel syndrome due to food intolerance. Clin Exp Allergy 1991;21:569–72.
[58] Madsen K, Cornish A, Soper P, McKaigney C, Jijon H, Yachimec C, Doyle J, Jewell L, De Simone C. Probiotic bacteria enhance murine and human intestinal epithelial barrier function. Gastroenterology 2001;121:580–91.
[59] Maier SF, Goehler LE, Fleshner M, Watkins LR. The role of the vagus nerve in cytokine-to-brain communication. Ann NY Acad Sci 1998;840:289–300.
[60] Main C, Blennerhassett P, Collins SM. Human recombinant interleukin 1beta suppresses acetylcholine release from rat myenteric plexus. Gastroenterology 1993;104:1648–54.
[61] Marshall JK, Thabane M, Borgaonkar MR, James C. Postinfectious irritable bowel syndrome after a food-borne outbreak of acute gastroenteritis attributed to a viral pathogen. Clin Gastroenterol Hepatol 2007;5:457–60.
[62] Marshall JK, Thabane M, Garg AX, Clark W, Meddings J, Collins SM. Intestinal permeability in patients with irritable bowel syndrome after a waterborne outbreak of acute gastroenteritis in Walkerton, Ontario. Aliment Pharmacol Ther 2004;20:1317–22.
[63] Matthews PJ, Aziz Q, Facer P, Davis JB, Thompson DG, Anand P. Increased capsaicin receptor TRPV1 nerve fibres in the inflamed human oesophagus. Eur J Gastroenterol Hepatol 2004;16:897–902.

[64] Maxwell PR, Rink E, Kumar D, Mendall MA. Antibiotics increase functional abdominal symptoms. Am J Gastroenterol 2002;97:104–8.

[65] Mazmanian SK, Liu CH, Tzianabos AO, Kasper DL. An immunomodulatory molecule of symbiotic bacteria directs maturation of the host immune system. Cell 2005;122:107–18.

[66] McKay DM, Singh PK. Superantigen activation of immune cells evokes epithelial (T84) transport and barrier abnormalities via IFN-gamma and TNF alpha: inhibition of increased permeability, but not diminished secretory responses by TGF-beta2. J Immunol 1997;159:2382–90.

[67] Mearin F, Pérez-Oliveras M, Perelló A, Vinyet J, Ibañez A, Coderch J, Perona M. Dyspepsia and irritable bowel syndrome after a Salmonella gastroenteritis outbreak: one-year follow-up cohort study. Gastroenterology 2005;129:98–104.

[68] Melke J, Landén M, Baghei F, Rosmond R, Holm G, Björntorp P, Westberg L, Hellstrand M, Eriksson E. Serotonin transporter gene polymorphisms are associated with anxiety-related personality traits in women. Am J Med Genet 2001;105:458–63.

[69] Menard S, Candalh C, Bambou JC, Terpend K, Cerf-Bensussan N, Heyman M. Lactic acid bacteria secrete metabolites retaining anti-inflammatory properties after intestinal transport. Gut 2004;53:821–8.

[70] Mendall MA, Kumar D. Antibiotic use, childhood affluence and irritable bowel syndrome (IBS). Eur J Gastroenterol Hepatol 1998;10:59–62.

[71] Montalto M, Maggiano N, Ricci R, Curigliano V, Santoro L, Di Nicuolo F, Vecchio FM, Gasbarrini A, Gasbarrini A. Lactobacillus acidophilus protects tight junctions from aspirin damage in HT-29 cells. Digestion 2004;69:225–8.

[72] Morotti RA, Kaufman SS, Fishbein TM, Chatterjee NK, Fuschino ME, Morse DL, Magid MS. Calicivirus infection in pediatric small intestine transplant recipients: pathological considerations. Hum Pathol 2004;35:1236–40.

[73] Motomura Y, Ghia JE, Wang H, Akiho H, El-Sharkawy RT, Collins M, Wan Y, McLaughlin JT, Khan WI. Enterochromaffin cell and 5-hydroxytryptamine responses to the same infectious agent differ in Th1 and Th2 dominant environments. Gut 2008;57:475–81.

[74] Neal KR, Hebden J, Spiller R. Prevalence of gastrointestinal symptoms six months after bacterial gastroenteritis and risk factors for development of the irritable bowel syndrome: postal survey of patients. BMJ 1997;314:779–82.

[75] Neunlist M, Aubert P, Toquet C, Oreshkova T, Barouk J, Lehur PA, Schemann M, Galmiche JP. Changes in chemical coding of myenteric neurones in ulcerative colitis. Gut 2003;52:84–90.

[76] Niv E, Naftali T, Hallak R, Vaisman N. The efficacy of Lactobacillus reuteri ATCC 55730 in the treatment of patients with irritable bowel syndrome-a double blind, placebo-controlled, randomized study. Clin Nutr 2005;24:925–31.

[77] Nobaek S, Johansson ML, Molin G, Ahrne S, Jeppsson B. Alteration of intestinal microflora is associated with reduction in abdominal bloating and pain in patients with irritable bowel syndrome. Am J Gastroenterol 2000;95:1231–8.

[78] O'Brien SM, Scully P, Scott LV, Dinan TG. Cytokine profiles in bipolar affective disorder: focus on acutely ill patients. J Affect Disord 2006;90:263–7.

[79] O'Mahony L, McCarthy J, Kelly P, Hurley G, Luo F, Chen K, O'Sullivan GC, Kiely B, Collins JK, Shanahan F, Quigley EM. Lactobacillus and Bifidobacterium in irritable bowel syndrome: symptom responses and relationship to cytokine profiles. Gastroenterology 2005;128:541–51.

[80] O'Sullivan M, Clayton N, Breslin NP, Harman I, Bountra C, McLaren A, O'Morain CA. Increased mast cells in the irritable bowel syndrome. Neurogastroenterol Motil 2000;12:449–57.

[81] Penders J, Thijs C, Vink C, Stelma FF, Snijders B, Kummeling I, van den Brandt PA, Stobberingh EE. Factors influencing the composition of the intestinal microbiota in early infancy. Pediatrics 2006;118:511–21.

[82] Pfeiffer CJ, Qiu B, Lam SK. Reduction of colonic mucus by repeated short-term stress enhances experimental colitis in rats. J Physiol Paris 2001;95:81–7.

[83] Piche T, Saint-Paul MC, Dainese R, Marine-Barjoan E, Iannelli A, Montoya ML, Peyron JF, Czerucka D, Cherikh F, Filippi J, et al. Mast cells and cellularity of the colonic mucosa correlated with fatigue and depression in irritable bowel syndrome. Gut 2008;57:468–73.

[84] Pollard M, Sharon N. Responses of the Peyer's patches in germ-free mice to antigenic stimulation. Infect Immun 1970;2:96–100.

358   R. Spiller and F. Shahanan

[85] Pronio A, Montesani C, Butteroni C, Vecchione S, Mumolo G, Vestri A, Vitolo D, Boirivant M.
      Probiotic administration in patients with ileal pouch-anal anastomosis for ulcerative colitis is
      associated with expansion of mucosal regulatory cells. Inflamm Bowel Dis 2008;14:662–8.
[86] Rao SSC, Edwards CA, Austen CJ, Bruce C, Read NW. Impaired colonic fermentation of carbo-
      hydrate after ampicillin. Gastroenterology 1988;94:928–32.
[87] Raqib R, Lindberg AA, Wretlind B, Bardhan PK, Andersson U, Andersson J. Persistence
      of local cytokine production in shigellosis in acute and convalescent stages. Infect Immun
      1995;63:289–96.
[88] Rousseaux C, Thuru X, Gelot A, Barnich N, Neut C, Dubuquoy L, Dubuquoy C, Merour E,
      Geboes K, Chamaillard M, et al. *Lactobacillus acidophilus* modulates intestinal pain and induces
      opioid and cannabinoid receptors. Nat Med 2007;13:35–7.
[89] Santos J, Saperas E, Nogueiras C, Mourelle M, Antolin M, Cadahia A, Malagelada JR. Re-
      lease of mast cell mediators into the jejunum by cold pain stress in humans. Gastroenterology
      1998;114:640–8.
[90] Santos J, Saunders PR, Hanssen NP, Yang PC, Yates D, Groot JA, Perdue MH. Corticotropin-
      releasing hormone mimics stress-induced colonic epithelial pathophysiology in the rat. Am J
      Physiol 1999;277:G391–9.
[91] Santos J, Yang PC, Soderholm JD, Benjamin M, Perdue MH. Role of mast cells in chronic stress
      induced colonic epithelial barrier dysfunction in the rat. Gut 2001;48:630–6.
[92] Schmitz H, Fromm M, Bentzel CJ, Scholz P, Detjen K, Mankertz J, Bode H, Epple HJ, Riecken
      EO, Schulzke JD. Tumor necrosis factor-alpha (TNFalpha) regulates the epithelial barrier in the
      human intestinal cell line HT-29/B6. J Cell Sci 1999;112:137–46.
[93] Schultz M, Linde HJ, Lehn N, Zimmermann K, Grossmann J, Falk W, Schölmerich J. Immu-
      nomodulatory consequences of oral administration of Lactobacillus rhamnosus strain GG in
      healthy volunteers. J Dairy Res 2003;70:165–73.
[94] Seth A, Yan F, Polk DB, Rao RK. Probiotics ameliorate the hydrogen peroxide-induced epithelial
      barrier disruption by a PKC and MAP kinase-dependent mechanism. Am J Physiol Gastrointest
      Liver Physiol 2008;294:G1060–9.
[95] Simpson J, Sundler F, Humes DJ, Jenkins D, Wakelin D, Scholefield JH, Spiller RC. Prolonged
      elevation of galanin and tachykinin expression in mucosal and myenteric enteric nerves in trini-
      trobenzene sulphonic acid colitis. Neurogastroenterol Motil 2008;20:392–406.
[96] Sjolund K, Alumets J, Berg NO, Hakanson R, Sundler F. Enteropathy of coeliac disease in adults:
      increased number of enterochromaffin cells the duodenal mucosa. Gut 1982;23:42–8.
[97] Smiley JR, Chang KO, Hayes J, Vinje J, Saif LJ. Characterization of an enteropathogenic bovine
      calicivirus representing a potentially new calicivirus genus. J Virol 2002;76:10089–98.
[98] Söderholm JD, Yang PC, Ceponis P, Vohra A, Riddell R, Sherman PM, Perdue MH. Chronic
      stress induces mast cell-dependent bacterial adherence and initiates mucosal inflammation in
      rat intestine. Gastroenterology 2002;123:1099–108.
[99] Söderholm JD, Yates DA, Gareau MG, Yang PC, MacQueen G, Perdue MH. Neonatal maternal
      separation predisposes adult rats to colonic barrier dysfunction in response to mild stress. Am J
      Physiol Gastrointest Liver Physiol 2002;283:G1257–63.
[100] Spiller RC, Jenkins D, Thornley JP, Hebden JM, Wright T, Skinner M, et al. Increased rectal
      mucosal enteroendocrine cells, T lymphocytes, and increased gut permeability following acute
      Campylobacter enteritis and in post-dysenteric irritable bowel syndrome. Gut 2000;47:804–11.
[101] Stefanini GF, Prati E, Albini MC, Piccinini G, Capelli S, Castelli E, Mazzetti M, Gasbarrini G.
      Oral disodium cromoglycate treatment on irritable bowel syndrome: an open study on 101 sub-
      jects with diarrheic type. Am J Gastroenterol 1992;87:55–7.
[102] Steidler L, Hans W, Schotte L, Neirynck S, Obermeier F, Falk W, Fiers W, Remaut E. Treatment
      of murine colitis by *Lactococcus lactis* secreting interleukin-10. Science 2000;289:1352–5.
[103] Stoyanova II, Gulubova MV. Mast cells and inflammatory mediators in chronic ulcerative colitis.
      Acta Histochem 2002;104:185–92.
[104] Sudo N, Sawamura S, Tanaka K, Aiba Y, Kubo C, Koga Y. The requirement of intestinal bacterial
      flora for the development of an IgE production system fully susceptible to oral tolerance induc-
      tion. J Immunol 1997;159:1739–45.
[105] Szentkuti L, Riedesel H, Enss ML, Gaertner K, Von EW. Pre-epithelial mucus layer in the colon
      of conventional and germ-free rats. Histochem J 1990;22:491–7.

[106] Thornley JP, Jenkins D, Neal K, Wright T, Brough J, Spiller RC. Relationship of *Campylobacter* toxigenicity in vitro to the development of postinfectious irritable bowel syndrome. J Infect Dis 2001;184:606–9.

[107] Van Kerkhoven LA, Laheij RJ, Jansen JB. Meta-analysis: a functional polymorphism in the gene encoding for activity of the serotonin transporter protein is not associated with the irritable bowel syndrome. Aliment Pharmacol Ther 2007;26:979–86.

[108] Vandenbroucke K, Hans W, Van Huysse J, Neirynck S, Demetter P, Remaut E, Rottiers P, Steidler L. Active delivery of trefoil factors by genetically modified *Lactococcus lactis* prevents and heals acute colitis in mice. Gastroenterology 2004;127:502–13.

[109] Velin AK, Ericson AC, Braaf Y, Wallon C, Soderholm JD. Increased antigen and bacterial uptake in follicle associated epithelium induced by chronic psychological stress in rats. Gut 2004;53:494–500.

[110] Verdú EF, Bercik P, Verma-Gandhu M, Huang XX, Blennerhassett P, Jackson W, Mao Y, Wang L, Rochat F, Collins SM. Specific probiotic therapy attenuates antibiotic induced visceral hypersensitivity in mice. Gut 2006;55:182–90.

[111] Vergnolle N. Clinical relevance of proteinase activated receptors (pars) in the gut. Gut 2005;54:867–74.

[112] Verma-Gandhu M, Verdu EF, Cohen-Lyons D, Collins SM. Lymphocyte-mediated regulation of beta-endorphin in the myenteric plexus. Am J Physiol Gastrointest Liver Physiol 2007;292: G344–8.

[113] Wallon C, Yang PC, Keita AV, Ericson AC, McKay DM, Sherman PM, Perdue MH, Söderholm JD. Corticotropin-releasing hormone (CRH) regulates macromolecular permeability via mast cells in normal human colonic biopsies in vitro. Gut 2008;57:50–8.

[114] Wang H, Steeds J, Motomura Y, Deng Y, Verma-Gandhu M, El-Sharkawy RT, McLaughlin JT, Grencis RK, Khan WI. CD4+ T cell-mediated immunological control of enterochromaffin cell hyperplasia and 5-hydroxytryptamine production in enteric infection. Gut 2007;56:949–57.

[115] Wang H, Yu M, Ochani M, Amella CA, Tanovic M, Susarla S, Li JH, Wang H, Yang H, Ulloa L, et al. Nicotinic acetylcholine receptor alpha7 subunit is an essential regulator of inflammation. Nature 2003;421:384–8.

[116] Wang LH, Fang XC, Pan GZ. Bacillary dysentery as a causative factor of irritable bowel syndrome and its pathogenesis. Gut 2004;53:1096–101.

[117] Watanabe T, Kubota Y, Muto T. Substance P containing nerve fibers in rectal mucosa of ulcerative colitis. Dis Colon Rectum 1997;40:718–25.

[118] Wheatcroft J, Wakelin D, Smith A, Mahoney CR, Mawe G, Spiller R. Enterochromaffin cell hyperplasia and decreased serotonin transporter in a mouse model of postinfectious bowel dysfunction. Neurogastroenterol Motil 2005;17:863–70.

[119] Wheeler JG, Sethi D, Cowden JM, Wall PG, Rodrigues LC, Tompkins DS, Hudson MJ, Roderick PJ. Study of infectious intestinal disease in England: rates in the community, presenting to general practice, and reported to national surveillance. The Infectious Intestinal Disease Study Executive. BMJ 1999;318:1046–50.

[120] Whorwell PJ, Altringer L, Morel J, Bond Y, Charbonneau D, O'Mahony L, Kiely B, Shanahan F, Quigley EM. Efficacy of an encapsulated probiotic Bifidobacterium infantis 35624 in women with irritable bowel syndrome. Am J Gastroenterol 2006;101:1581–90.

[121] Xia Y, Hu HZ, Liu S, Ren J, Zafirov DH, Wood JD. IL-1beta and IL-6 excite neurons and suppress nicotinic and noradrenergic neurotransmission in guinea pig enteric nervous system. J Clin Invest 1999;103:1309–16.

[122] Yeo A, Boyd P, Lumsden S, Saunders T, Handley A, Stubbins M, Knaggs A, Asquith S, Taylor I, Bahari B, et al. Association between a functional polymorphism in the serotonin transporter gene and diarrhoea predominant irritable bowel syndrome in women. Gut 2004;53:1452–8.

[123] Yiangou Y, Facer P, Dyer NH, Chan CL, Knowles C, Williams NS, Anand P. Vanilloid receptor 1 immunoreactivity in inflamed human bowel. Lancet 2001;357:1338–9.

[124] Yoshioka H, Iseki Ki, Fujita K. Development and differences of intestinal flora in the neonatal period in breast-fed and bottle-fed infants. Pediatrics 1983;72:317–21.

[125] Zoetendal EG, Akkermans AD, De Vos WM. Temperature gradient gel electrophoresis analysis of 16s rRNA from human fecal samples reveals stable and host-specific communities of active bacteria. Appl Environ Microbiol 1998;64:3854–9.

[126] Zund G, Madara JL, Dzus AL, Awtrey CS, Colgan SP. Interleukin-4 and interleukin-13 differentially regulate epithelial chloride secretion. J Biol Chem 1996;271:7460–4.
[127] Zyrek AA, Cichon C, Helms S, Enders C, Sonnenborn U, Schmidt MA. Molecular mechanisms underlying the probiotic effects of *Escherichia coli* Nissle 1917 involve ZO-2 and PKCzeta redistribution resulting in tight junction and epithelial barrier repair. Cell Microbiol 2007;9:804–16.

Correspondence to: Robin Spiller, MD, FRCP Nottingham Digestive Diseases Centre, Biomedical Research Unit, School of Medical and Surgical Sciences, Queen's Medical Centre, Nottingham NG7 2UH, United Kingdom. Email: robin. spiller@nottingham.ac.uk.

Visceral Hypersensitivity

17

Fernando Cervero[a] and G.F. Gebhart[b]

[a]Anesthesia Research Unit and Alan Edwards Centre for Research on Pain,
McGill University, Montreal, Quebec, Canada; [b]Department of Anesthesiology,
Center for Pain Research, University of Pittsburgh, Pittsburgh, Pennsylvania, USA

The neuroanatomical complexity and characteristic features of visceral pain are unique among tissues of the body. In addition, the viscera are associated with a large number of functional disorders characterized by hypersensitivity in the absence of a pathobiological explanation for the discomfort and pain that patients experience. Typically, patients with functional visceral disorders have relatively lower thresholds for response to provocative visceral stimuli (e.g., balloon distension of hollow organs). They also show increased sensitivity during normal organ function and exhibit increased tenderness in expanded areas of somatic referral. These features of functional visceral disorders suggest nervous system alterations in the processing of visceral stimuli and their central interpretation. Experimental investigations have thus addressed the contributions of both peripheral and central components of visceral sensory processing, revealing roles for the peripheral sensory innervation of the viscera as well as for spinal and supraspinal sites of processing of visceral sensory information.

Visceral Sensory Innervation

Each internal organ is innervated by two nerves that share some functions, but have significant differences in function as well. Differences in the location, distribution, and sensitivities of receptive endings in viscera are more complex than in skin, muscle, or joints. Moreover, accumulating evidence suggests significant differences in response to experimental inflammation between the two nerves innervating the same organ. In consequence, targeting one nerve innervating an organ as opposed to the other may provide more appropriate strategies for management of discomfort and pain.

The viscera are also characterized by having an intrinsic innervation. This intrinsic innervation has been most widely documented and studied for the gastrointestinal (GI) tract (i.e., the enteric nervous system). The enteric nervous system of the GI tract is important in normal motility, secretion, and absorption, but also in gastric and colonic reflexes. It has long been assumed that the extrinsic sensory innervation and intrinsic innervation of organs interact, but the relationship and interaction between these independent nervous systems is not well understood, either anatomically or functionally. Accordingly, despite what is likely to be a contribution from the intrinsic nervous system to the extrinsic sensory events arising from the viscera, there is little information on the potential role of the intrinsic innervation in either the development or maintenance of visceral hypersensitivity.

Visceral Nociceptors

There is a long and interesting history to our present-day appreciation of the characteristics of the sensory innervation of the viscera. Several points bear emphasis. First, most of the information conveyed to the central nervous system (CNS) by the visceral afferent innervation is not consciously appreciated. Input from the heart, lungs, vasculature, and GI tract that is associated with normal function is not commonly perceived. Visceral events that are associated with awareness include nausea, dyspnea, bloating, fullness, and organ filling or distension. Second, it is assumed that only a small proportion of the visceral afferent innervation conveys information of potential nociceptive character, but the encoding properties and sensitization of the visceral innervation suggest that the proportion of afferents that contribute to discomfort and pain may include a larger proportion of the visceral innervation. The focus of much investigation has thus been on mechanosensation, with the use of stretch/tension or distending stimuli. It has been widely documented that most, if not all, mechanosensitive endings in the hollow organs that respond to stretch or distension also respond to chemical and/or thermal (hot or cold) stimuli and are thus polymodal in character. It is not known with the same degree of certainty whether visceral afferent endings that respond to nutrients, for example, also respond to either mechanical or thermal stimuli.

Mechanosensation

With respect to visceral nociception, and given the research focus on mechanosensation, it is clear that virtually all the hollow organs studied across a variety of animal species contain mechanosensitive nerve endings with both low and high thresholds for activation by stretch/distension. Studies that have supported this knowledge have typically employed teased fiber preparations, in which small filaments from visceral nerves (e.g., the pelvic nerve innervating the colon or bladder, or the splanchnic innervation of the small bowel) are teased apart with fine forceps until one or a few afferent fibers can be studied in response to stimuli applied to the organ (e.g., see Fig. 1). These studies have principally been carried out in situ, but in vitro and ex vivo preparations have also contributed to our understanding of visceral mechanosensitivity.

The accumulated evidence suggests that 70–80% of the mechanosensitive innervation of the organs studied have low thresholds for response. That is, response thresholds are in the physiological (filling) range, usually 2 or 3 mm Hg distension. Interestingly, many low-threshold mechanosensitive visceral afferents continue to encode mechanical stimulus intensity well into the noxious range (typically at intensities greater than 30 mm Hg distension; see [57]). The smaller proportion of mechanosensitive visceral afferent fibers (20–30%) have high thresholds for response, typically in the noxious range (i.e., at or greater than 30 mm Hg distension). These high-threshold mechanosensitive fibers also continue to encode

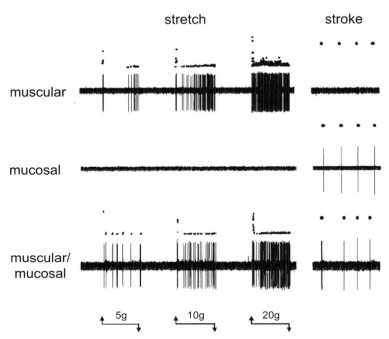

Fig. 1. Examples of mechanosensitive urinary bladder afferents recorded from the mouse pelvic nerve. About 60% of afferents, designated "muscular," respond to graded stretch of the bladder, 10% respond to stroking of the mucosal surface (but not to stretch), and 15% respond to both stretch and mucosal stroking, designated "muscular/mucosal." Adapted from Xu and Gebhart [66], with permission. Similar muscular, muscular/mucosal, and mucosal afferent endings have been recorded in the pelvic nerve innervation of the mouse colon (see Brierley et al. [10]).

stimulus intensity in the noxious range. One can imagine that the low-threshold mechanosensitive proportion of the population is involved in contributing input to the CNS at low filling pressures that may not be consciously perceived; however, as organ filling continues, input from these visceral afferent fibers is consciously perceived. With respect to the smaller proportion of high-threshold afferent fibers within the mechanosensitive population, it is supposed that they play a role in acute discomfort and pain arising from the viscera.

It may seem unusual that low-threshold mechanosensitive endings in the viscera encode into the noxious range, but so too do afferents that innervate joints and skin, including human skin (e.g., see [63]). Thus, it is becoming increasingly evident that a proportion of cutaneous nociceptors have low thresholds for response to mechanical stimuli that are clearly non-noxious, but also encode well into the noxious range and are nociceptors (see reference [12] for review).

Sensitization and Sleeping Nociceptors

A distinguishing characteristic of cutaneous nociceptors is their ability to become sensitized. By sensitization is meant an increase in response to a noxious intensity of stimulation, frequently associated with a decrease in response threshold, and occasionally with development of ongoing or spontaneous activity. Non-nociceptors do not become sensitized. Interestingly, many, if not most, of the low-threshold mechanosensitive afferents in the viscera, as well as the high-threshold afferents, exhibit the property of sensitization (see Figs. 2 and 3). This finding suggests that visceral hypersensitivity, and thus discomfort and pain, depend in part on mechanosensitive endings that have either low or high thresholds for response.

A third potential contributor to discomfort and pain associated with visceral hypersensitivity is the "silent" or "sleeping" nociceptor. Silent nociceptors are those that are mechanically insensitive, even to high intensities of mechanical stimulation, but awaken or become active in the presence of tissue insult. In this circumstance, they acquire mechanosensitivity as well as ongoing activity, and their potential contribution to visceral sensation is significant. In human skin, approximately 20% of C-fiber nociceptors are of the silent variety [63]. If approximately one-fifth of the afferent C-fiber input is normally silent, tissue insult that awakens these nociceptors has the potential to contribute a significant amount of new information to nociceptive processing in the CNS. Between 35% and 80% of the visceral afferent population is estimated to be of the silent or sleeping variety. These estimates suggest that the proportion of silent afferents within the visceral afferent population is greater than among cutaneous afferent nociceptors. However, a rigorous and unbiased strategy to study visceral silent nociceptors has yet to be presented. Thus, while the potential exists for visceral silent afferents to contribute disproportionately to visceral pain, relative to the contribution of silent afferents in the skin to cutaneous pain, it remains to be established whether the proportion of silent visceral afferents is as great as current estimates suggest.

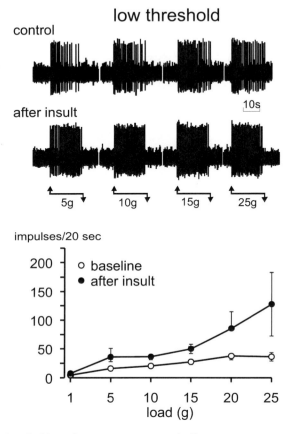

Fig. 2. Low-threshold mechanosensitive visceral afferents sensitize. An example from the pelvic nerve innervation of the urinary bladder is presented at the top, and a data summary is given below. Note that low-threshold responses to stretch in this in vitro preparation are apparent at an applied load of 1 g. Responses before (control/baseline) and 5 minutes after exposure for 2 minutes of the afferent terminal to an inflammatory soup illustrate that response magnitude is significantly increased by exposure to the chemical soup. Adapted from Xu and Gebhart [66], with permission.

Because many low- and high-threshold mechanosensitive visceral afferents can encode into the noxious range and also become sensitized, their contribution to the development of visceral hypersensitivity appears to be significant. Additional contributions to visceral hypersensitivity in functional bowel disorders may arise from "awakened" silent visceral afferents.

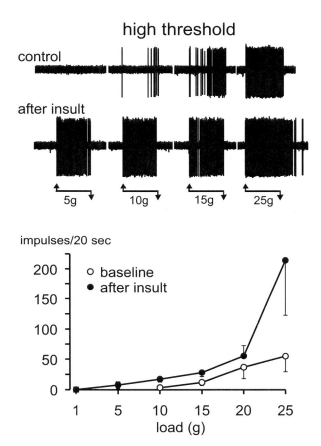

Fig. 3. High-threshold mechanosensitive visceral afferents sensitize. An example from the pelvic nerve innervation of the urinary bladder is presented at the top, and a data summary is given below. Note that high-threshold responses to stretch in this in vitro preparation are not apparent until a load of 10 g is applied. Responses before (control/baseline) and 5 minutes after exposure for 2 minutes of the afferent terminal to an inflammatory soup illustrate that response magnitude is significantly increased by exposure to the chemical soup. Adapted from Xu and Gebhart [66], with permission.

Functional Differences

Mechanosensitivity has been the focus of study of visceral afferents and is the foundation of most of our understanding to date. Relatively little is know about chemosensation, at least with respect to visceral nociceptive mechanisms. Accordingly, considerable effort has been directed toward investigating potential mediators and modulators of visceral mechanosensation and visceral hypersensitivity. With respect to mechanosensitivity, and to a lesser extent chemosensitivity, it is becoming clear that the two nerves innervating the same organ, although they have overlapping functions, also clearly have distinct functions. For example, studies of mouse bladder and mouse colon have shown that the topographical distribution of receptive endings in the organs differs between the splanchnic and pelvic nerve innervations and that the proportions of mechanosensitive receptive endings similarly differ between the two pathways [10,66]. In the splanchnic innervation of the mouse colon, receptive endings are predominantly located on the mesenteric attachment and in the serosa; receptive endings responsive to circumferential stretch are relatively few. In contrast, there are no receptive endings on the mesenteric attachment in the pelvic nerve innervation of the mouse colon, and circumferential stretch activates nearly half of the mechanosensitive afferents studied. In the mouse urinary bladder, similar differences were reported between the splanchnic and pelvic innervations of the organ (see Fig. 1 for examples).

Whereas mechanical stimuli commonly produce pain and discomfort in the GI and urinary tracts, lower-airway and cardiac pain is primarily initiated by chemical stimuli. A variety of chemicals that have been studied in the GI tract—including bradykinin, adenosine triphosphate (ATP), serotonin (5-HT), and capsaicin—are reported to activate serosal and mesenteric receptive endings in the splanchnic innervation of the colon, but they do not generally affect afferent endings in the pelvic innervation of the colon. For example, Brierley et al. [9] reported that 40% of serosal splanchnic afferents in the mouse colon responded to application of 1 mM α,β-methylene adenosine 5-triphosphate (α,β-meATP) to the receptive ending, an effect that was concentration-dependent and reversed by 100 µM of the nonselective P2X antagonist pyridoxl 5-phosphate 6-azophenyl-2,4-disulphonic acid (PPADS). Significantly fewer pelvic nerve serosal afferents (7%) responded to α,β-meATP. Capsaicin (3 µM) excited serosal afferents in both the splanchnic (61%) and pelvic (47%) innervation of the colon. Brierley et al. also noted that α,β-meATP or capsaicin recruited mechanically insensitive serosal afferents, almost exclusively in the splanchnic innervation. In the rat, Coldwell et al. [14] reported that

58% of colonic serosal and mesenteric afferents responded to application of 5-HT (10^{-4} M), a percentage that increased to 88% during acute colonic inflammation. Undem's laboratory has studied mechanisms and mediators of lower-airway pain (e.g., [26,36,39,61]); Pan, Longhurst, and colleagues have examined mechanisms of ischemia- and hypoxia-driven pain (e.g., [47–49]); and Holzer's group has provided evidence of vagal chemonociception (e.g., [29,30,64]; see also [7,25] for additional discussion).

Because mechanosensitivity has been a focus of study, molecules that contribute to visceral mechanosensitivity have come to the forefront of research attention. Such research has been driven in large part by the availability of mice with genetic deletions of voltage- or ligand-gated channels of presumed importance to either mechanosensation or hypersensitivity. Researchers have studied the transient receptor potential vanilloid 1 (TRPV1) receptor and TRPV4 receptors, as well as acid-sensing ion channels (ASICs), purinergic P2X receptors, protease-activated receptors, and voltage-gated sodium channels. Generally, knockout strategies have produced mice in which either mechanosensitivity to organ stimulation is reduced or sensitization is altered, or both. For example, TRPV1 knockout mice exhibit reduced responses to colon distension and correspondingly reduced responses of afferent fibers to circumferential stretch [35]. Deletion of TRPV1 also impairs afferent fiber detection of mechanical stimuli in the jejunum [52] and urinary bladder [8]. Similarly, TRPV4 knockout mice show attenuated afferent fiber mechanosensitivity and reduced responses to colon distension [11]. In support of these findings, application of TRPV1 or TRPV4 agonists or antagonists to receptive endings in the colon activated or antagonized, respectively, responses in these experiments.

Studies of ASICs have established that the absence of ASIC3 diminishes mechanosensitivity in gastroesophageal afferents [46] and causes reduced responses to colon distension as well as sensitization of stretch-sensitive pelvic nerve afferent fibers innervating the mouse colon [35]. ASICs 1 and 2 have been investigated as well, but results are less consistent than with ASIC3. For example, the absence of ASIC1a increases mechanosensitivity, whereas the absence of ACIC2 has differential effects depending upon the target within the GI tract.

The role of P2X receptors has been most widely studied in association with the urinary bladder. Micturition reflexes and response to bladder inflammation are attenuated in P2X3 and P2X2/3 knockout mice. P2X receptors are also important in colon mechanosensitivity and hypersensitivity [65], and P2X3 knockout mice show reduced sensitivity to colon distension [59].

Another major target has been the voltage-gated sodium channel $Na_V1.8$, which appears to have a distribution limited to nociceptor cell bodies in dorsal root ganglia. Laird et al. [37] have reported deficits in visceral nociception in $Na_V1.8$ knockout mice, as shown by reduced responses to intracolonic capsaicin or mustard oil administration as well as changes in referred hypersensitivity. In other studies, $Na_V1.8$ knockout mice did not exhibit increases in visceral sensory neuron excitability following jejunitis, but they did show the expected increase in excitability when a different voltage-gated sodium channel, $Na_V1.9$, was knocked out [28].

Central Mechanisms of Visceral Hypersensitivity

Every form of visceral pain produces an additional form of discomfort characterized by increased pain sensitivity in a remote, and usually superficial, area from the damaged or inflamed viscus. These areas of referred hyperalgesia are maintained by the enhanced afferent drive from the primary focus and are the consequence of altered sensory processing by the CNS. The patterns of referred hyperalgesia are closely associated with the originating focus and are therefore a valuable clinical tool for the diagnosis of many forms of visceral disease.

The most popular interpretation of the mechanisms of referred hyperalgesia is based on the idea of central sensitization, whereby CNS neurons become sensitized by the enhanced afferent drive from the primary focus. The consequences of this hyperexcitability would be enhanced pain sensitivity from the originating viscus, a general increase in motor and autonomic reactions, and the appearance of areas of hyperalgesia in the somatic areas whose afferent innervation converges with that of the damaged viscus in the spinal cord. Central sensitization is the result of synaptic plasticity and is a memory trace of previous painful stimuli (for review, see [33,54]). A number of potential molecular targets have recently been associated with the process of CNS sensitization and synaptic plasticity. Some of them have been specifically identified as being related to the development of viscerally induced hyperalgesic states.

Potentiation of spinal nociceptive transmission by synaptic delivery of AMPA (GluR1) receptors, via a pathway dependent on N-methyl-D-aspartate (NMDA) receptors and Ca^{2+}/calmodulin-dependent protein kinase II (CaMKII), may underlie certain forms of hyperalgesia. Galan et al. [21] have described a delivery of GluR1 receptors to the membrane of dorsal horn neurons following stimulation of visceral nociceptive afferents (Fig. 4A). They observed that this trafficking requires CaMKII activity, just like the process of long-term potentiation in hippocampal neurons [15,43]. In addition, blockade of the exocytotic process responsible for the trafficking of GluR1 receptors also reduced the referred abdominal hyperalgesia induced by the intracolonic instillation of capsaicin [21]. Therefore, trafficking of GluR1 receptors is a prime candidate for the enhancement of synaptic transmission in the spinal cord induced by a visceral noxious stimulus as well as for the resulting referred hyperalgesia.

Mitogen-activated protein (MAP) kinases, also known as extracellular signal-regulated kinases (ERKs), are members of a family of serine/threonine protein kinases that mediate intracellular signal transduction in response to a variety of stimuli. Current evidence suggests a role for ERKs in nociceptive processing in the spinal cord in models of somatic pain as well as in persistent hyperalgesic states [22,32,53]. ERKs also play an important role in spinal processing of visceral pain, particularly in the development of referred visceral hyperalgesia [20]. Intracolonic instillation of capsaicin, a process that generates robust and prolonged referred abdominal hyperalgesia [38], induces a rapid activation of ERK1/2 in the lumbosacral spinal cord (Fig. 4B). ERK activation induced by intracolonic capsaicin correlates well with the expression of hyperalgesia because treatment with the ERK inhibitor U0126 produces a dose-dependent inhibition of referred hyperalgesia but not of the

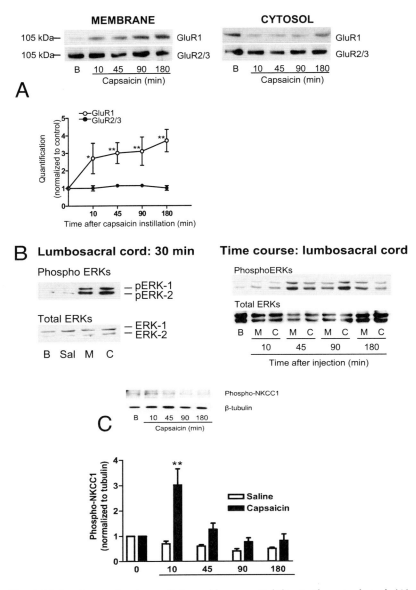

Fig. 4. Molecular mechanisms of visceral hyperexcitability in the spinal cord. (A) AMPA trafficking induced by a visceral noxious stimulus. Top: Time course of subcellular distribution of the AMPA receptors GluR1 and GluR2/3 in the plasma membrane fraction and in the cytosolic fraction. The graph below shows quantification of GluR1 and GluR2/3 normalized to levels detected in control spinal tissue. Asterisks indicate groups that were significantly different from control levels (*P < 0.05, **P < 0.01). Data from Galan et al.

spontaneous pain response induced by capsaicin instillation [20]. These data show that ERK activation plays an important and specific role in the transcriptional events underlying the maintenance of referred visceral hyperalgesia.

Recently, several studies have suggested a role for the homeostasis of chloride ions in primary afferents and spinal cord neurons in the generation and maintenance of hyperalgesic states, including those of visceral origin [50]. Changes in the intracellular concentration of chloride in neurons of the nociceptive pathway can transform the actions of GABA from inhibitory (when the intracellular concentration of chloride is low) to excitatory (when the concentration is higher). The intracellular chloride concentration is regulated by chloride cotransporters, which have now become the object of scientific scrutiny as potential candidates for manipulation of pain sensitivity and especially of hyperalgesic states. Galan and Cervero [19] found that intracolonic capsaicin induces in vivo trafficking of the NKCC1 (Na^+-K^+-$2Cl^-$-1) cotransporter from the cytosol to the plasma membrane of neurons in the spinal cord of adult mice. The peak times of such trafficking correspond to the plateau phase of the referred mechanical hyperalgesia evoked in the abdominal region by the visceral stimulus [38]. Galan and Cervero [19] also showed that intracolonic capsaicin evokes a fast and transient phosphorylation of the NKCC1 cotransporter 10 minutes after the stimulus, which returns toward basal levels 90 minutes after treatment (Fig. 4C). Therefore, phosphorylation and trafficking of NKCC1 could contribute to the initial development and subsequent maintenance of capsaicin-induced visceral hyperalgesia, respectively.

[21]. (B) Role of extracellular signal-regulated kinases (ERKs) in visceral hyperalgesia. Left: Western blots of lumbosacral spinal tissue 30 minutes after intracolonic instillation of saline (Sal), mustard oil (M), or capsaicin (C). In all cases, the two bands shown represent ERK-1 (p44) and ERK-2 (p42). Right: Time course of pERK1/2 activation in lumbosacral segments after mustard oil or capsaicin instillation. Data from Galan et al. [20]. (C) Intracolonic capsaicin induces NKCC1 cotransporter phosphorylation. Representative Western blot from membrane protein extracts showing the time course of NKCC1 phosphorylation. Membranes were re-incubated with β-tubulin as a loading control. The graph below shows the quantification of phospho-NKCC1 normalized to β-tubulin values after intracolonic capsaicin. Asterisks indicate groups that were significantly different from control levels (**P < 0.01). Data from Galan et al. [19]. In all immunoblots, the lane marked "B" contains control (basal) tissue.

Central Hypersensitivity and Functional Abdominal Pain

There are two kinds of visceral pain: organic and functional. Organic pain is the consequence of a traumatic, inflammatory, or degenerative lesion of the viscera or is produced by tumors that impinge on an organ's sensory innervation. This kind of pain is due to sensitization of the local sensory afferents, and to the processing of these enhanced signals by CNS mechanisms that amplify them and maintain an increased excitability of central neurons [4]. On the other hand, functional pain appears in the absence of demonstrable pathology of the viscera or of their associated nerves. It is particularly prevalent in women and tends to be located in the abdominal and pelvic regions [13,17]. Patients complain of discomfort, bloating, or pain, but after extensive clinical investigations nothing is found in the abdominal viscera that could explain the sensory symptoms.

Functional pain is commonly interpreted as a consequence of hypersensitivity of visceral nociceptive pathways, either of the sensory receptors in the periphery or of the central neurons [1]. However, the pathophysiology of visceral hypersensitivity is far from clear, and there is ongoing discussion as to whether there is a peripheral focus that can be identified at the origin of visceral hypersensitivity [6] or if the process is due to cognitive and affective factors that alter central processing of visceral sensory signals [5]. Because functional abdominal pain conditions are highly prevalent in women, it has been suggested that the pain correlates with the levels of circulating estrogens rather than with an organic disease of an abdominal or pelvic organ [2,40].

There is some controversy in the literature as to whether estrogen has pronociceptive or antinociceptive properties in humans and animals. It is well documented that there are gender differences in pain sensitivity, with females showing increased sensitivity to pain and a higher incidence of certain chronic pain syndromes [18]. These observations have led some investigators to believe that estrogen is a pronociceptive hormone, responsible for the increased pain sensitivity seen in females. However, this notion has been difficult to prove in women because the data have generally shown an antinociceptive action of estrogen, both in normal females and in those suffering from chronic pain [31,60,68]. A comprehensive review of the literature on the relationship between the menstrual cycle and pain sensitivity in humans [58] determined that numerous methodological inconsistencies made it difficult to draw conclusions about the relationship of female sex hormones with pain perception.

Animal studies have also produced contradictory results regarding the effects of estrogen on pain sensitivity. Studies using a variety of acute noxious stimuli and acute administration of estrogen have reported an increase in the visceromotor and neuronal responses to colorectal distension [34], a sensitization of visceral afferents that innervate the uterine cervix [42,62], and an amplification of pain responses to uterine cervical distension [67]. On the other hand, there are also reports of increases in pain sensitivity in ovariectomized (OVX) rats that could be reversed or reduced by exogenous administration of estrogen. Gaumond et al [23,24] observed an antihyperalgesic effect of 17β-estradiol implanted pellets on the interphase between phase 1 and phase 2 of the formalin test in OVX rats, a result that was confirmed and extended in a recent report from another laboratory [45], which also used the formalin test. These latter authors concluded that estradiol replacement in OVX rats is antihyperalgesic rather than antinociceptive, because 17β-estradiol does not change acute pain thresholds in normal animals [44]. Another study found that the selective estrogen receptor-β agonist ERB-041 is antihyperalgesic in rat models of chemical and inflammatory pain [41]. At a more mechanistic level, studies have shown that estradiol administration to OVX rats increases the concentration of μ-opioid receptor protein in the hypothalamus, as demonstrated with both immunohistochemistry and mRNA [16,27,51]. Similar increases in enkephalin mRNA expression have been reported in rats shortly after estrogen administration [3], which, taken together with the previous reports, would indicate that estrogen can increase endogenous antinociception and thus reduce pain sensitivity.

Over the last few years we have developed an animal model of functional abdominal pain in OVX adult mice [55,56]. These animals develop a chronic abdominal hyperalgesic state after ovariectomy (Fig. 5), characterized by mechanical hyperalgesia and allodynia restricted to the abdominal and pelvic regions and to the hind limbs but sparing the rest

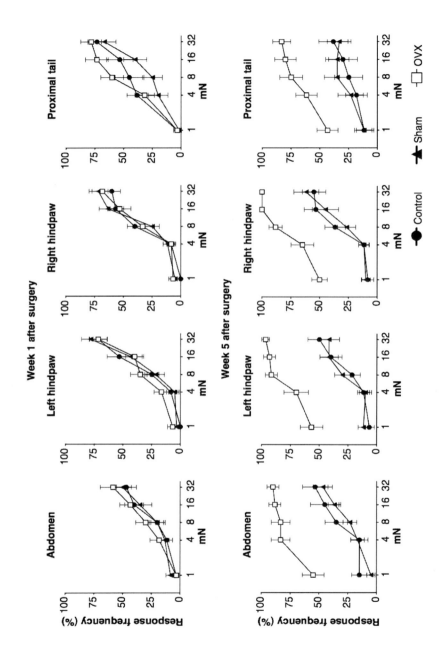

A

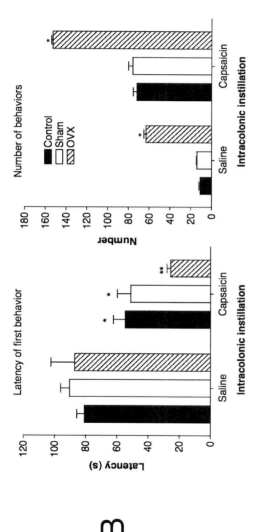

Fig. 5. Abdominal hyperalgesia induced by ovariectomy in adult mice. (A) Responses to mechanical stimulation (with von Frey hairs) of the abdomen, hindpaws, and proximal tail in ovariectomized (OVX), sham-operated (Sham), and control mice. The same animals were tested 1 week (top graphs) and 5 weeks (bottom graphs) after surgery. Significant differences ($P < 0.05$) were detected on week 5 after surgery between OVX animals and the other two groups. (B) Visceral pain and hyperalgesia. Latency of the first behavior (left) and number of behavioral reactions (right) (licking of the abdomen, stretching, and abdominal retractions) evoked by intracolonic instillation of saline (0.9%) or capsaicin (0.1%). Asterisks on the latency graph indicate the groups that were significantly different from their respective saline-treated control (*$P < 0.05$, **$P < 0.01$). The asterisks on the number of behaviors graph indicate that OVX animals showed a significantly higher ($P < 0.05$) number of behaviors when compared to sham and control mice. Data from Sanoja and Cervero [55].

of the body. Thermal and visceral hyperalgesia are also present in these animals. This hyperalgesic state appears 4 to 5 weeks after ovariectomy and persists for several weeks thereafter. A particularly prominent feature of this model is a robust visceral hyperalgesia of early onset and long duration (Fig. 5).

A striking aspect of the OVX-induced hyperalgesic state is its sensitivity to estrogen replacement therapy. Administration of exogenous estrogens to OVX animals by means of slow-release pellets containing 17-β estradiol can either prevent the development of the hyperalgesic state or reverse it back to normal once it has developed (Fig. 6). Because of the clinical features of the hyperalgesia and its sensitivity to exogenous estrogen, we have suggested that OVX-induced hyperalgesia mimics the process that underlies functional abdominal pain disorders in women, particularly those in which no primary lesion of an abdominal or pelvic organ can be found and which have slow onset, hormonal modulation, and a trend toward chronification [55,56]).

A detailed examination of the literature suggests that acute administration of estrogen tested against an acute noxious procedure results in enhanced nociception, whereas long-term loss of estrogen—such as after OVX—produces an hyperalgesic state that can be prevented and reversed by exogenous estrogen. Perhaps these different effects could be mediated by the different types of estrogen receptor described in the brain and the spinal cord. The chronic effects could thus be the result of the genomic effects of nuclear estrogen receptors, and the acute actions could be

Fig. 6. Estrogen dependency of the hyperalgesic state induced by ovariectomy (OVX). ⟶
Top graphs: Responses to mechanical stimulation (von Frey hairs) of the abdomen in ovariectomized mice to which slow-release pellets containing 17β-estradiol (OVX+17β-estradiol) or the vehicle only (OVX) had been implanted 1 week after surgery. The same animals were tested 1 week and 5 weeks after surgery. Note that estrogen replacement after ovariectomy prevents the development of the hyperalgesic state. Bottom graphs: Estrogen reversal of mechanical hyperalgesia. Data are presented as the responses to mechanical stimulation of the abdomen (with von Frey hairs), in control, sham-operated, and OVX mice to which slow release pellets containing 17β-estradiol (OVX + estrogen) or the vehicle only (OVX) had been implanted at the end of week 5 after OVX. The same animals were tested 1, 5, 6, and 10 weeks after surgery. Note that all OVX mice develop a hyperalgesic state by week 5 after OVX. However, the group treated with estrogen at the end of week 5 (but not those treated with placebo) reverts to normal within 1 week. Data from Sanoja and Cervero [56].

Abdominal mechanical hyperalgesia: estrogen prevention

Abdominal mechanical hyperalgesia: estrogen reversal

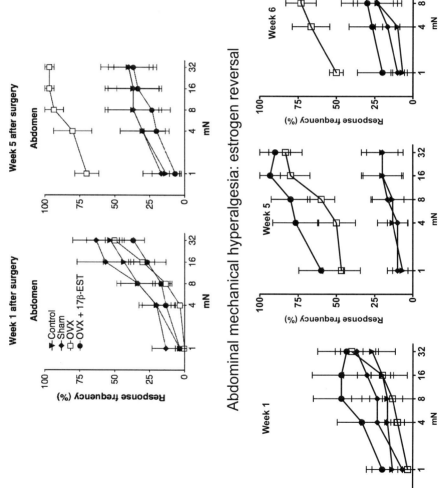

mediated by faster estrogen membrane receptors coupled to intracellular second-messenger pathways.

Concluding Remarks

All forms of visceral pain include the development of a robust hyperalgesic state that originates from the internal organ that has been damaged or inflamed and is referred to a remote and superficial region of the body. Hyperalgesia is the most prominent feature of the visceral pain process and is the expression of hypersensitivity of the pain pathway induced by the sensitization of the peripheral receptors that signal visceral sensory events or of the neurons that transmit and process this sensory information to the CNS. All kinds of visceral sensory receptors can be sensitized, acquiring enhanced, and sometimes novel, responsiveness to peripheral stimuli. On the other hand, a process of synaptic plasticity, of which several molecular components have already been identified, mediates the central amplification of the visceral afferent signals that leads to the hypersensitivity of central neurons.

In addition to the hyperalgesia triggered as a consequence of the injury or inflammation of an internal organ, there are also functional pain states, characterized by pain reported from the abdominal or pelvic cavities but in the absence of a demonstrable peripheral cause. Although not much is known about the causes of such states, it is thought that hypersensitivity of peripheral sensory receptors or an enhanced responsiveness of central visceral pathways may be responsible for the pain. Circulating sex hormones, particularly estrogen, may also have a role in the development and maintenance of functional pain syndromes in women.

References

[1]   Al-Chaer ED, Traub RJ. Biological basis of visceral pain: recent developments. Pain 2002;96:221–5.

[2]   Aloisi AM, Craft RM, Marchand S. The effects of gonadal hormones on pain. In: Flor H, Kaslo E, Dostrovsky JO, editors. Proceedings of the 11th World Congress on Pain. Seattle: IASP Press; 2006. p. 301–9.

[3]   Amandusson A, Hallbeck M, Hallbeck AL, Hermanson O, Blomqvist A. Estrogen-induced alterations of spinal cord enkephalin gene expression. Pain 1999;83:243–8.

[4]   Anand P, Aziz Q, Willert R, van Oudenhove L. Peripheral and central mechanisms of visceral sensitization in man. NeurogastroenterolMotil 2007;19:29–46.

[5]   Aziz Q. Visceral hypersensitivity: fact or fiction. Gastroenterology 2006;131:661−4.
[6]   Bercik P, Verdu EF, Collins SM. Is irritable bowel syndrome a low-grade inflammatory bowel disease? Gastroenterol Clin North Am 2005;34:235−7.
[7]   Bielefeldt K, Gebhart GF. Visceral pain: basic mechanisms. In: Koltzenburg M, McMahon SB, editors. Textbook of pain, 5th edition. London: Churchill-Livingstone; 2005. p. 721−36.
[8]   Birder LA, Nakamura Y, Kiss S, Nealen ML, Barrick S, Kanai AJ, Wang E, Ruiz G, De Groat WC, Apodaca G, et al. Altered urinary bladder function in mice lacking the vanilloid receptor TRPV1. NatNeurosci 2002;5:856−60.
[9]   Brierley SM, Carter R, Jones W, III, Xu LJ, Robinson DR, Hicks GA, Gebhart GE, Blackshaw LA. Differential chemosensory function and receptor expression of splanchnic and pelvic colonic afferents in mice. J Physiol 2005;567:267−81.
[10] Brierley SM, Jones RCW, III, Gebhart GF, Blackshaw LA. Splanchnic and pelvic mechanosensory afferents signal different qualities of colonic stimuli in mice. Gastroenterology 2004;127:166−78.
[11] Brierley SM, Page AJ, Hughes PA, Adam B, Liebregts T, Cooper NJ, Holtmann G, Liedtke W, Blackshaw LA. Selective role for TRPV4 ion channels in visceral sensory pathways. Gastroenterology 2008;134:2059−69.
[12] Cervero F. Sensory innervation of the viscera: peripheral basis of visceral pain. Physiol Rev 1994;74:95−138.
[13] Clouse RE, Mayer EA, Aziz Q, Drossman DA, Dumitrascu DL, Mînnikes H, Naliboff BD. Functional abdominal pain syndrome. Gastroenterology 2006;130:1492−7.
[14] Coldwell JR, Phillis BD, Sutherland K, Howarth GS, Blackshaw LA. Increased responsiveness of rat colonic splanchnic afferents to 5-HT after inflammation and recovery. J Physiol 2007;579:203−13.
[15] Contractor A, Heinemann SF. Glutamate receptor trafficking in synaptic plasticity. Sci STKE 2002;156:RE14.
[16] Dondi D, Limonta P, Maggi R, Piva F. Effects of ovarian hormones on brain opioid binding sites in castrated female rats. Am J Physiol 1992;263:E507−11.
[17] Drossman DA. Functional abdominal pain syndrome. Clin Gastroenterol Hepatol 2004;2:353−65.
[18] Fillingim RB, Ness TJ. Sex-related hormonal influences on pain and analgesic responses. Neurosci Biobehav Rev 2000;24:485−501.
[19] Galan A, Cervero F. Painful stimuli induce in vivo phosphorylation and membrane mobilization of mouse spinal cord NKCC1 co-transporter. Neuroscience 2005;133:245−52.
[20] Galan A, Cervero F, Laird JM. Extracellular signaling-regulated kinase-1 and -2 (ERK 1/2) mediate referred hyperalgesia in a murine model of visceral pain. Brain Res Mol Brain Res 2003;116:126−34.
[21] Galan A, Laird JMA, Cervero F. In vivo recruitment by painful stimuli of AMPA receptor subunits to the plasma membrane of spinal cord neurons. Pain 2004;112:315−23.
[22] Galan A, Lopez-Garcia JA, Cervero F, Laird JMA. Activation of spinal extracellular signaling-regulated kinase-1 and -2 by intraplantar carrageenan in rodents. Neurosci Lett 2002;322:37−40.
[23] Gaumond I, Arsenault P, Marchand S. The role of sex hormones on formalin-induced nociceptive responses. Brain Res 2002;958:139−45.
[24] Gaumond I, Arsenault P, Marchand S. Specificity of female and male sex hormones on excitatory and inhibitory phases of formalin-induced nociceptive responses. Brain Res 2005;1052:105−11.
[25] Gebhart GF, Bielefeldt K. Visceral pain. In: Bushnell MC, Basbaum AI, editors. The senses: a comprehensive reference, Vol. 5. Pain. San Diego: Academic Press; 2008. p. 543−70.
[26] Gracely RH, Undem BJ, Banzett RB. Cough, pain and dyspnoea: similarities and differences. Pulm Pharmacol Ther 2007;20:433−7.
[27] Hammer RP, Jr., Bridges RS. Preoptic area opioids and opiate receptors increase during pregnancy and decrease during lactation. Brain Res 1987;420:48−56.
[28] Hillsley K, Lin JH, Stanisz A, Grundy D, Aerssens J, Peeters PJ, Moechars D, Coulie B, Stead RH. Dissecting the role of sodium currents in visceral sensory neurons in a model of chronic hyperexcitability using $Na_v1.8$ and $Na_v1.9$ null mice. J Physiol 2006;576:257−67.
[29] Holzer P. Role of visceral afferent neurons in mucosal inflammation and defense. Curr Opin Pharmacol 2007;7:563−9.

[30] Holzer P. Taste receptors in the gastrointestinal tract. V. Acid sensing in the gastrointestinal tract. Am J Physiol Gastrointest Liver Physiol 2007;292:G699–705.

[31] Houghton LA, Lea R, Jackson N, Whorwell PJ. The menstrual cycle affects rectal sensitivity in patients with irritable bowel syndrome but not healthy volunteers. Gut 2002;50:471–4.

[32] Ji RR, Befort K, Brenner GJ, Woolf CJ. ERK MAP kinase activation in superficial spinal cord neurons induces prodynorphin and NK-1 upregulation and contributes to persistent inflammatory pain hypersensitivity. J Neurosci 2002;22:478–85.

[33] Ji RR, Kohno T, Moore KA, Woolf CJ. Central sensitization and LTP: do pain and memory share similar mechanisms? Trends Neurosci 2003;26:696–705.

[34] Ji YP, Murphy AZ, Traub RJ. Estrogen modulates the visceromotor reflex and responses of spinal dorsal horn neurons to colorectal stimulation in the rat. J Neurosci 2003;23:3908–15.

[35] Jones RCW III, Xu L, Gebhart GF. The mechanosensitivity of mouse colon afferent fibers and their sensitization by inflammatory mediators require transient receptor potential vanilloid 1 and acid-sensing ion channel 3. J Neurosci 2005;25:10981–9.

[36] Kollarik M, Undem BJ. Mechanisms of acid-induced activation of airway afferent nerve fibres in guinea-pig. J Physiol 2002;543:591–600.

[37] Laird JM, Souslova V, Wood JN, Cervero F. Deficits in visceral pain and referred hyperalgesia in Na$_v$1.8 (SNS/PN3)-null mice. J Neurosci 2002;22:8352–6.

[38] Laird JMA, Martinez-Caro L, Garcia-Nicas E, Cervero F. A new model of visceral pain and referred hyperalgesia in the mouse. Pain 2001;92:335–42.

[39] Lee MG, Undem BJ. Basic mechanisms of cough: current understanding and remaining questions. Lung 2008;186 Suppl 1:S10–6.

[40] LeResche L, Mancl L, Sherman JJ, Gandara B, Dworkin SF. Changes in temporomandibular pain and other symptoms across the menstrual cycle. Pain 2003;106:253–61.

[41] Leventhal L, Brandt MR, Cummons TA, Piesla MJ, Rogers KE, Harris HA. An estrogen receptor-β agonist is active in models of inflammatory and chemical-induced pain. Eur J Pharmacol 2006;553:146–8.

[42] Liu BG, Eisenach JC, Tong CY. Chronic estrogen sensitizes a subset of mechanosensitive afferents innervating the uterine cervix. J Neurophysiol 2005;93:2167–73.

[43] Malinow R, Malenka RC. AMPA receptor trafficking and synaptic plasticity. Annu Rev Neurosci 2002;25:103–26.

[44] Mannino CA, South SM, Inturrisi CE, Quinones-Jenab V. Pharmacokinetics and effects of 17β-estradiol and progesterone implants in ovariectomized rats. J Pain 2005;6:809–16.

[45] Mannino CA, South SM, Quinones-Jenab V, Inturrisi CE. Estradiol replacement in ovariectomized rats is antihyperalgesic in the formalin test. J Pain 2007;8:334–42.

[46] Page AJ, Brierley SM, Martin CM, Price MP, Symonds E, Butler R, Wemmie JA, Blackshaw LA. Different contributions of ASIC channels 1a, 2, and 3 in gastrointestinal mechanosensory function. Gut 2005;54:1408–15.

[47] Pan HL, Chen SR. Myocardial ischemia recruits mechanically insensitive cardiac sympathetic afferents in cats. J Neurophysiol 2002;87:660–8.

[48] Pan HL, Longhurst JC. Ischaemia-sensitive sympathetic afferents innervating the gastrointestinal tract function as nociceptors in cats. J Physiol 1996;492:841–50.

[49] Pan HL, Longhurst JC, Eisenach JC, Chen SR. Role of protons in activation of cardiac sympathetic C-fibre afferents during ischaemia in cats. J Physiol 1999;518:857–66.

[50] Price TJ, Cervero F, de KY. Role of cation-chloride-cotransporters (CCC) in pain and hyperalgesia. Curr Top Med Chem 2005;5:547–55.

[51] Quinones-Jenab V, Jenab S, Ogawa S, Inturrisi C, Pfaff DW. Estrogen regulation of mu-opioid receptor mRNA in the forebrain of female rats. Brain Res Mol Brain Res 1997;47:134–8.

[52] Rong WF, Hillsley K, Davis JB, Hicks G, Winchester WJ, Grundy D. Jejunal afferent nerve sensitivity in wild-type and TRPV1 knockout mice. J Physiol 2004;560:867–81.

[53] Sammons MJ, Raval P, Davey PT, Rogers D, Parsons AA, Bingham S. Carrageenan-induced thermal hyperalgesia in the mouse: role of nerve growth factor and the mitogen-activated protein kinase pathway. Brain Res 2000;876:48–54.

[54] Sandkuhler J. Learning and memory in pain pathways. Pain 2000;88:113–8.

[55] Sanoja R, Cervero F. Estrogen-dependent abdominal hyperalgesia induced by ovariectomy in adult mice: a model of functional abdominal pain. Pain 2005;118:243–53.

[56] Sanoja R, Cervero F. Estrogen modulation of ovariectomy-induced hyperalgesia in adult mice. Eur J Pain 2008;12:573–81.
[57] Sengupta JN, Gebhart GF. Mechanosensitive afferent fibers in the gastrointestinal and lower urinary tracts. In: Gebhart GF, editor. Visceral pain: progress in pain research and management. Vol. 5. Seattle: IASP Press; 1995. p. 75–98.
[58] Sherman JJ, LeResche L. Does experimental pain response vary across the menstrual cycle? A methodological review. Am J Physiol Regul Integr Comp Physiol 2006;291:R245–56.
[59] Shinoda M, Ohtsuka E, Gebhart GF. Role of P2X receptors in colon hypersensitivity in the mouse. J Pain 2008;9:3.
[60] Smith YR, Stohler CS, Nichols TE, Bueller JA, Koeppe RA, Zubieta JK. Pronociceptive and anti-nociceptive effects of estradiol through endogenous opioid neurotransmission in women. J Neurosci 2006;26:5777–85.
[61] Taylor-Clark T, Undem BJ. Transduction mechanisms in airway sensory nerves. J Appl Physiol 2006;101:950–9.
[62] Tong C, Ma W, Shin SW, James RL, Eisenach JC. Uterine cervical distension induces cFos expression in deep dorsal horn neurons of the rat spinal cord. Anesthesiology 2003;99:205–11.
[63] Torebjörk HE, Schmelz M, Handwerker HO. Functional properties of human cutaneous nociceptors and their role in pain and hyperalgesia. In: Belmonte C, Cervero F, editors. Neurobiology of nociceptors. Oxford: Oxford University Press; 1996. p. 349–69.
[64] Wultsch T, Painsipp E, Shahbazian A, Mitrovic M, Edelsbrunner M, Lazdunski M, Waldmann R, Holzer P. Deletion of the acid-sensing ion channel ASIC3 prevents gastritis-induced acid hyper-responsiveness of the stomach-brainstem axis. Pain 2008;134:245–53.
[65] Wynn G, Rong W, Xiang Z, Burnstock G. Purinergic mechanisms contribute to mechanosensory transduction in the rat colorectum. Gastroenterology 2003;125:1398–409.
[66] Xu L, Gebhart GF. Characterization of mouse lumbar splanchnic and pelvic nerve urinary bladder mechanosensory afferents. J Neurophysiol 2008;99:244–53.
[67] Yan T, Liu B, Du D, Eisenach JC, Tong C. Estrogen amplifies pain responses to uterine cervical distension in rats by altering transient receptor potential-1 function. Anesth Analg 2007;104:1246–50.
[68] Zubieta JK, Smith YR, Bueller JA, Xu Y, Kilbourn MR, Jewett DM, Meyer CR, Koeppe RA, Stohler CS. Mu-opioid receptor-mediated antinociceptive responses differ in men and women. J Neurosci 2002;22:5100–7.

Correspondence to: Prof. Fernando Cervero, MD, PhD, DSc, Anesthesia Research Unit, McGill University, McIntyre Medical Building, Room 1207, 3655 Promenade Sir William Osler, Montreal, Quebec, Canada H3G 1Y6. Tel: +1-514-398-5764; fax: +1-514-398-8241; email: fernando.cervero@mcgill.ca.

Brain Correlates of Psychological Amplification of Pain

Jürgen Lorenz[a] and Irene Tracey[b]

[a]Hamburg University of Applied Sciences, Faculty of Life Sciences, Laboratory of Human Biology and Physiology, Hamburg, Germany; [b]Centre for Functional Magnetic Resonance Imaging of the Brain, John Radcliffe Hospital, University of Oxford, Departments of Anaesthetics and Clinical Neurology, Oxford, United Kingdom

Pain is a complex subjective phenomenon that is influenced by the physical attributes of the painful stimulus, the pathophysiological condition of the body, and the psychological context in which it occurs. The close link between attention and pain can serve either to augment or reduce pain intensity, a phenomenon that can best be understood from an evolutionary viewpoint. Directing attention to a noxious event improves perceptual and behavioral reactivity to danger and is adaptive because it guarantees survival. The aversive quality of the experience also promotes learning, ideally to avoid pain in the future. However, active guidance of attention away from pain also can be of vital importance if an injured individual needs to fight against a predator or escape from a threatening situation without being incapacitated by pain. Attention has no such benefit when pain becomes inescapable, as is the case in the chronic pain state.

The mechanisms by which pain becomes chronic are still poorly understood, but they are likely to involve both physical and psychological processes. One of the greatest challenges is to understand how these processes interact in a given type of clinical pain in order to explain why pain can sometimes occur without an adequate correlate of tissue damage. Such knowledge will clearly aid decisions regarding the targeting of treatments, such as whether to use pharmacological, surgical, or cognitive behavioral therapy. Many research groups have therefore directed their focus of interest to the brain correlates of pain perception and to psychological modulation of pain.

Functional Brain Imaging for the Study of Pain

Recently a number of functional brain imaging studies have shown localized effects of psychological factors such as attention, emotion, cognitive appraisal, and mood on pain processing in various brain areas. We will first briefly describe the basic principles of these methodologies. Functional imaging techniques applied for the study of pain are positron emission tomography (PET), functional magnetic resonance imaging (fMRI), multichannel electroencephalography (EEG), and magnetoencephalography (MEG). PET measures cerebral blood flow, glucose metabolism, or neurotransmitter kinetics through injection of radiotracers. The most common use of O^{15}-water injection in pain studies allows visualization of the regional cerebral blood flow response (rCBF) as an indicator of neuronal activity. Usually, scans during painful stimulation are statistically compared with scans during the resting state or during nonpainful stimulation (blocked design) and plotted as three-dimensional color-coded t- or Z-score statistical maps. Functional MRI images blood oxygenation with a technique called BOLD (blood oxygenation level-dependent) that exploits the phenomenon that oxygenated and deoxygenated hemoglobin possess different magnetic properties, resulting in different relaxation behavior of protons in water following radiofrequency pulses inside the magnet. Both the rCBF method using O^{15}-water PET and the BOLD technique rely on neurovascular coupling mechanisms that are not yet fully understood, but which overcompensate for local oxygen consumption, thus causing a flow of oxygenated blood into neuronally active brain areas to provide oxygen in excess of that utilized [28].

   EEG and MEG are non-invasive neurophysiological techniques that measure the respective electrical potentials and magnetic fields generated by neuronal activity of the brain and propagated to the surface of the skull, where they are picked up with EEG electrodes, or in the case of MEG, received by SQUID (supra-conducting quantum interference device) sensors located outside the skull. Compared with PET and fMRI, EEG and MEG are direct indicators of neuronal activity and yield a higher temporal resolution, yet with significantly lower spatial acuity of investigated brain function. The spatial distributions of EEG potentials and MEG fields at characteristic time points following noxious stimulation are analyzed using an inverse mathematical modeling approach called equivalent current dipole (ECD) reconstruction. An ECD evoked by painful stimuli hence represents a source model of pain-relevant activity within the brain [10].

The Cerebral Signature of Pain

Because pain is a complex, multifactorial subjective experience, a large distributed brain network is accessed during nociceptive processing [60]. According to the relay of spinal nociceptive pathways in either lateral or medial thalamic nuclei, the "pain matrix" is simplistically divided into the lateral system, which subserves sensory-discriminative functions and is governed by the primary (S1) and secondary somatosensory (S2) cortices and posterior parts of the insula, and the medial system, which subserves affective-motivational functions and is governed by the anterior cingulate cortex (ACC), anterior parts of the insula, and the prefrontal cortex (PFC). Other regions, such as the basal ganglia, cerebellum, amygdala, hippocampus, and areas within the parietal and temporal cortices, can also be active, depending on the particular experimental or clinical pain conditions. Therefore, a cerebral signature for pain is perhaps a more useful term than the conventional "pain matrix" concept, especially when considering the neural representation of psychological phenomena that interact with different types of pain [61].

The Bodily Context of Pain

Normally, if a stimulus is intense enough to activate nociceptors, multiple areas of the brain—such as the thalamus, the primary (S1) and secondary (S2) somatosensory cortices, posterior and anterior parts of the insula, and the ACC—respond to this input in a manner correlated with perceived intensity [14]. In pathological pain states, inflammation or nerve lesions can exaggerate the sensitivity to painful stimuli (hyperalgesia) or cause pain following warm or touch stimuli (allodynia). In comparing equally intense contact heat stimuli across normal and capsaicin-treated skins, Lorenz et al. [39] demonstrated that tissue sensitization causes a specific activation in forebrain areas of the medial pain system, comprising the medial thalamus, rostral ACC, anterior insula, and dorsolateral prefrontal and orbitofrontal cortices (Fig. 1). Notably, although the perceived intensity was equal in the two skin conditions, pain on sensitized skin (heat allodynia) yielded greater negative affect, consistent with intrinsically stronger affective pain experiences during pathological tissue states.

Furthermore, the involvement of cerebral motor systems differs between normal and sensitized tissue conditions. Normal pain recruits the "motor loop" of the basal ganglia, which involves brain structures such as the putamen, motor and premotor cortex, and cerebellum, suited to govern an immediate and spatially guided defense or withdrawal due to their somatotopic organization [6,7]. On the other hand, sensitized pain conditions engage the ventral caudate and nucleus accumbens, which are part of a limbic basal ganglia loop relevant for motivational drive of behavior rather than for motor execution.

Overall, these results substantiate suggestions that different projection systems originating in the dorsal horn of the spinal cord mediate normal pain, as well as pain during neurogenic inflammation [33]. In

Fig. 1. Comparison of O^{15}-water positron emission tomography (PET) scans during equally painful contact heat stimuli elicited on capsaicin-treated (A) and normal (B) skin at the left forearm of 14 healthy volunteers. Rows A and B indicate the subtraction maps against the rest condition with normal skin, and the bottom row illustrates the direct subtraction map A minus B. The four columns represent different horizontal slice levels relative to the line between the anterior and posterior commissure (AC-PC) indicated at the top. Note that areas such as the posterior insula (Post INS), dorsal striatum (Dors striat), and lateral thalamus (Lat Tha) are equally activated by the two stimuli and therefore disappear in the direct comparison. In contrast, areas such as the anterior insula (Ant INS), ventral striatum (Vent striat), perigenual anterior cingulate cortex (Perig ACC), orbitofrontal cortex (OFC), dorsolateral prefrontal cortex (DLPFC), medial thalamus (Med Tha), and dorsomedial (Dm) midbrain are significantly more activated in the sensitized than in the normal skin condition and appear contrasted in the direct comparison A minus B (used with permission from Lorenz and Casey [38]; data from Lorenz et al. [39]).

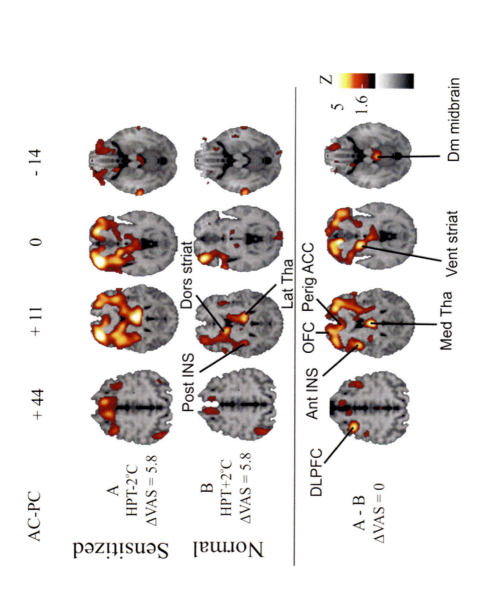

differentiating the bodily context of pain according to its origin from either outside or inside the body, the brain may engage different behavioral adaptations (e.g., withdrawal or quiescence) according to the meaning of the threat in relation to the physiological status of the body. The shift from mid-anterior cingulate to perigenual cingulate and from posterior insula to anterior insula during capsaicin-induced neurogenic heat sensitization in direct comparison with equally intense normal heat pain appears to model quite well pathological types of clinical pain [54]. Notably, this shift also appears during anticipated pain [48], empathic pain [57], or imagined pain when compared with real sensory pain (Fairhurst M, Fairhurst K, Renella CB, Tracey I, unpublished manuscript). Thus, augmented pain in a chronic state may involve the heightened interoceptive awareness of the bodily state reflected by an exaggeration of limbic brain areas that is otherwise only transiently more strongly engaged during acute tissue injury or inflammation. It is, therefore, possible that the brain "unlearns" the differentiation of the bodily from the psychological context of pain in the chronic state. However, pain is real regardless of whether it is generated by bodily or psychological processes. Many studies have shown that pain can exist when there is no measurable nociceptive input [15,51,57]. The following section will review the evidence that psychological factors exert powerful influences on brain structures engaged in the human pain experience.

The Psychological Context of Pain

Attentional modulation of pain has been documented thoroughly in laboratory settings using psychophysical [12,58], behavioral [18], and electrophysiological [40] methods in human volunteers. Functional neuroimaging studies focusing on the relationship of pain and attention have incorporated attention-related phenomena, such as anticipation [48,53], anxiety [47], hypnotic suggestions [51], placebo conditions [8,46,67], distraction [1,62], or habituation [8].

Vigilance, Attention, and Habituation

The painfulness of repetitive noxious stimulation typically diminishes over time, a phenomenon that is often referred to as a time-dependent decline of vigilance [5,10] or to habituation [12,36] Although the brain network regulating vigilance is well described by the variety of ascending pathways from the brainstem [49], the brain mechanisms underlying short- or long-term fluctuations of vigilance during wakefulness and the associated loss of efficiency of behavioral control are unknown [50]. More recent work [20] suggests that prior to performance lapses during mental tasks of long duration, there is a maladaptive relative increase in activation of a synaptic network (involving the precuneus, retrosplenial, and anterior medial frontal cortex) that governs a default mode of awake brain function. The study identified brain processes associated with maintaining task effort in the anterior cingulate and right prefrontal cortex. Given a similar importance of these latter brain areas for heightened awareness of pain and maintenance of task effort, one may postulate that "hypervigilance" to pain (according to, e.g., [18]) may represent a failure of default mode brain regions to disengage from pain. This possibility would be compatible with the notion that enhanced focused attention over prolonged periods of time can amplify some chronic clinical pain states [66].

The close relationship between pain and the control of attention is of fundamental importance for any type of experimental or clinical pain. Pain is a salient stimulus that draws one's attention for extended periods [17]. The manipulation of attention by distraction or focused attention has been used as a therapeutic intervention for several years [43]. Patients with chronic pain problems seem to selectively attend to pain, and the degree by which pain distracts attention from concurrent tasks appears to depend upon the evaluation of pain stimuli as threatening or worrying [18]. In tasks that require attentional shifts, anxious patients exhibit difficulty disengaging from painful stimuli [64]. Although some degree of modulation by selective attention has been reported of the primary somatosensory cortex (S1) [13,32], the secondary somatosensory cortex (S2) shows more consistent attention-dependent processing of nociceptive input [41,53].

More recent studies using EEG and MEG have concentrated on cortical synchronization processes as indicators of selective attention of sensory input. Mainly derived from experiments with non-painful stimuli it is proposed that selective attention may act by modulating sub-threshold oscillations in sensory assemblies and by enhancing the gain of oscillatory responses to stimuli that match stored contextual information [21,31]. Fig. 2 shows the results of a recent study indicating that during selective attention to pain, the S2 cortices bilaterally yield enhanced oscillatory activity in the gamma bandwidth of MEG (120 Hz rhythms) and show a stronger inter-regional degree of synchronization as a sign of increased neuronal communication between the two S2 cortices [29]. One possible neuronal correlate of abnormal attentional amplification may therefore be suspected in an "oversynchronization" among pain-related cortical areas, leading to an uncontrolled spread of signals even in the case of weak or absent nociceptive inputs. Thus, the dynamic control of neuronal signal flow might be disturbed, preventing an appropriate context-dependent modulation of the gain of neural signals, and reducing the capacity for descending control of nociceptive afferent inputs. As assumed for states of chronic pain, such an "oversynchronization" might be viewed as the result of central neuroplastic changes underlying a learning process [23].

Although habituation can be difficult to experimentally differentiate from a vigilance decrement or a temporary fluctuation of focused attention, it most likely represents a distinct phenomenon. Functional MRI experiments on the mechanisms of habituation to pain have revealed decreases of activation in major pain-processing areas, including the thalamus, insula, S2, and putamen. Similarly, amplitudes of pain-relevant evoked potentials after electrical stimuli, painful chemical stimulation of the nasal mucosa, and laser stimulation are strongly attenuated by habituation and decreases of vigilance over time [40]. Notably, an increase of activation was observed in the rostral ACC [9]. One possible mechanism could be the involvement of the endogenous opioidergic pain control system. In an animal model of habituation, naloxone sufficiently prevents habituation to repeated electrical pain stimuli [34]. It is, however, questionable

Fig. 2. Pain modulation by attention. Attention to pain (pain attention) was induced by having subjects count rare electrical pain stimuli at one finger, while ignoring frequent pain stimuli at the other finger (pain ignored) within a random series (oddball paradigm). Electrophysiological signals were recorded using magnetoencephalography (MEG). After time-frequency transformation, neuronal oscillations around 120 Hz (gamma band) and with latencies around 500 ms indicated a difference for attention. This effect was localized in sensory-motor areas. Furthermore, increased communication (imaginary coherence, IMC) between the sensory-motor sites of both hemispheres was observed during attention (from [29]).

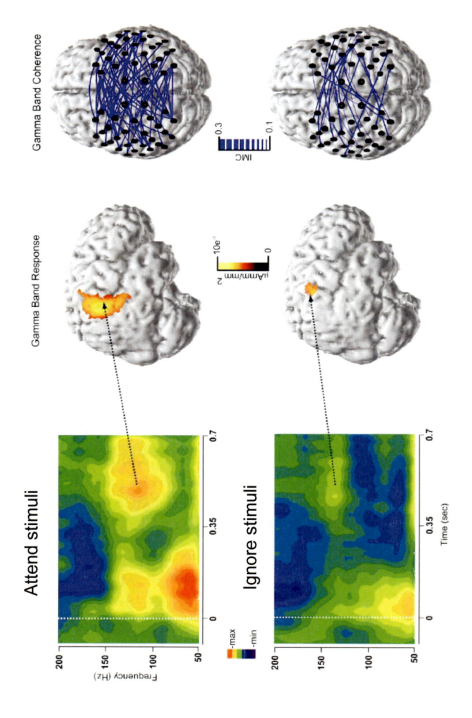

Attend stimuli

Gamma Band Response

Gamma Band Coherence

Ignore stimuli

Frequency (Hz)

Time (sec)

that habituation represents a uniform entity. It is more likely to involve processes that are unique within a given sensory modality, such as glutamatergic habituation of olfaction, which occur similarly in all sensory modalities, such as habituation during the learning phase of conditioning. There are important interindividual differences in the strength of habituation over repetitive painful stimulation that are not well understood; these differences might be relevant to the observation that some chronic pain patients show an impairment of habituation [16,24,45,63]. Thus, amplified pain perception in some patients might pertain either to an altered interaction of pain processes with the network regulating vigilance within the brain or to a lack of both pain and vigilance systems of normal inhibitory control. This view would be compatible with the coincidence of chronic pain and sleep disturbances in some functional pain disorders such as fibromyalgia [52].

Self-Control of Pain

Top-down mechanisms, driven by the prefrontal cortex, are assumed to primarily mediate disengagement from prepotent perceptions such as pain to pursue superordinate behavioral goals [42]. The ability to cope with pain and reduce pain-directed anxiety varies among individuals according to the degree to which they perceive pain as controllable and to what extent the anterolateral prefrontal cortex is recruited [68]. A key phenomenon of self-control over pain is the placebo effect, which can be attributed to different psychological mechanisms including expectation, Pavlovian conditioning, and reduction of anxiety [2]. Work in humans has helped provide a framework to explain the ways in which the placebo effect and subsequent analgesia are mediated. Again, the brainstem is critically involved in mediating placebo analgesia. Descending influences from the diencephalon, hypothalamus, amygdala, ACC, and the insular and prefrontal cortex, which inhibit or facilitate nociceptive transmission via brainstem structures, are thought to occur during placebo analgesia. Using PET, Petrovic et al. [46] confirmed that both opioid and placebo analgesia are associated with increased activity in the rostral ACC; they also observed a covariation between the activity in the rostral ACC and the brainstem during both opioid and placebo analgesia, but not during pain alone.

Wager and colleagues [67] extended these observations to consider whether or not placebo treatments produce analgesia by altering expectations. Using a conditioning design, the authors found that placebo analgesia was related to decreased brain activity in classic pain-processing brain regions (the thalamus, insula, and ACC), but was additionally associated with increased activity during anticipation of pain in the PFC, an area involved in maintaining and updating internal representations of expectations. Stronger PFC activation during anticipation of pain was found to correlate with greater placebo-induced pain relief and reductions in neural activity within pain regions. Furthermore, placebo-increased activation of the PAG region was found during anticipation. This activity in the PAG correlated significantly with dorsolateral PFC (DLPFC) activity. This finding is consistent with the concept that prefrontal mechanisms can trigger opioid release within the brainstem and thereby influence the descending pain-modulatory system to regulate pain perception during the placebo effect. For instance, during placebo analgesia it was observed that subjects who were good responders to real opioid injections were also the better placebo responders, implying individual variance in engaging endogenous opioid networks during placebo analgesia [46].

In analogy to the concept of "placebo" (i.e., expect a positive outcome), a negative expectation of pain, other aversive symptoms, or side effects of drugs is nowadays often referred to as the "nocebo" effect (i.e., expect a negative outcome). The neurobiological mechanisms of the nocebo effect have been less thoroughly investigated. Just as the expectation of pain relief biases perception toward hypoalgesia during placebo trials, the expectation of pain, or of stronger pain than is actually presented, biases perception toward hyperalgesia, which is associated with changes in brain activation of different regions including the S2/posterior insula area [35,37,41,53]. Expectation and conditioning mechanisms, which are similar and opposite to those of the placebo counterpart, are thought to be involved [4]. Nocebo hyperalgesia can be prevented by pretreatment with proglumide, a nonspecific cholecystokinin (CCK) antagonist for both CCK-A and CCK-B receptors, suggesting the possible involvement of CCKergic systems in the nocebo effect [3]. By using selective CCK-A and CCK-B receptor antagonists, several studies in animals and humans have shown the important role of CCKergic systems in the modulation of anxiety and in the link between anxiety and hyperalgesia [30].

Anxiety, Depression, and Decision Making

The nocebo phenomenon indicates that expectation of the worst is closely coupled with anxiety. Clinical and experimental experience confirms that being anxious about pain can exacerbate the pain experienced. Furthermore, the normally adaptive benefit that anticipatory mechanisms bring, via learned associations between pain and pain-related cues to avoid injury, becomes highly maladaptive in the chronic pain state. The patient cannot avoid a known cue-pain association and therefore experiences fear, leading to avoidance, helplessness, and anxiety. Furthermore, predictive learning of pain relief becomes impossible because the "cost" of pain as an aversive experience dominates over the "reward" of an expected termination of pain [56], giving rise to poor decision-making processes such as catastrophizing.

Studies aimed at understanding how anticipation and anxiety cause a heightened pain experience have been performed using imaging methods and novel paradigm designs [60]. Critical regions involved in amplifying or exacerbating the pain experience include the entorhinal complex, amygdalae, anterior insula, and prefrontal cortices. The entorhinal complex and amygdalae are not commonly found to be active in pain studies, and therefore activity in these regions strongly indicates anxiety as a critical factor in a subject's pain experience. More recent studies confirm the role of these brain regions in amplifying pain in patients with somatoform pain disorder [27] and rheumatoid arthritis [55] and have sought to identify how activity within these regions produces increased pain intensity [22].

With regard to mood, depressive disorders clearly accompany persistent pain [65]. Although the exact relationship between depression and pain is unknown, and debate continues regarding whether one condition leads to the other or if an underlying diathesis exists, studies have attempted to isolate brain regions that may mediate their interaction [44]. One fMRI study showed that activation in the amygdala and anterior insula differentiated patients with fibromyalgia with and without major depression, confirming limbic involvement in the emotional augmentation of the pain experience [25]. Another study on fibromyalgia patients found that pain catastrophizing [59], independently of the influence of depression, was significantly associated with increased activity in brain areas related to anticipation of pain (the medial frontal cortex and cerebellum), attention to pain (the dorsal ACC and DLPFC), emotional aspects of pain (the claustrum, closely connected to the amygdala), and motor control [26]. The construct of catastrophizing incorporates magnification of pain-related symptoms, rumination about pain, feelings of helplessness, and pessimism about pain-related outcomes [19]. In a more recent study in rheumatoid arthritis patients, the medial prefrontal cortex was shown to possibly mediate the increased processing in limbic regions that accounts for depression-related augmentation of clinical pain [55].

What is apparent from these and other studies is that amplification of the pain experience via central mechanisms related to emotional aspects is significant and measurable. Measures of emotion-related pain amplification could possibly be used in future studies as diagnostic readouts and biomarkers to monitor over the course of therapy, be it pharmacological or behavioral. Providing patients with evidence that their mood really does influence the pain experienced has the potential to be a powerful means to encourage and support them to use strategies of self-control of pain.

Conclusions

Over the past 10 years, we have advanced our understanding of the brain correlates involved in psychological amplification and attenuation of the pain experience. Key regions include those listed in our summary Fig. 3. Confirmation of the causal relevance of these brain regions for driving changes in the pain experience will come from longitudinal studies in patients undergoing psychological interventions aimed at alleviating components specific to these aspects of amplification, such as anxiety and catastrophizing. Future studies that combine the use of novel, noninvasive magnetic resonance tractography methods to determine white matter connections between brain regions with functional connectivity analyses,

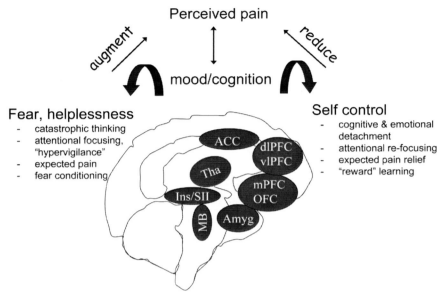

Fig. 3. Summary figure of main brain regions determined to be relevant in the psychological amplification and reduction of the pain experience based on bodily or psychological context. ACC = anterior cingulate cortex; Amyg = amygdala; dlPFC = dorsolateral prefrontal cortex; Ins = insular cortex; MB = midbrain; mPFC = medial prefrontal cortex; OFC = orbitofrontal cortex; SII = secondary somatosensory cortex; Tha = Thalamus; vlPFC = ventrolateral prefrontal cortex.

such as dynamic causal modeling, will facilitate the development of a network model to describe how recruitment of these regions produces the observed behavioral effect on pain perception. Important for this work, particularly for patient studies, will be to combine information related to possible widespread plasticity, re-representation of activity, and possible gray matter atrophy that will no doubt affect these networks and how they function in the diseased state.

References

[1]   Bantick SJ, Wise RG, Ploghaus A, Clare S, Smith SM, Tracey I. Imaging how attention modulates pain in humans using functional MRI. Brain 2002;125:310–9.
[2]   Benedetti F. Mechanisms of placebo and placebo-related effects across diseases and treatments. Annu Rev Pharmacol Toxicol 2008;48:33–60.
[3]   Benedetti F, Amanzio M, Vighetti S, Asteggiano G. The biochemical and neuroendocrine bases of the hyperalgesic nocebo effect. J Neurosci 2006;26:12014–22.

[4] Benedetti F, Pollo A, Lopiano L, Lanotte M, Vighetti S, Rainero I. Conscious expectation and unconscious conditioning in analgesic, motor, and hormonal placebo/nocebo responses. J Neurosci 2003;23:4315–23.

[5] Beydoun A, Morrow TJ, Shen JF, Casey KL. Variability of laser-evoked potentials: attention, arousal and lateralized differences. Electroenceph Clin Neurophysiol 1993;88:173–81.

[6] Bingel U, Gläscher J, Weiller C, Büchel C. Somatotopic representation of nociceptive information in the putamen: an event-related fMRI study. Cereb Cortex 2004;14:1340–5.

[7] Bingel U, Lorenz J, Glauche V, Knab R, Gläscher J, Weiller C, Büchel C. Somatotopic organization of human somatosensory cortices for pain: a single trial fMRI study. Neuroimage 2004;23:224–32.

[8] Bingel U, Lorenz J, Schoell E, Weiller C, Büchel C. Mechanisms of placebo analgesia: rACC recruitment of a subcortical antinociceptive network. Pain 2006;120:8–15.

[9] Bingel U, Schoell E, Herken W, Buchel C, May A. Habituation to painful stimulation involves the antinociceptive system. Pain 2007;131:21–30.

[10] Bromm B, Lorenz J. Neurophysiological evaluation of pain. Electroenceph Clin Neurophysiol 1998;107:227–53.

[11] Bromm B, Scharein E. Response plasticity of pain evoked reactions in man. Physiol Behav 1982; 28:109–16.

[12] Bushnell MC, Duncan GH, Dubner R, Jones RL, Maixner W. Attentional influences on noxious and innocuous cutaneous heat detection in humans and monkeys. J Neurosci 1985;5:1103–10.

[13] Bushnell MC, Duncan GH, Hofbauer RK, Ha B, Chen JI, Carrier B. Pain perception: is there a role for primary somatosensory cortex? Proc Natl Acad Sci USA 1999;96:7705–9.

[14] Coghill RC, Sang CN, Maisog JM, Iadarola MJ. Pain intensity processing within the human brain: a bilateral, distributed mechanism. J Neurophysiol 1999;82:1934–43.

[15] Derbyshire SW, Whalley MG, Stenger VA, Oakley DA. Cerebral activation during hypnotically induced and imagined pain. Neuroimage 2004;23:392–401.

[16] Demirci S, Savas S. The auditory event related potentials in episodic and chronic pain sufferers. Eur J Pain 2002;6:239–44.

[17] Downar J, Mikulis DJ, Davis KD. Neural correlates of the prolonged salience of painful stimulation. Neuroimage 2003;20:1540–51.

[18] Eccleston C, Crombez G. Pain demands attention: a cognitive-affective model of the interruptive function of pain. Psychol Bull 1999;125:356–66.

[19] Edwards R, Bingham CO 3rd, Bathon J, Haythornthwaite JA. Catastrophizing and pain in arthritis, fibromyalgia, and other rheumatic diseases. Arthritis Rheum 2006;15:325–32.

[20] Eichele T, Debener S, Calhoun VD, Specht K, Engel AK, Hugdahl K, von Cramon DY, Ullsperger M. Prediction of human errors by maladaptive changes in event-related brain networks. Proc Natl Acad Sci USA 2008;105:6173–8.

[21] Engel AK, Fries P, Singer W. Dynamic predictions: oscillations and synchrony in top-down processing. Nat Rev Neurosci 2001;2:704–16.

[22] Fairhurst M, Wiech K, Dunckley P, Tracey I. Anticipatory brainstem activity predicts neural processing of pain in humans. Pain 2007;128:101–10.

[23] Flor H, Diers M. Limitations of pharmacotherapy: behavioral approaches to chronic pain. Handb Exp Pharmacol 2007; 177:415–27.

[24] Flor H, Diers M, Birbaumer N. Peripheral and electrocortical responses to painful and nonpainful stimulation in chronic pain patients, tension headache patients and healthy controls. Neurosci Lett 2004;361:147–50.

[25] Giesecke T, Gracely RH, Williams DA, Geisser ME, Petzke FW, Clauw DJ. The relationship between depression, clinical pain, and experimental pain in a chronic pain cohort. Arthritis Rheum 2005;52:1577–84.

[26] Gracely RH, Geisser ME, Giesecke T, Grant MA, Petzke F, Williams DA, Clauw DJ. Pain catastrophizing and neural responses to pain among persons with fibromyalgia. Brain 2004;127:835–43.

[27] Gündel H, Valet M, Sorg C, Huber D, Zimmer C, Sprenger T, Tölle TR. Altered cerebral response to noxious heat stimulation in patients with somatoform pain disorder. Pain 2008;137:413–21.

[28] Gusnard DA, Raichle ME, Raichle ME. Searching for a baseline: functional imaging and the resting human brain. Nat Rev Neurosci 2001;2:685–94.

[29] Hauck M, Lorenz J, Engel AK. Attention to painful stimulation enhances gamma-band activity and synchronization in human sensorimotor cortex. J Neurosci 2007;27:9270–7.

[30] Hebb AL, Poulin JF, Roach SP, Zacharko RM, Drolet G. Cholecystokinin and endogenous opioid peptides: interactive influence on pain, cognition, and emotion. Prog Neuropsychopharmacol Biol Psychiatry 2005;29:1225–38.

[31] Herrmann CS, Munk MH, Engel AK. Cognitive functions of gamma-band activity: memory match and utilization. Trends Cogn Sci 2004;8:347–55.

[32] Hofbauer RK, Rainville P, Duncan GH, Bushnell MC. Cortical representation of the sensory dimension of pain. J Neurophysiol 2001;86:402–11.

[33] Hunt SP, Mantyh PW. The molecular dynamics of pain control. Nat Rev Neurosci 2001;2:83–91.

[34] Janicki P, Libich J, Gumulka W. Lack of habituation of pain evoked potentials after naloxone. Pol J Pharmacol Pharm 1979;31:201–5.

[35] Keltner JR, Furst A, Fan C, Redfern R, Inglis B, Fields HL. Isolating the modulatory effect of expectation on pain transmission: a functional magnetic resonance imaging study. J Neurosci 2006;26:4437–43.

[36] Kobal G, Hummel T. Cerebral chemosensory evoked potentials elicited by chemical stimulation of the human olfactory and respiratory nasal mucosa. Electroenceph Clin Neurophysiol 1988;71:241–50.

[37] Koyama T, McHaffie JG, Laurienti PJ, Coghill RC. The subjective experience of pain: where expectations become reality. Proc Natl Acad Sci USA 2005;102:12950–5.

[38] Lorenz J, Casey KL. Imaging of acute versus pathological pain in humans. Eur J Pain 2005;9:163–5.

[39] Lorenz J, Cross DJ, Minoshima S, Morrow TJ, Paulson PE, Casey KL. A unique representation of heat allodynia in the human brain. Neuron 2002;35:383–93.

[40] Lorenz J, Garcia-Larrea L. Contribution of attentional and cognitive factors to laser evoked brain potentials. Neurophysiol Clin 2003;33:293–301.

[41] Lorenz J, Hauck M, Paur RC, Nakamura Y, Zimmermann R, Bromm B, Engel AK. Cortical correlates of false expectations during pain intensity judgments: a possible manifestation of placebo/nocebo cognitions. Brain Behav Immun 2005;19:283–95.

[42] Lorenz J, Minoshima S, Casey KL. Keeping pain out of mind: the role of the dorsolateral prefrontal cortex in pain modulation. Brain 2003;126:1079–91.

[43] McCracken LM, Turk DC. Behavioral and cognitive-behavioral treatment for chronic pain: outcome, predictors of outcome, and treatment process. Spine 2002;27:2564–73.

[44] Neugebauer V, Li W, Bird GC, Han JS. The amygdala and persistent pain. Neuroscientist 2004;10:221–34.

[45] Peters ML, Schmidt AJ, Van den Hout MA. Chronic low back pain and the reaction to repeated acute pain stimulation. Pain 1989;39:69–76.

[46] Petrovic P, Kalso E, Petersson KM, Ingvar M. Placebo and opioid analgesia: imaging a shared neuronal network. Science 2002;295:1737–40.

[47] Ploghaus A, Narain C, Beckmann CF, Clare S, Bantick S, Wise R, Matthews PM, Rawlins JN, Tracey I. Exacerbation of pain by anxiety is associated with activity in a hippocampal network. J Neurosci 2001;21:9896–903.

[48] Ploghaus A, Tracey I, Gati JS, Clare S, Menon RS, Matthews PM, et al. Dissociating pain from its anticipation in the human brain. Science 1999;284:1979–81.

[49] Posner MI, Petersen SE. The attention system in the human brain. Annu Rev Neurosci 1990;13: 25–42.

[50] Parasuraman R, Warm JS, See JE. Brain systems of vigilance. In: Parasuraman R, editor. The attentive brain. Harvard: MIT Press; 1998. pp. 221–56.

[51] Raij TT, Numminen J, Närvänen S, Hiltunen J, Hari R. Brain correlates of subjective reality of physically and psychologically induced pain. Proc Natl Acad Sci USA 2005;102:2147-51.

[52] Russell IJ, Raphael KG. Fibromyalgia syndrome: presentation, diagnosis, differential diagnosis, and vulnerability. CNS Spectr 2008;13(3 Suppl 5):6–11.

[53] Sawamoto N, Honda M, Okada T, Hanakawa T, Kanda M, Fukuyama H, Konishi J, Shibasaki H. Expectation of pain enhances responses to nonpainful somatosensory stimulation in the anterior cingulate cortex and parietal operculum/posterior insula: an event-related functional magnetic resonance imaging study. J Neurosci 2000;20:7438–45.

[54] Schweinhardt P, Glynn C, Brooks J, McQuay H, Jack T, Chessell I, Bountra C, Tracey I. An fMRI study of cerebral processing of brush-evoked allodynia in neuropathic pain patients. Neuroimage 2006;32:256–65.

[55] Schweinhardt P, Kalk N, Wartolowska K, Chessell I, Wordsworth P, Tracey I. Investigation into the neural correlates of emotional augmentation of clinical pain. Neuroimage 2008;40:759–66.

[56] Seymour B, O'Doherty JP, Koltzenburg M, Wiech K, Frackowiak R, Friston K, Dolan R. Opponent appetitive-aversive neural processes underlie predictive learning of pain relief. Nat Neurosci 2005;8:1234–40.

[57] Singer T, Seymour B, O'Doherty J, Kaube H, Dolan RJ, Frith CD. Empathy for pain involves the affective but not sensory components of pain. Science 2004;303:1157–62.

[58] Spence C, Bentley DE, Phillips N, McGlone FP, Jones AKP. Selective attention to pain: a psychophysical investigation. Exp Brain Res 2002;145:395–402.

[59] Sullivan MJ, Thorn B, Haythornthwaite JA, Keefe F, Martin M, Bradley LA, Lefebvre JC. Theoretical perspectives on the relation between catastrophizing and pain. Clin J Pain 2001;17:52–64.

[60] Tracey I. Imaging pain. Br J Anaesth 2008;101:32–9.

[61] Tracey I, Mantyh PW. The cerebral signature for pain perception and its modulation. Neuron 2007;55:377–91.

[62] Tracey I, Ploghaus A, Gati JS, Clare S, Smith S, Menon RS, Matthews PM. Imaging attentional modulation of pain in the periaqueductal gray in humans. J Neurosci 2002;22:2748–52.

[63] Valeriani M, de Tommaso M, Restuccia D, Le Pera D, Guido M, Iannetti GD, Libro G, Truini A, Di Trapani G, Puca F, Tonali P, Cruccu G. Reduced habituation to experimental pain in migraine patients: a CO_2 laser evoked potential study. Pain 2003;105:57–64.

[64] Van Damme S, Crombez G, Eccleston C, Goubert L. Impaired disengagement from threatening cues of impending pain in a crossmodal cueing paradigm. Eur J Pain 2004;8:227–36.

[65] Villemure C, Bushnell MC. Cognitive modulation of pain: how do attention and emotion influence pain processing? Pain 2002;95:195–9.

[66] Vlaeyen JW, Linton SJ. Fear-avoidance and its consequences in chronic musculoskeletal pain: a state of the art. Pain. 2000;85:317–32.

[67] Wager TD, Rilling JK, Smith EE, Sokolik A, Casey KL, Davidson RJ, et al. Placebo-induced changes in FMRI in the anticipation and experience of pain. Science 2004;303:1162–7.

[68] Wiech K, Kalisch R, Weiskopf N, Pleger B, Stephan KE, Dolan RJ. Anterolateral prefrontal cortex mediates the analgesic effect of expected and perceived control over pain. J Neurosci 2006;26:11501–9.

Correspondence to: Jürgen Lorenz, Dr med, Hamburg University of Applied Sciences, Faculty of Life Sciences, Laboratory of Human Biology and Physiology, Lohbrügger Kirchstrasse 65, 21033 Hamburg, Germany. Email: juergen.lorenz@ ls.haw-hamburg.de.

Part V

Environment-Gene Interactions and Chronic Pain

The Genetics of Pain

Jeanette Papp and Eric Sobel

*Department of Human Genetics, David Geffen School of Medicine,
University of California-Los Angeles, Los Angeles, California, USA*

Pain is an adaptive response to adverse stimuli. There is great variability in individual response to pain, in pain modulation (inhibition and facilitation of pain), and in analgesia. Functional chronic pain syndromes comprise a family of complex multifactorial disorders, which typically combine persistent pain, psychological and emotional symptoms, and possibly shared pathophysiological mechanisms. Examples of chronic pain disorders include musculoskeletal forms such as fibromyalgia (FM), temporomandibular joint disorder (TMD), and chronic back pain, as well as visceral forms such as irritable bowel syndrome (IBS), chronic pelvic pain, and interstitial cystitis/painful bladder syndrome (IC/PBS). Chronic pain syndromes are common, with some estimates of prevalence as high as 4% for FM, 12% for TMD, 20% for chronic back pain, and 15% for IBS. Many chronic pain disorders are more prevalent in women; female/male ratios of 3 to 1 or higher are not uncommon [48,78]. Chronic pain disorders are often comorbid with each other [14], and with other neuropsychiatric disorders such as anxiety, panic disorder, and depression [57].

Some of the observed variation in pain sensitivity and response has a genetic basis. This conclusion is drawn from several types of evidence—twin

Functional Pain Syndromes: Presentation and Pathophysiology
edited by Emeran A. Mayer and M. Catherine Bushnell
IASP Press, Seattle, © 2009

and family studies of chronic pain syndromes, such as IC/PBS [26,92], IBS [64], FM [71], and TMD [56]; rare inherited forms of pain sensitivity [5,40,83]; and animal studies. Animal studies report heritabilities ranging from 28% to 76% [60]. Reliable estimates of heritability for chronic pain syndromes in humans are difficult to obtain due to the complexity of the gene-environment interaction and comorbidities with other psychiatric conditions [52,79,85]. Estimates of around 50% heritability have been reported for IBS [6]. Over 200 candidate genes for pain response have emerged from animal studies [49], but of these candidates only a few have been associated with pain phenotypes in humans.

It is only fairly recently that an understanding of the genetics of pain has begun to emerge. Most of the candidate genes implicated in human pain pathways have been published since the turn of the 21st century. From our emerging understanding of the genetics of pain, what seems most certain is that pain response and chronic pain syndromes are phenotypically very diverse, often with intermediate phenotypes or comorbid conditions. It is probable that pain, in its many manifestations, is influenced by highly complex genetics. Multiple genes can be expected to be involved, with gene-gene and gene-environment interactions playing a strong role as well, confounded by psychological and emotional factors. Gene-by-sex interactions are implicated by differences in response to pain analgesia between male and female mice [61,67,82], and have been described in men and women with mutations in the same analgesia pathway [63]. While some of the individual genetic polymorphisms implicated in chronic pain disorders may be common in the healthy population, interactions with other genes and with environmental factors can result in chronic pain. Individual small effects from multiple genes may cross a threshold and cause a pain disorder. There is also evidence for environmental triggers such as early life or adult psychological stress [45]. Genetics may predispose an individual to a pain disorder, which can develop if triggered by environmental factors. However, from this complexity, some patterns are beginning to emerge. A number of gene candidates have been implicated in pain disorders, and there appears to be evidence for shared, genetically determined vulnerabilities among chronic pain disorders [23].

Genes Implicated in Chronic Pain Syndromes

Animal studies, and in particular mouse knockouts (mice with a particular gene selectively inactivated), have played a large role in identifying candidate genes influencing pain [62]. A list of the over 200 proposed candidate genes for pain modulation can be found in the Pain Genes Database (http://paingeneticslab.ca/4105/06_02_pain_genetics_database.asp) [49]. However, although the list of candidates is long, a relatively small number are found to be associated with pain phenotypes in humans. The strongest evidence of the contribution of genetics to human chronic pain syndromes are from the following genes, which have been implicated in a number of studies from different research groups: (1) adrenergic genes such as genes expressing the adrenoreceptors, and catechol-O-methyl transferase (COMT); (2) monoaminergic genes such as the serotonin transporter gene; and (3) genes involved with ion channels such as those for transport of Na, Ca, and K.

Adrenergic Genes

Variation in the *COMT* gene is one of the best-characterized genetic mechanisms proposed to have a role in pain physiology. COMT is one of several enzymes that metabolize catecholamines and catecholamine-containing drugs. Catecholamine neurotransmitters such as dopamine, epinephrine, and norepinephrine are associated with stress, and have been implicated in experimental pain sensitivity [24,99], in morphine response in cancer pain treatment [74,75], and in chronic pain syndromes such as TMD [24] and FM [35,86]. *COMT* is also important in a number of psychiatric disorders such as depression [72,95], anxiety [39], and schizophrenia [94].

The human *COMT* gene is located on the long arm of chromosome 22. Five single nucleotide polymorphisms (SNPs) within *COMT* have been demonstrated to be associated with pain disorders: rs4646312, rs6269, rs4633, rs4680, and rs4818 [54]. Functional polymorphisms in the *COMT* gene can result in a 3- to 15-fold reduction in COMT activity [24,53], and decreases in COMT activity in animal studies have in turn been associated with increases in pain sensitivity through a β-adrenergic mechanism [65]. A common *COMT* functional SNP (approximately 50%

minor allele frequency), rs4680, causes the substitution of the amino acid valine (val) for methionine (met). The met allele *COMT* gene product has lower thermostability and decreased enzymatic activity. Individuals homozygous for the met allele show decreased response to opioid analgesics and higher pain sensitivity than val homozygotes, and heterozygotes have an intermediate response [99]. Three *COMT* haplotypes, comprising six SNPs, were identified as influencing pain sensitivity in TMD patients. The haplotypes were labeled low pain sensitivity (LPS), average pain sensitivity (APS), and high pain sensitivity (HPS). The presence of even one LPS allele increased *COMT* activity and reduced the risk of TMD by as much as 2.3-fold [24]. In addition to *COMT,* common variants of the human β_2-adrenoceptor gene, coding for differences in receptor expression and internalization, are associated with the development of TMD [22,65].

Monoaminergic Genes

The serotonin (5-HT) transporter gene *SLC6A4,* on chromosome 17q11.2, codes for the monoamine serotonin transporter protein (SERT). Serotonin acts as a short-range neurotransmitter in the central nervous system, and it also mediates long-range signaling, particularly in the gut. Polymorphisms in the serotonergic transport system have been implicated in FM [9], IBS [44,70,96], and TMD [38]. Like COMT, SERT is also important in a number of psychiatric disorders such as depression [8,27,97], anxiety [51], and bipolar disorder [17,77]. A number of polymorphisms of *SLC6A4* have been identified, both intronic and exonic. *5-HTTLPR* is a 44-base pair insertion/deletion polymorphism in the regulatory region of *SLC6A4* with two forms: a short allele, S, and a long allele, L. The L allele can be further subdivided into two allelic functional variants designated as L_A and L_G. Carriers of the L_G and S alleles have reduced transcriptional efficiency, lower concentrations of 5-HT transporters, and thus higher concentrations of synaptic 5-HT. These individuals also have a greater probability of developing chronic pain disorders and psychiatric disorders, particularly in conjunction with early life stress. 5-HT appears to be critical for the early development of emotional circuitry in the brain, and even transient alterations in 5-HT homeostasis during early development modify brain circuits implicated in mood disorders and cause permanent elevations in anxiety-related behaviors during adulthood, according to both human [13] and animal studies [2,11,12]. Norepinephrine and dopamine signaling systems are other monoaminergic systems implicated in chronic pain. Drugs that target monoaminergic systems have shown effectiveness in treatment of IC/PBS, IBS, FM [9], migraine, and TMD. However, there are contradictory reports on the association of *SLC6A4* (SERT) gene polymorphisms and chronic pain disorders. A meta-analysis by Van Kerkhoven et al. [90] of eight published studies found no association between *5-HTTLPR* and IBS. Some of the failure to replicate findings within and between chronic pain syndromes may be due to insufficient sample sizes, given the modest effects of any single locus in complex traits, and to failure to control for environmental factors such as psychological trauma and adverse early life events [89].

Ion Channel Genes

A number of voltage-gated ion channels have been implicated in the pathophysiology of pain. Sodium, calcium, and potassium channels are all reported to play a part in the pain response. The role of sodium ion channels was first identified through rare, single gene pain disorders. Mutations in the *SCN9A* gene, which codes for the $Na_V1.7$ sodium channel, can result in hyper- or hyposensitivity syndromes [25,31]. Mutant $Na_V1.7$ subunits have a lower activation threshold for channel opening, as well as slower inactivation. Inflammatory mediators, such as prostaglandin, adenosine, and serotonin, affect the electrophysiological properties of voltage-gated ion channels and enhance the rates of channel activation and inactivation, sensitizing nociceptive neurons and resulting in the pain associated with inflammation [29]. In animal studies, mutations of the $Na_V1.7$ coding gene resulted in a resistance to pain or hypersensitivity in response to inflammatory stimuli, without affecting sensitivity to neuropathic pain (chronic pain resulting from injury to the nervous system). $Na_V1.7$ may act to set the inflammatory pain threshold [66].

A number of rare Mendelian pain disorders are caused by mutations in genes coding for ion channels. Erythromelalgia, a rare, idiopathic chronic pain disorder that includes burning pain in the extremities, is an

autosomal dominant sodium channel disorder caused by missense mutations in *SCN9A* [29]. Paroxysmal extreme pain disorder, a disorder that
includes rectal, ocular, and submaxillary pain, is another autosomal dominant sodium channel disorder caused by missense mutations in *SCN9A*
that impair inactivation of the A subunit of the $Na_v1.7$ channel [31]. Familial hemiplegic migraine (FHM), a rare hereditary migraine, has three
forms known to be related to mutations in different voltage-gated ion
channels [21]: FHM1 is caused by mutations in *CACNA1A*, a gene coding for the α_{1a}-subunit of a voltage-gated calcium channel [69]; FHM2
is caused by mutations in *ATP1A2*, the gene coding for Na^+/K^+-ATPase
[30]; and FHM3 is caused by mutations in *SCN1A*, the gene coding for the
$Na_v1.1$ sodium channel [81].

RUNX1 is a transcription factor gene that regulates the expression of many ion channels and receptors, including transient receptor
potential (TRP) class thermal receptors [55]; Na^+-gated, adenosine triphosphate (ATP)-gated, and H^+-gated channels; and the μ-opioid receptor. *RUNX1* knockout mice are deficient in thermal and neuropathic
pain [15].

Analgesia

Analgesia is known to be influenced by genetics. The genes implicated
can vary depending on the drug, the type of pain, and the sex of the
individual. Sensitivity to analgesics is affected by drug metabolism mediated by cytochrome P-450 (*CYP2D6*).Variations in this enzyme affect
the metabolism of a wide variety of drugs [7]. Analysis of these variations
resulted in the first DNA microarray device approved by the U.S. Food
and Drug Administration to help physicians make treatment decisions
regarding drug and dosage. Polymorphisms in the *CYP2D6* gene can enhance or reduce responses to codeine, tramadol, and selective serotonin
reuptake inhibitors [33]. SNPs within a number of other genes have also
been shown to affect analgesia sensitivity: *ABCB1/MDR1* codes for the
efflux transporter P-glycoprotein and affects the bioavailability of opioid
analgesics [10]; *OPRM1* codes for the μ-opioid receptor and affects binding of opioid analgesics [10]; and *MCIR* codes for the melanocortin-1

receptor and causes decreased sensitivity to pain and increased sensitivity to opioid analgesia [63]. Animal studies suggest high heritability of sensitivity to gabapentin and pregabalin, drugs used to treat chronic pain [16].

Hyposensitivity to Pain

Congenital insensitivity to pain (CIP) is a rare syndrome that has been reported in a number of families around the world. These cases are caused by rare single gene mutations. Although rare, these idiopathic pain disorders can help elucidate the pathophysiology of pain, with far-reaching impact on the study and treatment of pain disorders. Over 40 different mutations have been reported that can lead to CIP [41,42,88]. A few of the genes responsible for hyposensitivity to pain are the gene encoding serine palmitoyltransferase, which causes CIP/hereditary sensory neuropathy type I [19]; neurotrophic tyrosine kinase receptor type 1 (*NTRK1*), a receptor in the neurotrophin signaling pathway, which causes CIP/hereditary sensory neuropathy type IV [88,91]; and *SCN9A*, which codes for the $Na_v1.7$ sodium ion channel, and with non-sense mutations causes channelopathy-associated insensitivity to pain [19].

Why Do Genes for Chronic Pain Syndromes Persist?

Chronic pain syndromes cause significant physical and emotional suffering and loss of productivity. Why do these deleterious variations in genes persist in the human population? There are several possible explanations:. (1) Many chronic pain syndromes are late- onset diseases that do not influence reproductive success. (2) It is probable that multiple genes with small individual effects cause chronic pain syndromes. Each mutation may be only slightly deleterious or may be beneficial in another context (pleiotropy). (3) Chronic pain syndromes often require environmental stimuli to trigger the disorder. The modern environment may create different pressures than those affecting the gene through most of human evolutionary history. (4) Some pain genes may reside in mutational "hot spots" (chromosomal regions with high mutation rates) so that new mutations appear fairly often. (5) Finally, for large outbred populations, genetic drift may allow slightly deleterious mutations to persist for many generations.

Future Research Directions

Although there are some strong candidates for pain-mediating genes, notably *COMT* and *SLC6A4,* there is still much work to be done to obtain a thorough understanding of the genetics of chronic pain syndromes. Contradictory results and lack of replication in studies of genes proposed to contribute to chronic pain highlight the need for more research and new strategies. Future research on pain genetics should include the following lines of inquiry.

Large-Scale Association Studies

The genetics of Mendelian disorders have been studied using linkage analysis. Linkage analysis follows the transmission of chromosomal regions through individuals within families to identify an interval linked to the trait. This method has been very successful at mapping the genes of simple, monogenic traits. However, most common genetic disorders are thought to be the result of interactions of many genes having minor effects, with other genes and with the environment. In order to obtain sufficient power to identify causative genes with small effects, larger sample populations are required than are typically available in linkage studies. Association testing is less effective than linkage analysis for identifying rare disease-causing variants, but because common traits such as chronic pain are thought to be caused by common variants, association testing is appropriate [76]. Association testing of unrelated cases and controls is a study design that allows collection of the necessary sample sizes with a practical expenditure of time and money. Association analysis tests whether a particular allele at a chromosomal locus appears more or less frequently in the cases than in the controls. Association studies can be less powerful than linkage studies for equal sample sizes, but it is so much easier and cheaper to collect large numbers of unrelated cases and controls than large family data sets that association studies have become the preferred study design. Family-based data, when available, can also be used in association studies [50]. Two types of association design can be employed, often in conjunction or in a two-staged approach: genome-wide scans and candidate gene studies.

Genome-Wide Association Studies

Genome-wide association studies with large, often multicenter, sample populations are today's preferred method to identify genes with subtle effects. Because this design tests all regions of the genome for association with the trait, it is considered a hypothesis-free strategy [47]. This approach has begun to yield results revolutionizing the genetic studies of common traits, from age-related macular degeneration [46] to schizophrenia [43]. Whole-genome association strategies are most effective with very large sample sizes and very dense marker maps. Statistical estimates of the sample sizes required for sufficient power to detect commonly observed effect sizes are in the thousands of individuals, typed at tens of thousands to millions of loci. Fortunately, genotyping costs have decreased precipitously in the last decade, and today a DNA sample can be genotyped at a million SNPs in a few hours for a few hundred U.S. dollars. Collecting the samples and phenotypes is now the rate-limiting step in both time and expense. And while rapid and accurate determination of genotypic data has become straightforward, acquiring precise phenotypic data is a challenging yet critical component in analysis of highly complex disorders such as the chronic pain syndromes, which may have many genetically important intermediate phenotypes and subphenotypes.

Candidate Gene Studies

While genome-wide, hypothesis-free association studies are useful, one can also test specific genes, or chromosomal regions containing genes that are believed to influence pain disorders. This is also called a "candidate gene" approach. Gene candidates can be suggested from many sources: genome-wide association studies, family-based linkage studies, or functional or pathway analysis of known genes [76]. In addition, animal studies have identified a large number of candidate genes, that now need to be evaluated for their relevance to human pain syndromes. For candidate gene studies, as with whole-genome scans, association analysis is the pre-ferred analysis tool due to the large population samples required to detect the small effect sizes of many genes involved with pain disorders.

Quantitative Trait Locus Mapping

If the pain disorder phenotype can be reliably quantified, analysis based on dichotomizing the trait to affected and unaffected loses considerable information. Significant power can be gained by using a statistical genetics method designed to locate quantitative trait loci (QTL). For QTL linkage analysis, the variance components method has been very successful [4]. For QTL association testing, the measured genotype approach holds great promise [50].

Sequencing to Identify Rare Variants

A widely held hypothesis is that common gene variants cause common disorders such as chronic pain syndromes. However, in highly complex syndromes such as pain disorders, there may be many genes that make small contributions to the trait, with no one gene being either necessary or sufficient. Under this mechanism, rare variants may play a role in some forms of common disease [28]. With the recent appearance on the mar-ket of massively parallel sequencing machines, deep resequencing for rare variants has become economically and practically feasible.

Epigenetic Variations

Epigenetic variations create stable genetic modifications that result in changes in gene expression and function without altering DNA sequence. Epigenetic changes can explain the mechanisms behind cell differentiation and show how patterns of gene expression are passed from a cell to its de-scendants and how environmental changes affect gene expression. Epigen-etic changes can result in expression of different phenotypes when there are no genotypic differences, and they may explain some of the difficulty in determining and reproducing the genetic causes of chronic pain syn-dromes. Chromatin modifications, DNA methylation, and micro-RNAs are some of the epigenetic phenomena being studied. DNA methylation may play a role in schizophrenia and bipolar disorder [1,18,59]. Abdol-maleky et al. report hypomethylation of the membrane-bound COMT promoter in patients with schizophrenia and bipolar disorder that may increase *COMT* expression and enrich for the val allele in the *val158met* polymorphism [1]. These epigenetic changes may mediate the observed effect of early life events on adult phenotypes such as chronic pain.

Copy Number Variants

Chromosomal gains and loses on the order of ten thousand to five million nucleotides are known as copy number variants. It is now known that these types of large-scale variation are more common than was previously understood. In humans, the genomic variation due to these large-scale differences may be on an order similar to the variation contained in SNPs. An individual can have multiple copies of the same gene, and this may have implications for disease susceptibility. Copy number variants have been reported to affect predisposition to glomerulonephritis [3] and autism [93]. Copy number variation has not yet been extensively studied with regard to chronic pain syndromes, but this will be an important area of research in the future.

Gene Expression Profiling, Gene Networks, and Systematics

To begin to understand how disease-associated genetic variation leads to disease, it will be valuable to use systems biology methods that combine information from a variety of types of data. An example of a systems approach that shows promise for explaining the mechanisms of neuro-genetic syndromes is gene coexpression analysis. This method uses gene expression levels in affected tissue to build networks of coexpressed genes. These gene networks can then be partitioned into modules of highly connected genes that exhibit functional significance. The coexpression data can then be integrated with genotypic data to look for important "hub" genes within modules [98]. This method has been used to study brain networks [68] and chronic fatigue syndrome [73], a syndrome that may be a comorbid phenotype of some chronic pain disorders (see Chapter 12 by Lange and Natelson).

Endophenotypes

The genetic etiology of common traits can be complex, with many minor, single gene effects and subtle gene-gene and gene-environment interactions. A promising approach to penetrate this complexity is to subdivide a disease into endophenotypes, that is, specific, well-defined, biologically significant traits that may be mediated by a small subset of genes [32,34]. For example, there are a wide variety of general pain measures, including pressure pain, cold pain, heat pain, ischemic pain, muscle pain due to hypertonic saline, and analgesic response. Rather than use these general measures of pain response as the phenotype to analyze, one might use neuroimaging data to describe detailed neurological phenotypes underlying the pain response. These more specific neuroimaging phenotypes have a good chance of being under the control of just a few genes, each with a reasonably large effect. A larger effect implies more power to discover those genes.

Comorbid Phenotypes

There is a large body of clinical evidence associating chronic pain disorders with mood and anxiety disorders [80,87] (see also Chapter 9 by Naliboff and Rhudy on anxiety in functional pain disorders, and Chapter 10 by Schatzberg on depression). In addition, it is thought that exposure to adverse events, particularly in early life, can result in lifelong alterations in stress responsiveness and pain sensitivity when superimposed on a genetic background predisposing the individual to chronic pain. Promising approaches aim to identify differences among chronic pain patients in the central mechanisms involved in emotional arousal and affective pain modulation, and to identify possible associations with candidate gene polymorphisms and early life experience. A number of susceptibility genes may be active in establishing brain circuits early in life that may mediate symptoms and behaviors in the adult. Genetic variability by itself may not be sufficient to produce the adult phenotypic traits. Environmental influences at the time of circuit formation may be of critical importance. This may be one reason why studies on the genetics of chronic pain syndromes have proven difficult to replicate. It will be valuable to study genes known to associate with psychological phenotypes such as post-traumatic stress disorder, chronic fatigue syndrome, panic disorder [84], social anxiety disorder, and depression, and the interactions of these genes and phenotypes and early life environment with chronic pain.

Rare Disease Forms

The study of rare, idiopathic pain disorders, including both hyper- and hypo-sensitivity syndromes, has yielded valuable insights into the pathways of nociception and can continue to shed light on possible contributing mechanisms in the more common forms of pain disorder. Examples of this approach are studies of the rare diseases familial hemiplegic migraine, and congenital insensitivity to pain syndrome.

Animal Models

Animal models and transgenic animals can give great insight into the genetics of human disease [62]. Animal models for a phenotype can be selected and bred. Mouse strains with a homogeneous genetic background on which to study a phenotype are readily available. Crosses between model mouse strains and well-characterized mouse strains can yield information about the genes and genotypes contributing to traits. Candidate genes can be studied in transgenic animals. It is possible to selectively knock out, knock in, or upregulate specific genes in model organisms, simplifying the study of effects of gene mutations [49]. Short interfering RNAs can be used as tools for precise silencing of specific genes or portions of genes [36,37,58].

Treatment and Prevention

A goal of the study of pain genetics is to find ways to affect pain sensitivity. Chronic pain syndromes affect large numbers of people and are the cause of much suffering and loss of productivity. Understanding the genetics of pain sensitivity and chronic pain can inform treatment in a number of ways. Genetics clearly affects individual responsiveness to drug treatment and analgesia. Testing a patient's genotype at a number of pain loci could allow individualization of treatment in both drug choice and dosage. Understanding the underlying pathways may allow the development of novel drugs to target specific points in the pain mediation pathway. Pharmacogenetic strategies may allow the design of drugs for particular targets, conferring pain relief while sparing other neuronal functions. An example might be small-molecule therapy and channel blockers for ion channelopathies. Finally, an understanding of the gene-environment interactions and effects of early life adverse events could help prevent chronic pain in later life.

References

[1] Abdolmaleky HM, Cheng KH, Faraone SV, Wilcox M, Glatt SJ, Gao F, Smith CL, Shafa R, Aeali B, Carnevale J, et al. Hypomethylation of MB-COMT promoter is a major risk factor for schizophrenia and bipolar disorder. Hum Mol Genet 2006;15:3132–45.
[2] Adamec R, Burton P, Blundell J, Murphy DL, Holmes A. Vulnerability to mild predator stress in serotonin transporter knockout mice. Behav Brain Res 2006;170:126–40.
[3] Aitman TJ, Dong R, Vyse TJ, Norsworthy PJ, Johnson MD, Smith J, Mangion J, Roberton-Lowe C, Marshall AJ, Petretto E, et al. Copy number polymorphism in Fcgr3 predisposes to glomerulonephritis in rats and humans. Nature 2006;439:851–5.
[4] Almasy L, Blangero J. Contemporary model-free methods for linkage analysis. Adv Genet 2008;60:175–93.
[5] Bednarek N, Arbuès AS, Motte J, Sabouraud P, Plouin P, Morville P. Familial rectal pain: a familial autonomic disorder as a cause of paroxysmal attacks in the newborn baby. Epileptic Disord 2005;7:360–2.
[6] Bengtson MB, Rønning T, Vatn MH, Harris JR. Irritable bowel syndrome in twins: genes and environment. Gut 2006;55:1754–9.
[7] Bertz RJ, Granneman GR. Use of in vitro and in vivo data to estimate the likelihood of metabolic pharmacokinetic interactions. Clin Pharmacokinet 2008;32:210–58.
[8] Bozina N, Peles AM, Sagud M, Bilusic H, Jakovljevic M. Association study of paroxetine therapeutic response with SERT gene polymorphisms in patients with major depressive disorder. World J Biol Psychiatry 2007;30:1–8.
[9] Buskila D, Sarzi-Puttini P, Ablin JN. The genetics of fibromyalgia syndrome. Pharmacogenomics 2007;8:67–74.
[10] Campa D, Gioia A, Tomei A, Poli P, Barale R. Association of ABCB1/MDR1 and OPRM1 gene polymorphisms with morphine pain relief. Clin Pharmacol Ther 2008;83:559–66.
[11] Carola V, Frazzetto G, Pascucci T, Audero E, Puglisi-Allegra S, Cabib S, Lesch KP, Gross C. Identifying molecular substrates in a mouse model of the serotonin transporter × environment risk factor for anxiety and depression. Biol Psychiatry 2008;63:840–6.
[12] Carroll JC, Boyce-Rustay JM, Millstein R, Yang R, Wiedholz LM, Murphy DL, Holmes A. Effects of mild early life stress on abnormal emotion-related behaviors in 5-HTT knockout mice. Behav Genet 2007;37:214–22.
[13] Caspi A, Sugden K, Moffitt TE, Taylor A, Craig IW, Harrington H, McClay J, Mill J, Martin J, Braithwaite A, Poulton R. Influence of life stress on depression: moderation by a polymorphism in the 5-HTT gene. Science 2003;301:386–9.
[14] Chang L, Mayer EA, Johnson T, FitzGerald L, Naliboff B. Differences in somatic perception in female patients with irritable bowel syndrome with and without fibromyalgia. Pain 2000;84:297–307.
[15] Chen CL, Broom DC, Liu Y, de Nooij JC, Li Z, Cen C, Samad OA, Jessell TM, Woolf CJ, Ma Q. Runx1 determines nociceptive sensory neuron phenotype and is required for thermal and neuropathic pain. Neuron 2006;49:365–77.

[16] Chesler EJ, Ritchie J, Kokayeff A, Lariviere WR, Wilson SG, Mogil JS. Genotype-dependence of gabapentin and pregabalin sensitivity: the pharmacogenetic mediation of analgesia is specific to the type of pain being inhibited. Pain 2003;106:325–35.

[17] Cho HJ, Meira-Lima I, Cordeiro Q, Michelon L, Sham P, Vallada H, Collier DA. Population-based and family-based studies on the serotonin transporter gene polymorphisms and bipolar disorder: a systematic review and meta-analysis. Mol Psychiatry 2005;10:771–81.

[18] Connor CM, Akbarian S. DNA methylation changes in schizophrenia and bipolar disorder. Epigenetics 2008;3:55–8.

[19] Cox JJ, Reimann F, Nicholas AK, Thornton G, Roberts E, Springell K, Karbani G, Jafri H, Mannan J, Raashid Y, et al. An SCN9A channelopathy causes congenital inability to experience pain. Nature 2006;444:894–8.

[20] Dawkins JL, Hulme DJ, Brahmbhatt SB, Auer-Grumbach M, Nicholson GA. Mutations in SPTLC1, encoding serine palmitoyltransferase, long chain base subunit-1, cause hereditary sensory neuropathy type I. Nat Genet 2001;27:309–12.

[21] De Vries B, Haan J, Frants RR, Van den Maagdenberg AM, Ferrari MD. Genetic biomarkers for migraine. Headache 2006;46:1059–68.

[22] Diatchenko L, Nackley AG, Slade GD, Fillingim RB, Maixner W. Idiopathic pain disorders: pathways of vulnerability. Pain 2006;123:226–30.

[23] Diatchenko L, Nackley AG, Tchivileva IE, Shabalina SA, Maixner W. Genetic architecture of human pain perception. Trends Genet 2007;23:605–13.

[24] Diatchenko L, Slade GD, Nackley AG, Bhalang K, Sigurdsson A, Belfer I, Goldman D, Xu K, Shabalina SA, Shagin D, et al. Genetic basis for individual variations in pain perception and the development of a chronic pain condition. Hum Mol Genet 2005;14:135–43.

[25] Dib-Hajj SD, Cummins TR, Black JA, Waxman SG. From genes to pain: Na$_v$1.7 and human pain disorders. Trends Neurosci 2007;30:555–63.

[26] Dimitrakov JD. A case of familial clustering of interstitial cystitis and chronic pelvic pain syndrome. Urology 2001;58:281.

[27] Dorado P, Peñas-Lledó EM, González AP, Cáceres MC, Cobaleda J, Llerena A. Increased risk for major depression associated with the short allele of the serotonin transporter promoter region (5-HTTLPR-S) and the CYP2C9*3 allele. Fundam Clin Pharmacol 2007;21:451–3.

[28] Doris PA. Hypertension genetics, single nucleotide polymorphisms, and the common disease: common variant hypothesis. Hypertension 2002;39:323–31.

[29] Drenth JP, Waxman SG. Mutations in sodium-channel gene SCN9A cause a spectrum of human genetic pain disorders. J Clin Invest 2007;117:3603–9.

[30] Fernandez DM, Hand CK, Sweeney BJ, Parfrey NA. A novel ATP1A2 gene mutation in an Irish familial hemiplegic migraine kindred. Headache 2008;48:101–8.

[31] Fertleman CR, Baker MD, Parker KA, Moffatt S, Elmslie FV, Abrahamsen B, Ostman J, Klugbauer N, Wood JN, Gardiner RM, Rees M. SCN9A mutations in paroxysmal extreme pain disorder: allelic variants underlie distinct channel defects and phenotypes. Neuron 2006;52:767–74.

[32] Flint J, Munafo MR. The endophenotype concept in psychiatric genetics. Psychol Med 2007;37:163–80.

[33] Foster A, Mobley E, Wang Z. Complicated pain management in a CYP450 2D6 poor metabolizer. Pain Pract 2007;7:352–6.

[34] Gottesman II, Gould TD. The endophenotype concept in psychiatry: etymology and strategic intentions. Am J Psychiatry 2003;160:636–45.

[35] Gürsoy S, Erdal E, Herken H, Madenci E, Alaşehirli B, Erdal N. Significance of catechol-O-methyltransferase gene polymorphism in fibromyalgia syndrome. Rheumatol Int 2003;23:104–7.

[36] Hannon GJ. RNA interference. Nature 2002;418:244–51.

[37] Hasuwa H, Kaseda K, Einarsdottir T, Okabe M. Small interfering RNA and gene silencing in transgenic mice and rats. FEBS Lett 2002;532:227–30.

[38] Herken H, Erdal E, Mutlu N, Barlas O, Cataloluk O, Oz F, Güray E. Possible association of temporomandibular joint pain and dysfunction with a polymorphism in the serotonin transporter gene. Am J Orthod Dentofacial Orthop 2001;120:308–13.

[39] Hettema JM, An SS, Bukszar J, van den Oord EJ, Neale MC, Kendler KS, Chen X. Catechol-O-methyltransferase contributes to genetic susceptibility shared among anxiety spectrum phenotypes. Biol Psychiatry 2008;64:302–10.

[40] Higashimoto T, Baldwin EE, Gold JI, Boles RG. Reflex sympathetic dystrophy: complex regional pain syndrome type I in children with mitochondrial disease and maternal inheritance. Arch Dis Child 2008;93:390–7.

[41] Huehne K, Zweier C, Raab K, Odent S, Bonnaure-Mallet M, Sixou JL, Landrieu P, Goizet C, Sarlangue J, Baumann M, et al. Novel missense, insertion and deletion mutations in the neurotrophic tyrosine kinase receptor type 1 gene (*NTRK1*) associated with congenital insensitivity to pain with anhidrosis. Neuromuscul Disord 2008;18:159–66.

[42] Indo Y. Molecular basis of congenital insensitivity to pain with anhidrosis (CIPA): mutations and polymorphisms in *TRKA* (*NTRK1*) gene encoding the receptor tyrosine kinase for nerve growth factor. Hum Mutat 2001;18:462–71.

[43] Irmansyah, Schwab SG, Heriani, Handoko HY, Kusumawardhani A, Widyawati I, Amir N, Nasrun MW, Holmans P, Knapp M, Wildenauer DB. Genome-wide scan in 124 Indonesian sib-pair families with schizophrenia reveals genome-wide significant linkage to a locus on chromosome 3p26-21. Am J Med Genet B Neuropsychiatr Genet 2008; Epub Apr 30.

[44] Jarrett ME, Kohen R, Cain KC, Burr RL, Poppe A, Navaja GP, Heitkemper MM. Relationship of *SERT* polymorphisms to depressive and anxiety symptoms in irritable bowel syndrome. Biol Res Nurs 2007;9:161–9.

[45] Kendler KS, Kuhn JW, Vittum J, Prescott CA, Riley B. The interaction of stressful life events and a serotonin transporter polymorphism in the prediction of episodes of major depression: a replication. Arch Gen Psychiatry 2005;62:529–35.

[46] Klein RJ, Zeiss C, Chew EY, Tsai JY, Sackler RS, Haynes C, Henning AK, Sangiovanni JP, Mane SM, Mayne ST, et al. Complement factor H polymorphism in age-related macular degeneration. Science 2005;308:385–9.

[47] Kruglyak L. The road to genome-wide association studies. Nat Rev Genet 2008;9:314–8.

[48] Kumano H, Kaiya H, Yoshiuchi K, Yamanaka G, Sasaki T, Kuboki T. Comorbidity of irritable bowel syndrome, panic disorder, and agoraphobia in a Japanese representative sample. Am J Gastroenterol 2004;99:370–6.

[49] LaCroix-Fralish ML, Ledoux JB, Mogil JS. The Pain Genes Database: an interactive web browser of pain-related transgenic knockout studies. Pain 2007;131:1–4.

[50] Lange K, Sinsheimer JS, Sobel E. Association testing with Mendel. Genet Epidemiol 2005;29:36–50.

[51] Lesch KP, Bengel D, Heils A, Sabol SZ, Greenberg BD, Petri S, Benjamin J, Muller CR, Hamer DH, Murphy DL. Association of anxiety-related traits with a polymorphism in the serotonin transporter gene regulatory region. Science 1996;274:1527–31.

[52] Levy RL, Jones KR, Whitehead WE, Feld SI, Talley NJ, Corey LA. Irritable bowel syndrome in twins: heredity and social learning both contribute to etiology. Gastroenterology 2001;121:799–804.

[53] Lotta T, Vidgren J, Tilgmann C, Ulmanen I, Melén K, Julkunen I, Taskinen J. Kinetics of human soluble and membrane-bound catechol O-methyltransferase: a revised mechanism and description of the thermolabile variant of the enzyme. Biochemistry 1995;34:4202–10.

[54] Lötsch J, Geisslinger G. Current evidence for a modulation of nociception by human genetic polymorphisms. Pain 2007;132:18–22.

[55] Macpherson LJ, Xiao B, Kwan KY, Petrus MJ, Dubin AE, Hwang S, Cravatt B, Corey DP, Patapoutian A. An ion channel essential for sensing chemical damage. J Neurosci 2007;27:11412–5.

[56] Matsuka Y, Nagamatsu C, Itoh S, Tomonari T, Makki A, Minakuchi H, Maekawa K, Kanyama M, Kuboki T. Comparison of inter-twin concordance in symptoms of temporomandibular disorders: a preliminary investigation in an adolescent twin population. Cranio 2007;25:23–92.

[57] Mayer EA, Craske MG, Naliboff BD. Depression, anxiety and the gastrointestinal system. J Clin Psychiatry 2001;62:28–36.

[58] McManus MT, Sharp PA. Gene silencing in mammals by small interfering RNAs. Nat Rev Genet 2002;3:737–47.

[59] Mill J, Tang T, Kaminsky Z, Khare T, Yazdanpanah S, Bouchard L, Jia P, Assadzadeh A, Flanagan J, Schumacher A, Wang SC, Petronis A. Epigenomic profiling reveals DNA-methylation changes associated with major psychosis. Am J Hum Genet 2008;82:696–711.

[60] Mogil JS. The genetic mediation of individual differences in sensitivity to pain and its inhibition. Proc Natl Acad Sci USA 1999;96:7744–51.

[61] Mogil JS, Chesler EJ, Wilson SG, Juraska JM, Sternberg WF. Sex differences in thermal nociception and morphine antinociception in the rodent depend on genotype. Neurosci Biobehav Rev 2000;24:375–89.

[62] Mogil JS, Grisel JE. Transgenic studies of pain. Pain 1998;77:107–28.

[63] Mogil JS, Ritchie J, Smith SB, Strasburg K, Kaplan L, Wallace MR, Romberg RR, Bijl H, Sarton EY, Fillingim RB, Dahan A. Melanocortin-1 receptor gene variants affect pain and mu-opioid analgesia in mice and humans. J Med Genet 2005;42:583–7.

[64] Morris-Yates A, Talley NJ, Boyce PM, Nandurkar S, Andrews G. Evidence of a genetic contribution to functional bowel disorder. Am J Gastroenterol 1998;93:1311–7.

[65] Nackley AG, Tan KS, Fecho K, Flood P, Diatchenko L, Maixner W. Catechol-O-methyltransferase inhibition increases pain sensitivity through activation of both beta2- and beta3-adrenergic receptors. Pain 2007;128:199–208.

[66] Nassar MA, Stirling LC, Forlani G, Baker MD, Matthews EA, Dickenson AH, Wood JN. Nociceptor-specific gene deletion reveals a major role for $Na_V1.7$ (PN1) in acute and inflammatory pain. Proc Natl Acad Sci USA 2004;101:12706–11.

[67] Nemmani KVS, Grisel JE, Stowe JR, Smith-Carliss R, Mogil JS. Modulation of morphine analgesia by site-specific N-methyl-D-aspartate receptor antagonists: dependence on sex, site of antagonism, morphine dose, and time. Pain 2004;109:274–83.

[68] Oldham MC, Horvath S, Geschwind DH. Conservation and evolution of gene co-expression networks in human and chimpanzee brain. Proc Natl Acad Sci USA 2006;103:17973–8.

[69] Ophoff RA, Terwindt GM, Vergouwe MN, van Eijk R, Oefner PJ, Hoffman SM, Lamerdin JE, Mohrenweiser HW, Bulman DE, Ferrari M, et al. Familial hemiplegic migraine and episodic ataxia type-2 are caused by mutations in the Ca^{2+} channel gene *CACNL1A4*. Cell 1996;87:543–52.

[70] Park MI, Camilleri M. Genetics and genotypes in irritable bowel syndrome: implications for diagnosis and treatment. Gastroenterol Clin North Am 2005;34:305–17.

[71] Pellegrino MJ, Waylonis GW, Sommer A. Familial occurrence of primary fibromyalgia. Arch Phys Med Rehabil 1989;70:61–3.

[72] Pezawas L, Meyer-Lindenberg A, Drabant EM, Verchinski BA, Munoz KE, Kolachana BS, Egan MF, Mattay VS, Hariri AR, Weinberger DR. *5-HTTLPR* polymorphism impacts human cingulate-amygdala interactions: a genetic susceptibility mechanism for depression. Nat Neurosci 2005;8:828–34.

[73] Presson AP, Sobel EM, Papp JC, Suarez CJ, Whistler T, Rajeevan MS, Vernon SD, Horvath S. Integrated weighted gene co-expression network analysis with an application to chronic fatigue syndrome. BMC Systems Biol 2008;2:95.

[74] Rakvåg TT, Klepstad P, Baar C, Kvam TM, Dale O, Kaasa S, Krokan HE, Skorpen F. The *Val-158Met* polymorphism of the human catechol-O-methyltransferase (COMT) gene may influence morphine requirements in cancer pain patients. Pain 2005;116:73–8.

[75] Reyes-Gibby CC, Shete S, Rakvåg T, Bhat SV, Skorpen F, Bruera E, Kaasa S, Klepstad P. Exploring joint effects of genes and the clinical efficacy of morphine for cancer pain: OPRM1 and COMT gene. Pain 2007;130:25–30.

[76] Risch N, Merikangas K. The future of genetic studies of complex human diseases. Science 1996;273:1516–7.

[77] Saleem Q, Ganesh S, Vijaykumar M, Reddy YC, Brahmachari SK, Jain S. Association analysis of 5HT transporter gene in bipolar disorder in the Indian population. Am J Med Genet 2000;96:170–2.

[78] Saito YA, Schoenfeld P, Locke GR 3rd. The epidemiology of irritable bowel syndrome in North America: a systematic review. Am J Gastroenterol 2002;97:1910–5.

[79] Schur EA, Afari N, Furberg H, Olarte M, Goldberg J, Sullivan PF, Buchwald D. Feeling bad in more ways than one: comorbidity patterns of medically unexplained and psychiatric conditions. J Gen Intern Med 2007;22:818–21.

[80] Slade GD, Diatchenko L, Bhalang K, Sigurdsson A, Fillingim RB, Belfer I, Max MB, Goldman D, Maixner W. Influence of psychological factors on risk of temporomandibular disorders. J Dent Res 2007;86:1120–5.

[81] Stam AH, van den Maagdenberg AM, Haan J, Terwindt GM, Ferrari MD. Genetics of migraine: an update with special attention to genetic comorbidity. Curr Opin Neurol 2008;21:288–93.

[82] Sternberg WF, Chesler EJ, Wilson SG, Mogil JS. Acute progesterone can recruit sex-specific neurochemical mechanisms mediating swim stress-induced and kappa-opioid analgesia in mice. Horm Behav 2004;46:467–73.

[83] Stych B, Dobrovolny D. Familial cold auto-inflammatory syndrome (FCAS): characterization of symptomatology and impact on patients' lives. Curr Med Res Opin 2008;24:1577–82.

[84] Talati A, Ponniah K, Strug LJ, Hodge SE, Fyer AJ, Weissman MM. Panic disorder, social anxiety disorder, and a possible medical syndrome previously linked to chromosome 13. Biol Psychiatry 2008;63:594–601.

[85] Talley NJ. Environmental versus genetic risk factors for irritable bowel syndrome: clinical and therapeutic implications. Rev Gastroenterol Disord 2005;5:82–8.

[86] Torpy DJ, Papanicolaou DA, Lotsikas AJ, Wilder RL, Chrousos GP, Pillemer SR. Responses of the sympathetic nervous system and the hypothalamic-pituitary-adrenal axis to interleukin-6: a pilot study in fibromyalgia. Arthritis Rheum 2000;43:872–80.

[87] Tunks ER, Crook J, Weir R. Epidemiology of chronic pain with psychological comorbidity: prevalence, risk, course, and prognosis. Can J Psychiatry 2008;53:224–34.

[88] Tüysüz B, Bayrakli F, Diluna ML, Bilguvar K, Bayri Y, Yalcinkaya C, Bursali A, Ozdamar E, Korkmaz B, Mason CE, et al. Novel *NTRK1* mutations cause hereditary sensory and autonomic neuropathy type IV: demonstration of a founder mutation in the Turkish population. Neurogenetics 2008;9:119–25.

[89] Uher R, McGuffin P. The moderation by the serotonin transporter gene of environmental adversity in the aetiology of mental illness: review and methodological analysis. Mol Psychiatry 2008;13:131–46.

[90] Van Kerkhoven LA, Laheij RJ, Jansen JB. Meta-analysis: a functional polymorphism in the gene encoding for activity of the serotonin transporter protein is not associated with the irritable bowel syndrome. Aliment Pharmacol Ther 2007;26:979–86.

[91] Verpoorten N, Claeys KG, Deprez L, Jacobs A, Van Gerwen V, Lagae L, Arts WF, De Meirleir L, Keymolen K, Ceuterick-de Groote C, et al. Novel frameshift and splice site mutations in the neurotrophic tyrosine kinase receptor type 1 gene (*NTRK1*) associated with hereditary sensory neuropathy type IV. Neuromuscul Disord 2006;16:19–25.

[92] Warren JW, Jackson TL, Langenberg P, Meyers DJ, Xu J. Prevalence of interstitial cystitis in first-degree relatives of patients with interstitial cystitis. Urology 2004;63:17–21.

[93] Weiss LA, Shen Y, Korn JM, Arking DE, Miller DT, Fossdal R, Saemundsen E, Stefansson H, Ferreira MA, Green T, et al.; Autism Consortium. Association between microdeletion and microduplication at 16p11.2 and autism. N Engl J Med 2008;358:667–75.

[94] Williams HJ, Owen MJ, O'Donovan MC. Is *COMT* a susceptibility gene for schizophrenia? Schizophr Bull 2007;33:635–41.

[95] Wray NR, James MR, Dumenil T, Handoko HY, Lind PA, Montgomery GW, Martin NG. Association study of candidate variants of *COMT* with neuroticism, anxiety and depression. Am J Med Genet B Neuropsychiatr Genet 2008; Epub Apr 2.

[96] Yeo A, Boyd P, Lumsden S, Saunders T, Handley A, Stubbins M, Knaggs A, Asquith S, Taylor I, Bahari B, et al. Association between a functional polymorphism in the serotonin transporter gene and diarrhoea-predominant irritable bowel syndrome in women. Gut 2004;53:1452–8.

[97] Young KA, Bonkale WL, Holcomb LA, Hicks PB, German DC. Major depression, *5HT-TLPR* genotype, suicide and antidepressant influences on thalamic volume. Br J Psychiatry 2008;192:285–9.

[98] Zhang B, Horvath S. A general framework for weighted gene co-expression network analysis. Stat Appl Genet Mol Biol 2005;4:Article 17.

[99] Zubieta JK, Heitzeg MM, Smith YR, Bueller JA, Xu K, Xu Y, Koeppe RA, Stohler CS, Goldman D. *COMT val158met* genotype affects mu-opioid neurotransmitter responses to a pain stressor. Science 2003;299:1240–3.

Correspondence to: Jeanette Papp, Department of Human Genetics, David Geffen School of Medicine at UCLA, 695 Charles E. Young Drive South, Los Angeles, CA 90095-7088, USA. Tel: 1-310-825-6204; fax: 1-310-794-5446; email: jcpapp@ucla.edu.

Early Life Trauma and Chronic Pain

Elie D. Al-Chaer[a] and Shelley A. Weaver[b]

[a]Center for Pain Research, Departments of Pediatrics, Internal Medicine-Gastroenterology,
Neurobiology and Developmental Sciences, University of Arkansas for Medical Sciences,
Little Rock, Arkansas, USA; [b]Quintiles, Parsippany, New Jersey, USA

Interindividual variability exists in pain sensitivity, efficacy of analgesics, and susceptibility to developing chronic pain conditions. Sources of such variability can be intrinsic or extrinsic to the individual. Intrinsic organismic variables include gender, age, hormonal status, genetic variability, and interactions among these factors, the effects of which have been elucidated by carefully controlled laboratory studies (see [25,99,100] for reviews). Indeed, investigations of genetically based variability in pain behavior (and analgesia) have indicated a high degree of heritability of such traits; a substantial portion of variability in these traits can be accounted for by differences in genes. However, there is much unexplained variance, even in pain-related traits with substantial heritability.

On the other hand, extrinsic environmental factors can also contribute to variability in pain-related traits. Of course, these factors operate on a background of genetic variability, but certain identifiable environmental factors—such as social environment, stressful conditions, or light cycle—can affect the observation of pain behavior in experimental subjects.

Prenatal and postnatal stages of development form a critical window for the programming of physiological responses by environmental factors. The purpose of early-life programming is to tip the scales in favor of survival, especially when conditions are suboptimal. Less desirable outcomes occur when there is a mismatch between the pre- and postnatal environments and those that will be experienced later in life. For example, malnutrition during early prenatal life will program metabolic efficiencies in the offspring that increase the likelihood of survival when food is scarce but lead to obesity when food is abundant [71,118]. The chronology of these critical windows depends on the physiological system, the species, and to some extent, the current environment. With respect to the nociceptive system, environmental factors encountered early in life are involved in programming future pain sensitivity.

A potential source of variability in the pain experience in adulthood is the individual's life history of environmental factors such as noxious stimuli and stress. Pain experience early in life, theoretically, can shape the developing nervous system during the period of heightened plasticity that characterizes early postnatal development. Overproduction of neurons and synapses is the rule during gestational development; postnatal experience refines and prunes those connections, such that only those that are used are retained. What is less clear, in somatosensory systems, is how the principle of use-dependence influences the integrity and competence of peripheral afferents and central modulatory circuitry.

Similarly, abuse during childhood is the hallmark of postnatal environmental adversity in humans, and there is evidence for an association between childhood abuse and chronic pain later in life [123,152]. For example, fibromyalgia is associated with early-life adversity, including physical and sexual abuse or impaired parental bonding [70,91]. Furthermore, individuals who report abuse during childhood report more pain symptoms and chronic pain disorders as adults, and individuals with chronic pain are more likely to report abuse or neglect in childhood [45,56]. However, studies on early-life trauma and pain sensitivity in humans are usually limited to retrospective data due to logistic and ethical considerations, so that animal models become crucial in understanding the programming of the nociceptive axis.

This chapter considers the long-term effects of early noxious stimulation and stress on pain behavior (and related behaviors) using animal models. The neonatal rodent represents a useful model for investigation of the long-term consequences of early pain or stress in humans, for a number of reasons. The pain system is understandably highly conserved across species due to its crucial role in survival: the thermal-pain threshold for rats is identical to that in humans (45°C) [19]. We can also model early-life adversity in animals during both prenatal and postnatal life. Newborn pups are born in a comparatively immature state, with neurological equivalents of cortical areas estimated at the second trimester stage of human brain development [36]. Human neonates born at such an early stage of development require extensive medical intervention, much of which is likely to be noxious in nature. Therefore, the study of newborn rodents allows researchers to model the effects of painful manipulations in the neonatal intensive care unit on severely premature infants. Rodents are also useful for ease of study. Laboratory rodents yield large litters of pups after a brief (approximately 3-week) gestation, and they have a very quick postnatal maturation rate—they are weaned from the dam at approximately 20 days of age and reach sexual maturity at roughly 6 weeks of age. Adult testing typically begins at 10–12 weeks of age in most investigations. Thus, an experiment on long-term consequences of early pain or stress in the laboratory rodent can be accomplished in a few months, rather than the decades required to investigate the phenomenon in human subjects. As a result, animal models are a highly appropriate and necessary substitute for human studies when examining the relationship between early-life trauma and pain.

Overview of the Developing Nervous System

Early pain experience requires that the functional capacity of the pain-sensing circuitry be sufficiently well-developed in the subjects under study. There is ample behavioral and neurological evidence that nociceptive pathways are formed and functional at birth in humans and laboratory animals [8,9,93]. Indeed, there is even evidence that preterm humans and newborn rodents exhibit exaggerated nociceptive responses compared to either young (not neonatal) or adult animals [57].

Newborn rodents exhibit enhanced behavioral responses to von Frey hair stimulation [59], noxious chemical stimuli [144], and noxious thermal stimuli [54,57,139], when compared to adults or older juveniles. They also demonstrate reduced specificity of peripheral afferents: large-diameter Aβ fibers make synaptic contacts in spinal cord laminae involved in nociceptive processing in the neonate [39], whereas in the adult, these large-diameter afferents are not believed to be involved in direct nociceptive processing. Furthermore, it has been suggested that the enhanced pain behavior observed in neonatal rodents results from the immaturity of descending pain inhibitory pathways.

The sensation of pain is not simply the perceptual outcome of activity in peripheral afferents but also depends on modulatory mechanisms throughout the central nervous system (CNS) that can serve to alter the signal that is ultimately interpreted as pain by the brain. Among these modulatory mechanisms are plastic synapses in the spinal cord that are strengthened by use (providing a plausible mechanism for enhanced responses resulting from exposure to early pain), as well as inhibitory controls that attenuate the signal arising from peripheral afferents. These descending inhibitory controls originate in brainstem loci such as the central gray matter (periaqueductal gray), with synapses in the rostroventral medulla, and they project down the spinal cord in the dorsolateral funiculus to synapse on dorsal horn neurons. This circuitry serves to diminish the ascending signal that will reach the brain. Electrical stimulation of the dorsolateral funiculus produces analgesia in adult rodents and in prepubertal juveniles, but not in neonates [58]. Therefore, one possible mechanism for enhanced pain experience in the neonate is the relative timing of the development of ascending nociceptive versus descending inhibitory pathways.

Analgesic responses can be observed in the neonate following administration of various opioid receptor agonists as early as postnatal day P0 (the day of birth), with increases in analgesia occurring throughout the first week of life [22]. Morphine, the prototypical μ-opioid agonist, produces near-maximal analgesia on P0 in tests of nociceptive reflexes (tail-withdrawal test, mechanical withdrawal), although the analgesic response to supraspinally organized thermal pain responses [67] is modest on P0 and increases significantly during the first weeks of life [103,139]. As early as P2, substantial analgesia is observed following administration of δ-and κ-opioid agonists [88,89]. Given that descending analgesic circuitry is not fully developed in the early neonatal period, the analgesic effects are most likely due to the presence of spinal opioid receptors, which appear to be in place at birth. Neonates are also capable of mounting an analgesic response to other opioid ligands and non-opioid analgesics, such as meperidine, buprenorphine [92], and isoflurane [125]. In some experimental models, the long-term effects of neonatal exposure to painful stimuli (described in detail in the next section) are attenuated by concurrent administration of analgesic agents, highlighting the importance of effective analgesic treatment in the neonate [2,21,138].

Thus, the nociceptive and antinociceptive neural circuits undergo substantial synaptic change during the early neonatal period, and they are therefore vulnerable to the effects of sensory stimulation. It is during this time of synapse formation, rearrangement, and retention that neural pathways are most malleable, as illustrated in numerous studies of the long-term effects of early visual deprivation on adulthood visual capacity. Most studies investigating basic principles of experience-dependent sensory development involve sensory deprivation, rather than overstimulation. However, various somatosensory or viscerosensory experimental models have recently been developed to investigate the consequences of early noxious stimulation in laboratory rodents. The next section describes these experimental models.

Models of Neonatal Noxious Experience

Models of early-life incidents—such as repetitive pain, inflammation, skin wounding, visceral stimulation, and surgery—in rodents and other species have noted multiple alterations in the neonatal and adult nervous system, correlated with specific behavioral phenotypes that depend on the timing and nature of the insult. The general rule in sensation is that sensitivity declines with chronic stimulation (i.e., habituation). However, pain sensation is different from other sensory abilities on many levels, including the ways in which nociceptors respond to repeated stimulation (wind-up and sensitization). In response to high levels of activation in nociceptive afferents, CNS mechanisms serve to strengthen spinal synapses, leading to enhanced responsiveness to future afferent input. The nociceptive neuronal circuits are generally formed during embryonic and postnatal times, when painful stimuli are normally limited and the neural circuitry involved in pain modulation is not yet fully developed. Therefore, the occurrence of persistent inflammation and pain in the neonate may come as a novelty and is likely to have a strong impact on development across several critical time points. Although there are some discrepancies in the long-term consequences of pain, produced by using different animal models of neonatal pain, the consensus is that early periods of development are especially vulnerable to the long-term effects of brief or repetitive pain exposures.

Repeated Noxious Stimulation

Rat pups exposed to daily footshock from birth to 21 days of age, and reared with no manipulation afterwards, showed a significant increase in paw-lick latency and in antinociceptive effects of morphine (1.25, 2.5, and 5.0 mg/kg) after maturation (at 90–100 days of age) compared with two control groups. These results indicate that exposure to painful footshock during the preweanling period has a long-term effect on the sensitivity of rats to painful events [129]. In another study, neonatal rat pups were stimulated four times each day from P0 to P7 with either needle pricks or tactile stimuli. Decreased pain latencies were noted at P16 and P22 in the rats exposed to acute pain in the neonatal period, indicating some effect of repetitive neonatal pain on subsequent development of the pain system, although no significant differences were observed in the adult rats [10]. Despite the discrepancies in the results of the two studies, both indicate that brief or repetitive pain exposures during early periods of development can have a long-term effect on the behavior of the adult.

Inflammatory Noxious Stimuli

In adult rats that received a brief period of inflammation just after birth, the receptive fields (areas of skin) supplied by individual dorsal horn neurons decreased by more than 30% [113], implying permanent alterations in spinal nociceptive processing for these areas. In a similar model of short-lasting local inflammation (produced by injection of 0.25% carrageenan), a long-term hypoalgesia at baseline occurred equally in the previously injured and uninjured paws [81], suggesting centrally mediated mechanisms [87,113]. However, after re-inflammation, long-term hyperalgesia occurred in the neonatally injured paw, indicating a significant segmental involvement in the spinal processing of pain [114]. The critical window for generation of both of these long-term effects (global hypoalgesia and segmental hyperalgesia) occurred within the first postnatal week in rats, and the effects were also detectable in 120–125-day-old rats [114].

Subsequent experiments tested the effects of neonatal hindpaw inflammation at P3 or P14 on visceral and somatic pain sensitivity in adult rats. P3-treated rats showed a greater degree of inhibitory processing of somatic and visceral stimuli during adulthood, but no long-term consequences were noted in the P14-treated rats. However, inflammation in the adult rat, in previously uninjured tissue, reversed the relative hypoalgesia resulting from neonatal inflammation and evoked the normal hyperexcitability associated with tissue injury [153].

In an animal model of persistent inflammatory pain, neonatal rat pups were exposed to repeated formalin injections from days P1 to P7. The rats exhibited decreased alcohol preference and reduced locomotor activity in adulthood, suggesting that plasticity of the neonatal brain may be causing permanent changes in spinal cord or brain development, leading to these behavioral changes [21]. By comparison, neonatal rats treated with complete Freund's adjuvant, used to produce intense inflammation that lasts for a relatively prolonged period, exhibited as adults increased input onto spinal neuronal circuits, segmental changes in nociceptive primary afferent axons, and altered responses to sensory stimulation [121]. These rats also showed increased dorsal horn neuronal activity in response to both innocuous and noxious stimuli; the receptive fields were significantly larger in the treated group as compared to the controls [108].

Skin Wounding

In a model of surgical skin wounding, removal of a small piece of skin was followed by robust sprouting of the local sensory nerve terminals, resulting in cutaneous hyperinnervation that lasted into adulthood. This response was more pronounced when it occurred at birth in newborn rats as compared to older ages, and it continued to mediate a heightened sensitivity to pain, even into adulthood [116]. Neither hyperinnervation nor hypersensitivity were significantly altered by the application of a regional nerve block at the time of injury, suggesting that regional analgesia, used commonly in clinical practice, is unlikely to prevent the hyperinnervation that follows skin wounding [46].

Visceral Stimuli

Newborn rat pups exposed to nociceptive or inflammatory treatments of their colons exhibit altered sensory pathways circuitry and a stronger response to pain in adulthood [3]. Adult rats exposed to persistent neonatal colon inflammation (produced with 2% mustard oil, injected into the colon lumen at P8–P21) exhibited visceral hypersensitivity in response to colorectal distension and also showed signs of central neural sensitization in the dorsal horn neurons. Similarly, adult rats that received neonatal colorectal distension (a painful stimulus produced using an angioplasty balloon inflated inside the descending colon) showed visceral hypersensitivity associated with central sensitization [3]. The visceral hypersensitivity was also associated with sensitization of primary afferents [82] and other functional changes in sensory pathways, including changes in thalamospinal modulation of dorsal horn sensory processes. In adult rats that had received noxious stimulation of the colon as neonates (P8–P12), a shift in the role of the thalamus was observed. Thalamic stimulation in the region of the ventrobasal complex is known to inhibit nociceptive neuronal responses in the dorsal horn under normal conditions [130]; however, in adult rats exposed neonatally to noxious stimulation of the colon, thalamic stimulation had a largely facilitatory effect [122].

In addition to viscerosomatic hypersensitivity and neurophysiological plasticity, adult rats exposed to neonatal noxious colon stimulation showed changes in metabolic outcomes, characterized mainly by disturbances in colon motility and changes in fecal output (J. Wang, C. Gu, and E.D. Al-Chaer, unpublished manuscript). These symptoms were observed in the absence of colon inflammation. When combined, these observations mimic to a large extent the symptoms commonly seen in patients with irritable bowel syndrome (IBS) [4]. In fact, a recent study concluded that noxious stimulation caused by gastric suction at birth may promote the development of long-term visceral hypersensitivity and cognitive hypervigilance, leading to an increased prevalence of functional intestinal disorders in later life [11]. On the other hand, a decrease in exploratory activity was also seen in adults rats treated with neonatal noxious colon stimulation, who confined themselves to a limited area of an open field. The decrease in exploratory activity was aggravated by stress [68]. In general, voluntary exploratory behavior of animals in a new environment may be used as a measure of discomfort that may be associated with ongoing pain [107], distress and anxiety, sociosexual behavior [63], or adaptation to or fear of leaving a familiar place. This fear, clinically known as agoraphobia, is often a symptom comorbid with IBS. These symptoms were studied in male and female rats at different stages of the estrous cycle. Early results indicate a differential outcome in males and females, with female rats showing more sensitivity to nociceptive stimuli, particularly when their levels of circulating estrogen are elevated [154].

Such investigations substantiate a long-lasting impact of early postnatal events on the neural processing of sensory information. This impact includes alterations in the afferent pathways, hyperexcitability or sensitization of the receptive neurons, and possibly a shift in the dynamics of sensory channels and descending controls, which in turn determine the visceral sensitivity of the adult organism and predispose the adult to chronic visceral pain.

Surgery

A clinically relevant model of surgical injury in neonates employed a laparotomy under cold anesthesia on the day of birth, followed by morphine analgesia postoperatively (or a saline control) in mouse pups. Laparotomy produced increased ultrasonic distress vocalizations, but did not change maternal care for these pups. In adulthood, various tests for nociceptive sensitivity showed that neonatal surgery decreased pain behavior relative to the control groups; this effect was reversed by postoperative morphine treatment in the neonatal period [138].

Long-Term Effects of Neonatal Pain on Adult Pain Behavior

A growing body of literature indicates that repetitive neonatal pain causes profound and long-lasting changes in nociceptive thresholds and in subsequent patterns of nociceptive processing [8] and leads to changes in adult behavior in animal models. These changes range from hypoalgesic to hyperalgesic states, depending on the nature, time, and duration of the neonatal injury, and are often associated with plastic changes in sensory circuitry. Change in some of these behaviors may be attributable to long-term changes in the supraspinal processing of pain or altered stress responses [10]. However, changes are also seen in the peripheral nervous system and the spinal cord [82,83]. These widespread changes in behavioral and neuromotor functions imply that the long-term effects of repetitive or prolonged neonatal pain may pervade all parts of the brain, including those involved in mediating responses to stress. It is important to keep in mind that in the neonate, "pain is always stressful, but stress is not necessarily painful" [7].

Prenatal Stress and Long-Term Pain-Related Behavior

In rodents, prenatal stress can be induced by repeated exposure to inescapable stress during the last week of pregnancy. Prenatal stress in rodents leads to a number of persistent physiological perturbations in offspring, such as hypertension [78], delayed cognitive development [69,79], anxiety [110], and hyperactivity of the endocrine stress axis [44]. Prenatal stress also affects acute and sustained pain sensitivity in offspring both early and late in life.

Using the latency to withdraw a paw from a noxious (50–56°C) thermal stimulus (the hotplate test) as a measure of somatic pain sensitivity, a number of groups have reported reduced pain sensitivity in both male and female offspring of prenatally stressed dams compared to offspring of non-stressed dams [137,142]. In one study, the difference was evident only in female offspring of stressed dams [135]. When the spinally mediated tail-flick test was used, female offspring of prenatally stressed dams exhibited increased pain sensitivity compared to offspring of non-stressed dams, with no difference detected between male offspring in either group [76].

Other groups have measured the impact of prenatal stress on inflammatory pain during both acute and persistent phases. Persistent pain can be measured in the rat using formalin injections into the paw to induce a mild inflammation with a biphasic behavioral response to pain that is characterized by an initial acute reaction, as a result of peripheral nociceptor activation, and a second and longer response, as a consequence of the inflammation and sensitization [1,38].

Seven-day-old male offspring of prenatally stressed rats displayed a significantly greater number of flinches and shakes during the second-phase (persistent) response to a 10% formalin solution injected in the plantar pad of the left hindpaw compared to male offspring of non-stressed dams [28]; however, this difference was not evident in female offspring. This difference in the behavioral expression of persistent pain in the male prenatally stressed offspring was accompanied by a greater number of Fos-labeled neurons, indicating greater neuronal activity, in laminae I–V of the lumbar dorsal horn [27]. Interestingly, the second-phase response was absent in both male and female offspring of non-stressed dams, indicating a central sensitization in the male offspring of prenatally stressed rats that had not developed in P7 pups from non-stressed dams [27]. Thus, even as early as 7 days of age, prenatal stress can affect pain sensitivity.

As adult rats (90 days of age), both male and female offspring of prenatally stressed dams exhibited increased pain sensitivity in response to formalin injections during the second phase compared to offspring from non-stressed dams [29]. A greater expression of pain-related behaviors during the first (acute) phase of the response to formalin was also evident in the offspring of prenatally stressed rats; however, this finding was limited to female offspring [29].

In summary, evidence exists for a critical prenatal window for the development of the nociceptive system. The perturbations in subsequent development vary depending on gender, age, and the type and duration of noxious stimuli, thus providing evidence for the complexity of the interactions between prenatal events and nociception throughout the life of the affected offspring.

Postnatal Manipulations: Neonatal Handling and Maternal Separation

The most extensively researched model of adversity during development is the impact of postnatal treatments that alter maternal care. The quality and amount of maternal care is the most salient environmental factor determining survival for rodents. A plethora of data also supports the importance of maternal care to future physiological responses to the environment. Decreases in maternal care can therefore be considered a form of early-life adversity.

Brief repeated 15-minute separations of litters from mothers (neonatal handling treatment [HT]) led to rats with low stress reactivity exhibited by dampened corticosterone and adrenocorticotropic hormone (ACTH) responses to stress later in life [95]. Enhanced negative feedback effects of corticosterone due to increased hippocampal glucocorticoid receptors were responsible for the relative hypothalamic-pituitary-adrenal axis hyporeactivity of these rats [95,106]. The converse was true in litters that had been separated from their mothers for 3-hour periods over the first 2 weeks of life (maternal separation treatment [MST]): hippocampal glucocorticoid receptor levels were reduced, and high stress reactivity was exhibited by exaggerated corticosterone and ACTH responses to stress [111]. Mothers of HT litters engage in greater licking and grooming of pups [86], whereas mothers of MST litters exhibit decreased licking and grooming behavior [24]. These changes in "nurture" are involved in regulating hippocampal glucocorticoid receptor mRNA expression and, therefore, stress reactivity, and as such they drive the effects of HT and MST in offspring [86].

MST and HT rats differ in a number of behaviors and in biochemical signaling. Examples include fearfulness, learning, and memory [77,85, 101]; responses to drugs of abuse such as opioids [96,97] and alcohol [74]; and aggression [146]. Signaling systems in the CNS that are affected by MST and HT treatments include cholinergic [85], noradrenergic [15,84], dopaminergic [15,26], GABAergic [30,141], serotonergic [15,80,149], and opioidergic systems [64,155]. It is no surprise that with such a broad impact on the CNS, nociception is altered by MST and HT treatments.

Self-reported sensitivity to a painful stimulus varies dramatically between individuals [105] and is accompanied by objective differences in supraspinal processing of pain-related information [40]. Importantly, heightened pain sensitivity may be a diathesis for chronic pain disorders [48,51]. For example, individuals who report the most pain at the time of an injury have the greatest risk of developing a persistent pain disorder [109,132]. Interestingly, there is evidence for altered pain sensitivity as a consequence of HT and MST treatments.

In mice, a modified handling procedure (in which pups are housed individually during the 15-minute isolations) led to increased paw-lick latencies on a 56°C hotplate compared to pups from undisturbed dams (non-handled [NH] animals) [137]. In rats, in male HT offspring, tail-flick latencies were longer, and the animals spent significantly less time licking the injected paw in the formalin test (first phase) compared to NH rats [43]. Conversely, repeated 5-minute handling of two pups from each litter by experimenters led to shorter paw-lick latencies on a 50°C hotplate in male mice [37]. When HT rats were compared to MST rats, somatic pain sensitivity (on the hotplate test) was increased [133] or decreased in MST rats [41] or did not differ across treatments [72,73].

Gender Differences in Pain Tolerance and Sensitivity

In general, males have a higher pain tolerance across a number of species [20], and different physiology has been suggested to be involved in pain sensitivity in males and females [98]. Importantly, females have a greater risk of developing a chronic pain disorder [148]. Tests of pain sensitivity in MST and HT rats have mostly involved male offspring, although some studies have reported the effects of these treatments in female offspring.

Female MST rats have been reported to exhibit both increased [133] and similar [72,73] somatic pain sensitivity compared to female NH rats. In female Fischer rats, Stephan et al. [133] found longer paw-lick latencies on a 53°C hotplate in HT compared to NH rats, and in female

Lewis rats, these investigators found both longer latencies in HT rats and shorter latencies in MST rats compared to NH rats.

Given that pain sensitivity varies over the estrous cycle [62,75,150], variations due to estrous stage can confound measures of pain sensitivity in female animals, leading to discrepancies across studies. More recently, female MST rats have been shown to have significantly lower sensitivity to somatic pain, measured with a 50°C hotplate test, compared to HT rats, during the diestrous phase of their cycle [155]. Interestingly, in a human study, it was only in women that self-reported childhood abuse led to decreased sensitivity to noxious thermal stimuli, compared to subjects not reporting prior abuse [56]. Therefore, the reduced somatic pain sensitivity as a consequence of early-life adversity in MST female rat models is reminiscent of that seen in women. Interestingly, MST female rats in the diestrous phase exhibited increased μ-opioid receptors in the medial preoptic area of the hypothalamus [155], a brain region with links to opioid-mediated pain sensitivity [145]. In addition, the binding capacity of μ-opioid receptors in the medial preoptic area changes over the estrous cycle, with highest levels during met- and diestrous phases [66], when pain sensitivity is at its lowest in female rats [62,75,150].

The picture that emerges for somatic pain sensitivity in MST and HT rats is varied. This variation most likely arises from differences in the methodologies used across the studies. In order to avoid potential confounds, researchers must take several factors into consideration when designing studies that make use of manipulated neonatal environments. Maternal behavior is determined by many factors, including stimulation from the pups [119,134], gender distribution of the pups, litter size [102], and maternal experience [55]. Recent evidence has described increased maternal care induced by fostering [44]. Relevant to the impact on nociception is the report that male mice raised in litters composed of only male pups had shorter paw-lick latencies on a 55°C hotplate after treatment with 5 or 10 mg/kg morphine compared to male mice raised in litters containing male and female offspring [5]. Moreover, a substantial contribution of thermal challenge on the effects of handling has been demonstrated, thus emphasizing the critical role of the environment during the separations [47,126]. An important consideration is the statistical power of studies using MST and HT offspring. The treatment is applied to the litter as a whole; therefore, the experimental unit is the litter, rather than the individual. The use of small numbers of litters in this paradigm can result in litter effects being erroneously assigned to treatment effects.

Early-Life Stress and Visceral Pain

Visceral hypersensitivity in humans is characterized by increased visceromotor responses to distension and by reports of pain in response to distension pressures not considered painful in healthy subjects [156]. There is some evidence for an association between IBS and early-life trauma [124,143]. Several animal studies have investigated visceral sensitivity in HT and MST rats. In rats, electromyographic recordings of abdominal muscle contractions in response to graded colorectal distension are used as a surrogate measure of visceral pain [104,156].

In a number of studies, MST rats exhibited hypersensitivity to rectal distension, as reflected in greater visceromotor responses to distension of noxious intensity (>40 mm Hg) compared to NH rats [17,41,115,156]. The visceral response to colorectal distension in MST rats was greater in female compared to male MST rats [120]. Interestingly, tail-flick latencies were significantly longer in MST rats, suggesting decreased somatic pain sensitivity in the face of visceral hyperalgesia [41]. In fact, visceral hyperalgesia along with somatic hypoalgesia has been reported in women with IBS [31].

This enhanced visceral sensitivity in MST rats was accompanied by greater Fos-IR in ascending nociceptive pathways, including laminae I, II, and V–VI of the lumbosacral spinal cord [34,115], along with the paraventricular thalamic nucleus, the cingulate cortex, and the central nucleus of the amygdala [34]. In addition, increased expression of tyrosine receptor kinase A (TrkA, the receptor for nerve growth factor) was evident in MST compared to NH rats in laminae I–III and laminae V–VI at rest and after colorectal distension [35], thus implicating an important role of nerve growth factor in the enhanced visceral pain sensitivity of MST rats.

We can conclude that maternal separation is associated with enhanced visceral sensitivity to noxious colorectal distension and that this behavioral indicator of increased visceral pain sensitivity is accompanied by changes at a variety of levels of the nociceptive axis. Importantly, stress is known to be linked to an increase in the severity of IBS symptoms [131], and in fact there are important interactions between stress and pain that may play a role in the differential nociceptive sensitivity found in MST, HT, and NH rats.

Relationship between Stress and Pain Behavior

Antinociceptive effects of acute stress would be beneficial to survival in situations such as successful flight from a predator after an injury. In fact, acute stress applied immediately prior to pain testing does have an antinociceptive effect [147]. Links between stress and pain are apparent in the following clinical examples: the high rates of chronic pain in combat veterans with post-traumatic stress disorder [18], the correlation of cortisol levels with morning pain in fibromyalgia patients [94], the positive association between serum cortisol concentrations and chronic widespread pain [90], and the fact that patients with herpes zoster who reported psychosocial stress at disease onset had more severe pain during the acute phase of the infection and were more likely to develop postherpetic neuralgia than patients without such stress [53]. Moreover, the onset of many chronic pain disorders is characterized by a preceding or concurrent exposure to stress [12,61]. Thus, an examination of the impact of MST and HT treatments on pain sensitivity cannot exclude a discussion of potential interactions between differential stress reactivity and stress prior to or during the measurement of pain sensitivity.

Importantly, HT and MST rats have antipodal differences in stress reactivity, with MST rats showing hyperreactivity and HT rats exhibiting hyporeactivity [60,95,111,112]. Therefore, an important confounding variable in studies of pain sensitivity in MST rats is whether stress-induced analgesia is playing a role. Corticotropin-releasing hormone (CRH) delivered into the central nucleus of the amygdala increased hindpaw withdrawal latency to a 52°C hotplate in rats [42]. MST rats have an increased density of CRH receptors in the amygdala and greater CRH release in response to stress, suggestive of greater stress-induced analgesia and reduced pain sensitivity in these rats compared to NH rats [111,112].

Tail-flick latencies were significantly longer in male MST compared to NH rats acclimated to loose restraint for 40 minutes prior to testing [41]. Exposure to more severe 1-hour water avoidance stress led to increases in tail-flick latencies in both MST and NH rats; however, the increase was significantly greater in NH compared to MST male rats [41]. In another study, repeated exposure to a hotplate kept at room temperature led to an exponential decrease in fecal boli in female HT rats, but no such relationship was found in MST or NH female rats. In that study, the MST rats had longer paw-lick latencies during the hotplate test compared to HT rats [155]. Stress-induced analgesia could conceivably drive the increased paw-lick latencies in the event that these rats remained appreciably distressed by the hotplate testing procedure [155].

There are two types of stress-induced analgesia, each recruiting different neural circuitry: one is mediated by β-endorphin and the other by neurotensin. The type of stress-induced analgesia expressed depends on the severity of the stress. More severe stressors lead to analgesia that is not eliminated by blocking the action of the opioid β-endorphin but can be abolished by blocking the actions of neurotensin. Conversely, milder stressors lead to an opioid-dependent analgesia that can be eliminated by blocking the effects of β-endorphin [50,128].

Weaver and colleagues measured the paw-lick latency for HT and MST male rats that were placed on a 50°C hotplate 30 minutes after a 3-minute forced swim in 3°C water (unpublished data). Analysis of covariance (with paw temperature as the covariate) revealed that MST rats had significantly smaller ($F_{2,27}$ = 6.83, P = 0.02) analgesic effects of the forced swim stressor compared to HT rats. This difference in acute stress-induced analgesia was not due to differences in stimulus intensity between MST and HT rats, since reductions in core temperature (t_{28} = 0.38, P = 0.71] and paw temperature [t_{28} = 0.212, P = 0.84) did not differ between MST and HT rats. Importantly, this difference in acute stress-induced analgesia between MST and HT rats was not evident when the forced swim was conducted in 32°C water (t_{28} = 0.072, P = 0.24), which suggests perturbations in the neurotensin system.

In a study examining opioid-based stress-induced analgesia, naloxone treatment at the end of water avoidance stress eliminated the resulting stress-induced analgesia, as measured by the spinal reflexive tail-flick test in NH rats, in comparison with a saline control treatment in NH rats. The same experiment in MST rats showed that while stress-induced analgesia was attenuated by naloxone, it was still present. The authors concluded that MST rats may have an inability to activate the opioidergic pain inhibitory systems that normally mediate stress-induced analgesia [41].

The link between stress and visceral pain sensitivity in MST rats has been explored with respect to the animals' responses to colorectal distension. One hour of water avoidance stress led to stress-induced visceral hyperalgesia to graded colorectal distension, even at non-noxious intensities, in MST rats, whereas stress did not alter the responses in NH rats [41]. In a subsequent study, the same investigators reported that HT rats showed a significant decrease in visceral sensitivity immediately after a 1-hour water avoidance stress, and the MST rats now had increased responses (compared to both HT and NH rats) that were only suggested in the previous study, with no changes being detected in male NH rats [127]. Twenty-four hours after stress, both MST and NH rats had significantly greater visceromotor responses to colorectal distension that were significantly greater in MST compared to HT rats [127]. The acute and delayed (24 hours after the stress) visceral hyperalgesia in MST rats, compared to HT rats, appeared to depend on exaggerated activity in the CRH system, because hyperalgesia in MST rats could be blocked by CRH receptor 1 [127].

In Wistar rats, restraint stress did not lead to increased visceral sensitivity in male NH or MST rats, but it did increase responses in female NH and MST rats, with higher levels in MST compared to NH rats. Thus, females were sensitive to the stress-induced visceral hyperalgesia, whereas males appeared immune to any such effects [120]. Other studies examining only males have found substantial stress-induced visceral hyperalgesia, but the maternal separation procedures differed among studies [41,127,156]. Restraint stress is a milder stress compared to the 1-hour water avoidance stressor used in the other studies, and this difference in stressor severity may account for the discrepancy between studies.

Taken together, the research indicates that early-life adversity does contribute to individual differences in pain sensitivity, and the effect is modified by stress to a different degree in MST and HT rats, thus implicating the importance of the effects of early handling and maternal separation on stress reactivity and indicating their potential impact on measures of pain behavior.

Response to Analgesics

The relationship between early-life trauma, nociceptive programming, and analgesic effectiveness is of relevance to the clinical treatment of patients with chronic pain disorders. Studies in adult mice have shown that the threshold for the analgesic effects of morphine was greater in HT mice compared to NH mice when measured during the peak analgesic actions of morphine, 30 minutes post-injection, based on tail-flick latencies [43]. Both male and female mice subjected to a modified handling procedure (in which they were housed in isolation during the 15-minute separations) exhibited a greater percentage of maximum possible effect (%MPE) in response to 10 mg/kg morphine [137]. In a previous study in rats, the %MPE in response to a cumulative dosing regime for morphine did not differ among female MST, HT, and NH rats (in which the estrous phase was not monitored), but the estimated median effective dose (ED_{50}) (based on %MPE values) was higher in MST rats [73]. Other studies have reported a higher ED_{50} in MST rats based on the %MPE values, but this result was accompanied by a significantly lower %MPE in MST compared to HT rats given a single 5 mg/kg dose of morphine [155]. Greater sensitivity to noxious thermal stimuli correlated with a greater dose of morphine required to produce analgesia [52,155]. These observations may give the appearance that morphine was less potent in the more pain-sensitive HT rats compared to the more pain-tolerant MST rats. However, when the paw-lick latency prior to morphine administration was taken into account—by calculating the %MPE of morphine and determining the ED_{50} from this figure—the value was substantially higher in MST compared to HT rats. Thus, the relative potency of morphine is in fact lower in the MST rat.

These studies demonstrate the potential interactions between the effectiveness of a traditional analgesic (morphine) and early-life adversity.

It may be that these early-life experiences contribute to the wide range of opioid doses required for pain relief efficacy across the population.

Mediating Effects of Maternal Behavior

Although early stressful or noxious experience appears to be capable of producing long-term alterations in physiology that manifest as altered nociceptive sensitivity, the possibility remains that the dam is the key mediator of these long-term changes, as has been demonstrated in the HT and MST models. However, it is not clear whether the models of neonatal pain experience that have been developed produce alterations in maternal care.

Walker et al. [151] illustrated a transient increase in maternal care following a neonatal repeated heel stick procedure (designed to mimic the experience of infants under medical care). Neonatal hindpaw inflammation produced an increase in maternal care during the period of active inflammation; however, this increase was followed (and perhaps, offset) by a subsequent reduction in care following recovery [13]. Neonatal abdominal surgery produced no obvious alterations in maternal care during the first 90 minutes following reunion [138]. In a more thorough observation of maternal behavior, dams were observed for a period of at least 360 minutes, spanning light and dark cycles, following their return to the nest of a mixed litter of P0 pups—half of which had received an injection of formalin, the other half an injection of saline to one hindpaw. Maternal care did not vary among the pups in the litter receiving saline or formalin injections, although the amount of care given (to all pups) was much increased during the light cycle compared to the dark cycle (due largely to an increase in time spent nursing the entire litter of pups during the light cycle) (see [136]). Thus, although maternal care may be responsive to pup distress, it is not clear whether dams are capable of directing attention to individual pups within the litter that have undergone particular treatments. More research is clearly necessary (on both dams and adult offspring) to determine the role of maternal care (and the state of littermates) in producing the long-term consequences of early pain. The importance of maternal care and its potential analgesic role are discussed in more detail below.

Steps that Can be Taken to Minimize Pain Experience in the Neonate

It is important to anticipate painful experiences while a child is hospitalized or receiving medical treatment. "Most acute pain experiences in medical settings can be prevented or substantially relieved" [6, p. 794].

The American Academy of Pediatrics, in conjunction with the Canadian Paediatric Society and the American Pain Society, have developed policy statements addressing the need to minimize painful or stressful procedures and eliminate pain-associated suffering in pediatric care facilities [6,7]. The goals of the project may include initiating policy changes to standardize pharmacological interventions, increasing the availability of nonpharmacological pain relief interventions, implementing a standing order for EMLA (eutectic mixture of lidocaine and prilocaine), and considering research initiatives to support evidence-based pain management [33]. Increasing the clinical staff's knowledge of pain assessment and management strategies is an essential component.

Use of Oral Sucrose

The administration of sucrose or the combination of sucrose with non-nutritive sucking is one of the most frequently studied nonpharmacological interventions for the relief of procedural pain in neonates [140]. Research demonstrates that sucrose can safely and effectively provide analgesia for young infants receiving heel lancings and other painful procedures. It is thought that the analgesic effect of sucrose works on opioid receptors, because in animal studies this effect can be blocked by naloxone [23]. The age dependency of oral sucrose analgesia may be the result of developmental changes in the interaction between gustatory and pain pathways [14]. The unique response of the neonate to an oral sucrose solution allows for a very safe and effective measure in minimizing procedural pain.

Kangaroo Care and Neonatal Cuddling

Kangaroo care (KC) is skin-to-skin contact between an infant and parent, where the infant is usually held chest-to-chest in an upright prone position. It is a very simple, beneficial developmental intervention for both baby and parent, as demonstrated in the literature, but many parents and health care professionals are not aware of the technique, its benefits, or how to perform it [49]. In its initial form, KC served as an alternative to standard inpatient care for stable low-birth-weight infants. However, with experience and a better understanding of the benefits of this method, its place in clinical practice has expanded [65]. It is now widely considered to be the most feasible, most readily available, and preferred intervention for decreasing neonatal morbidity and mortality in developing countries [32]. KC is seen to complement the standard care of stable low-birth-weight infants, thus allowing for better use of limited, expensive resources such as incubators. Intermittent KC can even be practiced in intensive care units, for example while the infant is being ventilated. Increased education for health care providers should lead to increased routine use of this beneficial intervention [49].

Conventional cuddling care (CCC) differs from KC mainly in that contact between parent and child in CCC takes place through normal clothing. However, both types of contact are equally beneficial to the infant. In a study that compared CCC to KC, infants in both groups experienced an equivalent maintenance of or rise in temperature while out of the incubators, as well as equal weight gain, a comparable length of stay in the hospital, and the same duration of breastfeeding [117]. A number of studies have proven that KC has a major positive impact on babies and their parents.

Facilitated tucking by parents (where a parent holds the infant in a flexed position) has also been shown to be an effective and safe pain management method during endotracheal/pharyngeal suctioning of preterm infants [16].

In a recent study in rats, Al-Chaer and colleagues showed that neonatal cuddling given to rats around the time of colon inflammation (on postnatal days 8, 10 and 12) prevented the development of long-term visceral hypersensitivity observed otherwise in adult rats that had experienced neonatal colon inflammation without cuddling [2].

Conclusion

Whereas controlled experimental studies on neonatal stress in rodents have been available for some time, similar studies of the long-term consequences of early pain are relatively recent additions to the literature, spurred in part by long-overdue clinical attention to the problem of pain in the neonatal intensive care unit. The research reviewed above suggests that early pain or stress experience may indeed account for a portion of the variability in adult pain behavior (including both hyperalgesia at the site of injury and overall sensitivity), as well as stress behavior and its underlying neuroendocrine substrates. The research described in this chapter highlights the responsiveness of the developing nervous system to stimulation during an early critical period following birth. As profound as some of these consequences are, the guiding principle for clinical care of the neonate should not be the long-term effects of pain or stress experience, but rather the recognition of the potential for suffering in the individual experiencing pain or stress at the time of the procedure. The best pain management approach includes avoiding pain by critical judgment of the need for any painful procedure, clustering the procedures, and performing the procedures smoothly. Whenever possible, nonpharmacological pain management methods should be considered to avoid or at least reduce the adverse effects of pharmacological treatments.

Acknowledgments

The authors would like to thank Ms. Kirsten Garner for administrative assistance with the manuscript. This work was supported in part by NIH grants DK077733 and RR020146.

References

[1]   Abbott FV, Franklin KB, Westbrook RF. The formalin test: scoring properties of the first and second phases of the pain response in rats. Pain 1995;60:91–102.
[2]   Al-Chaer ED, Gu C, Soni P, Garner KN, Fann A, Wang J. Neonatal cuddling prevents the development of adverse consequences of neonatal injury in rats. Pediatric Academic Societies Meeting, Honolulu, Hawaii, 2008, No. 4454.14.
[3]   Al-Chaer ED, Kawasaki M, Pasricha PJ. A new model of chronic visceral hypersensitivity in adult rats induced by colon irritation during postnatal development. Gastroenterology 2000;119:1276–85.

[4]   Al-Chaer ED, Traub RJ. Biological basis of visceral pain: recent developments. Pain 2002;96:221–5.
[5]   Alleva E, Caprioli A, Laviola G. Postnatal social environment affects morphine analgesia in male mice. Physiol Behav 1986;36:779–81.
[6]   American Academy of Pediatrics and American Pain Society. The assessment and management of acute pain in infants, children, and adolescents. Pediatrics 2001;108:793–7.
[7]   American Academy of Pediatrics and Canadian Paediatric Society. Prevention and management of pain and stress in the neonate. Pediatrics 2000;105:454–61.
[8]   Anand KJ. Effects of perinatal pain and stress. Prog Brain Res 2000;122:117–29.
[9]   Anand KJ. Consensus statement for the prevention and management of pain in the newborn. Arch Pediatr Adolesc Med 2001;155:173–80.
[10] Anand KJ, Coskun V, Thrivikraman KV, Nemeroff CB, Plotsky PM. Long-term behavioral effects of repetitive pain in neonatal rat pups. Physiol Behav 1999;66:627–37.
[11] Anand KJ, Runeson B, Jacobson B. Gastric suction at birth associated with long-term risk for functional intestinal disorders in later life. J Pediatr 2004;144:449–54.
[12] Ang DC, Peloso PM, Woolson RF, Kroenke K, Doebbeling BN. Predictors of incident chronic widespread pain among veterans following the first Gulf War. Clin J Pain 2006;22:554–63.
[13] Anseloni VC, He F, Novikova SI, Turnbach Robbins M, Lidow IA, Ennis M, Lidow MS. Alterations in stress-associated behaviors and neurochemical markers in adult rats after neonatal short-lasting local inflammatory insult. Neuroscience 2005;131:635–45.
[14] Anseloni VC, Weng HR, Terayama R, Letizia D, Davis BJ, Ren K, Dubner R, Ennis M. Age-dependency of analgesia elicited by intraoral sucrose in acute and persistent pain models. Pain 2002;97:93–103.
[15] Arborelius L, Eklund MB. Both long and brief maternal separation produces persistent changes in tissue levels of brain monoamines in middle-aged female rats. Neuroscience 2007;145:738–50.
[16] Axelin A, Salanterä S, Lehtonen L. 'Facilitated tucking by parents' in pain management of preterm infants–a randomized crossover trial. Early Hum Dev 2006;82:241–7.
[17] Barreau F, Cartier C, Ferrier L, Fioramonti J, Bueno L. Nerve growth factor mediates alterations of colonic sensitivity and mucosal barrier induced by neonatal stress in rats. Gastroenterology 2004;127:524–34.
[18] Beckham JC, Crawford AL, Feldman ME, Kirby AC, Hertzberg MA, Davidson JR, Moore SD. Chronic posttraumatic stress disorder and chronic pain in Vietnam combat veterans. J Psychosom Res 1997;43:379–89.
[19] Bennett GJ. Experimental neuropathic pain in animals: models and mechanisms. In: Justins DM, editor. Pain 2005: An updated review. Seattle: IASP Press; 2005. pp 97–119.
[20] Berkley KJ. Sex differences in pain. Behav Brain Sci 1997;20:371–80; discussion 435–513.
[21] Bhutta AT, Rovnaghi C, Simpson PM, Gossett JM, Scalzo FM, Anand KJ. Interactions of inflammatory pain and morphine in infant rats: long-term behavioral effects. Physiol Behav 2001;73:51–8.
[22] Blass EMC, Catherine P, Fanselow MS. The development of morphine-induced antinociception in neonatal rats: A comparison of forepaw, hindpaw, and tail retraction from a thermal stimulus. Pharmacol Biochem Behav 1993;44:643–9.
[23] Blass E, Fitzgerald E, Kehoe P. Interactions between sucrose, pain and isolation distress. Pharmacol Biochem Behav 1987;26:483–9.
[24] Boccia ML, Pedersen CA. Brief vs. long maternal separations in infancy: contrasting relationships with adult maternal behavior and lactation levels of aggression and anxiety. Psychoneuroendocrinology 2001;26:657–72.
[25] Bodnar RJ, Romero MT, Kramer E. Organismic variables and pain inhibition: roles of gender and aging. Brain Res Bull 1988;21:947–53.
[26] Brake WG, Zhang TY, Diorio J, Meaney MJ, Gratton A. Influence of early postnatal rearing conditions on mesocorticolimbic dopamine and behavioural responses to psychostimulants and stressors in adult rats. Eur J Neurosci 2004;19:1863–74.
[27] Butkevich IP, Barr GA, Mikhailenko VA, Otellin VA. Increased formalin-induced pain and expression of fos neurons in the lumbar spinal cord of prenatally stressed infant rats. Neurosci Lett 2006;403:222–6.

[28] Butkevich IP, Barr GA, Vershinina EA. Sex differences in formalin-induced pain in prenatally stressed infant rats. Eur J Pain 2007;11:888–94.

[29] Butkevich IP, Mikhailenko VA, Leonteva MN. Sequelae of prenatal serotonin depletion and stress on pain sensitivity in rats. Neurosci Behav Physiol 2005;35:925–30.

[30] Caldji C, Francis D, Sharma S, Plotsky PM, Meaney MJ. The effects of early rearing environment on the development of GABA$_A$ and central benzodiazepine receptor levels and novelty-induced fearfulness in the rat. Neuropsychopharmacology 2000;22:219–29.

[31] Chang L, Mayer EA, Johnson T, FitzGerald LZ, Naliboff B. Differences in somatic perception in female patients with irritable bowel syndrome with and without fibromyalgia. Pain 2000;84:297–307.

[32] Charpak N, Ruiz JG, Zupan J, Cattaneo A, Figueroa Z, Tessier R, Cristo M, Anderson G, Ludington S, Mendoza S, Mokhachane M, Worku B. Kangaroo mother care: 25 years after. Acta Paediatr 2005;94:514–22.

[33] Children's Medical Center Dallas. Pain Free Initiative. Children's Medical Center Dallas, 2000.

[34] Chung EK, Zhang X, Li Z, Zhang H, Xu H, Bian Z. Neonatal maternal separation enhances central sensitivity to noxious colorectal distention in rat. Brain Res 2007;1153:68–77.

[35] Chung EK, Zhang XJ, Xu HX, Sung JJ, Bian ZX. Visceral hyperalgesia induced by neonatal maternal separation is associated with nerve growth factor-mediated central neuronal plasticity in rat spinal cord. Neuroscience 2007;149:685–95.

[36] Clancy B, Darlington RB, Finlay BL. Translating developmental time across mammalian species. Neuroscience 2001;105:7–17.

[37] Clausing P, Mothes HK, Opitz B, Kormann S. Differential effects of communal rearing and preweaning handling on open-field behavior and hot-plate latencies in mice. Behav Brain Res 1997;82:179–84.

[38] Coderre TJ, Fundytus ME, McKenna JE, Dalal S, Melzack R. The formalin test: a validation of the weighted-scores method of behavioural pain rating. Pain 1993;54:43–50.

[39] Coggeshall RE, Jennings EA, Fitzgerald M. Evidence that large myelinated primary afferent fibers make synaptic contacts in lamina II of neonatal rats. Brain Res Dev Brain Res 1996;92:81–90.

[40] Coghill RC, McHaffie JG, Yen YF. Neural correlates of interindividual differences in the subjective experience of pain. Proc Natl Acad Sci USA 2003;100:8538–42.

[41] Coutinho SV, Plotsky PM, Sablad M, Miller JC, Zhou H, Bayati AI, McRoberts JA, Mayer EA. Neonatal maternal separation alters stress-induced responses to viscerosomatic nociceptive stimuli in rat. Am J Physiol Gastrointest Liver Physiol 2002;282:G307–16.

[42] Cui XY, Lundeberg T, Yu LC. Role of corticotropin-releasing factor and its receptor in nociceptive modulation in the central nucleus of amygdala in rats. Brain Res 2004;995:23–8.

[43] D'Amato FR, Mazzacane E, Capone F, Pavone F. Effects of postnatal manipulation on nociception and morphine sensitivity in adult mice. Brain Res Dev Brain Res 1999;117:15–20.

[44] Darnaudery M, Maccari S. Epigenetic programming of the stress response in male and female rats by prenatal restraint stress. Brain Res Rev 2008;57:571–85.

[45] Davis DA, Luecken LJ, Zautra AJ. Are reports of childhood abuse related to the experience of chronic pain in adulthood? A meta-analytic review of the literature. Clin J Pain 2005;21:398–405.

[46] De Lima J, Alvares D, Hatch DJ, Fitzgerald M. Sensory hyperinnervation after neonatal skin wounding: effect of bupivacaine sciatic nerve block. Br J Anaesth 1999;83:662–4.

[47] Denenberg VH, Brumaghim JT, Haltmeyer GC, Zarrow MX. Increased adrenocortical activity in the neonatal rat following handling. Endocrinology 1967;81:1047–52.

[48] Diatchenko L, Slade GD, Nackley AG, Bhalang K, Sigurdsson A, Belfer I, Goldman D, Xu K, Shabalina SA, Shagin D, Max MB, Makarov SS, Maixner W. Genetic basis for individual variations in pain perception and the development of a chronic pain condition. Hum Mol Genet 2005;14:135–43.

[49] DiMenna L. Considerations for implementation of a neonatal kangaroo care protocol. Neonatal Netw 2006;25:405–12.

[50] Dobner PR. Neurotensin and pain modulation. Peptides 2006;27:2405–14.

[51] Edwards RR. Individual differences in endogenous pain modulation as a risk factor for chronic pain. Neurology 2005;65:437–43.

[52] Elmer GI, Pieper JO, Negus SS, Woods JH. Genetic variance in nociception and its relationship to the potency of morphine-induced analgesia in thermal and chemical tests. Pain 1998;75:129–40.

[53] Engberg IB, Grondahl GB, Thibom K. Patients' experiences of herpes zoster and postherpetic neuralgia. J Adv Nurs 1995;21:427–33.
[54] Falcon M, Guendellman D, Stolberg A, Frenk H, Urca G. Development of thermal nociception in rats. Pain 1996;67:203–8.
[55] Featherstone RE, Fleming AS, Ivy GO. Plasticity in the maternal circuit: effects of experience and partum condition on brain astrocyte number in female rats. Behav Neurosci 2000;114:158–72.
[56] Fillingim RB, Edwards RR. Is self-reported childhood abuse history associated with pain perception among healthy young women and men? Clin J Pain 2005;21:387–97.
[57] Fitzgerald M, Gibson S. The postnatal physiological and neurochemical development of peripheral sensory C fibres. Neuroscience 1984;13:933–44.
[58] Fitzgerald M, Koltzenburg M. The functional development of descending inhibitory pathways in the dorsolateral funiculus of the newborn rat spinal cord. Brain Res 1986;389:261–70.
[59] Fitzgerald M, Shaw A, MacIntosh N. Postnatal development of the cutaneous flexor reflex: comparative study of preterm infants and newborn rat pups. Dev Med Child Neurol 1988;30:520–6.
[60] Francis DD, Diorio J, Plotsky PM, Meaney MJ. Environmental enrichment reverses the effects of maternal separation on stress reactivity. J Neurosci 2002;22:7840–3.
[61] Fries E, Hesse J, Hellhammer J, Hellhammer DH. A new view on hypocortisolism. Psychoneuroendocrinology 2005;30:1010–6.
[62] Frye CA, Cuevas CA, Kanarek RB. Diet and estrous cycle influence pain sensitivity in rats. Pharmacol Biochem Behav 1993;45:255–60.
[63] Griebel G, Perrault G, Sanger DJ. Limited anxiolytic-like effects of non-benzodiazepine hypnotics in rodents. J Psychopharmacol 1998;12:356–65.
[64] Gustafsson L, Oreland S, Hoffmann P, Nylander I. The impact of postnatal environment on opioid peptides in young and adult male Wistar rats. Neuropeptides 2008;42:177–91.
[65] Hall D, Kirsten G. Kangaroo mother care: a review. Transfus Med 2008;18:77–82.
[66] Hammer RP, Jr. Mu-opiate receptor binding in the medial preoptic area is cyclical and sexually dimorphic. Brain Res 1990;515:187–92.
[67] Hargreaves K, Dubner R, Brown F, Flores C, Joris J. A new and sensitive method for measuring thermal nociception in cutaneous hyperalgesia. Pain 1988;32:77–88.
[68] Hinze CL, Lin C, Al-Chaer ED. Estrous cycle and stress related variations of open field activity in adult female rats with neonatal colon irritation (CI). Soc Neurosci Abstracts 2002;155.14.
[69] Huizink AC, Robles de Medina PG, Mulder EJ, Visser GH, Buitelaar JK. Stress during pregnancy is associated with developmental outcome in infancy. J Child Psychol Psychiatry 2003;44:810–8.
[70] Imbierowicz K, Egle UT. Childhood adversities in patients with fibromyalgia and somatoform pain disorder. Eur J Pain 2003;7:113–9.
[71] Jackson AA, Langley-Evans SC, McCarthy HD. Nutritional influences in early life upon obesity and body proportions. Ciba Found Symp 1996;201:118–29; discussion 29–37, 88–93.
[72] Kalinichev M, Easterling KW, Holtzman SG. Early neonatal experience of Long-Evans rats results in long-lasting changes in morphine tolerance and dependence. Psychopharmacology (Berl) 2001;157:305–12.
[73] Kalinichev M, Easterling KW, Holtzman SG. Repeated neonatal maternal separation alters morphine-induced antinociception in male rats. Brain Res Bull 2001;54:649–54.
[74] Kawakami SE, Quadros IM, Takahashi S, Suchecki D. Long maternal separation accelerates behavioural sensitization to ethanol in female, but not in male mice. Behav Brain Res 2007;184:109–16.
[75] Kayser V, Berkley KJ, Keita H, Gautron M, Guilbaud G. Estrous and sex variations in vocalization thresholds to hindpaw and tail pressure stimulation in the rat. Brain Res 1996;742:352–4.
[76] Kinsley CH, Mann PE, Bridges RS. Prenatal stress alters morphine- and stress-induced analgesia in male and female rats. Pharmacol Biochem Behav 1988;30:123–8.
[77] Kosten TA, Lee HJ, Kim JJ. Neonatal handling alters learning in adult male and female rats in a task-specific manner. Brain Res 2007;1154:144–53.
[78] Langley-Evans SC. Hypertension induced by foetal exposure to a maternal low-protein diet, in the rat, is prevented by pharmacological blockade of maternal glucocorticoid synthesis. J Hypertens 1997;15:537–44.
[79] Laplante DP, Barr RG, Brunet A, Galbaud du Fort G, Meaney ML, Saucier JF, Zelazo PR, King S. Stress during pregnancy affects general intellectual and language functioning in human toddlers. Pediatr Res 2004;56:400–10.

[80] Lee JH, Kim HJ, Kim JG, Ryu V, Kim BT, Kang DW, Jahng JW. Depressive behaviors and decreased expression of serotonin reuptake transporter in rats that experienced neonatal maternal separation. Neurosci Res 2007;58:32–9.

[81] Lidow MS, Song ZM, Ren K. Long-term effects of short-lasting early local inflammatory insult. Neuroreport 2001;12:399–403.

[82] Lin C, Al-Chaer ED. Long-term sensitization of primary afferents in adult rats exposed to neonatal colon pain. Brain Res 2003;971:73–82.

[83] Lin C and Al-Chaer ED. Differential effects of glutamate receptor antagonists on dorsal horn neurons responding to colorectal distension in a neonatal colon irritation rat model. World J Gastroenterol 2005;11:6495–502.

[84] Liu D, Caldji C, Sharma S, Plotsky PM, Meaney MJ. Influence of neonatal rearing conditions on stress-induced adrenocorticotropin responses and norepinephrine release in the hypothalamic paraventricular nucleus. J Neuroendocrinol 2000;12:5–12.

[85] Liu D, Diorio J, Day JC, Francis DD, Meaney MJ. Maternal care, hippocampal synaptogenesis and cognitive development in rats. Nat Neurosci 2000;3:799–806.

[86] Liu D, Diorio J, Tannenbaum B, Caldji C, Francis D, Freedman A, Sharma S, Pearson D, Plotsky PM, Meaney MJ. Maternal care, hippocampal glucocorticoid receptors, and hypothalamic-pituitary-adrenal responses to stress. Science 1997;277:1659–62.

[87] Liu J, Rovnaghi C, Garg S, Anand K. Hyperalgesia in young rats associated with opioid receptor desensitization in the forebrain. Eur J Pharmacol 2004;491:127–36.

[88] Marsh D, Dickenson A, Hatch D, Fitzgerald M. Epidural opioid analgesia in infant rats I: mechanical and heat responses. Pain 1999;82:23–32.

[89] Marsh D, Dickenson A, Hatch D, Fitzgerald M. Epidural opioid analgesia in infant rats II: Responses to carrageenan and capsaicin. Pain 1999;82:33–38.

[90] McBeth J, Chiu YH, Silman AJ, Ray D, Morriss R, Dickens C, Gupta A, Macfarlane GJ. Hypothalamic-pituitary-adrenal stress axis function and the relationship with chronic widespread pain and its antecedents. Arthritis Res Ther 2005;7:R992–R1000.

[91] McBeth J, Macfarlane GJ, Benjamin S, Morris S, Silman AJ. The association between tender points, psychological distress, and adverse childhood experiences: a community-based study. Arthritis Rheum 1999;42:1397–404.

[92] McLaughlin CR, Dewey WL. A comparison of the antinociceptive effects of opioid agonists in neonatal and adult rats in phasic and tonic nociceptive tests. Pharmacol Biochem Behav 1994;49:1017–23.

[93] McLaughlin CR, Lichtman AH, Fanselow MS, Cramer CP. Tonic nociception in neonatal rats. Pharmacol Biochem Behav 1990;36:859–62.

[94] McLean SA, Williams DA, Harris RE, Kop WJ, Groner KH, Ambrose K, Lyden AK, Gracely RH, Crofford LJ, Geisser ME, Sen A, Biswas P, Clauw DJ. Momentary relationship between cortisol secretion and symptoms in patients with fibromyalgia. Arthritis Rheum 2005;52:3660–9.

[95] Meaney MJ, Aitken DH, Viau V, Sharma S, Sarrieau A. Neonatal handling alters adrenocortical negative feedback sensitivity and hippocampal type II glucocorticoid receptor binding in the rat. Neuroendocrinology 1989;50:597–604.

[96] Michaels CC, Holtzman SG. Enhanced sensitivity to naltrexone-induced drinking suppression of fluid intake and sucrose consumption in maternally separated rats. Pharmacol Biochem Behav 2007;86:784–96.

[97] Michaels CC, Holtzman SG. Early postnatal stress alters place conditioning to both mu- and kappa-opioid agonists. J Pharmacol Exp Ther 2008;325:313–8.

[98] Mogil JS. The genetic mediation of individual differences in sensitivity to pain and its inhibition. Proc Natl Acad Sci USA 1999;96:7744–51.

[99] Mogil JS, Chesler EJ, Wilson SG, Juraska JM, Sternberg WF. Sex differences in thermal nociception and morphine antinociception in rodents depend on genotype. Neurosci Biobehav Rev 2000;24:375–89.

[100] Mogil JS, Sternberg WF, Marek P, Sadowski B, Belknap JK, Liebeskind JC. The genetics of pain and pain inhibition. Proc Natl Acad Sci USA 1996;93:3048–55.

[101] Moles A, Rizzi R, D'Amato FR. Postnatal stress in mice: does "stressing" the mother have the same effect as "stressing" the pups? Dev Psychobiol 2004;44:230–7 .

[102] Moore CL, Morelli GA. Mother rats interact differently with male and female offspring. J Comp Physiol Psychol 1979;93:677–84.
[103] Nandi R, Fitzgerald M. Opioid analgesia in the newborn. Eur J Pain 2005;9:105–8.
[104] Ness TJ, Gebhart GF. Colorectal distension as a noxious visceral stimulus: physiologic and pharmacologic characterization of pseudaffective reflexes in the rat. Brain Res 1988;450:153–69.
[105] Nielsen CS, Price DD, Vassend O, Stubhaug A, Harris JR. Characterizing individual differences in heat-pain sensitivity. Pain 2005;119:65–74.
[106] O'Donnell D, Larocque S, Seckl JR, Meaney MJ. Postnatal handling alters glucocorticoid, but not mineralocorticoid messenger RNA expression in the hippocampus of adult rats. Brain Res Mol Brain Res 1994;26:242–8.
[107] Palecek J, Paleckova V, Willis WD. The roles of pathways in the spinal cord lateral and dorsal funiculi in signaling nociceptive somatic and visceral stimuli in rats. Pain 2002;96:297–307.
[108] Peng YB, Ling QD, Ruda MA, Kenshalo DR. Electrophysiological changes in adult rat dorsal horn neurons after neonatal peripheral inflammation. J Neurophysiol 2003;90:73–80.
[109] Perkins FM, Kehlet H. Chronic pain as an outcome of surgery. A review of predictive factors. Anesthesiology 2000;93:1123–33.
[110] Phillips NK, Hammen CL, Brennan PA, Najman JM, Bor W. Early adversity and the prospective prediction of depressive and anxiety disorders in adolescents. J Abnorm Child Psychol 2005;33:13–24.
[111] Plotsky PM, Meaney MJ. Early, postnatal experience alters hypothalamic corticotropin-releasing factor (CRF) mRNA, median eminence CRF content and stress-induced release in adult rats. Brain Res Mol Brain Res 1993;18:195–200.
[112] Plotsky PM, Thrivikraman KV, Nemeroff CB, Caldji C, Sharma S, Meaney MJ. Long-term consequences of neonatal rearing on central corticotropin-releasing factor systems in adult male rat offspring. Neuropsychopharmacology 2005;30:2192–204.
[113] Rahman W, Fitzgerald M, Aynsley-Green A, Dickenson A. The effects of neonatal exposure to inflammation and/or morphine on neuronal responses and morphine analgesia in adult rats. In: Jensen TS, Turner JA, Wiesenfeld-Hallin Z, editors. Proceedings of the 8th World Congress on Pain. Seattle: IASP Press; 1997. pp 783–94.
[114] Ren K, Anseloni V, Zou SP, Wade EB, Novikova SI, Ennis M, Traub RJ, Gold MS, Dubner R, Lidow MS. Characterization of basal and re-inflammation-associated long-term alteration in pain responsivity following short-lasting neonatal local inflammatory insult. Pain 2004;110:588–96.
[115] Ren TH, Wu J, Yew D, Ziea E, Lao L, Leung WK, Berman B, Hu PJ, Sung JJ. Effects of neonatal maternal separation on neurochemical and sensory response to colonic distension in a rat model of irritable bowel syndrome. Am J Physiol Gastrointest Liver Physiol 2007;292:G849–56.
[116] Reynolds ML, Fitzgerald M. Long-term sensory hyperinnervation following neonatal skin wounds. J Comp Neurol 1995;358:487–98.
[117] Roberts KL, Paynter C, McEwan B. A comparison of kangaroo mother care and conventional cuddling care. Neonatal Netw 2000;19:31–35.
[118] Roseboom T, de Rooij S, Painter R. The Dutch famine and its long-term consequences for adult health. Early Hum Dev 2006;82:485–91.
[119] Rosenblatt JS. Prepartum and postpartum regulation of maternal behaviour in the rat. Ciba Found Symp 1975;17–37.
[120] Rosztoczy A, Fioramonti J, Jarmay K, Barreau F, Wittmann T, Bueno L. Influence of sex and experimental protocol on the effect of maternal deprivation on rectal sensitivity to distension in the adult rat. Neurogastroenterol Motil 2003;15:679–86.
[121] Ruda MA, Ling QD, Hohmann AG, Peng YB, Tachibana T. Altered nociceptive neuronal circuits after neonatal peripheral inflammation. Science 2000;289:628–31.
[122] Saab CY, Park YC, Al-Chaer ED. Thalamic modulation of visceral nociceptive processing in adult rats with neonatal colon irritation. Brain Res 2004;1008:186–92.
[123] Sachs-Ericsson N, Kendall-Tackett K, Hernandez A. Childhood abuse, chronic pain, and depression in the National Comorbidity Survey. Child Abuse Negl 2007;31:531–47.
[124] Salmon P, Skaife K, Rhodes J. Abuse, dissociation, and somatization in irritable bowel syndrome: towards an explanatory model. J Behav Med 2003;26:1–18.
[125] Sanders RD, Patel N, Hossain M, Ma D and Maze M. Isoflurane exerts antinociceptive and hypnotic properties at all ages in Fischer rats. Br J Anaesth 2005;95:393–9.

[126] Schaefer T, Jr., Weingarten FS, Towne JC. Temperature change: the basic variable in the early handling phenomenon? Science 1962;135:41–2.

[127] Schwetz I, McRoberts JA, Coutinho SV, Bradesi S, Gale G, Fanselow M, Million M, Ohning G, Tache Y, Plotsky PM, Mayer EA. Corticotropin-releasing factor receptor 1 mediates acute and delayed stress-induced visceral hyperalgesia in maternally separated Long-Evans rats. Am J Physiol Gastrointest Liver Physiol 2005;289:G704–12.

[128] Seta KA, Jansen HT, Kreitel KD, Lehman M, Behbehani MM. Cold water swim stress increases the expression of neurotensin mRNA in the lateral hypothalamus and medial preoptic regions of the rat brain. Brain Res Mol Brain Res 2001;86:145–52.

[129] Shimada C, Kurumiya S, Noguchi Y, Umemoto M. The effect of neonatal exposure to chronic footshock on pain responsiveness and sensitivity to morphine after maturation in the rat. Behav Brain Res 1990;36:105–11.

[130] Sorkin LS, Westlund KN, Sluka KA, Dougherty PM, Willis WD. Neural changes in acute arthritis in monkeys. IV. Time-course of amino acid release into the lumbar dorsal horn. Brain Res Brain Res Rev 1992;17:39–50.

[131] Spiller R, Aziz Q, Creed F, Emmanuel A, Houghton L, Hungin P, Jones R, Kumar D, Rubin G, Trudgill N, Whorwell P. Guidelines on the irritable bowel syndrome: mechanisms and practical management. Gut 2007;56:1770–98.

[132] Stammberger U, Steinacher C, Hillinger S, Schmid RA, Kinsbergen T, Weder W. Early and long-term complaints following video-assisted thoracoscopic surgery: evaluation in 173 patients. Eur J Cardiothorac Surg 2000;18:7–11.

[133] Stephan M, Helfritz F, Pabst R, von Horsten S. Postnatally induced differences in adult pain sensitivity depend on genetics, gender and specific experiences: reversal of maternal deprivation effects by additional postnatal tactile stimulation or chronic imipramine treatment. Behav Brain Res 2002;133:149–58.

[134] Stern JM, Johnson SK. Ventral somatosensory determinants of nursing behavior in Norway rats. I. Effects of variations in the quality and quantity of pup stimuli. Physiol Behav 1990;47:993–1011.

[135] Sternberg WF. Sex differences in the effects of prenatal stress on stress-induced analgesia. Physiol Behav 1999;68:63–72.

[136] Sternberg WF, Al-Chaer ED. Long-term consequences of neonatal and infant pain from animal models. In: Anand, Stevens, McGrath, editors. Pain in neonates and infants, 3rd ed. Pain Research and Clinical Management. Edinburgh: Elsevier Churchill-Livingstone; 2007. pp 57–66.

[137] Sternberg WF, Ridgway CG. Effects of gestational stress and neonatal handling on pain, analgesia, and stress behavior of adult mice. Physiol Behav 2003;78:375–83.

[138] Sternberg WF, Scorr L, Smith LD, Ridgway CG, Stout M. Long-term effects of neonatal surgery on adulthood pain behavior. Pain 2005;113:347–53.

[139] Sternberg WF, Smith L, Scorr L. Nociception and antinociception on the day of birth in mice: sex differences and test dependence. J Pain 2004;5:420–6.

[140] Stevens B, Johnston C, Franck L, Petryshen P, Jack A, Foster G. The efficacy of developmentally sensitive interventions and sucrose for relieving procedural pain in very low birth weight neonates. Nurs Res 1999;48:35–43.

[141] Stevenson CW, Marsden CA, Mason R. Early life stress causes FG-7142-induced corticolimbic dysfunction in adulthood. Brain Res 2008;1193:43–50.

[142] Stohr T, Szuran T, Welzl H, Pliska V, Feldon J, Pryce CR. Lewis/Fischer rat strain differences in endocrine and behavioural responses to environmental challenge. Pharmacol Biochem Behav 2000;67:809–19.

[143] Talley NJ, Boyce PM, Jones M. Is the association between irritable bowel syndrome and abuse explained by neuroticism? A population based study. Gut 1998;42:47–53.

[144] Teng CJ, Abbott FV. The formalin test: a dose-response analysis at three developmental stages. Pain 1998;76:337–47.

[145] Tseng LF, Wang Q. Forebrain sites differentially sensitive to beta-endorphin and morphine for analgesia and release of Met-enkephalin in the pentobarbital-anesthesized rat. J Pharmacol Exp Ther 1992;261:1028–36.

[146] Veenema AH, Blume A, Niederle D, Buwalda B, Neumann ID. Effects of early life stress on adult male aggression and hypothalamic vasopressin and serotonin. Eur J Neurosci 2006;24:1711–20.

[147] Vendruscolo LF, Pamplona FA, Takahashi RN. Strain and sex differences in the expression of nociceptive behavior and stress-induced analgesia in rats. Brain Res 2004;1030:277–83.

[148] Verhaak PF, Kerssens JJ, Dekker J, Sorbi MJ, Bensing JM. Prevalence of chronic benign pain disorder among adults: a review of the literature. Pain 1998;77:231–9.

[149] Vicentic A, Francis D, Moffett M, Lakatos A, Rogge G, Hubert GW, Harley J, Kuhar MJ. Maternal separation alters serotonergic transporter densities and serotonergic 1A receptors in rat brain. Neuroscience 2006;140:355–65.

[150] Vincler M, Maixner W, Vierck CJ, Light AR. Estrous cycle modulation of nociceptive behaviors elicited by electrical stimulation and formalin. Pharmacol Biochem Behav 2001;69:315–24.

[151] Walker C-D, Kudreikis K, Sherrard A, Johnston CC. Repeated neonatal pain influences maternal behavior, but not stress responsiveness in rat offspring. Dev Brain Res 2003;140:253–61.

[152] Walsh CA, Jamieson E, Macmillan H, Boyle M. Child abuse and chronic pain in a community survey of women. J Interpers Violence 2007;22:1536–54.

[153] Wang G, Ji Y, Lidow MS, Traub RJ. Neonatal hind paw injury alters processing of visceral and somatic nociceptive stimuli in the adult rat. J Pain 2004;5:440–9.

[154] Wang J, Peng X, Al-Chaer ED. Sex-related differences in visceral sensitivity in adult rats with neonatal colon pain. Gastroenterology 2004;126(S1090):A-161.

[155] Weaver SA, Diorio J, Meaney MJ. Maternal separation leads to persistent reductions in pain sensitivity in female rats. J Pain 2007;8:962–9.

[156] Welting O, Van Den Wijngaard RM, De Jonge WJ, Holman R, Boeckxstaens GE. Assessment of visceral sensitivity using radio telemetry in a rat model of maternal separation. Neurogastroenterol Motil 2005;17:838–45.

Correspondence to: Elie D. Al-Chaer, MS, PhD, JD, University of Arkansas for Medical Sciences, Biomedical Research Center, Building II, Suite 406-2, 4301 West Markham Street, Slot 842, Little Rock, AR 72205, USA. Tel: 1-501-526-7828; fax: 1-501-526-7862; email: ealchaer@uams.edu.

Genetically Driven Interactions in the Brain: Lessons from Depression

Lukas Pezawas[a,b] and Andreas Meyer-Lindenberg[a,c]

[a]Genes, Cognition and Psychosis Program, National Institute of Mental Health, National Institutes of Health, Bethesda, Maryland, USA; [b]Division of Biological Psychiatry, Medical University of Vienna, Vienna, Austria; [c]Central Institute of Mental Health, Mannheim, Germany

Lessons from Depression

Several lines of evidence suggest that depression and functional pain syndromes such as irritable bowel syndrome (IBS), fibromyalgia, migraine, and many others have overlapping disease pathways, which are reflected at the clinical, cellular, genetic, and pharmacological level. Epidemiological studies indicate a significant longitudinal comorbidity of depression with functional pain syndromes such as IBS, fibromyalgia, tension headache, and migraine [14]. Clinical studies in depressive subjects further underline this association by revealing altered pain perception, such as hypoalgesia, in this patient sample [15]. A common pathophysiological pathway is further suggested by shared pharmacological treatment strategies for chronic pain syndromes such as antidepressive drug therapy with agents inhibiting serotonin and norepinephrine transporters as well as treatment with membrane-stabilizing antiepileptic drugs. Opioids, which are frequently used as drug therapy for pain, were also once used to treat depression prior to the emergence of tricyclic antidepressants. On a brain systems level, it is intriguing that pain perception converges in brain regions that are associated with the processing of negative mood, such as the anterior cingulate gyrus and the ventromedial prefrontal cortex [17,24]. Apart from this remarkable overlap on a clinical, pharmacological, and neurobiological level, functional pain syndromes also share genetic features with depression.

Multiple Phenotypes Caused by a Single Gene

The introduction of knockout mouse models for classic depression genes such as the serotonin (5-HT) transporter gene has been crucial for the understanding of functional pain disorders and their clinically observed comorbidity [15]. Such models have revealed that pleiotropy, which is defined as the occurrence of multiple phenotypes caused by a single gene, is a major feature of this gene. 5-HT transporter gene knockouts exhibit a broad variety of phenotypes, including traits such as anxiety-like behavior, hypoalgesia, hypoactivity, bladder dysfunction, gut hypermobility, late-onset obesity, stress susceptibility, REM-sleep disorder, depression, and low aggressiveness [15]. Therefore, it seems reasonable to suggest that functional pain syndromes might be genetically related to other clinical phenotypes such as depression. Furthermore, this proposed relationship opens up the possibility of applying knowledge of gene effects acquired within the framework of depression, mostly in healthy subjects [18], to functional pain syndromes, which this chapter will attempt to do.

Gene Discovery Efforts

Despite major research efforts over the past years, the genetic mechanisms of functional pain syndromes and depression are largely unknown. However, recent progress has been made in genome-wide association studies [1,23], mainly due to appropriately powered samples of clinical populations, the availability of linkage disequilibrium and genome-wide variation patterns within the International HapMap resource, and access to dense genotyping chips containing most of the single nucleotide polymorphisms of the human genome. Those studies have highlighted the importance of several genes that have been found to be relevant for human vulnerability to depression in imaging genetics studies and have also been associated with functional pain syndromes in animal studies.

The Serotonin System

The pharmacological inhibition of 5-HT and norepinephrine transporters by serotonin-norepinephrine reuptake inhibitors (SNRIs) is clinically proven to be superior to the inhibition of 5-HT transporters by selective 5-HT reuptake inhibitors (SSRIs). However, evidence shows that the 5-HT system is involved in pathways that play a role in functional pain syndromes [22]. One model proposes that descending serotonergic neurons, originating in the raphe nuclei, directly inhibit activity of dorsal horn neurons via 5-HT_{1B} and 5-HT_{1D} receptors, resulting in an inhibition of somatic input generated in the muscles and gut. Therefore, insufficient inhibition by serotonergic neurons might result in the perception of irrelevant somatic sensations [22].

Further support for this idea stems from studies of the 5-HT system in the developing brain. Serotonergic neurons are among the first neurons to be generated, and even nonserotonergic neurons such as glutamatergic projection neurons may transiently express 5-HT transporters (5-HTT). These transporters, which are the target of SSRI treatment, are critical for 5-HT turnover within the anterior cingulate cortex, a region associated with pain perception and processing of negative mood. This pattern of expression in nonserotonergic neurons within a specific temporal window is hypothesized to underlie the formation and fine-tuning of specific connectivity patterns, possibly through regulation of synaptogenesis and growth cone motility. Therefore, 5-HT appears to be critical for the development of specific brain circuitries. In fact, even transient alterations in 5-HT homeostasis during early developmental stages in animals can modify neural connections [5].

Genetics of the Serotonin Transporter

A variable number of tandem repeats in the 5′ promoter region (5-HTTL-PR) of the human serotonin transporter gene (*SLC6A4*) has been shown in both in vitro and in vivo studies to influence transcriptional activity and subsequent availability of the 5-HTT. Specifically, the 5-HTTLPR short (S) allele has reduced transcriptional efficiency in comparison to the long (L) allele, and individuals carrying the S allele tend to have increased anxiety-related temperamental traits [10], which represent a risk factor for depression and a comorbid symptom in many functional pain disorders [22]. In depressive patients, the presence of the S allele can adversely affect the clinical outcome of SSRI treatment. Furthermore, among patients with IBS, S-allele carriers exhibit increased pain sensation and increased rectal compliance, which is unlikely to be related to increased pain sensation ratings in this genetic risk group [2].

Over the last decade, neuroimaging techniques have made great strides, and recently it has become possible to detect subtle changes introduced by the 5-HTTLPR. Using functional magnetic resonance imaging (fMRI), a pioneering study found that healthy, nondepressed S-allele carriers showed an exaggerated amygdala response to threatening visual stimuli in comparison to individuals with the L-allele genotype, suggesting a possible link between variation in the gene and a basic brain mechanism involved in the regulation of negative emotion [7]. This finding was subsequently confirmed in several independent studies, confirming that S-allele carriers show exaggerated amygdala responses to potentially threatening stimuli.

A broader perspective evolved when anatomical and functional neuroimaging techniques investigated 5-HTTLPR effects on both a local and brain systems level [18]. As predicted from preclinical work, anatomical human imaging data in healthy controls were able to demonstrate that the S allele leads to a significant decrease of gray matter volume in the amygdala and specifically in the rostral subgenual portion of the anterior cingulate cortex (rACC). This finding is in accordance with evidence from other neuroimaging and neuropathological studies suggesting a key regulatory role of the rACC in pain perception, depression, induced sadness, antidepressant response, efficacy of therapeutic sleep deprivation, and it also agrees with anecdotal reports of therapeutic response in therapy-refractory depression and chronic pain to cingulotomy and, more recently, deep brain stimulation. Remarkably, the region showing the greatest effect of the 5-HTTLPR genotype is located within the phylogenetically older archicortical portion of the cingulate cortex, a region that displays the highest density of 5-HTT terminals within the human cortex and is a target zone of dense projections from the amygdala via the uncinate bundle [12]. Studies on a brain systems level revealed simultaneously with both functional and anatomical data that the S allele of 5-HTTLPR leads to a decrease in coupling between the amygdala and the rACC, resulting in increased amygdala reactivity. The investigators found that the measure of coupling predicted normal variation in temperamental measures of harm avoidance, a temperamental dimension that is linked to risk for depression and is frequently associated with functional pain syndromes [18]. These genotype-related alterations in anatomy and in the function of an amygdala-cingulate feedback circuitry critical for emotional and pain regulation have been implicated in a developmental, systems-level mechanism underlying emotional reactivity and genetic susceptibility for anxiety and depression [18]. Given that this circuitry is also involved in pain perception, the findings of this study (which was performed in healthy controls) might also apply to functional pain syndromes.

However, associations of 5-HTTLPR with clinical phenotypes such as depression or functional pain syndromes are contradictory, which makes it unlikely that 5-HTTLPR by itself causes these clinical conditions. Research in this field suggests that this genotype contributes to vulnerability to these disorders, which might be reflected on a clinical level in anxious temperament and probably in gut hypermobility and pain hypersensitivity [15]. In contrast, clinical observations and preclinical experiments report that stressful environmental triggers can induce phenotypes such as depression and pain syndromes [8], underlining the importance of environmental factors in the emergence of those clinical phenotypes. A recent pioneering study [3] demonstrated how 5-HTTLPR might contribute to the clinical phenotype of depression. This study showed that environmental adversity translates into the clinical phenotype only in the presence of genetic risk factors such as the S allele. In other words, this study reported a clinically relevant gene by environment interaction, which offers a model for future studies in the field of functional pain syndromes.

Brain-Derived Neurotrophic Factor

Human and animal evidence supports the idea that brain-derived neurotrophic factor (BDNF) modulates pain [13] as well as hippocampal-dependent learning and memory [4]. The specific role of BDNF in learning and memory has been related to the modulation of synaptic transmission and plasticity, particularly long-term potentiation, but also to its importance in mediating long-term developmental effects such as neuronal survival, migration, and differentiation, as well as activity-dependent refinement of synaptic architecture [21]. The role of BDNF in pain perception has been studied less thoroughly, but animal studies indicate that this neurotrophin is an effective modulator of pain on a spinal and central level via mechanisms similar to those demonstrated in the biology of learning [13]. BDNF has also been implicated in mediating the trophic effects of serotonin signaling in development and also in the effects of antidepressant drugs [19].

A common single nucleotide polymorphism in the BDNF gene (*val66met*) in the 5′ signal domain has been shown to affect intracellular packaging and regulated secretion of BDNF, and also human hippocampal function and episodic memory [4,6], but it has not yet received sufficient study in pain disorder models. Cell cultures of hippocampal neurons transfected with met-BDNF show reduced depolarization-induced secretion and fail to localize BDNF to secretory granules and dendritic processes. In accordance with results of preclinical studies, normal met-allele carriers have been shown to exhibit poorer episodic memory performance and reduced hippocampal physiological engagement during memory tasks when studied with fMRI [6]. Similarly, anatomical imaging studies [21], which found bilateral hippocampus and dorsolateral prefrontal cortical volume reductions in met-BDNF carriers, suggest that effects of this polymorphism may reflect not only rapid, context-dependent plasticity in the hippocampal formation, but also a trait characteristic related to hippocampal and prefrontal development and morphology. It is noteworthy that none of the human imaging studies has revealed any effects of BDNF on the amygdala-rACC circuitry, which has been shown to be modulated by 5-HTTLPR.

Studies of the genetic association of BDNF with depression and pain disorders have produced mixed results. Imaging studies of BDNF *val-66met* in the context of pain or functional pain disorders are still missing. Evidence indicates that the BDNF gene, similar to 5-HTTLPR, also interacts with environmental stressors. Preclinical studies suggest that BDNF mediates the biological consequences of social defeat stress and underlies the antidepressive effects in most treatment modalities such as electroconvulsive therapy and drug treatment with 5-HT reuptake inhibitors and enhancers, as well as the effects of mood stabilizers such as lithium and valproate. It is noteworthy that all of those drugs have shown some efficacy in the management of chronic pain disorders [22].

Interaction of Serotonin and BDNF

Mechanisms of 5-HT neurotransmission during brain development are poorly understood, but recent studies indicate that BNDF, by mediating neuroplastic changes in response to 5-HT signaling, may be involved [19,20]. Most studies highlight the molecular relationship between 5-HT and BDNF, whose expression is partly mediated via the transcription factor cyclic adenosine monophosphate (cAMP) response element-binding protein (CREB), which is responsive to 5-HT-induced intracellular signaling. Further evidence suggests that BDNF promotes the development and function of 5-HT neurons. This evidence is also supported by a recent animal study demonstrating that fluoxetine treatment restores activity-dependent neuroplasticity in the visual cortex, whereas diazepam cotreatment blocks these effects [11].

This biological interaction of BDNF and 5-HT signaling also supports the idea of epistasis (gene by gene interaction) between 5-HTTLPR and *val66met* BDNF in biasing brain development toward susceptibility for depression and most likely functional pain syndromes. This idea has been explored to a limited degree in animals genetically engineered to be hypomorphic at both genes [16]. Results suggest that a loss of BDNF exacerbates brain 5-HT deficiencies and increases stress abnormalities in *SLC6A4* knockout mice. More compelling are data from a variant genetically humanized mouse model demonstrating that anxiety behavior in animals carrying met-BDNF alleles is unresponsive to SSRIs, which can be viewed as pharmacological analogues of 5-HTTLPR S alleles [9]. Further support stems from a recent anatomical imaging study [19,20], which expands on previously reported evidence that development of the amygdala-rACC mood circuitry is genetically modulated by 5-HTTLPR [19]. This study was able to demonstrate that *val66met* BDNF interacts epistatically with 5-HTTLPR, presumably affecting the development and integrity of this neural system, which is consistent with epistatic concepts of depression as well as with animal models of social defeat stress-related plasticity.

Summary

Depression and functional pain syndromes share an intriguing overlap on a biological and clinical level. Progress in genetic research over the last couple of years supports the idea that genes involving the serotonin and neurotrophin system exhibit pleiotropic phenotypes, which have been associated with depression and functional pain syndromes. Furthermore, studies have demonstrated that 5-HTTLPR and *val66met* BDNF interact with environmental stressors, thus translating into clinical phenotypes. The potential complexity of those clinical phenotypes is highlighted by studies demonstrating epistatic effects between those genotypes on a brain systems level, suggesting a sophisticated relationship between vulnerability and clinical phenotype. Although most genetic imaging or knockout mouse studies have been conducted within the framework of depression, in healthy human subjects or animals, there is little argument against the application of those findings to functional pain syndromes.

References

[1]   Baum AE, Hamshere M, Green E, Cichon S, Rietschel M, Noethen MM, Craddock N, McMahon FJ. Meta-analysis of two genome-wide association studies of bipolar disorder reveals important points of agreement. Mol Psychiatry 2008;13:466–7.
[2]   Camilleri M, Busciglio I, Carlson P, McKinzie S, Burton D, Baxter K, Ryks M, Zinsmeister AR. Candidate genes and sensory functions in health and irritable bowel syndrome. Am J Physiol Gastrointest Liver Physiol 2008; Epub May 29.

[3]   Caspi A, Sugden K, Moffitt TE, Taylor A, Craig IW, Harrington H, McClay J, Mill J, Martin J, Braithwaite A, Poulton R. Influence of life stress on depression: moderation by a polymorphism in the 5-HTT gene. Science 2003;301:386–9.

[4]   Egan MF, Kojima M, Callicott JH, Goldberg TE, Kolachana BS, Bertolino A, Zaitsev E, Gold B, Goldman D, Dean M, Lu B, Weinberger DR. The BDNF val66met polymorphism affects activity-dependent secretion of BDNF and human memory and hippocampal function. Cell 2003;112:257–69.

[5]   Gaspar P, Cases O, Maroteaux L. The developmental role of serotonin: news from mouse molecular genetics. Nat Rev Neurosci 2003;4:1002–12.

[6]   Hariri AR, Goldberg TE, Mattay VS, Kolachana BS, Callicott JH, Egan MF, Weinberger DR. Brain-derived neurotrophic factor val66met polymorphism affects human memory-related hippocampal activity and predicts memory performance. J Neurosci 2003;23:6690–4.

[7]   Hariri AR, Mattay VS, Tessitore A, Kolachana B, Fera F, Goldman D, Egan MF, Weinberger DR. Serotonin transporter genetic variation and the response of the human amygdala. Science 2002;297:400–3.

[8]   Khasar SG, Burkham J, Dina OA, Brown AS, Bogen O, Alessandri-Haber N, Green PG, Reichling DB, Levine JD. Stress induces a switch of intracellular signaling in sensory neurons in a model of generalized pain. J Neurosci 2008;28:5721–30.

[9]   Krishnan V, Han M-H, Graham DL, Berton O, Renthal W, Russo SJ, LaPlant Q, Graham A, Lutter M, Lagace DC, et al. Molecular adaptations underlying susceptibility and resistance to social defeat in brain reward regions. Cell 2007;131:391–404.

[10] Lesch KP, Bengel D, Heils A, Sabol SZ, Greenberg BD, Petri S, Benjamin J, Muller CR, Hamer DH, Murphy DL. Association of anxiety-related traits with a polymorphism in the serotonin transporter gene regulatory region. Science 1996;274:1527–31.

[11] Maya Vetencourt JF, Sale A, Viegi A, Baroncelli L, De Pasquale R, O'Leary OF, Castren E, Maffei L. The antidepressant fluoxetine restores plasticity in the adult visual cortex. Science 2008;320:385–8.

[12] Mega MS, Cummings JL, Salloway S, Malloy P. The limbic system: an anatomic, phylogenetic, and clinical perspective. J Neuropsychiatry Clin Neurosci 1997;9:315–30.

[13] Merighi A, Salio C, Ghirri A, Lossi L, Ferrini F, Betelli C, Bardoni R. BDNF as a pain modulator. Prog Neurobiol 2008;85:297–317.

[14] Merikangas KR, Merikangas JR, Angst J. Headache syndromes and psychiatric disorders: association and familial transmission. J Psychiatr Res 1993;27:197–210.

[15] Murphy DL, Lesch KP. Targeting the murine serotonin transporter: insights into human neurobiology. Nat Rev Neurosci 2008;9:85–96.

[16] Murphy DL, Uhl GR, Holmes A, Ren-Patterson R, Hall FS, Sora I, Detera-Wadleigh S, Lesch KP. Experimental gene interaction studies with SERT mutant mice as models for human polygenic and epistatic traits and disorders. Genes Brain Behav 2003;2:350–64.

[17] Petrovic P, Dietrich T, Fransson P, Andersson J, Carlsson K, Ingvar M. Placebo in emotional processing: induced expectations of anxiety relief activate a generalized modulatory network. Neuron 2005;46:957–69.

[18] Pezawas L, Meyer-Lindenberg A, Drabant EM, Verchinski BA, Munoz KE, Kolachana BS, Egan MF, Mattay VS, Hariri AR, Weinberger DR. 5-HTTLPR polymorphism impacts human cingulate-amygdala interactions: a genetic susceptibility mechanism for depression. Nat Neurosci 2005;8:828–34.

[19] Pezawas L, Meyer-Lindenberg A, Goldman AL, Verchinski BA, Chen G, Kolachana BS, Egan MF, Mattay VS, Hariri AR, Weinberger DR. Evidence of biologic epistasis between BDNF and SLC6A4 and implications for depression. Mol Psychiatry 2008;13:654, 709–16.

[20] Pezawas L, Meyer-Lindenberg A, Goldman AL, Verchinski BA, Chen G, Kolachana BS, Egan MF, Mattay VS, Hariri AR, Weinberger DR. MET BDNF protects against morphological S allele effects of 5-HTTLPR. Mol Psychiatry 2008;13:654.

[21] Pezawas L, Verchinski BA, Mattay VS, Callicott JH, Kolachana BS, Straub RE, Egan MF, Meyer-Lindenberg A, Weinberger DR. The brain-derived neurotrophic factor val66met polymorphism and variation in human cortical morphology. J Neurosci 2004;24:10099–102.

[22] Stahl SM. Stahl's essential psychopharmacology : neuroscientific basis and practical applications. 3rd ed. New York: Cambridge University Press; 2008.

[23] Wellcome Trust Case Control Consortium. Genome-wide association study of 14,000 cases of seven common diseases and 3,000 shared controls. Nature 2007;447:661–78.
[24] Vogt BA. Pain and emotion interactions in subregions of the cingulate gyrus. Nat Rev Neurosci 2005;6:533–44.

Correspondence to: Priv.Doz. Dr. Lukas Pezawas, Division of Biological Psychiatry, Medical University of Vienna, Waehringer Guertel 18-20, 1090 Vienna, Austria. Email: lukas.pezawas@meduniwien.ac.at.

Part VI

Treatment Strategies

Pharmacotherapy for Functional Somatic Conditions

22

R. Bruce Lydiard

Department of Psychiatry/Mental Health, Ralph H. Johnson VA Medical Center, Charleston, South Carolina, USA; Southeast Health Consultants, Mount Pleasant, South Carolina, USA

Pharmacotherapy can be a useful option for the treatment of pain in functional somatic conditions. Inadequate understanding of the pathophysiology of these conditions has limited the development of effective pharmacotherapy and fostered the use of many agents with little to no therapeutic value [1,13,14]. As discussed in detail elsewhere in this volume, a complex array of interacting factors affect the clinical manifestation of functional pain. These include hyperalgesia, neural sensitization at multiple levels [35,46,54], excessive inflammation and immune dysregulation [51,53,88,90], stress vulnerability/reactivity [12,22,24], comorbid functional pain [20,69] and psychiatric disorders [69,70,97,111,120], severe psychosocial stress (including sexual and physical abuse) [12,30,103,117,122], developmental adversity [34,40,59,83,122], personality [58], coping strategies [43], and gender [20,19,41]. Finally, clinician-patient interactions can affect patients' perceptions of the etiology of their painful symptoms, thus playing a central role in the treatment process [40,100].

There are multiple potential peripheral and central sites of action for pharmacotherapeutic agents [16,27,79,80]. Experts generally agree that the altered pain perception in the functional somatic visceral pain syndromes is associated with distorted processing of somatovisceral afferent information and amplification of central nervous system (CNS) responses to this input. Antidepressants, including tricyclic antidepressants (TCAs), selective serotonin reuptake inhibitors (SSRIs), and dual serotonin-norepinephrine reuptake inhibitors (SNRIs), have been the most extensively studied. Recently, researchers have given increased attention to the clinical value of targeting pain-related anxiety as well as comorbid depression [76,80,85,97].

This chapter will highlight drug treatments for two of the most common and best studied syndromes, fibromyalgia and irritable bowel syndrome (IBS), with emphasis on central actions, and will provide practical suggestions for treatment of coexisting psychiatric and functional somatic syndromes.

Stress Reactivity as a Target for Treating Functional Pain Syndromes

The observation that treatment with TCAs can benefit the seemingly different conditions discussed in this volume led Hudson et al. to hypothesize that some neurobiological features may be shared among this group of conditions [57]. Further evidence to support the concept of some common neurobiology comes from family studies showing that these "affective spectrum disorders" coaggregate within families [56].

Like anxiety and depression, the functional somatic pain conditions are perceived as unpredictable and uncontrollable. In addition to being worsened by stress, these conditions also act as stressors themselves by causing symptom-related stress [81], which is relevant to the treatment of pain in these conditions. In a significant percentage of antidepressant studies in functional somatic pain syndromes, improved global functioning and reduced illness-related distress have been observed more consistently than effects on pain or other core illness symptoms. These observations are consistent with the emerging consensus that abnormal sensory processing and stress reactivity in the CNS are key features of altered pain perception in the functional pain disorders [21,27,80,95,112,114,121,124].

Clinical and preclinical research suggests that antidepressants can attenuate or reverse the effects of stress and act as stress buffers via specific actions in the CNS [94].

One common, but not universal, neurobiological feature associated with various functional pain syndromes is persistent hypothalamic-pituitary-adrenal (HPA) dysregulation [21,74,104,105]. Raison and Miller reviewed the neuroendocrine studies from post-traumatic stress disorder, major depression, fibromyalgia, and chronic fatigue [96] and concluded that insufficient glucocorticoid signaling was a core feature in these disorders. Insufficient glucocorticoid signaling describes a neurophysiological state in which the capacity of glucocorticoids is inadequate to restrain relevant stress-responsive systems, either as a result of decreased hormone bioavailability (e.g., hypocortisolism) or because of attenuated glucocorticoid receptor responsiveness following sustained hypercortisolism. The predicted consequences of glucocorticoid signaling insufficiency have a remarkable resemblance to conditions observed in the functional pain syndromes. These include fatigue, cognitive dysfunction, depression, anxiety, impaired immune function, increased inflammatory cytokines, increased sympathetic outflow, and insulin resistance (Fig. 1).

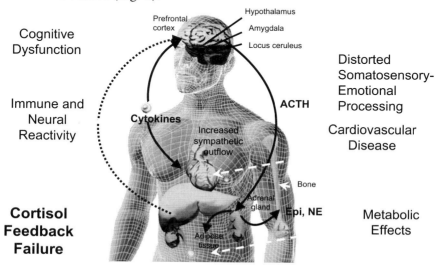

Fig. 1. Consequences of insufficient glucocorticoid signaling. ACTH = adrenocorticotropic hormone, Epi = epinephrine, NE = norepinephrine.

Antistress Actions of Antidepressants

Antidepressants can normalize or reverse cytokine-induced disruption of intracellular glucocorticoid receptor actions on gene transcription to improve glucocorticoid signaling efficiency, which is essential for termination of the stress response [23,88,92,96]. Corticotropin-releasing factor (CRF), the peptide that initiates the stress response, also plays an important role in the pathophysiology of anxiety disorders, depression, pain, and several chronic functional disorders [45,84,108,117]. Preclinical research has shown that all classes of antidepressants produce anti-CRF effects via reduced synthesis, release, receptor density, and postsynaptic response to CRF [94,104]. Interestingly, long-term alprazolam treatment produces similar anti-CRF effects [61,102]. Evidence indicates that individuals with functional somatic pain syndromes have elevated circulating pro-inflammatory cytokine levels and autonomic overactivity [4,53,65,96]. The resultant neural sensitization promotes the development of pain syndromes [62,73,95], as well as psychiatric disorders [64,72,82,106]. In depressed humans, effective antidepressant treatment lowers circulating proinflammatory cytokines [63,66,67,91,115].

Substantial preclinical evidence shows that antidepressants restore structural plasticity in the brain and spinal cord, restore adult neurogenesis in the brain, reverse stress-related neurodegenerative effects in brain centers critical for pain processing, and provide ongoing neuroprotection from future stressors [44,75,94]. For example, in severe post-traumatic stress disorder, long-term antidepressant treatment was associated with increased hippocampal volume and enhanced declarative memory [118]. See Fig. 2 for a diagram of the antistress effects of antidepressants.

Drug Treatment of Irritable Bowel Syndrome

Antidepressants

Antidepressants, especially low-dose TCAs (primarily amitriptyline), have been the most studied drug treatments in IBS. There is recent evidence that TCAs (but not SSRIs), in addition to their well-known effects on monoaminergic signaling systems, may exert antihyperalgesic effects via membrane Na^+ channel actions [36,37]. Morgan et al. [89] reported that

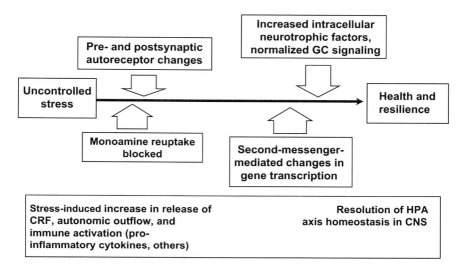

Fig. 2. Anti-stress effects of antidepressants. CNS = central nervous system, CRF = cortico-tropin-releasing hormone, GC = glucocorticoid, HPA = hypothalamic-pituitary-adrenal axis.

treatment with 50 mg amitriptyline for 1 month reduced perceived pain during rectal distension and the experimental psychological stress. The treatment also altered anterior cingulate cortex activation, suggesting at least partial activity on central pain-processing areas.

Clinical experience supports the utility of the TCAs [11,77], but the evidence for efficacy is still inadequate [16]. Inadequate sample size remains a major limitation. Other problems in studies conducted to date include variability in disorders included, outcome measures, and study duration; failure to account for psychiatric comorbidity; and use of different agents and dosage. Only one study [42] was adequately designed to empirically assess the efficacy of the TCA desipramine in women with IBS or other functional abdominal pain syndromes. Subjects received either desipramine (n = 137) (50–150 mg range, average 100 mg/day) or placebo (n = 72) for 12 weeks. Surprisingly, drug treatment failed to show statistical differences from placebo on the percentage of responders (60% desipramine; 47% placebo) in the intent-to-treat analysis. However, post hoc analysis showed that completers derived statistically significant benefits favoring the active drug over placebo (73% versus 49%). After the investigators excluded 13 completers with undetectable desipramine levels, they found an even more robust difference. Even though this study assessed for abuse history and psychiatric status, it did not measure anxiety specifically as an outcome variable, and therefore one cannot exclude a possible indirect effect on gastrointestinal (GI) symptoms via desipramine's anxiolytic effect.

Selective Serotonin Reuptake Inhibitors

The efficacy of SSRI treatment for IBS has been examined in several small studies. Like the majority of TCA studies, many are methodologically flawed; most often they were insufficiently powered to convincingly prove efficacy. One small placebo-controlled studies suggests clinical utility of citalopram [16], and another study in IBS patients who were unimproved after fiber treatment found that paroxetine was beneficial [107]. One large naturalistic study compared paroxetine (n = 86 subjects) with standard care (there was no placebo group) [29]. Half the patients dropped out by week 12. While the study found improvement in several outcome measures, it did not show sustained reduction of pain. A recent study comparing daily doses of 40 mg citalopram with 50 mg imipramine or placebo in a total of 51 IBS patients found no differences among them, most likely due to inadequate sample size [109]. There have been no placebo-controlled studies of the SNRIs in IBS.

In summary, empirical support for the effectiveness of antidepressants are IBS is lacking, largely because of inadequate study design. Preclinical research, as well as substantial clinical experience, supports their use, especially for patients with anxiety and depression. Clinical benefit can occur in the absence of psychiatric disorders, and the limited information suggests that all subtypes of IBS may benefit from paroxetine [29,42].

Agents Approved for IBS

Two drugs have been approved for treatment of IBS by the U.S. Food and Drug Administration (FDA), and are also available in some other countries.However, they are restricted to adult women with inadequate response to traditional treatment. Alosetron, a 5-HT_3 antagonist approved for diarrhea-predominant IBS, reduced both core and global IBS symptoms in large clinical trials in women [17,68] and more recently in men [19]. The use of a 5-HT_3 receptor antagonist originally selected to target gut receptors, but the therapeutic effects may have been mediated in part by central antinociceptive and anxiolytic mechanisms [78,80]. The second agent, lubiprostone, was recently approved for constipation-predominant IBS. It has been shown to benefit abdominal pain/discomfort [60]. These two agents fail to address the needs of a substantial majority of IBS patients. A summary of IBS drug treatments is shown in Table I.

Drug Treatment of Fibromyalgia

Fibromyalgia (FM) is characterized by unexplained widespread musculo-skeletal pain, nonrestorative sleep, fatigue, and tender points, as described in Chapter 1 by Clauw and Williams. Accumulating evidence implicates dysregulation of central pain processing as important in its pathogenesis [5,25,31,33,51,52]. There is significant overlap of FM with other functional somatic syndromes, including IBS [69] and interstitial cystitis [28,55,123]. Evidence suggests abnormal sympathetic and HPA axis function in FM [25,110]. In community studies and clinical samples, depression and anxiety disorders (including panic disorder and post-traumatic stress disorder) [15,97, 111,124] are commonly comorbid with FM, as is a history of prior victimization [3,30,101,117,119,122], cognitive dysfunction [27,49], and fatigue [27]. The TCA amitriptyline is the most studied agent for FM; about one-third of patients obtain short-term benefit, which in the only follow-up study [18] was lost by 26 weeks.

Several recent reviews and meta-analyses of peer-reviewed, published pharmacological treatment studies for FM note that the methodology of most studies was significantly flawed [1,26,50]. One review [116] excluded 134 of 167 antidepressant trials because they were duplicate publications. Lack of sufficient information on inclusion criteria, variable study duration, and different outcome measures were common problems, and sample size was most consistently problematic. A detailed review [116] of 26 antidepressant studies selected from the literature reported that only 9 of 19 studies that examined TCAs and 6 of 12 that examined SSRIs included a placebo. With few exceptions, the placebo-controlled studies that failed to show differences were substantially underpowered. Those trials in which significant differences were demonstrated included

Table I
Drug treatments for irritable bowel syndrome

Agent	Daily Dose	Effects on IBS	Tolerability	Comments	Evidence for Efficacy
Lubiprostone (Ca^{2+} channel blocker)	24 μg b.i.d.	Effective for constipation and abdominal discomfort	Dose-related diarrhea, nausea, headache, abdominal pain	Limited patient subgroup	Strong evidence; FDA approved; long-term data lacking; limited to women not responding to standard treatment for IBS
Tegaserod (5-HT$_4$ agonist)	6 mg b.i.d.	20% greater than placebo	Initial diarrhea, abdominal pain, rare cardiovascular ischemia	FDA approved; well-designed and powered; FM effect independent of mood effects	Strong evidence; FDA withdrew approval due to cardiovascular safety concerns
Loperamide (opioid agonist)	2–8 mg	Antidiarrheal	Diarrhea	Not approved; extensive clinical experience	Anecdotal evidence
Alosetron (5-HT$_3$ antagonist)	0.5–1 mg b.i.d.	Reduced motility	Constipation; rare ischemic colitis	Limited patient subgroup	Strong evidence; FDA approved; limited to women not responding to standard treatment for IBS

Drug	Dosage	Efficacy	Side effects	Study comments	Evidence
Amitriptyline (TCA)	25–50 mg at bedtime	Short-term improvement in most studies in pain and reduced sleep impairment	Anticholinergic; caution in elderly	Short-term treatment limits generalization; small samples	Moderate evidence; broad clinical experience; not tested adequately in RCTs
Desipramine (TCA)	50–150 mg	Early RCTs and recent large study show improved QOL and IBS core symptoms	Anticholinergic	Best-designed TCA study	Strong evidence
Selective serotonin reuptake inhibitors	Varies*	At 12 weeks, improvement in sleep and pain	Dry mouth, nausea, sleep disturbance	Two controlled studies; short duration limits generalization	Moderate to strong evidence; large RCT needed; independent of psychiatric disorder

Abbreviations: b.i.d. = twice daily; FDA = U.S. Food and Drug Administration; FM = fibromyalgia; IBS = irritable bowel syndrome; QOL = quality of life; RCT = randomized controlled trial; TCA = tricyclic antidepressant.

* Paroxetine 10–60 mg; citalopram 5–20 mg; fluoxetine 20–40 mg.

more than 100 subjects per group. All 26 excluded other functional somatic disorders and half excluded mental illness, but the methods used were generally not provided.

Agents Approved for Fibromyalgia

Pregabalin, an antiepileptic similar to gabapentin that binds the $\alpha_2\delta$ subunit of voltage-gated neuronal Ca^{2+} channels, was approved by the FDA for treatment of FM in June 2007. A second drug, duloxetine hydrochloride, was approved in June 2008 by the FDA. No medications are approved for FM in Europe at this time. Both of these compounds clearly exert their therapeutic effects via central mechanisms. Both are effective anxiolytics [2,47,98], which may be relevant to their efficacy. The clinical trials demonstrating efficacy in FM for duloxetine [8,9] and pregabalin [10,32,87] were well-designed and sufficiently powered for hypothesis testing.

Duloxetine

Duloxetine is an SNRI with proven efficacy in major depression and generalized anxiety disorder [2], neuropathic pain, and most recently, fibromyalgia [93]. Two large clinical trials evaluated its efficacy in individuals with FM with or without major depression. Arnold et al. treated 207 FM patients (25 men, 182 women) with 60 mg duloxetine daily or placebo over 12 weeks [8]. For both primary outcome measures—the Fibromyalgia Impact Questionnaire (FIQ) total score and the FIQ pain subscale total—and several secondary outcome measures, duloxetine was superior to placebo. This clinical trial was the first FM study to carefully document psychiatric comorbidity (allowing the participation of subjects with major depression but excluding subjects with anxiety disorders), and to control for the effects of depression on pain outcomes.

The second study [9], with a nearly identical design, compared 60 mg duloxetine twice daily with 60 mg daily or placebo in 364 women (men were excluded) with FM, with or without major depressive disorder. Both doses of duloxetine appeared to be efficacious, although the 60-mg dose was not significantly different from placebo on tender point ratings.

A third study was a 6-month, placebo-controlled study in 520 outpatients with FM with or without current major depression [99]. This study compared three doses of duloxetine (20 mg/day, 60 mg/day, or 120 mg/day) and placebo given once daily. The two primary outcome measures were the Brief Pain Inventory (BPI) and Patient Global Impression of Improvement (PGI-I) scores. All three doses were superior to placebo on most primary and secondary outcome measures at 3 and 6 months. Adverse effects were dose-related, and safety issues were similar among doses.

Pregabalin

Pregabalin is a novel agent that binds selectively at the $\alpha_2\delta$ subunit of voltage-gated neuronal Ca^{2+} channels [38,39] to reduce the release of norepinephrine, serotonin (5-HT), glutamate, and substance P. Pregabalin and its precursor gabapentin have analgesic, anxiolytic, and anticonvulsant effects in humans [48]. Pregabalin is rapidly absorbed, reaches steady-state levels in 24–48 hours, readily crosses the blood-brain barrier, does not bind to plasma proteins, and is excreted almost completely unchanged by the kidneys [38,39,48].

Two placebo-controlled, fixed-dose studies, one lasting 8 weeks [32] and one 14 weeks [10], examined pregabalin in doses ranging from 150 to 600 mg/day in a total of 529 subjects with FM. At least 100 subjects participated in each treatment cell. The primary outcome variable was average daily ratings of pain intensity. While doses of both 450 and 300 mg/day benefited most of the secondary outcome measures (sleep quality, fatigue, and global measures of change), the 450 mg/day dose most consistently reduced FM pain. Rates of discontinuation due to adverse events were similar across the three pregabalin and the placebo treatment groups. Another small study showed efficacy for gabapentin over placebo on most measures except tender point exam [7].

A 6-month [87] double-blind, placebo-controlled, randomized survival study evaluated the durability of effect of "optimized" pregabalin treatment on FM-related pain. In this study, subjects were initially treated with an optimized pregabalin dose of 300, 450, or 600 mg/day on an open-label basis. Those who experienced at least a 50% decrease in pain score on a visual analogue scale and a self-rating of "much" or "very much" improved on the Patient Global Impression of Change were randomized to placebo or to their pre-established optimal fixed dosage of pregabalin. The primary

Table II
Drug treatments for fibromyalgia

Agent	Daily Dose	Effects on FM	Tolerability	Comment	Evidence for Efficacy
Pregabalin ($\alpha_2\delta$ subunit of voltage-gated Ca^{2+} channel modulator)	450 mg (300–600 mg)	Positive effects for pain, sleep, most secondary measures	Dizziness, somnolence, fatigue; dose-related; well tolerated	Well-designed studies; 450-mg dose had most efficacy vs. side effects	Strong evidence; FDA approved; long-term data
Duloxetine (dual NE and 5-HT reuptake inhibitor)	60 or 120 mg	Positive effects on FIQ pain, tender points, most secondary outcome measures	Insomnia, nausea, dizziness, dry mouth, constipation; dose-related; more dropouts with duloxetine	Doses effective for depression and anxiety; well-designed and powered studies; FM effect independent of mood effects	Strong evidence; FDA approved; long-term data
Amitriptyline	25–50 mg at bedtime	Short-term improvement on pain and sleep	Dry mouth, sedation, urinary retention, constipation; caution in elderly	Short-term treatment limits generalization; small samples	Strong evidence
Cyclobenzaprine (muscle relaxant with tricyclic structure)	5–20 mg at bedtime	Short-term relief of pain and fatigue	Sedation		Moderate evidence; only one positive study

Drug	Dose	Efficacy	Side effects	Study comments	Evidence
Milnacipran (dual NE and 5-HT reuptake inhibitor)	100–200 mg daily	One RCT showed positive effects on pain and secondary outcome measures	Nausea, dizziness, dry mouth, constipation	Large, well-designed study; drug not available in U.S.	Strong evidence
Fluoxetine (selective 5-HT reuptake inhibitor)	10–80 mg, flexible; average 45 ± 25 mg	Improvement in sleep and pain FIQ, McGill Pain Questionnaire	Dry mouth, nausea, sleep disturbance	Two controlled studies; short duration limits generalization	Moderate evidence; other SSRIs inadequately studied
Tramadol + acetaminophen (weak NE-5HT reuptake inhibitor and mild μ-opioid agonist)	50 mg tramadol + acetaminophen	FIQ and pain improved over placebo	Nausea, dizziness, headache, somnolence; high dropout rates	Unusual designs; one parallel study positive (moderate)	Weak evidence; dependence/abuse liability
Combination of cyclobenzaprine + fluoxetine; fluoxetine + amitriptyline		Combination superior to either alone			Moderate to limited evidence
Zolpidem (nonbenzodiazepine hypnotic)	5–15 mg	Crossover, 4 nights each	N/A	No effect on FM; sleep improved	Not effective (inadequate duration)

outcome measure in this study was time to at least 30% reduction in pain (from the open-label baseline). Of 1051 patients entering the open-label study, 287 were randomized to placebo and 279 to pregabalin. At the end of double-blind treatment, 61% of the placebo patients vs. 32% of those taking pregabalin had either experienced a relapse or demonstrated sufficient loss of pain reduction according to predefined criteria.

Summary

The short-term studies for both new compounds were scientifically sound but sufficiently different to preclude direct comparisons. Inclusion of major depression in the duloxetine studies provided useful clinical information. The long-term studies had more important differences in design. For example, the long-term duloxetine study [99] was a parallel design measuring via changes in primary and secondary outcome variables including pain—a standard clinical trial design. In contrast, the long-term pregabalin trial [87] was "enriched" by subjects who were initially responders prior to randomization and measured the length of time until 30% of the improvement that occurred during the open-label treatment was lost over the 6-month double blind treatment.

All pregabalin studies excluded major depression. However, the long-term data provide a significant improvement over previous clinical trials. Table II provides a summary of agents used for the treatment of FM [86].

Treating Psychiatric Disorders in Patients with Functional Somatic Syndromes

Failure to detect and treat anxiety or depression may worsen the long-term outcome of IBS and FM [6,40]. Detailed evaluation of patients with functional pain disorders via extensive diagnostic interviews is impractical for nonpsychiatric practitioners. Because of the broad antidepressant and anxiolytic efficacy of the newer antidepressants, precision of diagnosis is less critical than detection of clinically significant levels of anxiety or depressive symptoms. The 14-item Hospital Anxiety and Depression Scale (HADS) [125] is a patient-rated scale that excludes somatic symptoms or pain, which makes it ideal for use with medical patients. The HADS is well suited both for screening and monitoring treatment in functional pain syndromes.

Practical Use of Psychotropics

In clinical practice, a critical part of psychotropic treatment is to assure an adequate medication dose for a minimum of 6 weeks, and preferably 8 weeks. Inadequate treatment intensity is the most common cause of psychotropic treatment failure. No agent is truly selective, due to multiple intermodulating connections on most neurons within the central and enteric nervous systems.

Antidepressants

Low-dose TCAs are frequently the first pharmacological step in treating patients with functional pain; for some patients tolerability of TCAs at doses of 50 mg or more can be problematic [42]. In these cases, combining a low-dose TCA with a full dose of an SSRI or SNRI may be useful [77].

Antidepressant classes and anxiolytics shown in Table III have been established as having efficacy via randomized, placebo-controlled clinical trials for the disorders shown. The SNRIs and SSRIs are generally considered to be equivalent in safety, efficacy, and tolerability. Both classes are broadly efficacious as antidepressants and anxiolytics. The relative advantages and disadvantages of each of the available treatments should be anticipated for the individual patient. It is important to address sleep disturbance, which is associated with more severe symptoms in IBS and overlapping disorders.,

Mirtazapine inhibits reuptake of 5-HT and norepinephrine and is a 5-HT_3 and 5-HT_{2C} antagonist with a low propensity for causing jitteriness and nausea during initiation. However, it can cause sedation and weight gain. Adding mirtazapine to an SSRI or SNRI during initiation of treatment can reduce unpleasant nausea and promote sleep. Bupropion, a dopamine-norepinephrine reuptake inhibitor, can be combined with SSRIs or SNRIs to improve treatment-related sexual dysfunction in the

Table III
Comparative efficacy for anxiety disorders and depression

Drug*	Panic Disorder	Post-traumatic Stress Disorder	Generalized Anxiety Disorder	Social Anxiety Disorder	Major Depression
TCAs	+	+	+	0	+
SSRIs †	+	+	+	+	+
SNRIs ‡	+	+	+	+	+
Mirtazapine	0	0	0	0	+
Trazodone	0	0	+	0	+
Bupropion	0	0	0	0	+
Benzodiazepines	+	0	+	+	0
Buspirone	0	0	+	0	0

Notes: 0 = not effective per at least one RCT; + = evidence from at least one RCT.
* Not all compounds within each class has received approval for each indication, but all have been approved for major depression and at least one anxiety disorder; paroxetine and sertraline are approved for all indications.
† Selective serotonin reuptake inhibitors (SSRIs) are consistently superior to tricyclic antidepressants (TCAs) for patients with atypical features (hyperphagia, weight gain, hypersomnia, carbohydrate craving, extreme fatigue, and interpersonal sensitivity).
‡ Venlafaxine is reflected in the table; duloxetine is a new serotonin-norepinephrine reuptake inhibitor (SNRI) that has been FDA approved for major depression, diabetes-related neuropathic pain, generalized anxiety disorder, and fibromyalgia.

30% to 40% of patients affected over the long term. Trazodone, a 5-HT reuptake inhibitor that also acts as a $5\text{-HT}_2/5\text{-HT}_{1C}$ receptor, postsynaptic α_1 receptor, and histamine-1 receptor antagonist, is most often used to promote sleep (in a 50–200 mg dose range), and it stops antidepressant and anxiolytic properties at higher dosages (300–600 mg).

Benzodiazepines

Benzodiazepines are safe and effective anxiolytics. Patients with prominent anxiety are often intolerant of antidepressants, and many can be treated with benzodiazepine monotherapy. The main disadvantage of benzodiazepines is a lack of reliable antidepressant efficacy. In open-label studies, alprazolam (2–8 mg/day) improves IBS in patients [70,113]. Due to its pharmacokinetic properties, alprazolam requires multiple daily dosing.

Clonazepam is as effective as alprazolam for anxiety, and its longer elimination half-life allows for once- or twice-daily dosing for most patients. Despite objective evidence to the contrary, patients and clinicians continue to worry that long-term treatment with benzodiazepines will lead to tolerance, potential abuse, and particularly, inability to discontinue the drug. Neither loss of efficacy nor abuse of benzodiazepines has been shown to be a significant clinical problem in anxious patients [71]. Assurance should be given that with proper supervision, any patient can stop benzodiazepines as long as an appropriate tapering rate is used. For patients who may benefit from long-term treatment, the rationale for continued use can be documented. Collateral information from a significant other that there has been no misuse and that the benzodiazepine is clearly beneficial is suggested. This process addresses the medicolegal concerns of the clinician and may allow patients who have derived significant benefits from benzodiazepine treatment to continue.

Buspirone is an azaspirodecanedione that acts as a partial 5-HT_{1A} receptor agonist, and it is the only marketed anxiolytic in its class. It has not been adequately studied in functional pain conditions, but it may have potential in those with generalized anxiety disorder [71].

Treatment Approach

As every practitioner knows, early in treatment, patients with visceral sensitivity tend to react strongly to side effects. Starting at a low dosage (e.g., 25% to 50% of the usual initial antidepressant dose) may help minimize exacerbation of preexisting GI symptoms or anxiety. Offering the patient the opportunity to pace the rate of advancement with the optimal therapeutic dose as the goal will provide patients with perceived and actual control, which can foster compliance.

Using a rating instrument, such as the HADS [125], can be a useful guide throughout the process of treatment. In general, any given agent prescribed at sufficient dosage should begin to show benefits within the first 6 weeks (Table IV). If a patient has shown a partial response to treatment it is prudent to increase the dose of that agent, reassessing response and tolerability every 4–6 weeks. Some patients benefit at doses either lower or higher than typical doses.

Table IV
Dosing guidelines for treatment
of depression and anxiety

Drug	Dose at 6–8 Weeks (mg)	Starting Dose (mg)
Tricyclic Antidepressants		
Imipramine	≥200	10
Desipramine	≥200	10
Clomipramine	≥50	2.5–10
SSRIs/SNRIs		
Sertraline	≥150	12.5–25
Paroxetine	≥40	5–10
Fluoxetine	≥40	2–5
Escitalopram	≥30	5
Citalopram	≥40	10
Fluvoxamine	≥150	25
Venlafaxine	≥225	18.75
Duloxetine	≥90	30
High-Potency Benzodiazepines		
Alprazolam	≥4	0.5–1 t.i.d.
Clonazepam	≥2	0.25–0.5 b.i.d.

Abbreviations: SSRIs = selective serotonin reuptake inhibitors; SSRIs = serotonin-norepinephrine reuptake inhibitors.

The "optimal dose" is a dose that controls the target symptoms (anxiety, depression, and/or stress reactivity) without unacceptable side effects or toxicity. With adequate dosage, some response in the first 6–8 weeks should be apparent, but remission may take several months. If there is no response at 6 weeks, and compliance and treatment intensity appear to be adequate, switching to another class may obviate the need for referral for psychiatric consultation. Whether to persist with treatment efforts or refer the patient to a psychiatric practitioner remains a clinical decision between the physician and patient. For some patients, the use of concomitant benzodiazepines for anxiety control may help with compliance and allow more optimal control of symptoms. Fig. 3 presents an

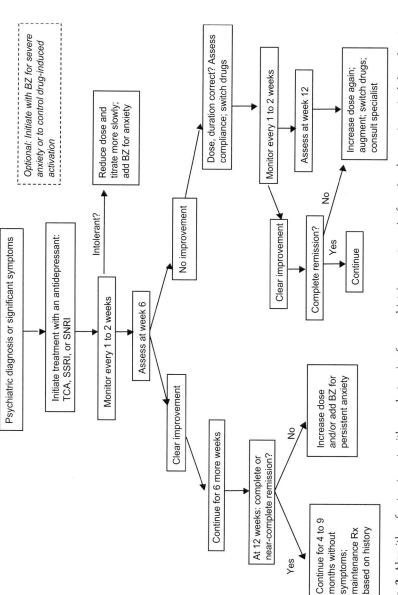

Fig. 3. Algorithm for treatment with psychotropics for psychiatric symptoms in functional gastrointestinal disorders in clinical practice. BZ = benzodiazepine; SNRI = serotonin-norepinephrine reuptake inhibitor; SSRI = selective serotonin reuptake inhibitor; TCA = tricyclic antidepressant.

algorithm for treating psychiatric symptoms in patients with functional GI disorders.

Summary

Clinically significant psychiatric symptoms in patients with functional somatic pain syndromes merit aggressive treatment. Antidepressants and anxiolytics may affect stress reactivity, a key factor in these syndromes. Confirmation of existing practices via scientifically sound randomized, controlled trials of the psychotropic agents such as the low-dose TCAs and SSRIs are needed in order bring this practice into the arena of evidence-based medicine.

References

[1] Abeles M, Solitar BM, Pillinger MH, Abeles AM. Update on fibromyalgia therapy. Am J Med 2008;121:555–61.

[2] Allgulander C, Hartford J, Russell J, Ball S, Erickson J, Raskin J, Rynn M. Pharmacotherapy of generalized anxiety disorder: results of duloxetine treatment from a pooled analysis of three clinical trials. Curr Med Res Opin 2007;23:1245–52.

[3] Amir M, Kaplan Z, Neumann L, Sharabani R, Shani N, Buskila D. Posttraumatic stress disorder, tenderness and fibromyalgia. J Psychosom Res 1997;42:607–13.

[4] Anisman H, Merali Z, Hayley S. Sensitization associated with stressors and cytokine treatments. Brain Behav Immun 2003;17:86–93.

[5] Arnold BS, Alpers GW, Suss H, Friedel E, Kosmutzky G, Geier A, Pauli P. Affective pain modulation in fibromyalgia, somatoform pain disorder, back pain, and healthy controls. Eur J Pain 2008;12:329–38.

[6] Arnold LM. Management of fibromyalgia and comorbid psychiatric disorders. J Clin Psychiatry 2008;69(Suppl 2):14–9.

[7] Arnold LM, Goldenberg DL, Stanford SB, Lalonde JK, Sandhu HS, Keck PE Jr, Welge JA, Bishop F, Stanford KE, Hess EV, Hudson JI. Gabapentin in the treatment of fibromyalgia: a randomized, double-blind, placebo-controlled, multicenter trial. Arthritis Rheum 2007;56:1336–44.

[8] Arnold LM, Lu Y, Crofford LJ, Wohlreich M, Detke MJ, Iyengar S, Goldstein DJ. A double-blind, multicenter trial comparing duloxetine with placebo in the treatment of fibromyalgia patients with or without major depressive disorder. Arthritis Rheum 2004;50:2974–84.

[9] Arnold LM, Rosen A, Pritchett YL, D'Souza DN, Goldstein DJ, Iyengar S, Wernicke JF. A randomized, double-blind, placebo-controlled trial of duloxetine in the treatment of women with fibromyalgia with or without major depressive disorder. Pain 2005;119:5–15.

[10] Arnold LM, Russell IJ, Diri EW, Duan WR, Young JP Jr, Sharma U, Martin SA, Barrett JA, Haig G. A 14-week, randomized, double-blinded, placebo-controlled monotherapy trial of pregabalin in patients with fibromyalgia. J Pain 2008;9:792–805.

[11] Azpiroz F, Bouin M, Camilleri M, Mayer EA, Poitras P, Serra J, Spiller RC. Mechanisms of hypersensitivity in IBS and functional disorders. Neurogastroenterol Motil 2007;19:62–88.

[12] Bennett EJ, Tennant CC, Piesse C, Badcock CA, Kellow JE. Level of chronic life stress predicts clinical outcome in irritable bowel syndrome. Gut 1998;43:256–61.

[13] Bradesi S, Tillisch K, Mayer EA. Emerging drugs for irritable bowel syndrome. Expert Opin Emerg Drugs 2006;11:293–313.

[14] Brandt LJ, Bjorkman D, Fennerty MB, Locke GR, Olden K, Peterson W, Quigley E, Schoenfeld P, Schuster M, Talley N. Systematic review on the management of irritable bowel syndrome in North America. Am J Gastroenterol 2002;97:S7–26.

[15] Buskila D, Cohen H. Comorbidity of fibromyalgia and psychiatric disorders. Curr Pain Headache Rep 2007;11:333–8.

[16] Camilleri M, Bueno L, de Ponti F, Fioramonti J, Lydiard RB, Tack J. Pharmacological and pharmacokinetic aspects of functional gastrointestinal disorders. Gastroenterology 2006;130:1421–34.

[17] Camilleri M, Northcutt AR, Kong S, Dukes GE, McSorley D, Mangel AW. Efficacy and safety of alosetron in women with irritable bowel syndrome: a randomised, placebo-controlled trial. Lancet 2000;355:1035–40.

[18] Carette S, Bell MJ, Reynolds WJ, Haraoui B, McCain GA, Bykerk VP, Edworthy SM, Baron M, Koehler BE, Fam AG, et al. Comparison of amitriptyline, cyclobenzaprine, and placebo in the treatment of fibromyalgia. A randomized, double-blind clinical trial. Arthritis Rheum 1994;37:32–40.

[19] Chang L, Ameen VZ, Dukes GE, McSorley DJ, Carter EG, Mayer EA. A dose-ranging, phase II study of the efficacy and safety of alosetron in men with diarrhea-predominant IBS. Am J Gastroenterol 2005;100:115–23.

[20] Chang L, Mayer EA, Johnson T, FitzGerald LZ, Naliboff B. Differences in somatic perception in female patients with irritable bowel syndrome with and without fibromyalgia. Pain 2000;84:297–307.

[21] Chang L, Sundaresh S, Elliott J, Anton PA, Baldi P, Licudine A, Mayer M, Vuong T, Hirano M, Naliboff BD, Ameen VZ, Mayer EA. Dysregulation of the hypothalamic-pituitary-adrenal (HPA) axis in irritable bowel syndrome. Neurogastroenterol Motil 2008; Epub Aug 5.

[22] Chapman CR, Tuckett RP, Song CW. Pain and stress in a systems perspective: reciprocal neural, endocrine, and immune interactions. J Pain 2008;9:122–45.

[23] Charmandari E, Tsigos C, Chrousos G. Endocrinology of the stress response. Annu Rev Physiol 2005;67:259–84.

[24] Charney DS. Psychobiological mechanisms of resilience and vulnerability: implications for successful adaptation to extreme stress. Am J Psychiatry 2004;161:195–216.

[25] Clauw DJ. Potential mechanisms in chemical intolerance and related conditions. Ann NY Acad Sci 2001;933:235–53.

[26] Clauw DJ. Pharmacotherapy for patients with fibromyalgia. J Clin Psychiatry 2008;69(Suppl 2):5–9.

[27] Clauw DJ, Chrousos GP. Chronic pain and fatigue syndromes: overlapping clinical and neuroendocrine features and potential pathogenic mechanisms. Neuroimmunomodulation 1997;4:134–53.

[28] Clauw DJ, Schmidt M, Radulovic D, Singer A, Katz P, Bresette J. The relationship between fibromyalgia and interstitial cystitis. J Psychiatr Res 1997;31:125–31.

[29] Creed F, Fernandes L, Guthrie E, Palmer S, Ratcliffe J, Read N, Rigby C, Thompson D, Tomenson B. The cost-effectiveness of psychotherapy and paroxetine for severe irritable bowel syndrome. Gastroenterology 2003;124:303–17.

[30] Crofford LJ. Violence, stress, and somatic syndromes. Trauma Violence Abuse 2007;8:299–313.

[31] Crofford LJ. Determining long-term efficacy for treatment of chronic pain in fibromyalgia patients. Pain 2008;138:473–4.

[32] Crofford LJ, Rowbotham MC, Mease PJ, Russell IJ, Dworkin RH, Corbin AE, Young JP Jr, LaMoreaux LK, Martin SA, Sharma U. Pregabalin for the treatment of fibromyalgia syndrome: results of a randomized, double-blind, placebo-controlled trial. Arthritis Rheum 2005;52:1264–73.

[33] Dadabhoy D, Crofford LJ, Spaeth M, Russell IJ, Clauw DJ. Biology and therapy of fibromyalgia. Evidence-based biomarkers for fibromyalgia syndrome. Arthritis Res Ther 2008;10:211.

[34] Devanux LD, Kerr JR. Chronic fatigue syndrome. J Clin Virol 2006;37:139–50.

[35] Dhabhar FS, McEwen BS. Acute stress enhances while chronic stress suppresses cell-mediated immunity in vivo: a potential role for leukocyte trafficking. Brain Behav Immun 1997;11:286–306.

[36] Dick IE, Brochu RM, Purohit Y, Kaczorowski GJ, Martin WJ, Priest BT. Sodium channel blockade may contribute to the analgesic efficacy of antidepressants. J Pain 2007;8:315–24.

[37] Dickenson AH, Ghandehari J. Anti-convulsants and anti-depressants. Handb Exp Pharmacol 2007;145–77.

486   R.B. Lydiard

[38] Dooley DJ, Donovan CM, Meder WP, Whetzel SZ. Preferential action of gabapentin and prega-balin at P/Q-type voltage-sensitive calcium channels: inhibition of K+-evoked [3H]-norepineph-rine release from rat neocortical slices. Synapse 2002;171–90.
[39] Dooley DJ, Taylor CP, Donevan S, Feltner D. Ca2+ channel alpha2delta ligands: novel modula-tors of neurotransmission. Trends Pharmacol Sci 2007;28:75–82.
[40] Drossman DA, Camilleri M, Mayer EA, Whitehead WE. AGA technical review on irritable bowel syndrome. Gastroenterology 2002;123:2108–31.
[41] Drossman DA, McKee DC, Sandler RS, Mitchell CM, Cramer EM, Lowman BC, Burger AL. Psychosocial factors in the irritable bowel syndrome. A multivariate study of patients and non-patients with irritable bowel syndrome. Gastroenterology 1988;95:701–8.
[42] Drossman DA, Toner BB, Whitehead WE, Diamant NE, Dalton CB, Duncan S, Emmott S, Prof-fitt V, Akman D, Frusciante K, et al. Cognitive-behavioral therapy versus education and desip-ramine versus placebo for moderate to severe functional bowel disorders. Gastroenterology 2003;125:19–31.
[43] Drossman DA, Whitehead WE, Toner BB, Diamant N, Hu YJ, Bangdiwala SI, Jia H. What de-termines severity among patients with painful functional bowel disorders? Am J Gastroenterol 2000;95:974–80.
[44] Duman RS. Role of neurotrophic factors in the etiology and treatment of mood disorders. Neu-romolecular Med 2004;5:11-25.
[45] Duman RS, Monteggia LM. A neurotrophic model for stress-related mood disorders. Biol Psy-chiatry 2006;59:1116–27.
[46] Eriksen HR, Ursin H. Subjective health complaints, sensitization, and sustained cognitive activa-tion (stress). J Psychosom Res 2004;56:445–8.
[47] Feltner D, Wittchen HU, Kavoussi R, Brock J, Baldinetti F, Pande AC. Long-term efficacy of pre-gabalin in generalized anxiety disorder. Int Clin Psychopharmacol 2008;23:18–28.
[48] Fink K, Dooley DJ, Meder WP, Suman-Chauhan N, Duffy S, Clusmann H, Gothert M. Inhibition of neuronal Ca(2+) influx by gabapentin and pregabalin in the human neocortex. Neuropharma-cology 2002;42:229–36.
[49] Glass JM. Fibromyalgia and cognition. J Clin Psychiatry 2008;69 Suppl 2:20–4.
[50] Goldenberg DL, Burckhardt C, Crofford L. Management of fibromyalgia syndrome. JAMA 2004;292:2388–95.
[51] Gur A, Karakoc M, Nas K, Remzi, Cevik, Denli A, Sarac J. Cytokines and depression in cases with fibromyalgia. J Rheumatol 2002;29:358–61.
[52] Harris RE, Sundgren PC, Pang Y, Hsu M, Petrou M, Kim SH, McLean SA, Gracely RH, Clauw DJ. Dynamic levels of glutamate within the insula are associated with improvements in multiple pain domains in fibromyalgia. Arthritis Rheum 2008;58:903–7.
[53] Hayley S, Anisman H. Multiple mechanisms of cytokine action in neurodegenerative and psychi-atric states: neurochemical and molecular substrates. Curr Pharm Des 2005;11:947–62.
[54] Hayley S, Merali Z, Anisman H. Stress and cytokine-elicited neuroendocrine and neurotrans-mitter sensitization: implications for depressive illness. Stress 2003;6:19–32.
[55] Hudson JI, Goldenberg DL, Pope HGJ, Keck PEJ, Schlesinger L. Comorbidity of fibromyalgia with medical and psychiatric disorders. Am J Med 1992;92:363–7.
[56] Hudson JI, Mangweth B, Pope HG Jr, De Col C, Hausmann A, Gutweniger S, Laird NM, Biebl W, Tsuang MT. Family study of affective spectrum disorder. Arch Gen Psychiatry 2003;60:170–7.
[57] Hudson JI, Pope HG, Jr. Affective spectrum disorder: does antidepressant response identify a family of disorders with a common pathophysiology? Am J Psychiatry 1990;147:552–64.
[58] Jarcho JM, Chang L, Berman SM, Suyenobu B, Naliboff BD, Lieberman MD, Ameen VZ, Man-delkern MA, Mayer EA. Neural and psychological predictors of treatment response in irritable bowel syndrome patients with a 5-HT3 receptor antagonist: a pilot study. Aliment Pharmacol Ther 2008; Epub Apr 21.
[59] Jarcho JM, Mayer EA. Stress and the irritable bowel syndrome. Prim Psychiatry 2007;1:74–8.
[60] Johanson JF, Drossman DA, Panas R, Wahle A, Ueno R. Clinical trial: phase 2 study of lubipros-tone for irritable bowel syndrome with constipation. Aliment Pharmacol Ther 2008;27:685–96.
[61] Kalogeras KT, Calogero AE, Kuribayiashi T, Kahn J, Gallucci WT, Kling MA, Chrousos GP, Gold PW. In vitro and in vivo effects of the triazolobenzodiazepine alprazolam on hypothalamic-pi-tuitary-adrenal function: pharmacological and clinical implications. J Clin Endocrinol Metab 1990;70:1642–71.

[62] Kaufmann I, Eisner C, Richter P, Huge V, Beyer A, Chouker A, Schelling G, Thiel M. Lymphocyte subsets and the role of TH1/TH2 balance in stressed chronic pain patients. Neuroimmunomodulation 2007;14:272–80.

[63] Kenis G, Maes M. Effects of antidepressants on the production of cytokines. Int J Neuropsychopharmacol 2002;5:401–12.

[64] Kim YK, Na KS, Shin KH, Jung HY, Choi SH, Kim JB. Cytokine imbalance in the pathophysiology of major depressive disorder. Prog Neuropsychopharmacol Biol Psychiatry 2007;31:1044–53.

[65] Kronfol A, Remick A. Cytokines and the brain: implications for clinical psychiatry. Am J Psychiatry 2000;157:683–94.

[66] Kubera M, Lin AH, Kenis G, Bosmans E, van Bockstaele D, Maes M. Anti-inflammatory effects of antidepressants through suppression of the interferon-gamma/interleukin-10 production ratio. J Clin Psychopharmacol 2001;21:199–206.

[67] Kubera M, Maes M, Holan V, Basta-Kaim A, Roman A, Shani J. Prolonged desipramine treatment increases the production of interleukin-10, an anti-inflammatory cytokine, in C57BL/6 mice subjected to the chronic mild stress model of depression. J Affect Disord 2001;63:171–8.

[68] Lembo T, Wright RA, Bagby B, Decker C, Gordon S, Jhingran P, Carter E. Alosetron controls bowel urgency and provides global symptom improvement in women with diarrhea-predominant irritable bowel syndrome. Am J Gastroenterol 2001;96:2662–70.

[69] Lubrano E, Iovino P, Tremolaterra F, Parsons WJ, Ciacci C, Mazzacca G. Fibromyalgia in patients with irritable bowel syndrome. An association with the severity of the intestinal disorder. Int J Colorectal Dis 2001;16:211–5.

[70] Lydiard RB. Irritable bowel syndrome, anxiety, and depression: what are the links? J Clin Psychiatry 2001;62(Suppl 8):38–45.

[71] Lydiard RB, Otto M, Milrod B. Panic disorder treatment. In: Gabbard GO, editor. Treatments of psychiatric disorders, 3rd ed (TPD-III). Washington, DC: American Psychiatric Press; 2001. p. 1447–83.

[72] Maes M. The cytokine hypothesis of depression: inflammation, oxidative & nitrosative stress (IO&NS) and leaky gut as new targets for adjunctive treatments in depression. Neuro Endocrinol Lett 2008;29:287–91.

[73] Maier SF. Bi-directional immune-brain communication: implications for understanding stress, pain, and cognition. Brain Behav Immun 2003;17:69–85.

[74] Maloney EM, Gurbaxani BM, Jones JF, de Souza Coelho L, Pennachin C, Goertzel BN. Chronic fatigue syndrome and high allostatic load. Pharmacogenomics 2006;7:467–73.

[75] Manji HK, Quiroz JA, Sporn J, Payne JL, Denicoff K, N AG, Zarate CA Jr, Charney DS. Enhancing neuronal plasticity and cellular resilience to develop novel, improved therapeutics for difficult-to-treat depression. Biol Psychiatry 2003;53:707–42.

[76] Matsuzawa-Yanagida K, Narita M, Nakajima M, Kuzumaki N, Niikura K, Nozaki H, Takagi T, Tamai E, Hareyama N, Terada M, Yamazaki M, Suzuki T. Usefulness of antidepressants for improving the neuropathic pain-like state and pain-induced anxiety through actions at different brain sites. Neuropsychopharmacology 2008;33:1952–65.

[77] Mayer EA. Clinical practice. Irritable bowel syndrome. N Engl J Med 2008;358:1692–9.

[78] Mayer EA, Bradesi S. Alosetron and irritable bowel syndrome. Expert Opin Pharmacother 2003;4:2089–98.

[79] Mayer EA, Bradesi S, Chang L, Spiegel BM, Bueller JA, Naliboff BD. Functional GI disorders: from animal models to drug development. Gut 2008;57:384–404.

[80] Mayer EA, Tillisch K, Bradesi S. Review article: modulation of the brain-gut axis as a therapeutic approach in gastrointestinal disease. Aliment Pharmacol Ther 2006;24:919–33.

[81] McEwen BS. Protective and damaging effects of stress mediators. N Engl J Med 1998;338:171–9.

[82] McEwen BS. Mood disorders and allostatic load. Biol Psychiatry 2003;54:200–7.

[83] McEwen BS, Wingfield JC. The concept of allostasis in biology and biomedicine. Horm Behav 2003;43:2–15.

[84] McLean SA, Williams DA, Stein PK, Harris RE, Lyden AK, Whalen G, Park KM, Liberzon I, Sen A, Gracely RH, et al. Cerebrospinal fluid corticotropin-releasing factor concentration is associated with pain but not fatigue symptoms in patients with fibromyalgia. Neuropsychopharmacology 2006;31:2776–82.

488

R.B. Lydiard

[85] McWilliams LA, Goodwin RD, Cox BJ. Depression and anxiety associated with three pain conditions: results from a nationally representative sample. Pain 2004;111:77–83.

[86] Mease P. Fibromyalgia syndrome: review of clinical presentation, pathogenesis, outcome measures, and treatment. J Rheumatol Suppl 2005;6–21.

[87] Mease PJ, Russell IJ, Arnold LM, Florian H, Young JP Jr, Martin SA, Sharma U. A randomized, double-blind, placebo-controlled, phase III trial of pregabalin in the treatment of patients with fibromyalgia. J Rheumatol 2008;35:502–14.

[88] Miller AH, Pariante CM, Pearce BD. Effects of cytokines on glucocorticoid receptor expression and function. Glucocorticoid resistance and relevance to depression. Adv Exp Med Biol 1999;461:107–16.

[89] Morgan V, Pickens D, Gautam S, Kessler R, Mertz H. Amitriptyline reduces rectal pain related activation of the anterior cingulate cortex in patients with irritable bowel syndrome. Gut 2005;54:601–7.

[90] Mullington JM, Hinze-Selch D, Pollmacher T. Mediators of inflammation and their interaction with sleep: relevance for chronic fatigue syndrome and related conditions. Ann NY Acad Sci 2001;933:201–10.

[91] O'Brien SM, Scott LV, Dinan TG. Cytokines: abnormalities in major depression and implications for pharmacological treatment. Hum Psychopharmacol 2004;19:397–403.

[92] Pariante CM, Makoff A, Lovestone S, Feroli S, Heyden A, Miller AH, Kerwin RW. Antidepressants enhance glucocorticoid receptor function in vitro by modulating the membrane steroid transporters. Br J Pharmacol 2001;134:1335–43.

[93] Perahia DG, Pritchett YL, Desaiah D, Raskin J. Efficacy of duloxetine in painful symptoms: an analgesic or antidepressant effect? Int Clin Psychopharmacol 2006;21:311–7.

[94] Pittenger C, Duman RS. Stress, depression, and neuroplasticity: a convergence of mechanisms. Neuropsychopharmacology 2008;33:88–109.

[95] Pontari MA, Ruggieri MR. Mechanisms in prostatitis/chronic pelvic pain syndrome. J Urol 2008;179:S61–7.

[96] Raison CL, Miller AH. When not enough is too much: the role of insufficient glucocorticoid signaling in the pathophysiology of stress-related disorders. Am J Psychiatry 2003;160:1654–65.

[97] Raphael KG, Janal MN, Nayak S, Schwartz JE, Gallagher RM. Psychiatric comorbidities in a community sample of women with fibromyalgia. Pain 2006;124:117–25.

[98] Rickels K, Pollack MH, Feltner DE, Lydiard RB, Zimbroff DL, Bielski RJ, Tobias K, Brock JD, Zornberg GL, Pande AC. Pregabalin for treatment of generalized anxiety disorder: a 4-week, multicenter, double-blind, placebo-controlled trial of pregabalin and alprazolam. Arch Gen Psychiatry 2005;62:1022–30.

[99] Russell IJ, Mease PJ, Smith TR, Kajdasz DK, Wohlreich MM, Detke MJ, Walker DJ, Chappell AS, Arnold LM. Efficacy and safety of duloxetine for treatment of fibromyalgia in patients with or without major depressive disorder: results from a 6-month, randomized, double-blind, placebo-controlled, fixed-dose trial. Pain 2008;136:432–44.

[100] Schmulson MJ, Valdovinos MA. Current and future treatment of chest pain of presumed esophageal origin. Gastroenterol Clin North Am 2004;33:93–105.

[101] Sherman JJ, Turk DC, Okifuji A. Prevalence and impact of posttraumatic stress disorder-like symptoms on patients with fibromyalgia syndrome. Clin J Pain 2000;16:127–34.

[102] Skelton K, Nemeroff CB, Knight DL, Owens MJ. Chronic administration of the triazolobenzodiazepine alprazolam produces opposite effects on corticotropin-releasing factor and urocortin neuronal systems. J Neurosci 2000;20:1240–8.

[103] Stam R, Akkermans LMA, Weigant VM. Trauma and the gut: interactions between stressful experience and intestinal function. Gut 1997;40:704–9.

[104] Stout SC, Owens MJ, Nemeroff CB. Regulation of corticotropin-releasing factor neuronal systems and hypothalamic-pituitary-adrenal axis activity by stress and chronic antidepressant treatment. J Pharmacol Exp Ther 2002;323:1–10.

[105] Sung IK. [Hypothalamic-pituitary-gut axis dysregulation in irritable bowel syndrome: plasma cytokines as a potential biomarker?]. Korean J Gastroenterol 2006;48:140–2.

[106] Szelenyi J, Vizi ES. The catecholamine cytokine balance: interaction between the brain and the immune system. Ann NY Acad Sci 2007;1113:311–24.

[107] Tabas G, Beaves M, Wang J, Friday P, Mardini H, Arnold G. Paroxetine to treat irritable bowel syndrome not responding to high-fiber diet: a double-blind, placebo-controlled trial. Am J Gastroenterol 2004;99:914–20.

[108] Tache Y, Martinez V, Million M, Wang L. Stress and the gastrointestinal tract III. Stress-related alterations of gut motor function: role of brain corticotropin-releasing factor receptors. Am J Physiol Gastrointest Liver Physiol 2001;280:G173–7.

[109] Talley NJ, Kellow JE, Boyce P, Tennant C, Huskic S, Jones M. Antidepressant therapy (imipramine and citalopram) for irritable bowel syndrome: a double-blind, randomized, placebo-controlled trial. Dig Dis Sci 2008;53:108–15.

[110] Tanriverdi F, Karaca Z, Unluhizarci K, Kelestimur F. The hypothalamo-pituitary-adrenal axis in chronic fatigue syndrome and fibromyalgia syndrome. Stress 2007;10:13–25.

[111] Thieme K, Turk DC, Flor H. Comorbid depression and anxiety in fibromyalgia syndrome: relationship to somatic and psychosocial variables. Psychosom Med 2004;66:837–44.

[112] Tillisch K, Mayer EA. Pain perception in irritable bowel syndrome. CNS Spectr 2005;10:877–82.

[113] Tollefson GD, Luxenberg M, Valentine R, Dunsmore G, Tollefson SL. An open label trial of alprazolam in comorbid irritable bowel syndrome and generalized anxiety disorder. J Clin Psychiatry 1991;52:502–8.

[114] Tsigos T, Chrousos GP. Hypothalamic–pituitary–adrenal axis, neuroendocrine factors and stress. J Psychosom Res 2002;53:865–71.

[115] Tuglu C, Kara SH, Caliyurt O, Vardar E, Abay E. Increased serum tumor necrosis factor-alpha levels and treatment response in major depressive disorder. Psychopharmacology (Berl) 2003;170:429–33.

[116] Uçeyler N, Häuser W, Sommer C. A systematic review on the effectiveness of treatment with antidepressants in fibromyalgia syndrome. Arthritis Rheum 2008;15:1279–98.

[117] Van Houdenhove B, Neerinckx E, Lysens R, Vertommen H, Van Houdenhove L, Onghena P, Westhovens R, D'Hooghe MB. Victimization in chronic fatigue syndrome and fibromyalgia in tertiary care: a controlled study on prevalence and characteristics. Psychosomatics 2001;42:21–8.

[118] Vermetten E, Vythilingam M, Southwick SM, Charney DS, Bremner JD. Long-term treatment with paroxetine increases verbal declarative memory and hippocampal volume in posttraumatic stress disorder. Biol Psychiatry 2003;54:693-702.

[119] Walker EA, Keegan D, Gardner G, Sullivan M, Bernstein D, Katon WJ. Psychosocial factors in fibromyalgia compared with rheumatoid arthritis: II. Sexual, physical, and emotional abuse and neglect. Psychosom Med 1997;59:572–7.

[120] Walker EA, Roy-Byrne PP, Katon WJ. Irritable bowel syndrome and psychiatric illness. Am J Psychiatry 1990;147:565–72.

[121] Watkins LR, Maier SF. The pain of being sick: implications of immune-to-brain communication for understanding pain. Annu Rev Psychol 2000;51:29–57.

[122] Weissbecker I, Floyd A, Dedert E, Salmon P, Sephton S. Childhood trauma and diurnal cortisol disruption in fibromyalgia syndrome. Psychoneuroendocrinology 2006;31:312–24.

[123] Whitehead WE, Palsson O, Jones KR. Systematic review of the comorbidity of irritable bowel syndrome with other disorders: what are the causes and implications? Gastroenterology 2002;122:1140–56.

[124] Yunus MB. Role of central sensitization in symptoms beyond muscle pain, and the evaluation of a patient with widespread pain. Best Pract Res Clin Rheumatol 2007;21:481–97.

[125] Zigmond A, Snaith RP. The Hospital Anxiety and Depression Scale. Acta Psychiatr Scand 1983;67:361–70.

Correspondence to: R. Bruce Lydiard, PhD, MD, Psychiatry/Mental Health, Ralph H. Johnson VA Medical Center, 109 Bee Street, Charleston, SC 29401-5799, USA. Email: lydiardb@mindyourhealth.net.

Cognitive-Behavioral Treatment of Functional Pain Disorders

Jeffrey M. Lackner[a] and Lance M. McCracken[b]

[a] University at Buffalo School of Medicine and Biomedical Sciences, State University of New York, Buffalo, New York, USA; [b]Centre for Pain Services, Royal National Hospital for Rheumatic Diseases and Centre for Pain Research, University of Bath, Bath, United Kingdom

Epidemiological data suggest that functional pain disorders are astonishingly common and disabling (e.g., [6]). Irritable bowel syndrome (IBS), arguably the most common of these disorders, affects 15% of the world's population at any given time. The addition of temporomandibular joint disorder, fibromyalgia syndrome, and chronic low back pain (with an estimated worldwide prevalence of around 10%, 3%, and 10–15%, respectively) makes functional pain syndromes a health problem of staggering proportions. Because they have no known etiology and mimic "organic" diseases whose symptoms are linearly related to nociceptive stimulation from the periphery, these pain disorders are a source of aggravation for physicians and of despair for patients and their families. Moreover, they are linked with skyrocketing medical expenses for health care systems teetering on the precipice of viability.

To make matters worse, there are no simple, satisfactory medical treatments for functional pain disorders. Physical therapy, massage, acupuncture, and other rehabilitative or palliative treatments have such limited empirical support that they are regarded as experimental options reserved for "when all else fails."

Functional Pain Syndromes: Presentation and Pathophysiology
edited by Emeran A. Mayer and M. Catherine Bushnell
IASP Press, Seattle, © 2009

In the meantime, millions of patients with functional pain disorders are struggling to piece together meaningful lives and cope with symptoms that exact a heavy toll on their mental and physical wellbeing. There is growing recognition that even for chronic illnesses resistant to medical therapies, patients can effectively manage the day-to-day burden of their symptoms by learning specific behavioral self-care skills including self-monitoring, goal setting and problem solving, educating themselves, and managing negative emotions and other aversive somatic states such as pain [78]. These skills form a significant part of a psychological treatment approach called cognitive-behavioral therapy (CBT). The overarching goal of CBT is to teach patients skills for taking a proactive role in controlling their symptoms, coping with the emotional unpleasantness of the symptoms, and improving their quality of life.

The term "cognitive-behavioral therapy" refers to a wide array of conceptually and technically different treatment techniques based on principles derived from experimental psychology and social learning theory [2]. Behavioral interventions are designed to enhance daily functioning directly by manipulating environmental influences on overt behavior. Cognitive interventions are designed to reduce unwanted emotions and somatic sensations, and to alter behavior patterns by modifying individual appraisal and thinking patterns. Both approaches share common assumptions about how behavior develops that distinguish them from other psychological therapies. The underlying assumption of CBT is that learning processes play an important role in the acquisition and regulation of both healthy and unhealthy behavior patterns. These learning processes can therefore be harnessed to create change in dysfunctional behavior and in negative emotional states. Cognitive and behavioral procedures are structured and comparatively brief, goal focused, and aimed, in part, at remediating skills deficits presumably underlying clinical symptoms. These skills are taught in the context of a collaborative therapeutic relationship and rehearsed through behavioral assignments in the context of the daily routines in which symptoms occur. Unlike other types of psychotherapy that view symptoms as physical manifestations of unconscious and resolved past conflicts [58,67], CBT views symptoms as important in their own right and targets the contemporaneous cognitive and behavioral processes maintaining them. CBT is often offered in 12 to 16 sessions, usually over 12 weeks. Treatment is usually delivered on an outpatient basis.

Theoretical Foundations of Cognitive-Behavioral Therapy

The principles and practice of contemporary cognitive-behavioral approaches for functional pain disorders derive from two major theories of human behavior—learning theory and cognitive theory. Cognitive theory emphasizes the role of faulty thinking processes in the development and maintenance of clinical problems. Cognitive therapies posit that clinical disorders involve habitual, automatic negative thoughts that must be identified and modified to change erroneous or unhelpful ways of thinking and related behaviors that maintain clinical symptoms. Traditional conditioning models attach greatest importance to observable behaviors because they are empirically verifiable (i.e., provide measurable information), are presumably more readily acquired, and are therefore easier to modify than "mental phenomena." Learning theory has its conceptual roots in the paradigms of Pavlovian classical conditioning [57] and Skinnerian operant learning [66]. These models have led to the development of most widely applied therapies for treating functional pain disorders.

Functional Pain Disorders as Faulty Conditioning

Operant learning refers to those behaviors that are increased in frequency by reinforcement from the consequences they produce [66]. Generally speaking, behaviors that result in either rewarding or positive outcomes or that allow an individual to avoid or escape aversive or negative consequences are likely to increase in frequency. If a patient with a functional pain disorder receives attention or overly solicitous offers of help after complaining of pain, and then complains more often, the attention would be considered a positive reinforcer of pain complaints [19]. These reinforcing consequences may maintain a display of pain behaviors (activity reduction, medication use, facial expression of pain, and altered gait) long after the normal healing time for injury [30]. Operant techniques are designed to increase the frequency of "well" behaviors by associating their occurrence with some form of positive consequence (e.g., verbal reinforcement). Contingencies that prompt and reinforce previously reinforced illness behaviors are weakened or "extinguished" by the withholding of reinforcement following their occurrence. Operant methods include contingency management (providing attention and feedback contingent on an increase in a specific activity), behavior contracting to prompt and reinforce frequent skills practice, daily self-monitoring of symptoms and their triggers, behavioral rehearsal of newly taught skills, functional analysis of controlling antecedents and consequences, and scheduling of pleasant events. Treatment may involve training the patient's spouse, whose responses to the patient are often the most influential.

More recently, theories from the operant tradition have emphasized the role of negative reinforcement (the strengthening of behavior by avoiding or terminating unpleasant experiences) in shaping the fear and avoidance symptoms of functional pain disorders. Negative reinforcement is believed to directly influence the cognitive aspects (perceptions of control), emotions (fear of pain), and behavioral features (situational avoidance) of pain experience [59,74,75], through reduction of anticipated aversive consequences (pain, anxiety, and reinjury). If an IBS patient feels anxious in a setting (e.g., a crowded football stadium) where belly pain is expected to act up, and leaving or avoiding these situations reduces this anxiety, then the patient is more likely to avoid or leave these situations because avoidance is "negatively reinforced" by reduction of anxiety or other anticipated negative consequences.

Avoidance responses can be overt, observable by others, or covert, observable only by the person who is making the response, such as cognitive avoidance in the form of rumination, distraction, or thought suppression. Avoidance can be a particularly troubling behavior pattern because of the ways in which it restricts healthy functioning and is self-perpetuating (e.g., [18]). When a feared situation is never confronted, it is difficult to learn a new behavior pattern related to that situation.

Given the crucial role of avoidance in clinical pain states, a number of pain researchers [3,59] recommend that behavioral treatments should be explicitly geared toward reducing avoidance behaviors through exposure procedures. These treatments involve confrontation with cues that are expected to elicit unpleasant consequences. Exposure-based treatments can differ in technique; however, they share a common goal of systematically guiding patients to confront aversive stimuli long enough to extinguish conditioned avoidance responses and strengthen patients' sense of personal mastery over a feared stimulus. Exposure can entail a face-to-face (in vivo) experience or an imaginal confrontation with stimuli that evoke excessive discomfort. Imaginal exposure involves the therapist describing the feared situation while the patient listens and vividly envisions the events as well as the accompanying thoughts, images, and feelings. This type of exposure is applied when real-life confrontation with the feared stimulus is impractical to carry out in a clinical setting, or else the fear involves hypothetical situations that do not exist in the "here and now." In vivo exposure has traditionally required the patient to physically confront an actual object or situation where an unpleasant consequence is expected to occur. For example, a patient with fibromyalgia may associate increased physical activity with pain and anxiously avoid exercises (e.g., working out on a treadmill) that may have therapeutic potential. The therapist and patient begin the process of exposure by generating a hierarchy of feared activities or situations that are rank-ordered on dimensions of anxiety, pain, distress, and avoidance potential. Treatment begins with exposure to the least provocative situation. Patients are instructed to face the feared stimulus until discomfort diminishes and the urge to avoid the situation is extinguished. As mastery for less anxiety-provoking stimuli is achieved and these situations no longer elicit distress, the patient progresses to face more provocative stimuli. Through the process of habituation, a patient works through the hierarchy of feared stimuli until the anxiety subsides and the most feared stimuli no longer provoke the urge for avoidance.

Over the past 20 years, experts have begun to recognize that for some patients the problem of avoidance is motivated by anxiety evoked not only by external situations but by internal bodily sensations as well, through the process of "interoceptive conditioning" [60]. Through interoceptive conditioning, previously neutral internal bodily sensations can acquire the ability to evoke anxiety and avoidance, responses normally associated with actually threatening situations [7]. Treatments to reduce these effects include deliberate confrontation with the previously neutral sensations. These procedures are called interoceptive exposure. Relevant bodily sensations are confronted first in session exercises and then through more naturalistic tasks that induce somatic sensations similar to the patient's clinical symptoms.

For example, for the IBS patient keenly sensitive to visceral sensations, the sensation induction exercise [DeCola JP, Craske M, Naliboff B, unpublished manuscript] may include holding a sit-up position, straining, and cinching a tight wide belt across the abdomen, applying a cold compress to the belly, or drinking a large amount of ice water quickly. Exercises for the patient with noncardiac chest pain may include cardiovascular challenges such as hyperventilating, spinning in a chair, breathing through a narrow straw, holding the breath, or running up the stairs. Tasks provoking distress (pain or anxiety) are ranked and repeatedly performed until the unpleasant sensations either diminish or are tolerated with minimal anxiety or discomfort.

During the induction exercise, the patient is told to experience the sensation as fully as possible without terminating the exercise or resorting to "safety behaviors" (maladaptive coping behaviors such as body checking, reassurance seeking, distraction, vigilance, or scanning the environment). The patient may have relied on these behaviors to ward off aversive outcomes, but they actually inhibit learning. With repeated exposure, patients learn that the sensations are not harmful and need not be feared, which interrupts the fear-pain cycle that is believed to maintain functional pain disorders [13].

Whereas operant approaches highlight the consequences of behavior, classical conditioning models of pain are most concerned with the stimuli that evoke behavioral response. According to the theory of classical conditioning, a previously neutral stimulus acquires the ability to trigger a response when it is paired repeatedly with an unconditioned stimulus (an event that that automatically elicits a response that is not learned). For example, the connection between the unconditioned stimulus (pain) and the unconditioned response (flexion of a muscle as part of a startle or "fright" reaction) is automatic, reflexive, and unlearned. The neutral stimulus (called a conditioned stimulus) can then acquire an ability to elicit a response (a conditioned response) similar to the unconditioned response when it is contiguously paired with an unconditioned stimuli. A traditional classical conditioning model argues that reduction in the conditioned responses necessitates a counterconditioning strategy that pairs the unconditioned stimulus (pain) with a response that is physiologically incompatible with it (e.g., relaxation). Provided that the latter is of greater intensity than the conditioned response, tension will presumably lessen [81]. Because muscle tension is regarded as pathogenetic for many functional pain states [17], tension reduction via relaxation training is believed to diminish pain intensity, and for that reason it is a staple of most CBT regimens for functional pain disorders.

The most common form of relaxation used with patients with functional pain disorders is progressive muscle relaxation, as originally formulated by Jacobson [26] and later abbreviated by Bernstein and Borkovec [5]. Biofeedback (using electromyography), relaxed or diaphragmatic breathing, imagery, autogenic training (self-instruction of warmth and heaviness to promote a state of deep relaxation) [62], and hypnosis are other respondent techniques used with patients with functional pain disorders [33,69,73,76,77]. These exercises presumably work by helping patients exert control over physiological responses and specifically regulate autonomic arousal. Most likely they work cognitively by strengthening perceptions of control, such as pain self-efficacy.

The notion that clinical relief comes about by unlearning old habits and by learning or relearning more effective ones is integral to the skills-based emphasis of behavioral pain treatments. Behavioral approaches assume that regardless of underlying organic pathology, a significant portion of patients' problems in the context of functional pain lies with their responses to symptoms, including their repertoire of skills to manage them. Skills deficits create negative emotions that worsen the experience of pain, prevent an individual from attaining reinforcing goals, provoke negative reactions from support networks, and undermine the effectiveness of coping with other challenges. Thus, when patients learn better skills to deal with stressful life experiences, they become more proficient in solving the problems and challenges emanating from a chronic functional pain disorder. Assertiveness and other communication skills help patients to achieve these outcomes and can be gained through formal training in listening, conflict negotiation, anger management, expressing feelings, and issuing requests. Such training includes instruction, therapist modeling, behavioral rehearsal, corrective feedback, reinforcement, and homework assignments.

Functional Pain Disorders as Faulty Thinking

Following developments in behavior therapy, the late 1960s saw an increased emphasis on the role of cognitive processes for understanding abnormal behavior. A general principle of these theories is that the problem of disorders such as pain, anxiety, and depression is embedded in maladaptive thought patterns and other cognitive factors *within* the individual rather than in events external to the individual. A core principle of CBT is that peoples' idiosyncratic appraisal of events, not the events per se, is responsible for the production of unwanted emotions, sensations, and feelings that aggravate clinical symptoms of functional pain syndromes.

To the extent that these cognitive processes contribute to symptoms, the goal of treatment is to challenge them and substitute more adaptive ways of thinking. Experts believe that once patients learn to process information in a "more accurate and reasonable fashion ... their symptoms will gradually improve" [50].

To this end, CBT-based approaches emphasize the technique of cognitive restructuring, as outlined originally by Beck [4] and Ellis [15] and later modified by Clark [10]. The goals of cognitive restructuring exercises are threefold: (1) to identify and understand how dysfunctional thoughts that occur during stressful or pain-provoking situations influence undesirable feelings, behaviors, and somatic reactions; (2) to evaluate the accuracy and/or usefulness of these thoughts; and (3) to develop alternative, more effective and rational ways of thinking that modulate the intensity and bothersomeness of pain.

Empirical Support for Cognitive-Behavioral Treatment for Chronic Pain, Including Functional Pain Syndromes

The results of an electronic database search, together with a search of reference lists in published papers, revealed nine meta-analyses of treatments for chronic pain conditions published between 1988 and 2008 related to low back pain, IBS, fibromyalgia, or chronic pain in general. The four earliest reviews concluded that psychological approaches are effective and are superior to comparison conditions for fibromyalgia [61], low back pain [11], and samples with mixed pain conditions [16,40]. These reviews, however, were limited because they predominantly included studies of low methodological quality, such as studies without randomization to conditions, without active treatment comparisons, or with a mix of treatment types, some of which were not primarily psychological.

The findings of the five more recent systematic reviews suggest that cognitive-behavioral methods are effective over the short term, including significant short-term improvements in pain intensity, with effect sizes ranging from 0.22 to 0.59, and functioning (e.g., daily activity, social functioning, disability, pain interference), with effect sizes from 0.23 to 0.60 for low back pain [22,25,55] and in samples with mixed pain conditions [52]. (Cohen's d effect size ranges: >0.2 = small; >0.05 = medium; >0.8 = large.) The systematic review of psychological treatments for IBS generally produced significant effect sizes for abdominal pain, bowel dysfunction, depression, and anxiety that ranged from 0.27 to 0.57 and yielded a number needed to treat for 50% reduction of symptoms of 2 [34].

Long-term maintenance of improvements following treatment is not well documented from the systematic reviews. The Hoffman et al. review [25], however, reported significant increases in long-term work status (>1 year after treatment) following multidisciplinary CBT treatment. Individual trials show significant long-term maintenance of improvements from multidisciplinary treatment in back or neck pain at a 3-year follow-up, especially in women [28], and in low back pain at a 13-year follow-up [56].

A further literature search revealed an additional 13 trials that included cognitive-behavioral methods for chronic pain that were not included in previous meta-analyses and are relevant to the focus of this chapter. Taken together, these studies demonstrated the effectiveness of cognitive-behavioral methods for chronic pain, across multiple outcome domains (e.g., pain, mood, and daily functioning), in groups of patients with fibromyalgia [35,64,68,80], low back pain [31,65], mixed musculoskeletal pain conditions [28,36,38], temporomandibular disorder pain [51,71], and vaginismus [72].

Developments in Cognitive-Behavioral Treatment in General

Clearly, the efficacy of CBT is well supported for a wide range of conditions such as depression and anxiety disorders (e.g., [9]), and for chronic pain. The models underlying CBT and methods that derive from these models, however, are constantly evolving. Some of the developments in the wider applications of CBT overall may signal directions that treatments for functional pain disorders may take in the future. For example, an earlier component analysis of CBT for depression ($N = 150$) showed that both the behavioral activation component of CBT (an approach to increasing behavior that yields a sense of pleasure and mastery) and combined components of behavioral activation and skills training for modifying automatic thoughts were as effective as the entire package of these components plus a component that focused on changing core cognitive schemas [27]. Also, the behavioral activation methods were as effective as the full set of components at altering dysfunctional thinking. These results suggest that a relatively simple treatment for depression aimed at direct behavior change, and not at changing the way people think, may be as effective as a more complex form of treatment that emphasizes cognitive change.

A randomized trial comparing behavioral activation to cognitive therapy and antidepressant medication ($N = 241$) found that, in severely depressed patients, behavioral activation produced better results than cognitive therapy [14]. The authors' opinion was that cognitive therapy may be more complicated to deliver because of its focus on patient behavior, beliefs, and attitudes, as opposed to the narrower, more straightforward focus on overt behavior included in behavioral activation. The authors suggested that a more limited focus is perhaps an advantage when the length of treatment is constrained.

Treatment component analyses and alternate treatment comparisons are concordant with results of process studies of CBT (e.g., [8]). A review of both CBT treatment component and process studies [39] concluded that "almost without exception, component studies found no difference in effectiveness between cognitive and behavioral elements of CBT" (p. 184). The authors found "little empirical support for the role of cognitive change as causal in the symptomatic improvements achieved in CBT" (p. 173).

The results and conclusions from more developed areas within CBT are relevant because many patients with functional pain disorders suffer from the types of anxiety and depressive disorders targeted by the treatments. The literature also suggests that we maintain a wider perspective on potential processes of change for patients with such disorders and that we continue to develop and apply methods of direct behavior change without necessarily being tied to the need to change what these patients feel or think.

Developments in Contextual Cognitive-Behavioral Therapy

Developments in cognitive and behavioral therapies over the past 40 years or so have been described as a series of "waves" [23]. The first wave was simply called behavior therapy, or, in the field of pain management, the "operant approach" [19]. The second wave is cognitive-behavioral therapy (e.g., [70]). The third wave includes approaches that fully integrate the behavioral and cognitive elements of the first two waves but also consider these within a conceptual framework that is nonmechanistic and contextual. The treatment processes that emerge within this wave include notions such as acceptance, mindfulness, and values. Examples of these third wave therapies include mindfulness-based stress reduction [29], dialectical behavior therapy [37], mindfulness-based cognitive therapy [63], acceptance and commitment therapy (ACT [24]), and an approach to chronic pain based on ACT called contextual cognitive-behavioral therapy (CCBT [42]).

The therapeutic model that derives from ACT and underlies CCBT includes six core processes: acceptance (e.g., willingness to have pain without struggling to control it), present-focused awareness (a feature of mindfulness), cognitive defusion (a loosening of verbal/cognitive processes that narrow behavioral options), committed action, self-as-context (a steady sense of self that is separate from thoughts, moods, and sensations), and value-based action [24]. A key overriding construct in this model is what is referred to as "psychological flexibility," which emerges from these separate processes. Psychological flexibility is a quality that allows behavior to persist or to change in line with long-term goals and values, relatively free from restrictions based on interactions between verbally based and direct (nonverbally based) influences.

Previous research has demonstrated that acceptance of pain is associated with lower pain intensity and with a healthier level of emotional, physical, and social functioning and medical care use. This research includes both retrospective (e.g., [43,54]) and prospective [44] studies in patients with heterogeneous pain problems. Acceptance has also been demonstrated as an important predictor of functioning in a sample including women with osteoarthritis (n = 36) and fibromyalgia (n = 86) [32], and in a sample with low back pain [41]. Additional studies have shown that mindfulness [45], values-based action [49], and general psychological flexibility [47] are, likewise, significantly related to key aspects of patient functioning.

Eight treatment outcome studies provide support for the benefits of treatment methods for chronic pain related to the ACT and CCBT model. Relatively small-scale quasi-randomized or randomized trials show that an 8-week mindfulness-based treatment can significantly reduce symptoms, anxiety, and depression and improve quality of life in women with fibromyalgia [21]. The same treatment reduced symptoms of depression in women with fibromyalgia [64] and increased pain acceptance and physical functioning in older adults with chronic back pain [53]. Each of these results is consistent with the generally positive results from meta-analyses of mindfulness-based treatments for a range of behavioral and health-related problems [1,20]. More inclusive packages of treatment methods (including exposure, mindfulness, values-based methods, and other methods to increase psychological flexibility) can yield significant results across a range of domains. Success has been demonstrated in samples of highly complex chronic pain patients with mostly nonspecific, diffuse musculoskeletal pain, based on a waiting-list controlled trial [48] and on analyses of clinical significance [46,47,79]. The most recent set of results, for example, includes mean effect sizes of 1.07 immediately after treatment ($N = 171$) and 0.89 at a 3-month follow-up ($N = 114$) for measures of pain, acceptance of pain, disability, depression, anxiety, and directly assessed physical performance following a 3- or 4-week course of interdisciplinary residential treatment in the United Kingdom [79]. One earlier published study [12] included a small randomized trial of participants "at risk" for work loss due to pain or stress; the results showed dramatically reduced sick days and medical treatment during the 6-month follow-up phase, after just 4 hours of treatment.

The particular value in acceptance-based, contextual, and mindfulness-based methods for highly distressed individuals with functional pain appears to arise from the specific inclusion of processes for addressing rumination, undermining avoidance, and reducing the impact of distressing and restricting influences from patterns of emotional thinking [24]. Although there are few trials, and much of the data comes from mixed samples, rather than from homogeneous groups with specific functional pain syndromes, the processes and results thus far appear generally applicable.

Summary and Conclusion

Functional pain syndromes, including fibromyalgia, IBS, TMD, IBS, and others such as noncardiac chest pain and vaginismus, entail significant personal suffering and a heavy burden on health care systems. Practically, by definition, these syndromes are not successfully treated by medical treatment methods designed for conditions with specific identifiable organic pathology. Increasingly, treatment of individuals with functional pain disorders falls into the hands of psychologists or multidisciplinary teams that provide treatment from a broadly cognitive-behavioral perspective.

Research results show that CBT significantly improves pain symptoms, daily functioning, and, in many cases, emotional functioning in patients with mixed pain disorders, low back pain, fibromyalgia, IBS, TMD, and vaginismus. Where data allow comparisons, it does not appear that patients with these disorders are any less likely than those with other chronic pain conditions to respond favorably to CBT.

CBT as it is usually practiced consists of packages of treatment methods, some of which are at least 25 years old. Alongside these methods, CBT continues to evolve, based on process and treatment component analyses, and other theoretical developments. Based in part on the notion that attempting to eliminate unwanted psychological experiences can cause increased suffering and life disruption, newer approaches advocate acceptance of—or willingness to experience—thoughts, memories, and feelings, without needing to change them or follow them. Other methods include mindfulness and values-based methods that help behavior to be more realistic and present-focused and more directed by what patients care most about, rather than by their symptoms. Several studies of these contextual CBT methods show encouraging results.

From a psychological standpoint, chronic pain, suffering, and restricted functioning are more or less the same whether they come in the form of a functional syndrome or a condition with a more firmly identified medical basis. This distinction is mostly a practical one and not a psychological one. The only exception to this is that those with functional pain disorders may experience the source of their pain as more mysterious and therefore frightening, may feel more disbelieved in their complaints, may meet with more medical investigation or treatment failures and more frustration from health care providers, and therefore they may experience more suffering from these experiences. The question is always the same: What are the manipulable social, verbal, and emotional influences on patient behavior that are most responsible for patients' restricted functioning and loss of vitality, and which of these influences can be most practically addressed with the greatest impact?

Acknowledgments

Preparation of this chapter was supported partly by NIH/NIDDK grants 67878 and 77738 (to J.M. Lackner).

References

[1]   Baer RA. Mindfulness training as a clinical intervention: a conceptual and empirical review. Clin Psychol Sci Pract 2003;10:125–143.

[2]   Bandura A. Social foundations of thought and action: a social cognitive theory. Englewood Cliffs, NJ: Prentice-Hall; 1986.

[3]   Bastiaenen CH, de Bie RA, Wolters PM, Vlaeyen JW, Bastiaanssen JM, Klabbers AB, Heuts A, van den Brandt PA, Essed GG. Treatment of pregnancy-related pelvic girdle and/or low back pain after delivery design of a randomized clinical trial within a comprehensive prognostic cohort study. BMC Public Health 2004;4:67.

[4]   Beck AT. Cognitive therapy and the emotional disorders. New York: Meridian; 1976.

[5]   Bernstein DA, Borkovec TD, et al. New directions in progressive relaxation training: a guidebook for helping professionals. Westport, CT: Praeger; 2000.

[6]   Blair HS, Elliott AM, Hannaford PC, Chambers WA, Smith WC. Factors related to the onset and persistence of chronic back pain in the community. Spine 2004;29:1032–1040.

[7]   Bouton ME, Mineka S, Barlow DH. A modern learning theory perspective on the etiology of panic disorder. Psychol Rev 2001;108:4–32.

[8]   Burns DD, Spangler DL. Do changes in dysfunctional attitudes mediate changes in depression and anxiety in cognitive behavioral therapy? Behav Ther 2001;32:337–369.

[9]   Butler AC, Chapman JE, Forman EM, Beck AT. The empirical status of cognitive-behavioral therapy: a review of meta-analyses. Clin Psychol Rev 2006;26:17–31.

[10] Clark DM. A cognitive approach to panic. Behav Res Ther 1986;24:461–470.

[11] Cutler RB, Fishbain DA, Rosomoff HL, Abdel-Moty E, Khahil TM, Rosomoff RS. Does nonsurgical pain center treatment of chronic pain return patients to work? Spine 1994;19:643–652.

[12] Dahl J, Wilson KG, Nilsson A. Acceptance and Commitment Therapy and the treatment of persons at risk for long-term disability resulting from stress and pain symptoms: a preliminary randomized trial. Behav Ther 2004;35:785–802.

[13] Dersh J, Polatin PB, Gatchel RJ. Chronic pain and psychopathology: research findings and theoretical considerations. Psychosom Med 2002;64:773–786.

[14] Dimidjian S, Hollon SD, Dobson KS, Schmaling KB, Kohlenberg RJ, Addis ME, Gallop R, McGlinchey JB, Markley DK, Gollan JK, et al. Randomized trial of behavioral activation, cognitive therapy, and antidepressant medication in the acute treatment of adults with major depression. J Consult Clin Psychol 2006;74:658–670.

[15] Ellis A. Reason and Emotion In Psychotherapy. New York: Lyle Stuart; 1962.

[16] Flor H, Fydrich T, Turk DC. Efficacy of multidisciplinary pain treatment centers: a meta-analytic review. Pain 1992;49:221–230.

[17] Flor H, Turk DC. Psychophysiology of chronic pain: do chronic pain patients exhibit symptom-specific psychophysiological responses? Psychol Bull 1989;105:215–59.

[18] Foa EB, Kozak MJ. Emotional processing of fear: exposure to corrective information. Psychol Bull 1986;99:20–35.

[19] Fordyce WE. Behavioural methods for chronic pain and illness. St Louis: Mosby; 1976.

[20] Grossman P, Niemann L, Schmidt S, Walach H. Mindfulness-based stress reduction and health benefits: a meta-analysis. J Psychosom Res 2004;57:35–43.

[21] Grossman P, Tiefenthaler-Gilmer U, Raysz A, Kesper U. Mindfulness training as an intervention for fibromyalgia: evidence of postintervention and 3-year follow-up benefits in well-being. Psychother Psychosom 2007;76:226–233.

[22] Guzman J, Esmail R, Karjalaainen K, Malmivaara A, Irvin E, Bombardier C. Multidisciplinary rehabilitation for chronic low back pain: systematic review. BMJ 2001;322:1511–1516.

[23] Hayes SC. Acceptance and Commitment Therapy, relational frame theory, and the third wave of behavior therapy. Behav Ther 2004;35:639–665.

[24] Hayes SC, Luoma JB, Bond FW, et al. Acceptance and Commitment Therapy: model, process and outcome. Behav Res Ther 2006;44:1–25.

[25] Hoffman BM, Papas RK, Chatkoff DK, Kerns RD. Meta-analysis of psychological interventions for chronic low back pain. Health Psychol 2007;26:1–9.

[26] Jacobson E. Progressive relaxation. Chicago: University of Chicago Press; 1938.

[27] Jacobson NS, Dobson KS, Traux PA, Addis ME, Prince SE. A component analysis of cognitive-behavioral treatment for depression. J Consult Clin Psychol 1996;64:295–304.

[28] Jensen IB, Bergstrom G, Ljungquist T, Bodin L. A 3-year follow-up of a multidisciplinary rehabilitation programme for back and neck pain. Pain 2005;115:273–283.

[29] Kabat-Zinn J. Full catastrophe living: using the wisdom of your body and mind to face stress, pain, and illness. New York: Dell; 1990.

[30] Keefe FJ, Dunsmore J. Behavioral and cognitive-behavioral approaches to chronic pain: recent advances and future directions. J Consult Clin Psychol 1992;60:528–536.

[31] Kole-Snijders AMJ, Vlaeyen JWS, Goosens MEJB, Rutten-van Molken MPMH, Heuts PHTG, van Breukelen G, van Eek H. Chronic low-back pain: what does cognitive coping skills training add to operant behavioral treatment methods? Results of a randomized clinical trial. J Consult Clin Psychol 1999;67:931–944.

[32] Kratz AL, Davis MC, Zautra AJ. Pain acceptance moderates the relationship between pain and negative affect in female osteoarthritis and fibromyalgia patients. Ann Behav Med 2007;33:291–301.

[33] Lackner JM. Controlling IBS the drug-free way: a 10-step plan for symptom relief. New York: Stewart, Tabori, and Chang; 2007.

[34] Lackner JM, Morley S, Dowzer C, Mesmer C, Hamilton S. Psychological treatments for irritable bowel syndrome: a systematic review and meta-analysis. J Consult Clin Psychol 2004;72:1100–1113.

[35] Lemstra M. Olszynski WPO. The effectiveness of multidisciplinary rehabilitation in the treatment of fibromyalgia. Clin J Pain 2005;21:166–174.

[36] Li EJQ, Li-Tsang CWP, Lam CS, Hui KYL, Chan CCH. The effect of a "training on work readiness" program for workers with musculoskeletal injuries: a randomized control trail (RCT) study. J Occup Rehabil 2006;16:529–541.

[37] Linehan MM. Cognitive-behavioral treatment of borderline personality disorder. New York: Guilford; 1993.

[38] Linton SJ, Ryberg M. A cognitive-behavioral group intervention as prevention for persistent neck and back pain in a non-patient population: a randomized controlled trial. Pain 2001;90:83–90.

[39] Longmore RJ, Worrell M. Do we need to challenge thoughts in cognitive behavior therapy? Clin Psychol Rev 2007;27:173–187.

[40] Malone MD, Strube MJ. Meta-analysis of non-medical treatment for chronic pain. Pain 1988;34:231–244.

[41] Mason VL, Mathias B, Skevington SM. Accepting low back pain: it is related to a good quality of life. Clin J Pain 2008;24:22–29.

[42] McCracken LM. Contextual cognitive-behavioral therapy for chronic pain. Progress in pain research and management, Vol. 33. Seattle: IASP Press; 2005.

[43] McCracken LM, Eccleston C. Coping or acceptance: what to do with chronic pain? Pain 2003;105:197–204.

[44] McCracken LM, Eccleston C. A prospective study of acceptance of pain and patient functioning with chronic pain. Pain 2005;118:164–169.

[45] McCracken, LM, Gauntlett-Gilbert J, Vowles KE. The role of mindfulness in a contextual cognitive-behavioral analysis of chronic pain-related suffering and disability. Pain 2007;131:63–69.

[46] McCracken LM, MacKichan F, Eccleston C. Contextual cognitive-behavioral therapy for severely disabled chronic pain sufferers: effectiveness and clinically significant change. Eur J Pain 2007;11:314–322.

[47] McCracken LM, Vowles KE. Psychological flexibility and traditional pain management strategies in relation to patient functioning with chronic pain: an examination of a revised instrument. J Pain 2007;8:700–707.

[48] McCracken LM, Vowles KE, Eccleston C. Acceptance-based treatment for persons with complex, long standing chronic pain: a preliminary analysis of treatment outcome in comparison to a waiting phase. Behav Res Ther 2005;43:1335–1346.

[49] McCracken LM, Yang S-Y. The role of values in a contextual cognitive-behavioral analysis of chronic pain. Pain 2006;123:137–145.

[50] McGinn LK, Sanderson WC. What allows cognitive behavioral therapy to be brief: overview, efficacy, and crucial factors facilitating brief treatment. Clin Psychol Sci Pract 2001;8:23–37.

[51] Mishra KD, Gatchel RJ, Gardea MA. The relative efficacy of three cognitive-behavioral treatment approaches to temporomandibular disorders. J Behav Med 2000;23:293–309.

[52] Morley S. Eccleston C, Williams A. Systematic review and meta-analysis of randomised controlled trials of cognitive behaviour therapy and behaviour therapy for chronic pain in adults, excluding headache. Pain 1999;80:1–13.

[53] Morone NE, Grecco CM, Weiner DK. Mindfulness meditation for the treatment of chronic low back pain in older adults: a randomized controlled pilot study. Pain 2008;134:310–319.

[54] Nicholas MK, Asgahari A. Investigating acceptance in adjustment to chronic pain: is acceptance broader than we thought? Pain 2006;124:269–279.

[55] Ostelo RWJG, van Tulder MW, Vlaeyen JWS, Linton SJ, Morley SJ, Assendelft WJJ. Behavioural treatment of chronic low-back pain. Cochrane Database Syst Rev 2005(1):CD002014.

[56] Patrick LE, Altmaier EM, Found EM. Long-term outcomes in multidisciplinary treatment of chronic low back pain: results of a 13-year follow-up. Spine 2004;29:850–855.

[57] Pavlov IP. Conditioned reflexes: an investigation of the physiological activity of the cerebral cortex. London: Oxford University Press; 1927.

[58] Perlman SD. Psychoanalytic treatment of chronic pain: the body speaks on multiple levels. J Am Acad Psychoanal 1996;24:257–271.

[59] Philips HC. Avoidance behavior and its role in sustaining chronic pain. Behav Res Ther 1987;25:273–280.

[60] Razran G. The observable unconscious and the inferable conscious in current Soviet psychophysiology: interoceptive conditioning, semantic conditioning, and the orienting reflex. Psychol Rev 1961;68:1–147.

[61] Rossy LA, Buckelew SP, Dorr N, Hagglund KJ, Thayer JF, McIntoch MJ, Hewett JE, Johnson JC. A meta-analysis of fibromyalgia treatment interventions. Ann Behav Med 1999;21:180–191.

[62] Schultz JH. Autogenic training: a psychophysiologic approach in psychotherapy. New York: Grune & Stratton; 1959.

[63] Segal ZV, Williams JMG, Teasdale JD. Mindfulness-based cognitive therapy for depression. New York: Guilford; 2002.

[64] Sephton SE, Salmon P, Weissbecker I, Ulmer C, Floyd A, Hoover K, Studts JL. Mindfulness meditation alleviates depressive symptoms in women with fibromyalgia. Arthritis Rheum 2007;57:77–85.

[65] Smeets RJEM, Vlaeyen JWS, Hidding A, Kester ADM, van der Heijden GJMG, van Geel ACM, Knotterus JA. Active rehabilitation for chronic low back pain: cognitive-behavioral, physical, or both? First direct post-treatment results from a randomized controlled trial. BMC Muskuloskelet Disord 2006;7:5.

[66] Skinner BF. Science and Human Behavior. New York: Free Press; 1953.

[67] Sperling M. A psychoanalytic study of migraine and psychogenic headache. Psychoanal Rev 1952;39:153–63.

[68] Thieme K, Flor H, Turk DC. Psychological pain treatment in fibromyalgia syndrome: efficacy of operant behavioural and cognitive behavioural treatments. Arthritis Res Ther 2006;8:R121.

[69] Turk DC, Flor H. Etiological theories and treatments for chronic back pain. II. Psychological models and interventions. Pain 1984;19:209–233.

[70] Turk DC, Meichenbaum D, Genest M. Pain and behavioral medicine: a cognitive-behavioral perspective. New York: Guilford; 1983.

508   J.M. Lackner and L.M. McCracken

[71] Turner JA, Mancl L, Aaron LA. Short- and long-term efficacy of brief cognitive-behavioral ther-
      apy for patients with chronic temporomandibular disorder pain: a randomized, controlled trial.
      Pain 2006;121:181–194.
[72] van Lankveld JJDM, ter Kuile MM, de Groot HE, Melles R, Nefs J, Zandbergen M. Cognitive-be-
      havioral therapy for women with lifelong vaginismus: a randomized waiting-list controlled trial
      of efficacy. J Consult Clin Psychol 2006;74:168–178.
[73] van Tulder MW, Ostelo R, Vlaeyen JW, Linton SJ, Morley SJ, Assendelft WJ. Behavioral treat-
      ment for chronic low back pain: a systematic review within the framework of the Cochrane Back
      Review Group. Spine 2000;25:2688–99.
[74] Vlaeyen JWS, de Jong J, Geilen M, Heuts PHTG, van Breukelen G. Graded exposure in vivo in
      the treatment of pain-related fear: a replicated single-case experimental design in four patients
      with chronic low back pain. Behav Res Ther 2001;39:151–166.
[75] Vlaeyen JW, de Jong J, Geilen M, Heuts PHTG, van Breukelen G. The treatment of fear of
      movement/(re)injury in chronic low back pain: further evidence on the effectiveness of exposure
      in vivo. Clin J Pain 2002;18:251–261.
[76] Vlaeyen JW, Haazen IW, Schuerman JA, Kole-Snijders AMJ, van Eek H. Behavioural rehabilita-
      tion of chronic low back pain: comparison of an operant treatment, an operant-cognitive treat-
      ment and an operant-respondent treatment. Br J Clin Psychol 1995;34:95–118.
[77] Vlaeyen JWS, Linton SJ. Fear-avoidance and its consequences in chronic musculoskeletal pain: a
      state of the art. Pain 2000;85:317–32.
[78] Von Korff MR, Gruman J, Schaefer J, Curry SJ, Wagner EH. Collaborative management of chron-
      ic illness. Ann Intern Med 1997;127:1097–102.
[79] Vowles KE, McCracken LM. Acceptance and values-based action in chronic pain: a study of ef-
      fectiveness and treatment process. J Consult Clin Psychol 2008;76:397–407.
[80] Williams DA, Cary MA, Groner KH, Chaplin W, Glazer LJ, Rodriguez AM, Clauw DJ. Improv-
      ing physical functional status in patients with fibromyalgia: a brief cognitive behavioral interven-
      tion. J Rheumatol 2002;29:1280–1286.
[81] Wolpe J. Reciprocal inhibition as the main basis of psychotherapeutic effects. AMA Arch Neurol
      Psychiatry 1954;72:205–26.

Correspondence to: Jeffrey M. Lackner, PsyD, Behavioral Medicine Clinic, Department of Medicine, University at Buffalo School of Medicine, SUNY, ECMC,
462 Grider Street, Buffalo, NY 14215, USA. Tel: 1-716-898-5671; fax: 1-716-898-
3040; email: lackner@buffalo.edu. Lance M. McCracken, PhD, Centre for Pain
Services, Royal National Hospital for Rheumatic Diseases, Bath BA1 1RL, United
Kingdom. Tel: 44-1225-473-403; fax: 44-1225-473-461; email: lance.mccracken@
rnhrd-tr.swest.nhs.uk.

Complementary Medicine and the Central Mediation of Functional Pain Disorders

Ginger Polich,[a] Jian Kong,[a,b] Vitaly Napadow,[b]
and Randy Gollub[a,b,c]

[a]Department of Psychiatry, [b]Athinoula A. Martinos Center for Biomedical Imaging,
[c]GCRC Biomedical Imaging Core, Massachusetts General Hospital, Charlestown,
Massachusetts, USA

Functional pain disorders represent a group of symptom-based diagnoses whose pathophysiological origins, at present, escape clear etiological definition. Although biomedicine continues to develop new pharmaceutical and surgical interventions to treat functional pain disorders, current therapies remain inadequate and often entail a steady burden of side effects [102]. As a result, many patients with such disorders seek out other treatment options, including complementary and alternative medicine (CAM), to augment any relief they already derive from conventional care [25,95,106].

CAM represents a diverse array of generally inexpensive, low-risk therapies [97], including acupuncture, massage, chiropractic, meditation, biofeedback, yoga, tai chi, qigong, spiritual healing, and herbal medicines. Although largely heterogeneous, most CAM therapies are process-oriented and experiential, engaging patients' experience and attention for extended periods of time. Other common CAM themes include a desire to enhance the body's endogenous healing capacity (in contrast to the pathophysiological focus of biomedicine), "holistic" treatment of the patient, and an optimistic and hopeful delivery of care.

Functional Pain Syndromes: Presentation and Pathophysiology
edited by Emeran A. Mayer and M. Catherine Bushnell
IASP Press, Seattle, © 2009

In regard to functional pain disorders, CAM therapies warrant consideration on two accounts—first because a preponderance of research studies evaluates them as effective, and second because of their mechanistic plausibility. Recent etiological hypotheses for functional pain disorders implicate a role for maladaptive neuroplasticity and aberrant processing at the level of the forebrain, in the same regions where CAM therapies may be exerting their effects.

To date, dozens of published peer-reviewed studies have espoused the benefits of CAM therapies for functional pain disorders. A review of the literature demonstrates biofeedback's usefulness in treating chronic low back pain [88], fibromyalgia [31,54], temporal mandibular joint disorder [23,37], chronic pelvic pain [22,83], and vulvodynia [40]. Meditation has reportedly improved symptoms in patients with chronic low back pain [17,51,82], fibromyalgia [43,52], irritable bowel syndrome [55], and cardiac syndrome X [24]. Yoga has improved symptoms of chronic low back pain [36,109] and irritable bowel syndrome [62,98]. Qigong has effectively treated fibromyalgia [45]. There is evidence for chiropractic as an effective treatment for chronic low back pain [44,47], fibromyalgia [19], and temporal mandibular joint disorder [27]. Massage has shown efficacy in treating fibromyalgia [12,33] and chronic low back pain [101]. Several studies report acupuncture as a useful treatment for chronic low back pain [16,46,76,80,99], temporal mandibular joint disorder [96], and chronic pelvic pain [18,70]. Overwhelmingly, the CAM research base reports treatment effectiveness for functional pain disorders.

Yet members of the wider scientific community frequently contest this affirmative body of CAM literature. Some researchers attribute the confirmatory results to a publication bias toward positive findings. Others disparage the studies for being observational or uncontrolled, criticizing that when sham controls are included, these studies frequently generate results in which both active and sham interventions show comparable improvements over wait-list controls.

To the contrary, this chapter will discuss the possibility that CAM therapies treat several aspects of functional pain disorders, and do so in ways that are consistent with our current scientific understanding of pain. Clinical and basic science studies of recent decades demonstrate the body's extensive modulation of nociceptive signaling via input from bottom-up peripheral nerves and top-down cortical and subcortical brain activity, and document how repeated nociception can sensitize and alter the structure of neurons over the long term [34,50,112]. Research indicates that maladaptive plasticity along nociceptive pathways, as well as negative cognitive and emotional states (context, anticipation, fear, and depression), may play a role in the development and maintenance of chronic pain. Put more simply, experience, attention, and affect could matter a great deal for patients suffering from functional pain disorders.

Process-oriented CAM therapies may be well primed to use experience, attention, and affect to redirect aberrant signaling in pain pathways. Evidence suggests that CAM treatments such as acupuncture can alter noxious peripheral inputs and change subcortical brain functioning [28] and that alternative treatments such as meditation and biofeedback can influence pain-related cortical and affective functioning [34]. Furthermore, given what we know about the complex presentation of pain, multimodal therapies that activate innate healing resources, engender positive expectations, and address psychosocial as well as physical concerns seem well suited to address the complexity of a functional pain disorder. Emerging neurobiological hypotheses have even begun to mechanistically account for the efficacy of these nonspecific effects [8,20,57,58].

In this chapter, CAM therapies will be discussed with respect to their potential influence along the neural axis of the pain pathway, particularly within the brain. The recent advent of minimally invasive neuroimaging modalities, such as positron emission tomography (PET) and noninvasive methods such as functional magnetic resonance imaging (fMRI) has advanced these speculations immensely. This chapter discusses three potential therapeutic aspects of CAM: their impact on maladaptive neuroplasticity, higher cortical modulation of pain, and salubrious "placebo effects." This chapter is neither exhaustive nor comprehensive in its selection of topics, and its emphasis on acupuncture reflects the authors' greater knowledge of the treatment and is not meant to imply superiority of this modality over others.

Reversing Maladaptive Plasticity in the Brain

Research indicates that sensations (including painful ones) do not always linearly correspond to peripheral input [79]. Functional pain disorders offer a demonstrative case, with patients exhibiting hypersensitivity to noxious and non-noxious stimuli, and experiencing pain even in the absence of stimulation [112].The latest neuroscientific investigations link this phenomenon with maladaptive changes in pain-responsive brain regions.

Scientific research is driving home the point that for chronic pain, experience matters. In response to repeated stimulation, "memories" of pain can become semi-permanently ingrained within the body and unconscious mind [34]. Framed mechanistically, repeated sensory input can reshape the spatial distribution and synaptic links of pain-processing neurons [79]. To accommodate prolonged noxious input over time, the brain can elaborate and entrench pain signals via cortical restructuring [35]. Functional pain disorders may thus be related to neuroplastic brain alterations, particularly within the primary somatosensory cortex area associated with the affected body part [34,75,86]. Physiological discriminative functioning may be downregulated in these brain regions [112].Validating fMRI studies demonstrate augmented and expanded cortical representation zones mapping to pain in patients with chronic low back pain [35,39], irritable bowel syndrome [67], or fibromyalgia [21,42].

If the dynamic processes leading to maladaptive plasticity can also work in reverse, CAM therapies such as acupuncture and biofeedback may provide relief by attenuating aberrant signaling in pain pathways. Through prolonged and carefully directed counterstimulation—regularly administered normal sensory input—CAM therapies may be able to interrupt or "reprogram" these habituated cycles [50].

Acupuncture has been well researched in this regard. This therapy has a 2,000-year Chinese medical history. Treatment involves a complex diagnostic procedure followed by insertion and stimulation (manual, electrical, or thermal) of fine needles through the skin and into underlying connective tissue at specific locations known as acupoints. Traditionally, needling aims to stimulate "qi" pervading the body, so as to regulate physiological balance and health [56].

Neuroimaging research shows acupuncture stimulation exerting complex effects on the brain of healthy adults, eliciting a diffuse and overlapping response within multiple cortical, subcortical/limbic, and brainstem areas [28,30,49,59,60,85]. A recent fMRI and acupuncture study has documented acupuncture's capacity to measurably reverse maladaptive brain plasticity in carpal tunnel syndrome patients [86]. Acupuncture modulated behavioral and mechanistic abnormalities in these patients, including characteristic sensorimotor hyperactivation and overlapping or blurred representation of adjacent fingers within the primary somatosensory cortex (S1) [86]. After 5 weeks of treatment, patients showed signs of clinical improvement, diminished hyperactivation, and greater separation in the S1 somatotopy of adjacent fingers (which was also correlated with improvement in median nerve conduction latency, an electrophysiological measure of peripheral dysfunction) (Fig. 1) [87]. While this study showed that acupuncture could partially restore peripheral nerve function and higher brain processing, no control stimulation group was included, and thus further research is warranted.

A closer understanding of the mechanisms underlying acupuncture's modulating effect on maladaptive neuroplasticity remains to be determined. Other speculative theories describing acupuncture efficacy via "counter-irritation analgesia," correction of connective tissue abnormalities, and synchronization of default mode brain networks may be relevant.

The "counter-irritation analgesia" theory grounds itself on the observation that counterstimulation, i.e., moderate pain, can sometimes alleviate prolonged, chronic pain [78]. Corroborating basic science research demonstrates that noxious nervous stimulation transmits to the brainstem and periaqueductal gray (PAG), inducing serotonin- and norepinephrine-mediated descending inhibitory control systems. Previous studies link activation of the midbrain, PAG, and surrounding areas with pain inhibition in patients suffering from pain disorders [5,48]. Acupuncture stimulation might be playing into this system. Acupuncture involves gross peripheral manipulation with a relatively coarse penetrating object (relative to the scale of a nerve receptor) that activates receptors innervated by multiple nerve fiber types [107]. Neuroimaging studies have shown needling-induced brain activity in the PAG [74,85]. This series of

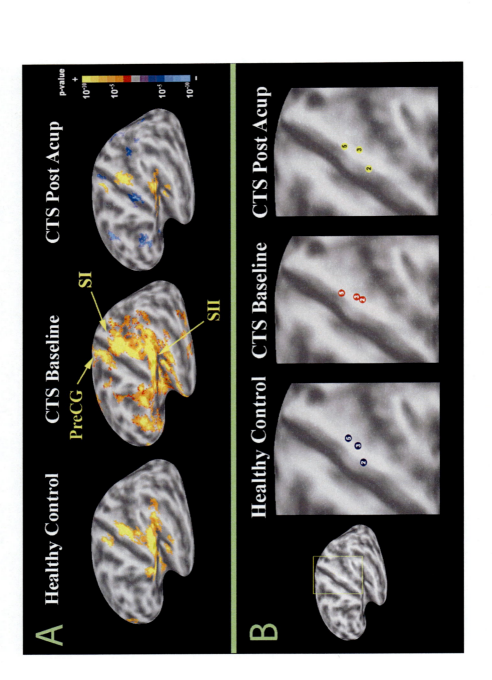

events may trigger the descending inhibition system to produce an analgesic effect [48,69].

By providing relief in the short term, acupuncture may also be enabling beneficial behavioral changes. Through "counter-irritation analgesia," the body returns to a temporary state of normalcy during which patients may be more likely to increase their day-to-day physical activity, producing steady patterns of normal sensory input. Over the long term, this normal input may interrupt the recurrence of abnormal pain processing in the brain [78].

The benefits of acupuncture may also derive through correction of maladaptive connective tissue biomechanics, caused in the first place by increased tissue stress (due to strain or inflammation) or decreased tissue stress (due to underuse) [65]. Basic science research reveals a dynamic responsiveness of connective tissue to acupuncture [66]. Acupuncture needle rotation can deform fibroblasts at cell-matrix focal adhesion sites and initiate cytoskeletal responses [64]. Acupuncture may induce connective tissue matrix remodeling [65] by changing local connective tissue biomechanics, as well as by altering the milieu of sensory afferent fibers innervating the tissue. Modulation of sensory afferent input from connective tissue could then lead to neuroplastic changes in areas of the central nervous system representing deep tissue proprioception and nociception.

Acupuncture may also exert its therapeutic effect on functional pain by eliciting changes in the default mode network (DMN), a network of functionally connected brain regions that is more active during rest than in a task condition and also exhibits spontaneous connectivity during a resting state [14,92]. The DMN, shown to respond differently across groups of healthy adults and low back pain patients [4], may prove to be disrupted in patients with functional pain as well. A recent publication found acupuncture to modulate resting connectivity in the DMN [29].

← *Fig. 1.* Acupuncture modulates brain somatosensory processing in patients with carpal tunnel syndrome (CTS). (A) In CTS, primary somatosensory cortex (S1) hyperactivation was noted for innocuous stimulation of the third finger (median nerve innervated) of the affected hand. After a 5-week acupuncture (Acup) treatment, less hyperactivation and more focused S1 finger representation were noted. (B) Compared to healthy controls, CTS patients demonstrated less separation in S1 somatotopic representations for the second and third fingers (both innervated by the median nerve). Following acupuncture, the second and third finger representations were more separated, approximating those of healthy adults (adapted from [86]).

Following verum, but not sham, acupuncture, resting DMN connectivity increased in brain regions related to pain signaling (anterior cingulate cortex [ACC], PAG), pain-related affect (amygdala, ACC), and memory (hippocampal formation, middle temporal gyrus). Acupuncture may thus enhance the post-stimulation spatial extent of resting brain networks associated with modulation of nociception, memory, and affect. However, this theory remains speculative, and the relationship between DMN modulation, neuroplasticity, and clinical efficacy is yet to be determined.

Other CAM therapies may also have an impact on maladaptive neuroplasticity. Biofeedback, for example, may help reprogram aberrant pain-related brain patterns by providing regulated sensory input to a specific region of the brain. During biofeedback therapy, patients learn to monitor and modulate their physiological states through use of electronic instruments that translate, in real time, unconscious bodily activity into interpretable sounds, lights, or images. Targets may include global indicators of stress (blood pressure and skin temperature), musculoskeletal tension in painful regions, and even brain activity directly [26].

Biofeedback uses self-directed peripheral sensory stimulation to alter the signals entering a specific brain region [34]. With muscular disorders, for example, patients are trained to become subtly aware of localized bodily regions of tension or dysfunction. Patients then learn to use directed attention to relax or tone these regions, using "normal" input to interrupt pain signals traveling to the brain. In the short term, patients can gain some control over their symptoms, and in the long term, the normal input could outcompete abnormal processing and restore the brain to a natural state of processing. A more detailed investigation of the mechanistic underpinnings of these biofeedback-induced changes in the brain remains to be undertaken.

Higher Cortical Modulation of Pain Perception

Functional pain disorders are associated with a constellation of higher-order mind states spanning the spectrum from normal coping behaviors to major mental illnesses. These states may include present-moment feelings of fear and anticipation as well as longer-term comorbidities of anxiety and depression. Catastrophizing—involving magnification of pain and pain-related symptoms, pessimism, rumination, and helplessness—has also been implicated in this regard. These negative mind states can be predisposing, complicating, or secondary factors for functional pain.

What matters for individuals with functional pain disorders is not just the pain they feel each day, but also how they think and feel about it. Beyond invoking conscious suffering, negative mind states can exacerbate pain through activation of descending pathways of the brain. Some research even suggests that prolonged activation of these pathways contributes to the development and maintenance of chronic pain states [38,91].

Numerous clinical studies demonstrate that through modulation of cognition and affect, process-oriented CAM treatments such as meditation, yoga, tai chi, and qigong can improve detrimental mind states associated with chronic pain [11,94]. Many of these CAM therapies include a meditative component. Meditation practice is broadly characterized as intentional relaxation of the body (release of muscle tension, slowing of the breath), paired with active self-regulation of attention (suspension of analysis and reflection, avoidance of discursive thought) via sustained concentration or awareness [15].

One of meditation's immediate effects is to relieve stress of the body. Meditation has been described as inducing a physiological "relaxation response," a mechanistic counterbalance to the "fight-or-flight" stress response [9]. The relaxation response helps induce a bodily state of hypometabolism and heightened parasympathetic activity, characterized by reduced heart rate, blood pressure, respiratory rate, and musculoskeletal tension. As prolonged stress and excessive amounts of cortisol have been shown to destroy muscle and neural tissue, exacerbating chronic pain over time, these opposing physiological benefits of CAM may be of great importance to chronic pain patients.

Studies suggest that different but overlapping brain networks are involved in the sensory encoding and cognitive evaluation of pain intensity [61], and neuroimaging studies suggest a major role for the latter in chronic pain [3]. Calm focus of the meditating mind may also benefit sufferers of functional pain disorders through top-down regulation along the neural axis of pain. Many chronic pain patients exhibit clinical hypervigilance to pain and pain information [100], aberrant tendencies that manifest in the brain processing of pain-related input [63,104]. As one mechanism of relief, meditation's demand for sustained concentration or awareness may distract attention away from noxious stimulation. Correspondence between decreased attention to pain and pain reduction is well supported by behavioral and neurobiological literature [93,108]. Fittingly, an fMRI study on meditation revealed reduced activity in the thalamus and medial occipital cortex, indicating the mind's withdrawal from sensory processing (Newberg 2006, as cited in [89]). Distraction away from noxious stimuli may activate the inhibitory descending modulatory system of the brainstem [100]. A separate MRI study has found long-term meditation practice to reduce age-associated cortical thinning in the prefrontal cortex and right anterior insula, brain regions associated with attention, interoception, and sensory processing [68].

Beyond attention, other psychosocial factors such as context, associated memory, expectation, and mood affect pain perception as well. Meditation may be able to ameliorate pain by influencing these evaluative responses. In mindfulness meditation specifically, patients are taught to cultivate nonjudgmental moment-to-moment awareness through "detached observation," passively regarding pain-related thoughts and feelings as impermanent, valueless, and potentially inaccurate mental activities [111]. Learning to experience a pain sensation without being bothered is said to engender an "uncoupling of the sensory dimension of the pain experience from the affective/evaluative alarm reaction" [51]. Research supports meditation's ability to dissociate pain sensation from subjective pain evaluation. A behavioral study showed meditation to increase acute pain tolerance via emotional regulation—afterwards, sensations felt intense, but less bothersome [81]. An fMRI study showed meditation to reduce responses to experimentally administered pain in the thalamus, prefrontal cortex, and ACC, networks modulating the brain's emotional/motivational response to pain [89]. Meditation may be therapeutically beneficial in both the short and long term. By quieting pain-related cognitive/affective networks for an extended period of time, meditation could counteract centrally mediated hypersensitivity in the brain.

The benefits of mind-body therapies can also be viewed on the level of the whole person because they foster a set of mental skills applicable to everyday life. Through their active effort, patients learn to manage their own pain-related thoughts, feelings, and sensations. This achievement in turn cultivates self-empowerment and a sense of control over their disorder. These positive coping strategies also promote peaceful acceptance of one's condition [84]. Such changes in daily psychological functioning can mark profound transitions for those with chronic pain disorders.

Complementary and Alternative Medicine and the Neurobiology of Placebo Analgesia

In addition to therapeutic modulation along the pain pathway, CAM's efficacy may also derive from activation of endogenous healing resources. Controlled clinical investigations of CAM regularly point to this trend, with trials showing that while many CAM therapies provide greater benefits than no-treatment groups, their effects are often indistinguishable from sham control groups. This trend has been most dramatically highlighted in four major German RCTs involving thousands of patients being treated for migraine [72], tension-type headache [77], low back pain [13], and osteoarthritis of the knee [110]. Subjects in these studies were randomized to receive either genuine acupuncture, a sham control treatment, or assignment to a no-treatment wait-list control. Of these four trials, only the knee arthritis trial showed acupuncture to be superior to sham acupuncture. In the other three trials, in which the outcomes for verum and sham acupuncture were essentially the same, both were dramatically superior to the wait-list control. Some attribute this finding to lack of acupuncture point specificity. (Notably, within many pharmaceutical drug RCTs, the benefits of real interventions frequently have proven indistinguishable from the benefits of placebo interventions as well [32,103].)

An emerging field of "placebo research" is also trying to account for these interesting trends. Researchers are discovering the therapeutic value of several nonspecific components of the healing encounter, most notably patient expectations and an optimized doctor-patient relationship, which can benefit chronic pain patients with and without accompanying mental illnesses. Pooling data from the four German trials mentioned above, a recent meta-analysis compared patient expectations with treatment outcome to show that a positive attitude toward acupuncture and expected improvement predicted positive benefit from both verum and sham acupuncture [73].

A recent placebo study on IBS patients experimentally demonstrated the heightened benefits of a positive doctor-patient interaction [53]. Patients were divided into a wait-list group, a group receiving "limited" placebo acupuncture treatment administered by a neutral practitioner, and a group receiving an "augmented" placebo acupuncture treatment administered by a warm and attentive practitioner. Results showed graded result across the groups, with the augmented placebo group reporting the greatest benefits in overall improvements, adequate relief, symptom severity, and quality of life.

On the whole, the effects of both CAM and conventional therapies are enhanced by nonspecific effects, but CAM therapies might be better positioned to maximize these endogenous healing responses in patients suffering from functional pain disorders. In conventional treatment, diagnosis of a functional pain disorder is often accompanied by dismal expectations. Practitioners know the limitations of current biomedical therapies, and some may explicitly or implicitly communicate this pessimistic information to patients. In contrast, CAM practitioners often administer their therapies with an atmosphere of optimism and hope (whether warranted or not). Novel CAM therapies for which patients have no prior experience or positive or negative conditioning may be particularly successful at raising therapeutic expectations. CAM's valuing of "holism" or attention to the "whole patient" may also translate into a closer relationship between practitioner and patient. During treatment, CAM patients are often allowed to discuss their ailment at length, while receiving the sustained, empathetic attention of the practitioner. This hope, optimism, patience, and attention afforded by CAM therapies might induce real therapeutic effects.

How nonspecific effects of CAM therapies mechanistically translate into healing remains an interesting question. Until recently, understanding of placebo analgesia was primarily based on psychological theories, but now physiological definitions of placebo analgesia have begun to emerge.

A Anterior Insula

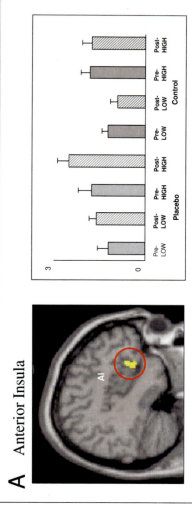

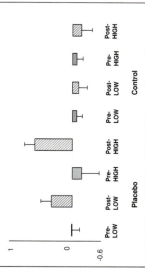

B Rostral Anterior Cingulate

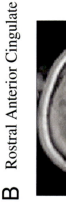

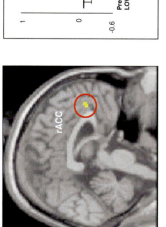

Fig. 2. Representative brain regions activated by expectancy-enhanced sham acupuncture. When comparing PRE- and POST-treatment brain activity for sham acupuncture administered on placebo and control sides for HIGH and LOW pain, increases occurred in (A) the anterior insula, a pain-responsive region (activation by HIGH pain is greater than LOW pain for pretreatment on both placebo and control sides; on the placebo but not control side, there is *greater* activity in the region despite a report of *less* pain), and (B) the rostral anterior cingulate cortex (rACC), a region that is not activated by pain, but is recruited during expectancy-induced analgesia. Adapted from [57]. The bar graphs show peak activation of each region for the fMRI contrast.

These neurobiological insights began with Levine and colleagues' finding [71] that placebo analgesia can be reversed by naloxone, an opioid antagonist. Subsequent experiments by Benedetti, Amanzio, and colleagues [2,6,7] provide validating evidence for the role of endogenous opioids in placebo analgesia. However, other studies show that placebo analgesia can occur without the involvement of endogenous opioids [1,41]. Such work suggests that multiple mechanisms underlie the phenomenon of placebo analgesia. It is speculated that placebo treatment can target the source of noxious information, the various mechanisms of pain sensation evaluation, or both processes [58]. Furthermore, the proportion of activity in these different neural circuits probably depends on circumstance, and it may even vary across different individuals.

Use of neuroimaging tools has provided new insight into the placebo effect [10,90,105,113]. For instance, Wager et al. found that after experimentally manipulating subjects to expect a positive outcome from a sham analgesia cream treatment, fMRI signal decreased in pain-sensitive regions, such as the thalamus, insula, and ACC, and increased in the dorsolateral prefrontal cortex [105]. A subsequent study by Kong et al., using a comparable paradigm for enhancing expectation from sham acupuncture, detected increased, not decreased, activations in pain-signaling regions including the right anterior insula, as well as activation in the bilateral rostral ACC (Fig. 2), regions associated with cognitive modulation of pain perception [57]. These diverse results suggest that placebo analgesia may be configured through multiple brain pathways and mechanisms.

Conclusion

A review of the research literature suggests that CAM therapies hold considerable therapeutic promise for treatment of functional pain disorders. Through the modulation of sensory experience, attention, and affect, some CAM therapies may be able to reverse maladaptive plasticity in networks of pain-related brain regions and improve pain-related cortical and affective functioning. Given what we know about the multifaceted presentation of pain, multimodal therapies that activate innate healing resources and address psychosocial as well physical aspects, while engendering positive expectations, seem well suited to address the complexity of functional pain disorders. However, further research is required to verify the effectiveness of these modalities and elucidate the role of placebo effects in CAM.

Acknowledgments

The authors would like to thank Dr. Ted Kaptchuk for his helpful discussions. Funding for this work came from: NIH (NCCAM) R21AT00949 to Randy Gollub, PO1-AT002048 to Project 3 Randy Gollub, KO1AT003883 to Jian Kong, K01-AT002166 to Vitaly Napadow, M01-RR-001066 for Mallinckrodt General Clinical Research Center Biomedical Imaging Core, and P41RR14075 for Center for Functional Neuroimaging Technologies from NCRR.

References

[1]   Amanzio M, Benedetti F. Neuropharmacological dissection of placebo analgesia: expectation-activated opioid systems versus conditioning-activated specific subsystems. J Neurosci 1999;19:484–94.
[2]   Amanzio M, Pollo A, Maggi G, Benedetti F. Response variability to analgesics: a role for nonspecific activation of endogenous opioids. Pain 2001;90:205–15.
[3]   Apkarian AV, Bushnell MC, Treede RD, Zubieta JK. Human brain mechanisms of pain perception and regulation in health and disease. Eur J Pain 2005;9:463–84.
[4]   Baliki MN, Apkarian AV. Neurological effects of chronic pain. J Pain Palliat Care Pharmacother 2007;21:59–61.
[5]   Baskin DS, Mehler WR, Hosobuchi Y, Richardson DE, Adams JE, Flitter MA. Autopsy analysis of the safety, efficacy and cartography of electrical stimulation of the central gray in humans. Brain Res 1986;371:231–6.
[6]   Benedetti F, Amanzio M, Baldi S, Casadio C, Maggi G. Inducing placebo respiratory depressant responses in humans via opioid receptors. Eur J Neurosci 1999;11:625–31.
[7]   Benedetti F, Arduino C, Amanzio M. Somatotopic activation of opioid systems by target-directed expectations of analgesia. J Neurosci 1999;19:3639–48.
[8]   Benedetti F, Mayberg HS, Wager TD, Stohler CS, Zubieta JK. Neurobiological mechanisms of the placebo effect. J Neurosci 2005;25:10390–402.
[9]   Benson H, Klipper MZ. The relaxation response. Avon Books; 1976.
[10] Bingel U, Lorenz J, Schoell E, Weiller C, Buchel C. Mechanisms of placebo analgesia: rACC recruitment of a subcortical antinociceptive network. Pain 2006;120:8–15.
[11] Bonadonna R. Meditation's impact on chronic illness. Holist Nurs Pract 2003;17:309–19.
[12] Brattberg G. Connective tissue massage in the treatment of fibromyalgia. Eur J Pain 1999;3:235–44.
[13] Brinkhaus B, Witt CM, Jena S, Linde K, Streng A, Wagenpfeil S, Irnich D, Walther HU, Melchart D, Willich SN. Acupuncture in patients with chronic low back pain: a randomized controlled trial. Arch Intern Med 2006;166:450–7.
[14] Buckner RL, Vincent JL. Unrest at rest: default activity and spontaneous network correlations. Neuroimage 2007;37:1091–6.
[15] Cardoso R, de Souza E, Camano L, Leite JR. Meditation in health: an operational definition. Brain Res Brain Res Protoc 2004;14:58–60.

[16] Carlsson CP, Sjolund BH. Acupuncture for chronic low back pain: a randomized placebo-controlled study with long-term follow-up. Clin J Pain 2001;17:296–305.

[17] Carson JW, Keefe FJ, Lynch TR, Carson KM, Goli V, Fras AM, Thorp SR. Loving-kindness meditation for chronic low back pain: results from a pilot trial. J Holist Nurs 2005;23:287–304.

[18] Chen R, Nickel JC. Acupuncture ameliorates symptoms in men with chronic prostatitis/chronic pelvic pain syndrome. Urology 2003;61:1156–9.

[19] Citak-Karakaya I, Akbayrak T, Demirturk F, Ekici G, Bakar Y. Short and long-term results of connective tissue manipulation and combined ultrasound therapy in patients with fibromyalgia. J Manipulative Physiol Ther 2006;29:524–8.

[20] Colloca L, Benedetti F. Placebos and painkillers: is mind as real as matter? Nat Rev Neurosci 2005 6:545–52.

[21] Cook DB, Lange G, Ciccone DS, Liu WC, Steffener J, Natelson BH. Functional imaging of pain in patients with primary fibromyalgia. J Rheumatol 2004;31:364–78.

[22] Cornel EB, van Haarst EP, Schaarsberg RW, Geels J. The effect of biofeedback physical therapy in men with chronic pelvic pain syndrome type III. Eur Urol 2005;47:607–11.

[23] Crider AB, Glaros AG. A meta-analysis of EMG biofeedback treatment of temporomandibular disorders. J Orofac Pain 1999;13:29–37.

[24] Cunningham C, Brown S, Kaski JC. Effects of transcendental meditation on symptoms and electrocardiographic changes in patients with cardiac syndrome X. Am J Cardiol 2000;85:653–5, A10.

[25] DeBar LL, Vuckovic N, Schneider J, Ritenbaugh C. Use of complementary and alternative medicine for temporomandibular disorders. J Orofac Pain 2003;17:224–36.

[26] deCharms RC, Maeda F, Glover GH, Ludlow D, Pauly JM, Soneji D, Gabrieli JD, Mackey SC. Control over brain activation and pain learned by using real-time functional MRI. Proc Natl Acad Sci USA 2005;102:18626–31.

[27] Devocht JW, Long CR, Zeitler DL, Schaeffer W. Chiropractic treatment of temporomandibular disorders using the activator adjusting instrument: a prospective case series. J Manipulative Physiol Ther 2003;26:421–5.

[28] Dhond RP, Kettner N, Napadow V. Neuroimaging acupuncture effects in the human brain. J Altern Complement Med 2007;13:603–16.

[29] Dhond RP, Yeh C, Park K, Kettner N, Napadow V. Acupuncture modulates resting state connectivity in default and sensorimotor brain networks. Pain 2008;136:407–18.

[30] Dougherty DD, Kong J, Webb JM, Bonab AA, Fischman AJ, Gollub RL. A combined [^{11}C]diprenorphine PET study and fMRI study of acupuncture analgesia. Behav Brain Res 2008; in press.

[31] Drexler AR, Mur EJ, Gunther VC. Efficacy of an EMG-biofeedback therapy in fibromyalgia patients. A comparative study of patients with and without abnormality in (MMPI) psychological scales. Clin Exp Rheumatol 2002;20:677–82.

[32] Fava M, Evins AE, Dorer DJ, Schoenfeld DA. The problem of the placebo response in clinical trials for psychiatric disorders: culprits, possible remedies, and a novel study design approach. Psychother Psychosom 2003;72:115–27.

[33] Field T, Diego M, Cullen C, Hernandez-Reif M, Sunshine W, Douglas S. Fibromyalgia pain and substance P decrease and sleep improves after massage therapy. J Clin Rheumatol 2002;8:72–6.

[34] Flor H. Cortical reorganisation and chronic pain: implications for rehabilitation. J Rehabil Med 2003;66–72.

[35] Flor H, Braun C, Elbert T, Birbaumer N. Extensive reorganization of primary somatosensory cortex in chronic back pain patients. Neurosci Lett 1997;224:5–8.

[36] Galantino ML, Bzdewka TM, Eissler-Russo JL, Holbrook ML, Mogck EP, Geigle P, Farrar JT. The impact of modified Hatha yoga on chronic low back pain: a pilot study. Altern Ther Health Med 2004;10:56–9.

[37] Gardea MA, Gatchel RJ, Mishra KD. Long-term efficacy of biobehavioral treatment of temporomandibular disorders. J Behav Med 2001;24:341–59.

[38] Gebhart GF. Descending modulation of pain. Neurosci Biobehav Rev 2004;27:729–37.

[39] Giesecke T, Gracely RH, Grant MA, Nachemson A, Petzke F, Williams DA, Clauw DJ. Evidence of augmented central pain processing in idiopathic chronic low back pain. Arthritis Rheum 2004;50:613–23.

[40] Glazer HI, Rodke G, Swencionis C, Hertz R, Young AW. Treatment of vulvar vestibulitis syndrome with electromyographic biofeedback of pelvic floor musculature. J Reprod Med 1995;40:283–90.

[41] Gracely RH, Dubner R, Wolskee PJ, Deeter WR. Placebo and naloxone can alter post-surgical pain by separate mechanisms. Nature 1983;306:264–5.

[42] Gracely RH, Petzke F, Wolf JM, Clauw DJ. Functional magnetic resonance imaging evidence of augmented pain processing in fibromyalgia. Arthritis Rheum 2002;46:1333–43.

[43] Grossman P, Niemann L, Schmidt S, Walach H. Mindfulness-based stress reduction and health benefits. A meta-analysis. J Psychosom Res 2004;57:35–43.

[44] Gudavalli MR, Cambron JA, McGregor M, Jedlicka J, Keenum M, Ghanayem AJ, Patwardhan AG. A randomized clinical trial and subgroup analysis to compare flexion-distraction with active exercise for chronic low back pain. Eur Spine J 2006;15:1070–82.

[45] Haak T, Scott B. The effect of qigong on fibromyalgia (FMS): a controlled randomized study. Disabil Rehabil 2007;1–9.

[46] Haake M, Muller HH, Schade-Brittinger C, Basler HD, Schafer H, Maier C, Endres HG, Trampisch HJ, Molsberger A. German acupuncture trials (GERAC) for chronic low back pain: randomized, multicenter, blinded, parallel-group trial with 3 groups. Arch Intern Med 2007;167:1892–8.

[47] Haas M, Groupp E, Kraemer DF. Dose-response for chiropractic care of chronic low back pain. Spine J 2004;4:574–83.

[48] Hosobuchi Y, Adams JE, Linchitz R. Pain relief by electrical stimulation of the central gray matter in humans and its reversal by naloxone. Science 1977;197:183–6.

[49] Hui KK, Liu J, Makris N, Gollub RL, Chen AJ, Moore CI, Kennedy DN, Rosen BR, Kwong KK. Acupuncture modulates the limbic system and subcortical gray structures of the human brain: evidence from fMRI studies in normal subjects. Hum Brain Mapp 2000;9:13–25.

[50] Jensen MP, Hakimian S, Sherlin LH, Fregni F. New insights into neuromodulatory approaches for the treatment of pain. J Pain 2008;9:193–9.

[51] Kabat-Zinn J. An outpatient program in behavioral medicine for chronic pain patients based on the practice of mindfulness meditation: theoretical considerations and preliminary results. Gen Hosp Psychiatry 1982;4:33–47.

[52] Kaplan KH, Goldenberg DL, Galvin-Nadeau M. The impact of a meditation-based stress reduction program on fibromyalgia. Gen Hosp Psychiatry 1993;15:284–9.

[53] Kaptchuk TJ, Kelley JM, Conboy LA, Davis RB, Kerr CE, Jacobson EE, Kirsch I, Schyner RN, Nam BH, Nguyen LT, et al. Components of placebo effect: randomised controlled trial in patients with irritable bowel syndrome. BMJ 2008;

[54] Kayiran S, Dursun E, Ermutlu N, Dursun N, Karamursel S. Neurofeedback in fibromyalgia syndrome. Agri 2007;19:47–53.

[55] Keefer L, Blanchard EB. The effects of relaxation response meditation on the symptoms of irritable bowel syndrome: results of a controlled treatment study. Behav Res Ther 2001;39:801–11.

[56] Kong J, Gollub R, Huang T, Polich G, Napadow V, Hui K, Vangel M, Rosen B, Kaptchuk TJ. Acupuncture de qi, from qualitative history to quantitative measurement. J Altern Complement Med 2007;13:1059–70.

[57] Kong J, Gollub RL, Rosman IS, Webb JM, Vangel MG, Kirsch I, Kaptchuk TJ. Brain activity associated with expectancy-enhanced placebo analgesia as measured by functional magnetic resonance imaging. J Neurosci 2006;26:381–8.

[58] Kong J, Kaptchuk TJ, Polich G, Kirsch I, Gollub RL. Placebo analgesia: findings from brain imaging studies and emerging hypotheses. Rev Neurosci 2007;18:173–90.

[59] Kong J, Kaptchuk TJ, Webb JM, Kong JT, Sasaki Y, Polich GR, Vangel MG, Kwong K, Rosen B, Gollub RL. Functional neuroanatomical investigation of vision-related acupuncture point specificity: a multisession fMRI study. Hum Brain Mapp 2007; Epub Nov 7.

[60] Kong J, Ma L, Gollub RL, Wei J, Yang X, Li D, Weng X, Jia F, Wang C, Li F, Li R, Zhuang D. A pilot study of functional magnetic resonance imaging of the brain during manual and electroacupuncture stimulation of acupuncture point (LI-4 Hegu) in normal subjects reveals differential brain activation between methods. J Altern Complement Med 2002;8:411–9.

[61] Kong J, White NS, Kwong KK, Vangel MG, Rosman IS, Gracely RH, Gollub RL. Using fMRI to dissociate sensory encoding from cognitive evaluation of heat pain intensity. Hum Brain Mapp 2006;27:715–21.

526

G. Polich et al.

[62] Kuttner L, Chambers CT, Hardial J, Israel DM, Jacobson K, Evans K. A randomized trial of yoga for adolescents with irritable bowel syndrome. Pain Res Manag 2006;11:217–23.
[63] Kwan CL, Diamant NE, Pope G, Mikula K, Mikulis DJ, Davis KD. Abnormal forebrain activity in functional bowel disorder patients with chronic pain. Neurology 2005;65:1268–77.
[64] Langevin HM, Bouffard NA, Churchill DL, Badger GJ. Connective tissue fibroblast response to acupuncture: dose-dependent effect of bidirectional needle rotation. J Altern Complement Med 2007;13:355–60.
[65] Langevin HM, Sherman KJ. Pathophysiological model for chronic low back pain integrating connective tissue and nervous system mechanisms. Med Hypotheses 2007;68:74–80.
[66] Langevin HM, Yandow JA. Relationship of acupuncture points and meridians to connective tissue planes. Anat Rec 2002;269:257–65.
[67] Lawal A, Kern M, Sidhu H, Hofmann C, Shaker R. Novel evidence for hypersensitivity of visceral sensory neural circuitry in irritable bowel syndrome patients. Gastroenterology 2006;130:26–33.
[68] Lazar SW, Kerr CE, Wasserman RH, Gray JR, Greve DN, Treadway MT, McGarvey M, Quinn BT, Dusek JA, Benson H, et al. Meditation experience is associated with increased cortical thickness. Neuroreport 2005;16:1893–7.
[69] Le Bars D, Dickenson AH, Besson JM. Opiate analgesia and descending control systems In: Bonica JJ, Lindblom U, Iggo A, editors. Advances in pain research and therapy. New York: Raven Press; 1983. p. 341–72.
[70] Lee SW, Liong ML, Yuen KH, Leong WS, Chee C, Cheah PY, Choong WP, Wu Y, Khan N, Choong WL, Yap HW, Krieger JN. Acupuncture versus sham acupuncture for chronic prostatitis/chronic pelvic pain. Am J Med 2008;121:79.e1–7.
[71] Levine JD, Gordon NC, Fields HL. The mechanism of placebo analgesia. Lancet 1978;2:654–7.
[72] Linde K, Streng A, Jurgens S, Hoppe A, Brinkhaus B, Witt C, Wagenpfeil S, Pfaffenrath V, Hammes MG, Weidenhammer W, et al. Acupuncture for patients with migraine: a randomized controlled trial. J Altern Complement Med 2005;293:2118–25.
[73] Linde K, Witt CM, Streng A, Weidenhammer W, Wagenpfeil S, Brinkhaus B, Willich SN, Melchart D. The impact of patient expectations on outcomes in four randomized controlled trials of acupuncture in patients with chronic pain. Pain 2007;128:264–71.
[74] Liu WC, Feldman SC, Cook DB, Hung DL, Xu T, Kalnin AJ, Komisaruk BR. fMRI study of acupuncture-induced periaqueductal gray activity in humans. Neuroreport 2004;15:1937–40.
[75] Maihofner C, Handwerker HO, Neundorfer B, Birklein F. Patterns of cortical reorganization in complex regional pain syndrome. Neurology 2003;61:1707–15.
[76] Manheimer E, White A, Berman B, Forys K, Ernst E. Meta-analysis: acupuncture for low back pain. Ann Intern Med 2005;142:651–63.
[77] Melchart D, Streng A, Hoppe A, Brinkhaus B, Witt C, Wagenpfeil S, Pfaffenrath V, Hammes M, Hummelsberger J, Irnich D, et al. Acupuncture in patients with tension-type headache: randomised controlled trial. BMJ 2005;331:376–82.
[78] Melzack R. Folk Medicine and the sensory modulation of pain. In: Wall PD, Melzack R, editors. Textbook of pain. London: Churchill Livingstone; 1994. p. 1209–17.
[79] Melzack R. From the gate to the neuromatrix. Pain 1999;Suppl 6:S121–6.
[80] Meng CF, Wang D, Ngeow J, Lao L, Peterson M, Paget S. Acupuncture for chronic low back pain in older patients: a randomized, controlled trial. Rheumatology (Oxford) 2003;42:1508–17.
[81] Mills WW, Farrow JT. The transcendental meditation technique and acute experimental pain. Psychosom Med 1981;43:157–64.
[82] Morone NE, Greco CM, Weiner DK. Mindfulness meditation for the treatment of chronic low back pain in older adults: a randomized controlled pilot study. Pain 2008;134:310–9.
[83] Nadler RB. Bladder training biofeedback and pelvic floor myalgia. Urology 2002;60:42–3; discussion 4.
[84] Naliboff BD, Frese MP, Rapgay L. Mind/body psychological treatments for irritable bowel syndrome. Evid Based Complement Alternat Med 2008;5:41–50.
[85] Napadow V, Dhond RP, Purdon P, Kettner N, Makris N, Kwong KK, Hui KKS. Correlating acupuncture fMRI in the human brainstem with heart rate variability. Conf Proc IEEE Eng Med Biol Soc 2005; 5:4496–9.
[86] Napadow V, Kettner N, Ryan A, Kwong KK, Audette J, Hui KK. Somatosensory cortical plasticity in carpal tunnel syndrome: a cross-sectional fMRI evaluation. Neuroimage 2006;31:520–30.

[87] Napadow V, Liu J, Li M, Kettner N, Ryan A, Kwong KK, Hui KK, Audette JF. Somatosensory cortical plasticity in carpal tunnel syndrome treated by acupuncture. Hum Brain Mapp 2007;28:159–71.
[88] Newton-John TR, Spence SH, Schotte D. Cognitive-behavioural therapy versus EMG biofeedback in the treatment of chronic low back pain. Behav Res Ther 1995;33:691–7.
[89] Orme-Johnson DW, Schneider RH, Son YD, Nidich S, Cho ZH. Neuroimaging of meditation's effect on brain reactivity to pain. Neuroreport 2006;17:1359–63.
[90] Petrovic P, Kalso E, Petersson KM, Ingvar M. Placebo and opioid analgesia: imaging a shared neuronal network. Science 2002;295:1737–40.
[91] Porreca F, Ossipov MH, Gebhart GF. Chronic pain and medullary descending facilitation. Trends Neurosci 2002;25:319–25.
[92] Raichle ME, MacLeod AM, Snyder AZ, Powers WJ, Gusnard DA, Shulman GL. A default mode of brain function. Proc Natl Acad Sci USA 2001;98:676–82.
[93] Seminowicz DA, Mikulis DJ, Davis KD. Cognitive modulation of pain-related brain responses depends on behavioral strategy. Pain 2004;112:48–58.
[94] Sephton SE, Salmon P, Weissbecker I, Ulmer C, Floyd A, Hoover K, Studts JL. Mindfulness meditation alleviates depressive symptoms in women with fibromyalgia: results of a randomized clinical trial. Arthritis Rheum 2007;57:77–85.
[95] Sherman KJ, Cherkin DC, Connelly MT, Erro J, Savetsky JB, Davis RB, Eisenberg DM. Complementary and alternative medical therapies for chronic low back pain: what treatments are patients willing to try? BMC Complement Altern Med 2004;4:9.
[96] Smith P, Mosscrop D, Davies S, Sloan P, Al-Ani Z. The efficacy of acupuncture in the treatment of temporomandibular joint myofascial pain: a randomised controlled trial. J Dent 2007;35:259–67.
[97] Tan G, Craine MH, Bair MJ, Garcia MK, Giordano J, Jensen MP, McDonald SM, Patterson D, Sherman RA, Williams W, Tsao JC. Efficacy of selected complementary and alternative medicine interventions for chronic pain. J Rehabil Res Dev 2007;44:195–222.
[98] Taneja I, Deepak KK, Poojary G, Acharya IN, Pandey RM, Sharma MP. Yogic versus conventional treatment in diarrhea-predominant irritable bowel syndrome: a randomized control study. Appl Psychophysiol Biofeedback 2004;29:19–33.
[99] Thomas KJ, MacPherson H, Thorpe L, Brazier J, Fitter M, Campbell MJ, Roman M, Walters SJ, Nicholl J. Randomised controlled trial of a short course of traditional acupuncture compared with usual care for persistent non-specific low back pain. BMJ 2006;333:623.
[100] Tracey I, Mantyh PW. The cerebral signature for pain perception and its modulation. Neuron 2007;55:377–91.
[101] Tsao JC. Effectiveness of massage therapy for chronic, non-malignant pain: a review. Evid Based Complement Alternat Med 2007;4:165–79.
[102] Turk DC. Clinical effectiveness and cost-effectiveness of treatments for patients with chronic pain. Clin J Pain 2002;18:355–65.
[103] Turner EH, Matthews AM, Linardatos E, Tell RA, Rosenthal R. Selective publication of antidepressant trials and its influence on apparent efficacy. N Eng J Med 2008;358:252–60.
[104] Verne GN, Himes NC, Robinson ME, Gopinath KS, Briggs RW, Crosson B, Price DD. Central representation of visceral and cutaneous hypersensitivity in the irritable bowel syndrome. Pain 2003;103:99–110.
[105] Wager TD, Rilling JK, Smith EE, Sokolik A, Casey KL, Davidson RJ, Kosslyn SM, Rose RM, Cohen JD. Placebo-induced changes in FMRI in the anticipation and experience of pain. Science 2004;303:1162–7.
[106] Wahner-Roedler DL, Elkin PL, Vincent A, Thompson JM, Oh TH, Loehrer LL, Mandrekar JN, Bauer BA. Use of complementary and alternative medical therapies by patients referred to a fibromyalgia treatment program at a tertiary care center. Mayo Clin Proc 2005;80:55–60.
[107] White A. Neurophysiology of acupuncture analgesia. In: Ernst E, White A, editors. Acupuncture: a scientific appraisal. Oxford: Reed Educational and Professional Publishing; 1999. p. 60–92.
[108] Wiech K, Seymour B, Kalisch R, Stephan KE, Koltzenburg M, Driver J, Dolan RJ. Modulation of pain processing in hyperalgesia by cognitive demand. Neuroimage 2005;27:59–69.
[109] Williams KA, Petronis J, Smith D, Goodrich D, Wu J, Ravi N, Doyle EJ Jr, Gregory Juckett R, Munoz Kolar M, Gross R, Steinberg L. Effect of Iyengar yoga therapy for chronic low back pain. Pain 2005;115:107–17.

[110] Witt C, Brinkhaus B, Jena S, Linde K, Streng A, Wagenpfeil S, Hummelsberger J, Walther HU, Melchart D, Willich SN. Acupuncture in patients with osteoarthritis of the knee: a randomised trial. Lancet 2005;366:136–43.

[111] Wooton J. Meditation and chronic pain. In: Audette J, Bailey A, editors. Integrative pain medicine: the science and practice of complementary and alternative medicine in pain management. Totowa: Humana Press; 2008. p. 195–209.

[112] Zhuo M. Cortical excitation and chronic pain. Trends Neurosci 2008;31:199–207.

[113] Zubieta JK, Bueller JA, Jackson LR, Scott DJ, Xu Y, Koeppe RA, Nichols TE, Stohler CS. Placebo effects mediated by endogenous opioid activity on mu-opioid receptors. J Neurosci 2005;25:7754–62.

Correspondence to: Randy Gollub, MD, PhD, Psychiatry Department, Massachusetts General Hospital, Building 149, 13th Street, Suite 2660, Charlestown, MA 02129, USA. Tel: 1-617-724-9602; fax: 1-617-726-4078; email: rgollub@partners.org.

Part VII

Synthesis

Functional Pain Disorders: Time for a Paradigm Shift?

Emeran A. Mayer[a] and M. Catherine Bushnell[b]

[a]Center for Neurobiology of Stress, Departments of Medicine, Physiology and Psychiatry, David Geffen School of Medicine, UCLA, Los Angeles, California, USA; [b]McGill Alan Edwards Centre for Research on Pain, Departments of Anesthesiology, Dentistry and Neurology, McGill University, Montreal, Quebec, Canada

A major aim of this book is to challenge the traditional concept of a multitude of unrelated, individual functional pain syndromes, which are the "property" of different medical and surgical subspecialties, represented by different patient organizations, investigated by funding coming from separate government funding agencies, and for which therapies are developed by distinct divisions within major pharmaceutical companies. There are legitimate historical reasons for each of the listed stakeholders to view individual syndromes as unique, separate disorders: for medical and surgical subspecialties, affected patients make up a significant portion of their practices and procedures; for patient advocacy organizations, the legitimization of symptoms as real (rather than imagined or psychological) requires the assignment of individual syndromes into medical and surgical (rather than psychiatric and psychological) subspecialties. Political pressure exerted by patient advocacy organizations on the leadership of different divisions of the U.S. National Institutes of Health and other research funding organizations has resulted into the silo model of research funding. This traditional separation into presumed end-organ-specific syndromes is deeply entrenched and defended by stakeholders in the health care profession as well as by affected patients. Nevertheless, the striking failure to develop novel and cost-effective treatments, together with emerging breakthroughs in the neurobiological understanding of these complex, symptom-based syndromes, have begun to challenge the old concepts and fostered the gradual acceptance of a more global view of these disorders.

This chapter synthesizes many of the recurring themes discussed in the individual chapters by (1) addressing the major differences in clinical presentation; (2) discussing the evidence supporting overlap and shared features; and (3) proposing a general conceptual neurobiological model that can incorporate many of the individual features of these syndromes, including both peripheral and central disease mechanisms.

Differences between Syndromes: The Specific End-Organ Concept

The main difference between individual syndromes is the fact that patients refer their predominant symptoms to different target organs. This concept has been supported by different types of reasoning. Elaborate systems of symptom-based classification have been developed for many of the syndromes, and these definitions (analogous to the DSM classification in psychiatry) have created a false framework of distinct syndromes, with specific end-organ-related pathophysiologies. By focusing on end-organ-specific symptoms while dismissing the other clinical manifestations as secondary "comorbidities," medical and surgical subspecialists have legitimized their respective approaches and have rejected a unifying view of all syndromes. However, many of the symptom-based constructs are not stable over time [38], and symptoms may manifest as different syndromes during the life of a patient while subthreshold symptoms of other syndromes are ignored. Despite studies demonstrating the instability of symptom-based syndromes over time, and the anecdotal reports from the astute clinician who obtains a history of other symptoms or syndromes preceding the index syndrome, there is only limited information to answer the question of how symptoms evolve over the patient's life. As long as we rely on cross-sectional studies for characterization of the index syndrome and comorbidities and ignore their temporal dimension, we will not understand whether there is a common underlying substrate shared by all disorders, which manifests as an apparent end-organ-specific syndrome later in life.

In a small number of patients, the onset of symptoms can be traced (generally retrospectively or less often prospectively) to a specific event and to an organ-specific site. The onset of irritable bowel syndrome (IBS) symptoms following a documented gastroenteric infection in about 10% of all patients (Chapter 17), the onset of fibromyalgia (FM) (Chapter 2) or chronic low back pain (Chapter 3) following a documented injury, or the onset of symptoms of interstitial cystitis/painful bladder syndrome (IC/PBS) following a urinary tract infection (Chapter 8). The problem with this argument is that the main risk factors for each of these clinical presentations include the presence of multiple somatic complaints (unrelated to the specific organ-related complaints) in an individual prior to the onset of the environmentally triggered syndrome, and that psychosocial factors (including major life events, trait anxiety, depression, and somatization) are some of the best predictors of symptom development (Chapter 17). In an attempt to attribute the new group of symptoms to a "legitimate," organic disorder, patients (and frequently investigators) ignore the preceding history and the risk factors around the time of the incident, and refer to the incident as the only causative factor.

In some patients, sophisticated diagnostic techniques have demonstrated biological or structural end-organ alterations, which are used as evidence that these changes play a causative role in symptom severity. However, as repeatedly illustrated by the poor correlation of such changes in chronic nonspecific low back pain (Chapter 3), in IBS [17], and in IC/PBS [39], such "biomarkers" cannot be considered the primary cause for any of these syndromes. Alternatively, non-specific changes such as increased mast cell counts in the urinary bladder or in the colon may be secondary manifestations of chronic alterations in autonomic control of these organs [30].

In some patients, there is significant improvement of symptoms following an end-organ-directed surgical or pharmacological therapy. The problem is the lack of high-quality randomized controlled clinical trials to support many of these claims, and in general it cannot be ruled out that the improvement is due to a placebo effect. This is of particular relevance for such invasive procedures as spine surgeries, implantation of electrical stimulators, or bladder overdistensions, which rarely can be evaluated in a placebo-controlled study. Nevertheless, it is conceivable that in a subset of patients with other risk factors to develop a chronic pain syndrome, organ-related pathologies (disk degeneration, latent bladder infections, altered intestinal microflora, mechanical temporomandibular joint changes) or a history of an acute organ-related injury may be required to produce the full clinical syndrome.

Before we can definitively answer the question of one or many syndromes, many gaps in our knowledge remain to be filled. For example, the question regarding the natural history and evolution of symptoms in a vulnerable individual can only be investigated in a long-term longitudinal study monitoring not just a particular syndrome, but the whole spectrum of symptoms from other functional pain disorders and affective disorders. For example, in the pediatric population, do symptoms of anxiety and depression precede the first onset of abdominal pain or vice versa? [14] Can these disorders be considered as part of a spectrum ("affective spectrum disorders") reflecting various degrees of breakdown of homeostatic mechanisms related to pain perception and general mental and physical well-being? More specifically, is there a severity and frequency gradient or progression of syndromes, with most individuals being affected by the mildest, least disruptive, and most easily treatable syndromes (stage I), and a progressively smaller number being affected by more severe syndromes (stage II)? Such a scenario would be reflected by patients at stage I showing the smallest prevalence of associated syndromes, with those at stage II showing the highest comorbidity. The prevalence figures of comorbid conditions shown in Table I of Chapter 6 might suggest that IBS could be considered one of the milder syndromes, because the prevalence of IBS in various other disorders appears to be higher than the presence of symptoms from other functional pain disorders in IBS patients. Future, more rigorously controlled studies should address this hypothesis.

In summary, the rationale and scientific evidence provided to support the specific end-organ model of chronic functional pain syndromes is weak, and it is unlikely to fully explain these syndromes in the majority of patients. This does not rule out the involvement of peripheral organs in "brain-body loops" (discussed in Chapter 14), where autonomically mediated (or HPA-axis-driven) changes in a specific organ may play a role in the maintenance of a chronic syndrome (see also the discussion at the end of this chapter). Major gaps in our knowledge of the natural history of these syndromes need to be addressed before a definitive answer can be given to the question of "one syndrome or many?"

Shared Epidemiological, Clinical, and Biological Features

Epidemiological and Clinical Features

Overlap of Patient and Healthy Populations

Most functional pain syndromes, as defined by symptom criteria, show a lack of a distinct boundary between the large number of healthy individuals in the general population who have experienced characteristic symptoms transiently, and the population in which characteristic chronic symptoms are present but are not severe enough, or do not interfere with an individual's quality of life sufficiently for this person to seek medical or surgical care. This situation is similar to findings with symptom-based psychiatric diagnoses, where it has been suggested that most psychopathology can be viewed as quantitative deviation along continuous trait dimensions that merge imperceptibly from "normalcy" into the "pathological" range [5]. It is only a minority of symptomatic individuals who seek health care, and an even smaller number who consult a subspecialist. Patient advocacy organizations as well as the pharmaceutical industry have generally emphasized the much larger number of individuals who meet symptom criteria (patients and nonpatients), rather than focusing on the smaller subset who consult a physician for these symptoms. Should the first category be considered healthy individuals, and only individuals in the second category be considered as having a clinical syndrome?

In terms of research and treatment, it may be less important to understand the physiology of symptoms in healthy individuals who never consult a physician, and more crucial to focus on the factors and mechanisms that underlie the transition to becoming a chronic patient. While the former (primary risk) factors may have more to do with differences in viscerosomatic sensitivity, peripheral and central sensitization, limbic system responsiveness, or autonomic nervous system activity, the latter (secondary risk) factors are likely to be shared across all the syndromes. These shared secondary risk factors may include such neurocognitive and uniquely human factors as selective attention to bodily sensations, catastrophizing, and symptom-related worries and illness behavior, in addition to psychological stressors. In contrast to the traditional view of the medical establishment and of many patients, who view such factors as psychological and not real (compared to "real," "organic" causes), cognitive neuroscience has made tremendous progress in identifying the neurobiological substrate of such neurocognitive factors. While primary risk factors may be primarily related to early gene-environment interactions and their influence on general stress responsiveness and homeostatic mechanisms (and may be modeled fairly accurately in various animal models), secondary risk factors may be more related to the shaping of prefrontal, neurocognitive mechanisms by the parental, cultural, and medical environment, including the medicalization of symptoms into distinct syndromes [3, 62]. Animal models for such factors generally do not exist.

Greater Prevalence in Women

Experts generally agree that in both population-based studies and patient-based studies, women are more likely affected by most chronic functional pain conditions, including migraine, burning mouth, temporomandibular joint disorder (TMJD), IC/PBS, IBS, and FM [57]. The mechanisms underlying the greater vulnerability of women remains incompletely understood. Despite the generally greater pain sensitivity of female experimental animals, in humans it has been difficult to reconcile the apparent discrepancy between the relatively small, and sometimes contradictory, sex-related differences observed in experimental pain studies in healthy control subjects and the robust differences seen in the prevalence of many chronic pain disorders [57]. One may speculate that this discrepancy results in part from the dominance of neurocognitive mechanisms (and their possible sex-related differences) in determining chronic symptom-related behavior and clinical symptom severity, whereas acute experimental stimuli aimed at testing traditional spinothalamic pain pathways do not address the primary symptom-related pathology.

History of Adverse Early Life Events and Stress Sensitivity

As emphasized by many chapters in this volume, and discussed in detail in Chapter 21, a history of adverse early life events poses a significant risk factor for many chronic functional pain syndromes, as well as for commonly comorbid anxiety, depression, and somatization. Even though much less information is available in humans on the interaction between sex of the patient, adverse early life events, and genes, it is likely that such interactions could produce a phenotype that is more vulnerable and shows less resilience to a variety of adverse environmental influences, including chronic stress, trauma, and injury. Given the relatively high prevalence of early adverse life events in psychiatric and in functional pain disorder patients, and the high prevalence of such disorders, such a phenotype may have been selected in evolution for its survival advantage in a dangerous and hostile environment, in which selective attention to physical, potentially life-threatening danger, vigilance, and harm avoidance were highly adaptive. For females, such behavioral characteristics as "interrupting foraging at the glimpse of a potential predator behind a tree" [6] would not only be protective for the mother, but also greatly increase chances for the survival of the offspring.

For individuals with such a phenotype living in the developed world of the 21st century, in which the environment in general has become much safer in terms of physical threats to survival but has seen a dramatic increase in terms of chronic psychological stress, uncertainties, and worries, these traits have become maladaptive, resulting in the unintended consequences of chronic pain syndromes and affective disorders. Consistent with such an interpretation is the shared increased stress sensitivity of patients with functional pain disorders. Based on anecdotal evidence and limited studies, symptoms seem to be less sensitive to physical stress posed by natural disasters (earthquakes, fires), compared to such psychological stressors as divorce, loss of a loved one, or struggling with insurance companies over damages following a disaster (Chapter 2).

Comorbidity with Disorders of Mood and Affect

As addressed in many of the preceding chapters, all functional pain disorders show a higher comorbidity than would be expected by chance with anxiety disorders, post-traumatic stress disorder (PTSD), depression, and somatization (Chapters 9–12). For IBS, an earlier suggestion was that the apparently high comorbidity in specialty clinic patient populations was an artifact due to the greater health-care-seeking behavior and the self-selection of patients with comorbid psychiatric disease into specialty clinics [29]. However, other population-based studies have confirmed the high comorbidity of IBS-like symptoms and various psychiatric disorders [76]. Furthermore, even those patients who do not meet DSM-IV criteria for anxiety or depression generally show higher scores (often within the normal range) on questionnaires for symptoms of anxiety and depression than healthy control subjects. Also, patients may be free from psychiatric symptoms at the time of diagnosis of their functional pain syndrome, but may have a personal or family history of disorders of mood and affect.

Response to Centrally Acting Therapies

As reflected in the various chapters, there is general agreement that centrally targeted therapies, either pharmacological (Chapter 23) or nonpharmacological (Chapters 24, 25), are effective in a subset of patients with functional pain disorders, and that their effectiveness is not limited to patients with comorbid psychiatric symptoms (Chapter 23). The limited number of high-quality randomized controlled trials (RCTs) reported in different types of functional pain disorders makes it difficult to determine the percentage of responders and the effect size in responders. The evidence from high-quality RCTs may be best for FM in terms of nonselective serotonin-norepinephrine reuptake inhibitors (duloxetine, milnacipran) and for the calcium channel blocker pregabalin (see Chapters 2 and 23), while in many disorders the quality of evidence to support the effectiveness of low-dose tricyclic antidepressants, selective serotonin reuptake inhibitors (SSRIs), and anxiolytics is much weaker. Even in the case of

FM, only about a third of patients show improvement on pharmacological treatments. Even though trials evaluating the effectiveness of cognitive-behavioral therapy (CBT) have been criticized for the lack of true control groups, effect sizes are at least comparable to currently available drug therapies. There are no reported high-quality RCTs for combined therapy with CBT and centrally acting drugs.

Evidence for Shared Biological Mechanisms

Evidence for Altered Pain Perception and Processing

Hypersensitivity to experimental stimuli. As shown throughout the specific syndrome-related chapters of this book, one line of evidence for similarities between the multiple functional pain syndromes is that patients categorized as having each syndrome also show hypersensitivity to experimental pain stimuli, and sometimes even to nonpainful stimuli in other modalities, including olfaction, gustation, and audition. Studies have shown heightened perception of noxious thermal and mechanical stimulation for patients with IBS [75,87], FM [27,31,32,79], vulvodynia [70], TMJD [52], and chronic back pain [33,81]. Sensory amplification in auditory, olfactory or gustatory modalities have been documented in patients with FM and chronic back pain [31,79,81]. Further, similar sensory amplification has been documented for patients with chronic fatigue and with major depressive disorders [32,47,84].

Compromised diffuse noxious inhibitory control (DNIC). Some studies have used psychophysical tests to examine a possible dysfunction in pain inhibitory systems. DNIC is a modulatory system involving the descending inhibition of the processing of a noxious input by the presence of another noxious input. The perceptual correlate of DNIC is termed "counterirritation." The DNIC system has been identified in humans and animals and has been characterized physiologically in extensive rodent studies. Several studies have shown that individuals with functional pain disorders, including FM, IBS, and vulvodynia [43,48,49,83,87], have a reduced or absent DNIC response. Thus, accumulating evidence suggests that one possible common mechanism underlying diverse functional pain syndromes is a dysfunction in descending pain modulatory systems.

Evidence from brain imaging studies of altered pain processing and modulation. Functional brain imaging studies now show that when patients report increased pain sensitivity, this perception is reflected in stimulus-evoked brain activations. For example, functional magnetic resonance imaging studies in FM, back pain, IBS, and vulvodynia patients show increased neural activation in response to mechanical or thermal experimental pain stimuli [2,33,35,36,55,71,80]. Abnormal responses to anticipating pain are also seen in some patients with functional disorders [4]. Positron emission tomography radioligand studies in patients with FM and burning mouth syndrome have begun to reveal abnormalities in pain modulatory neurotransmitters, including forebrain opioid and dopamine systems [37,40,88,89].

Evidence of Structural Brain Abnormalities

A number of anatomical imaging studies now show that individuals with chronic low back pain, FM, IBS, or headache show changes in gray matter density or cortical thickness [54]. Although the specific areas affected vary from study to study, the general tendency is for patients to show a reduction in gray matter in regions associated with affective and cognitive responses and stress, including the frontal cortex, cingulate cortex, insular cortex, hippocampus, and perihippocampal gyrus. The structural brain abnormalities observed in patients with functional pain syndromes are similar to those observed with other stress-related disorders, such as PTSD [13,46], as well as in depressed patients [85].

Evidence of Altered Neurocognitive Function

Many FM patients describe themselves as having "fibro-fog," in which they have trouble thinking and remembering. Experimental studies support the idea that FM patients have cognitive deficits, and one study now shows that some of these deficits correlate with gray matter loss [34,50,51,65,82]. Similarly, patients with chronic low back pain show impairments on an emotional decision-making task [1], and IBS patients show verbal IQ deficits [28]. The cognitive deficits associated with chronic pain are similar to those associated with PTSD and depression [41,85]. Such deficits indicate that structural brain abnormalities associated with chronic pain conditions have a functional consequence. Further, they show the similarity in long-term effects of functional pain syndromes on the central nervous system (CNS), no matter what end organ is involved.

Evidence of Increased Activity in Central Arousal Circuits and Sympathetic Nervous System Activity

Epidemiological studies show that many individuals with functional pain disorders have a history of early childhood stressful events or childhood behavioral characteristics such as excessive shyness, anxiety, or phobias that would make them excessively reactive to potentially stressful events (see Chapter 20). Thus, enhanced stress responsiveness has been implicated as a potential mechanism contributing to the pathophysiology of a number of functional pain syndromes, including FM, IBS, and TMJD. The possible importance of stress in these syndromes links them even more closely mechanistically to PTSD, chronic fatigue, and depression. Enhanced stress responsiveness should be reflected in altered function of the sympathetic nervous system, and less consistently in the hypothalamic-pituitary-adrenal (HPA) axis, and such changes are apparent in functional pain syndromes. Chapter 14 describes, in detail, overlapping autonomic dysfunction in FM and chronic fatigue. Chapter 16 shows further how chronic stress can alter immune responsiveness, affecting both the peripheral end organ (e.g., the gut) and the CNS.

Evidence of Common Genetic Susceptibility

As described in Chapters 3 and 17, there is now accumulating evidence that genetic variations can influence pain amplification and psychological distress. In fact, a number of genes have now been identified that are associated with both pain sensitivity and complex psychiatric disorders such as depression, anxiety, and panic disorder. Based on the evidence that functional pain disorders share common underlying pathophysiological mechanisms, researchers expect that a set of functional genetic variants will be associated with comorbid functional pain disorders and related signs and symptoms. Research into the genetic basis of chronic pain disorders is in its infancy, and the complex nature of the disorders as well as indications that many genes are involved make such research difficult. Nevertheless, an understanding of gene-environment interactions that lead to devastating chronic pain states is a reasonable goal for the next decade.

Dissecting Complex Clinical Phenotypes into Neurobiological Intermediate Phenotypes

Nearly unnoticed by the field of functional pain disorders, major advances in conceptualizing complex symptom-based disorders has occurred in other fields of neuroscience, in particular in psychiatry [12,15,60]. These advances have been largely driven by the realization that better conceptual approaches are needed to understand complex symptom-based syndromes such as schizophrenia, autism, or depression. Fig. 1 illustrates the basic concepts of the endophenotype approach to dissecting the complex symptom-based syndrome of schizophrenia.

When these advances are applied to the field of functional pain disorders, it is expected that clinical syndromes will be seen to be caused by numerous genetic and environmental factors, each of which has small effects individually. These factors only result in full disease expression in a given individual if their combined effects cross a "threshold of liability." For example, despite the presence of vulnerability genes, the threshold for a particular functional pain syndrome (e.g. IBS, FM, or noncardiac chest pain) may not be crossed in a generation, if the necessary environmental cofactors (for example, injury, early life trauma, and major life stress) are not present. However, the same genes may result in the expression of a different functional (or psychiatric) syndrome such as TMJD, low back pain, or panic attacks. The genes involved are likely to affect multiple neural systems that subserve a number of gastrointestinal, urological, pain-processing, affective, and neurocognitive functions. This concept is of particular relevance for functional gastrointestinal (GI) disorders because the CNS and the enteric nervous system share a large number of signaling mechanisms, including monoaminergic and neuropeptide-based signaling systems. As nicely demonstrated by various transgenic animals related to the serotonin signaling system, knockdowns of the serotonin transporter (SERT) affect not only CNS function, but also intestinal motility and secretion and a variety of seemingly unrelated physiological functions [63].

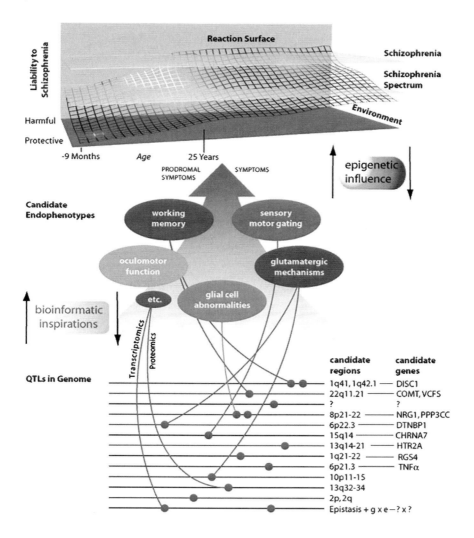

Fig. 1. Schematic illustration of the endophenotype approach to schizophrenia. Several neurobiological endophenotypes, or intermediate phenotypes (shown as colored ovals), lie in between the clinical phenotype (above) and several identified candidate genes. There may be a closer relationship between individual genes and intermediate biological phenotypes than between genes and the symptom-defined clinical syndrome. The influence of epigenetic factors during development further shapes the expression of the endophenotypes. A spectrum of clinical manifestations that may be produced by the interaction of the various endophenotypes will only manifest as the full clinical syndrome in certain individuals. QTLs = quantitative trait loci. Reproduced with permission from Braff [12].

Gene polymorphisms that affect the dopamine or noradrenergic signaling systems (such as COMT) affect pain sensitivity (Chapter 20) as well as neurocognitive functions (Chapter 22), and they are expected to contribute to symptom clusters that are not limited to a particular organ system. Such biological or behavioral subsystems that have strong effect sizes on the clinical phenotype are referred to as intermediate phenotypes or endophenotypes [60,77].

A key assumption of the endophenotype (or intermediate phenotype) approach is that the genetic determination of a particular system dysfunction (for example, a distinct mechanism underlying visceral or somatic hypersensitivity) in a particular disorder (e.g. in IBS, IC/PBS, or FM) is likely to be relatively less complex than that of the illness phenotype overall, given that the latter incorporates multiple neural system dysfunctions and summarizes the influences of all susceptibility genes as well as environmental etiological influences. In the particular case of the intermediate phenotype of "pain sensitivity," it must be emphasized that this endophenotype is still quite complex, with multiple more basic underlying endophenotypes, such as interoceptive sensitivity, attentional processes and emotional arousal circuits contributing to the overall human pain experience (Fig. 5). The consequence is the need to dissect the overall clinical syndrome into its more discretely inherited neurobehavioral subcomponents, or endophenotypes. Endophenotypes vary quantitatively among individuals at risk for the disorder, regardless of whether the illness is expressed phenotypically, making clinically unaffected relatives of affected patients informative for genetic linkage and association studies [15]. Fig. 2 illustrates how the phenomics approach can be applied to dissect various components of functional pain disorders and frequently comorbid psychiatric conditions.

What are the consequences of this endophenotype approach to functional pain disorders? The most obvious one is a need to abandon our false assumption that continued investigations into subspecialty-based symptom criteria will increase our pathophysiological understanding of the clinical syndromes. No matter how many revisions these criteria undergo, they will always miss the emerging reality of specialty- and syndrome-transcending genetically and environmentally determined endophenotypes, manifesting in multiple clinical domains. Moreover, there is an urgent need to identify robust human endophenotypes, related to the CNS (including brain circuit activity and connectivity and discrete aspects of pain processing and modulation), and possibly to certain end organs (for the GI tract, this would include the peristaltic or secretomotor reflex, or more complex motility patterns), which have high correlation coefficients with clinical endpoints such as abdominal pain or altered bowel habits. Robust human endophenotypes may in turn be related to gene polymorphisms and epigenetic factors (e.g., aversive early life events), which in turn can be modeled and studied in transgenic animals [63]. This translational endophenotype-based approach has been highly successful in unraveling the pathophysiology of such complex psychiatric syndromes as schizophrenia, and such approaches are a prerequisite for true scientific progress in the field of functional pain syndromes. The use of endophenotypes (intermediate phenotypes that form the causal links between genes and overt expression of disorders) promises to facilitate discovery of the genetic and environmental architecture of common functional GI disorders and thereby suggest novel strategies for intervention and prevention, based on an understanding of the molecular mechanisms underlying disease risk and manifestation.

Synthesis of Neurobiological Endophenotypes into a Comprehensive Model of Functional Pain Disorders and Comorbid Affective Disorders

The dissection of complex symptom-based disorders into neuropsychological and biological intermediate phenotypes—each of which may be influenced by sex, early environment, and a combination of several genes—provides a practical basis for studying these endophenotypes across different syndromes and for identifying vulnerability genes. Moreover, the synthesis of these endophenotypes into a comprehensive model makes it possible to test specific hypotheses regarding the pathophysiology and treatment responsiveness of these syndromes. Such a comprehensive

A

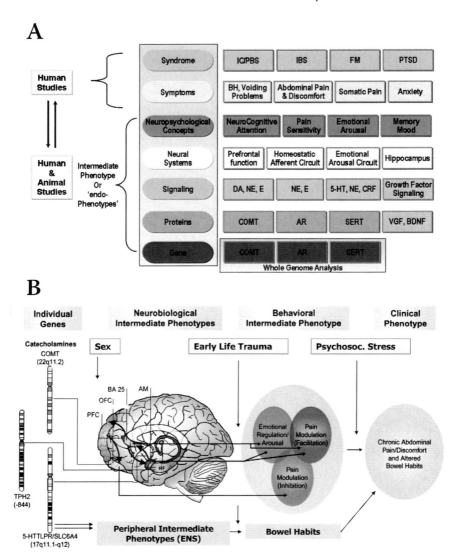

B

Fig. 2. The phenomics approach to functional pain disorders. (A) The first column shows a progression from the complex symptom-based clinical phenotype (top) all the way to the gene. In between, there are several intermediate phenotypes, some of which can be studied in animal models. The matrix on the right illustrates examples of intermediate phenotypes, some of which are relevant for more than one of the disorders listed in the top row. It is proposed that all the complex clinical syndromes are composed of aggregates of several shared intermediate phenotypes and related genes (modified from Sabb et al. [77]). Abbreviations: IC/PBS = interstitial cystitis/painful bladder syndrome, IBS = irritable

model should have reasonable face, construct, and predictive validity and should incorporate several processes thought to be relevant in variable degrees to symptom expression across the spectrum of functional disorders: (a) abnormal processing, modulation, or generation of interoceptive signals from different body regions, resulting in chronic pain and discomfort; (b) alterations in endogenous pain modulation (tonic and phasic inhibition and facilitation); and (c) abnormal responses of the emotional motor system in response to processes (a) and (b).

Abnormal Interoceptive Processing

The insula-centric model of interoception and homeostatic afferents originally proposed by Craig [22] and adapted by Paulus and Stein to anxiety disorders [66] and by Mayer et al. to functional GI disorders [58] is ideally suited to provide such a framework. Interoception can be defined in its most general form as one's sense of the physiological condition of the entire body [22]. In contrast to the earlier, much narrower definition of interoception to sensory signals arising from the viscera, the wider definition includes a wide range of sensations related to the overall homeostatic state of the body, such as temperature, pain, muscular and visceral sensations, hunger, thirst, taste, and air hunger. Interoception has long been thought to be critical for self-awareness because it provides the link between cognitive and affective processes and the current state of the body [21].

The neural system that underlies interoception can be conceptualized as a homeostatic afferent system that conveys signals from all aspects of the body encoded by small-diameter primary (vagal and spinal)

bowel syndrome, FM = fibromyalgia, PTSD = post-traumatic stress syndrome. AR = adrenergic receptor, BDNF = brain-derived neurotrophic factor, BH = bowel habit, COMT = catechol-O-methyltransferase, CRF = corticotropin-releasing factor, DA = dopamine, E = epinephrine, 5-HT = serotonin, NE = norepinephrine, SERT = serotonin transporter, VGF = vascular endothelial growth factor. (B) Illustration of the imaging genetics approach to functional gastrointestinal disorders. Candidate genes interact with early environmental factors and sex to shape the responsiveness of distinct brain circuits that interact to produce the characteristic symptom complex. Epigenetic modifications of the endophenotypes can occur throughout the life time of the individual. Genetic influences on brain circuits may be mirrored within the enteric nervous system, which shares the majority of transmitter systems with the brain. ENS = enteric nervous system. Modified from Meyer-Lindenberg and Weinberger [60].

afferents. Signals travel from the periphery to the brain via lamina I spinal afferents and a specific thalamocortical relay nucleus (VMpo) in the posterolateral thalamus (unique to humans and higher primates), ultimately creating an internal representation of the entire body in the posterior insula (pINS), the interoceptive cortex. In particular, ascending brain areas involved include the midbrain reticular nuclei, including the parabrachial nucleus and ventromedial and ventroposterior thalamus. Signals received in the pINS are re-represented ("remapped") progressively from the posterior to mid- and anterior insula (aINS), ultimately (but only for a fraction of interoceptive information) reaching the anterior insular cortex of the dominant (right) hemisphere [21,22]. As pointed out recently [58], the concept of homeostatic afferent input converging in a particular brain region (pINS), with a small fraction of this input reaching awareness in the aINS, is a particularly attractive way to explain the finding of increased perceptual sensitivity to a range of experimental stimuli, as well as the range of experiences and sensations reported by many functional pain patients during a detailed history. Their experiences are almost never restricted to a particular end organ, but almost always include both visceral and somatic sensations (including sensations of pain, heaviness, discomfort, bloating, early satiety, palpitations, and chest tightness), and alterations in temperature perception.

Several unique aspects of interoception and its neurobiological substrate in the brain have direct relevance for a comprehensive model of functional pain disorders (Fig. 3). First, during the re-representations of the interoceptive signal from the posterior to the anterior portions of the insula, the signal is integrated with other information about the context and the emotional state of the organism. Inputs from the amygdala

Fig. 3. Integration of interoceptive information in the insular cortex. (A) Interoceptive input from lamina I spinal neurons creates an internal representation of the entire body in the posterior insula (pINS), the interoceptive cortex. Signals from the thalamus (THA) received in the pINS are re-represented ("remapped") progressively from the posterior (pINS) to the mid- (mINS) and anterior insula (aINS), and activation of the latter is associated with interoceptive awareness. The signal is modulated by cognitive, affective, and reward circuit inputs at different stages of this remapping process. Processing of interoceptive information in the closely interconnected dorsal anterior cingulate cortex (dACC) is associated with the affective, motivational dimensions of the conscious experience. PFC = prefrontal cortex. (Modified from Craig [20].) (B) Interoceptive awareness

A

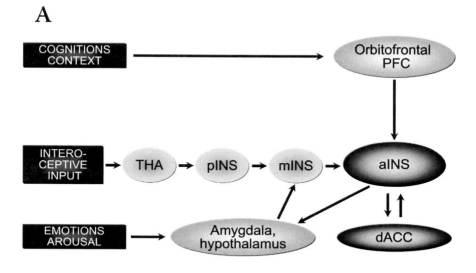

B

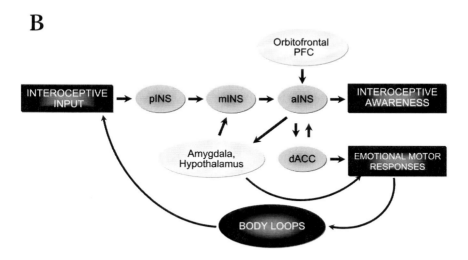

and emotional motor responses. Coprocessing of interoceptive information in the dACC associates the interoceptive awareness with a motor response (mediated by the output channels of the emotional motor system). These outputs in the form of skeletomotor, autonomic, and hypothalamic-pituitary-adrenal (HPA) axis responses can affect peripheral target cells, which in turn can change the nature and intensity of interoceptive input. Such "body loops" may be responsible for reported end-organ changes and may play an important role in the chronicity of symptoms.

and the nucleus accumbens to the mid-insula provide integration with evaluative and reward-related aspects of the organism, respectively, while inputs to the aINS from the prefrontal and orbitofrontal cortex provide integration with attentional and cognitive processes. Second, there are close interconnections between the aINS and the dACC, which provide for further integration with attentional processes, as well as linking interoception to circuits of the limbic motor cortex or emotional motor system [42].

Close Linkage of the Insula with the dACC Integrates Interoceptive Sensations with Attentional, Motivational, and Motor Responses

Interoceptive sensations are often associated with intense affective, autonomic, and motivational components, and these components are generally contingent on the context in which the sensations are experienced. For example, somatic pain or discomfort is immediately attributed to the object causing the pain and is associated with a strong skeletomotor response and withdrawal action. In contrast, visceral pain, which is more diffuse and rarely attributable to an object, is associated with a strong autonomic nervous system response. Greater sympathetic nervous system responses to a variety of experimental stimuli have been identified in many functional pain disorders, including IBS (Chapter 6) and FM (Chapters 2, 15).

The neuroanatomical basis for the close relationship between interoceptive feelings and affective, motivational, and autonomic responses lies in the close interactions between the aINS and the dACC, which have reciprocal connections, and both of which receive input from the ascending afferent lamina I pathway [22,25,26,44,72]. Primates and humans have a direct thalamocortical pathway that activates the dACC (by way of the ventral caudal part of the medial dorsal nucleus [MDvc]in the medial thalamus). Its interconnections with prefrontal cortex regions, insular regions, and ventral striatal regions, along with its strong descending projections to the brainstem, particularly the periaqueductal gray, strongly support the idea that it can be regarded generally as the limbic behavioral motor cortex, just as the insula can be regarded as the limbic sensory cortex [24,86].

Close Linkage of the Insula with the Amygdala and Emotional Arousal Circuits Integrates Arousal with Interoceptive Feelings

The insular cortex has bidirectional connections to the amygdala that provide information about the positive and negative valence of both external and internal stimuli, and about the state of arousal of the organism. Therefore, the insular cortex is centrally placed to receive information about the salience (both appetitive and aversive) and relative value of the stimulus environment and integrate this information with the effect that these stimuli may have on the body state. The assessment of the valence of the signal is highly dependent on the context and on the homeostatic state of the individual. For example, while light touching of the abdomen may be perceived as pleasant in a healthy individual, the same stimulus is typically perceived as uncomfortable or painful by a patient with abdominal pain. Vaginal stimulation is typically experienced as pleasure, but it is perceived as pain and discomfort in the patient with vulvodynia or dyspareunia. Food-induced gastric distension or intake of a high-fat meal is typically associated with pleasurable satiation, but it is associated with pain, discomfort, or nausea in an individual who has just finished a large meal, or in a patient with functional dyspepsia.

Role of Attentional Systems in Modulating Interoceptive Awareness

Threat-related attentional biases are characteristic of anxiety disorders as well as many functional pain disorders, and have been referred to as examples of hypervigilance [6] (see also the discussion of attentional processes in Chapter 19). Earlier views of threat-related attentional biases have centered on the dominant role of the amygdala [7]. Hyperactivity of the amygdala and associated emotional arousal circuits, including the locus ceruleus, provides a major input into the alerting network, one of several attentional networks proposed by Posner [69]. In IBS and in anxiety disorders, as well as in preclinical models of these syndromes, evidence has been reported for (a) increased activity of emotional arousal circuits and (b) upregulation of one of the cardinal chemical modulators of these circuits, the corticotropin-releasing factor (CRF) signaling system [53].

More recently, Bishop has provided evidence to support an alternative model that incorporates an influence of prefrontal cortical mechanisms in the early top-down control of selective attention to threat. According to her model, trait anxiety may be characterized by impaired recruitment of prefrontal mechanisms that are critical to the active control of attention to threat-related distractors when the task at hand does not fully govern the allocation of attention. When one's attention is fully absorbed by a given task, there is no longer competition with threat-related distracters [7]. When applied to functional pain disorders, the model would predict that patients show increased attention to various bodily sensations or related contexts when not absorbed by other attentional demands, but that this selective attentional bias disappears when there are other demands on one's attention. This mechanism may form the basis for the clinical observation that functional pain symptoms decrease when one's attention is absorbed by distraction (Chapter 19), by physically threatening circumstances (natural disasters) [18,19], or by attention-demanding situations such as a serious physical illness (e.g., cancer) or pregnancy. Bishop proposed that this deficit does not arise as a result of current anxiety (i.e., state anxiety), but instead reflects an underlying trait characteristic that influences attentional processing regardless of the presence or absence of threat-related stimuli [7]. This trait may interact with state anxiety influences on subcortical threat detection mechanisms (e.g., the amygdala and locus ceruleus) to account for the threat-related attentional biases associated with functional pain disorders and with clinical anxiety.

Even though they are not an explicit part of Bishop's model, the aINS and the closely connected dACC play a crucial part in the attentional processes outlined above. As proposed by Paulus and Stein [66], interoception involves monitoring the sensations that are important for the integrity of the internal body state (the insula) and connecting to systems that are important for allocating attention, evaluating context, and planning actions (the dACC). The dACC is thought to compute an error signal between a predicted and observed outcome to indicate the need for deployment of attentional resources in order to adjust behavior or cognition [9].

Error Processing, Learning, and Prediction

The ability to predict future body states (aversive and appetitive) is related to previous learning and memory formation about stimuli and contexts, and their association with future pleasant or aversive outcomes [78]. It has been proposed that processes analogous to reward learning [78] occur with aversive stimuli and that the insular cortex is critically involved in generating anticipatory signals that are important for learning about aversive outcomes [67]. We propose that similar to anxious individuals [66], patients with functional pain disorders focus on the likelihood or inevitability of a future aversive bodily state (such as pain or discomfort) in certain contexts. One may speculate that the common history of aversive early life events in the majority of functional pain syndromes (Chapter 20) as well as in anxiety disorders plays a role in the development of this learning process. The cognitive-behavioral conceptualization of anxiety and functional pain disorders is based on behavioral theories of fear conditioning and cognitive theories that highlight the role of ineffective cognitive strategies (such as catastrophizing or excessive worry) and anxious thinking (reviewed in Chapters 10, 24). In the literature on cognitive-behavioral theory, "anxiety sensitivity" is the construct used to describe the tendency of certain individuals to view interoceptive sensations as dangerous or threatening [73]. This tendency may be mediated through inputs from prefrontal circuits to the aINS that create a distorted body image, which does not match the actual body image created from afferent input in the posterior insula. This mismatch between actual and projected interoceptive image results in dACC activation, increased anxiety, and altered output from the emotional motor system (Fig. 4), in particular the autonomic nervous system, as it tries to decrease the mismatch between the actual and predicted interoceptive states.

One may speculate that in patients with functional pain disorders, the emotional motor responses are unable to correct the mismatch between the actual body state and the predicted state, resulting in chronically altered attentional processes, excessive worry, and maladaptive patterns of autonomic activity (e.g., tonically increased sympathetic tone, altered gastrointestinal function) and skeletomotor activity (chronic muscle tension). Panic disorder, which is frequently associated with IBS, IC/PBS, and other functional pain disorders, is thought to develop when exposure to panic attacks causes the conditioning of anxiety to exteroceptive and interoceptive cues, such as perception of signals arising within the cardiovascular system [10,23]. This mechanism is analogous to those that may play a role in patients with functional cardiac pain (Chapter 7). Based on the link between altered interoception and anxiety, it has been suggested that individuals who are prone to anxiety show an altered

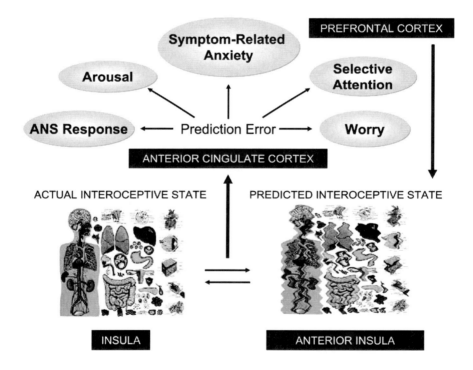

Fig. 4. Model of prefrontal/insular cortical interactions in the generation of a prediction error and secondary emotional and cognitive responses. The mismatch between the actual (representation of interoceptive input) and predicted (distortion by prefrontal influences) interoceptive states represented in the insular cortex results in a prediction error regarding the future state of the organism. This mismatch is associated with activation of the dorsal anterior cingulate cortex, hyperarousal, sympathetic nervous system hyperactivity, and increased anxiety. Prefrontal influences mediate excessive worry and selective attention to perceived threat. ANS = autonomic nervous system. Modified with permission from Paulus and Stein [66].

interoceptive prediction signal, i.e., they experience an augmented signaling of the difference between the observed and expected body states [66] (Fig. 4). When this concept is adapted to patients with functional pain disorders, a contextual or interoceptive stimulus (for example, physiological postprandial GI motility) previously associated with an aversive experience and predictive of an aversive outcome (abdominal, bladder, or cardiac pain or urinary or fecal urgency results) in an aversive body state prediction (distortion of the interoceptive representation of various organs), which is represented as a prediction signal in the aINS.

Paulus and Stein suggested that there are two possibilities of altered prediction signaling [66]. First, anxiety-prone individuals (and patients with functional pain disorders) may generate an error signal due to the mismatch between an *attenuated* baseline interoceptive state and a normal interoceptive expectation. Consistent with such a concept of attenuated interoceptive baseline sensitivity are several study reports in IBS patients. For example, women with a history of sexual abuse have *reduced* perception of experimental rectal distension [74], and a significant number of IBS patients have reduced perception of a slowly increasing rectal pressure stimulus [59], as well as of somatic pressure stimuli [16]. Alternatively, anxiety-prone individuals or individuals with low-grade immune activation or tissue irritation in a particular end organ may have a normal or even increased baseline interoceptive state but an exaggerated expected body state, also resulting in an error signal.

While the mismatch of baseline and expected interoceptive signal may be the primary process underlying increased feelings of anxiety and bodily discomfort, the autonomic, behavioral, and certain cognitive components are likely to be consequences of this altered prediction signal. It has been proposed that cognitive components (e.g., excessive worrying) and behaviors (e.g., avoidance) associated with this altered prediction signal are attempts to engage compensatory brain resources aimed to attenuate the difference between the observed and expected body state. For example, individuals who have a history of uncontrollable and unpredictable life stress may use a coping style of constant worry about possible bad outcomes or aversive and potentially dangerous body states as a cognitive avoidance response. Excessive worrying may function as a way to avoid unwanted internal experiences by attempting to determine ways of preventing envisioned future catastrophes [64] (Chapter 24). The suppression of emotional, autonomic, and interoceptive responses in individuals with excessive worry serves to reinforce the process of worry (avoidance) but also prevents extinction [8].

In contrast to proposed pathophysiological models based on a primary or exclusive role for pathologically enhanced interoceptive signals from a particular end organ (due to low-grade immune activation, altered gut flora, peripheral or central sensitization, or neuropathic signals), or on models of primary upregulation of amygdala-based arousal circuits (comorbid anxiety), we suggest that the interoception hypothesis proposed by Paulus and Stein provides a more comprehensive model. This model incorporates not only alterations in afferent signals from the body (interoception) and emotional arousal (related to the amygdala), but also a prominent role for top-down cognitive and attentional processes, such as selective attention to threat [7].

On the basis of this concept, there are several reasons to consider the notion that cortical processes may play a prominent role in functional pain disorders and in the commonly associated increased anxiety [66]. First, the neuroanatomical connections between the aINS and dACC place these regions at the center of altered interoceptive sensations, increased cognitive engagement, and increased emotional motor output, consistent with the characteristic finding of bodily discomfort and pain, sympathetic hyperarousal, and worry. Second, the focus on an altered prediction signal is consistent with the view of anxiety and functional pain disorders as a future-oriented cognitive and emotional characteristic. Third, the altered prediction signal generated by or modulated within the aINS provides a process by which learning and conditioned associations assume a crucial role in the development of pathological anxiety. Fourth, although the amygdala is critically involved in mediating anxiety, the complex and integrative nature of anxiety and functional pain disorders clearly points toward the involvement of cortical structures, including the insular, cingulate, and prefrontal cortices. One may speculate that such a prominent role of cortical mechanisms in the pathophysiology of functional pain disorders may explain the effectiveness of cognitive-behavioral strategies, the relatively disappointing results with centrally acting drugs such as SSRIs, and the poor predictive validity of animal models of these disorders [56].

Linkage of the Insula with the dACC and Amygdala Provides Pathways for Endogenous Pain Modulation

In addition to the mechanism of altered interoceptive awareness based on cognitive and limbic modulatory inputs to the aINS, there are multiple systems by which the CNS can up- and downregulate the amount of afferent information reaching the interoceptive cortex in the context of an aversive stimulus (see Fig. 5). For example, an extensive preclinical literature exists on tonic and phasic pain inhibition as well as pain facilitation systems [61,68] (see also Chapter 18). In addition to these descending corticolimbic pontine systems modulating the excitability of neurons in the dorsal horn, there is evidence for local modulation of brain regions by opioidergic mechanisms [90]. More recently, upregulation of spinal glia has been reported as a central mechanism maintaining a sensitized state (Chapter 16). Interestingly, such glial activation has been reported not only in response to peripheral nerve lesions, but also in response to chronic psychological stress, in the absence of any peripheral lesions [11].

Several questions remain to be answered before we can clearly implicate specific abnormalities in these pain modulation systems: (1) Are different functional pain syndromes characterized by a unique pain endophenotype or by multiple endophenotypes? (2) Is there evidence for a recruitment or failure of different pain modulation mechanisms over time? For example, could chronic hypervigilance and pain facilitation precede the development of neuroimmune abnormalities or the breakdown of serotonergic or noradrenergic endogenous pain inhibition systems? Could such a sequential involvement of different pain modulation mechanisms be correlated with a progression from increased levels of anxiety to depression? (3) Alternatively, do certain gene polymorphisms (such as *COMT*) affect several pain modulation systems at the same time? (4) Do somatizers have different pain modulation abnormalities than patients with depression?

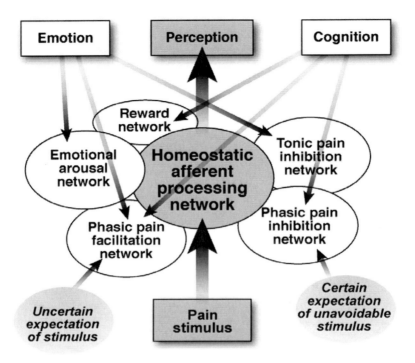

Fig. 5. Dissection of the human pain experience into distinct neurobiological components (overlapping processing and modulation networks). While interoceptive input is processed within the homeostatic afferent processing network, in particular the subregions of the insular cortex, several pain inhibitory and facilitatory networks modulate conscious perception of this input. These networks are engaged by cognitive, emotional, and contextual factors. Modified with permission from Mayer et al. [58].

Synthesis

The endophenotype approach to deconstructing complex symptom-based disorders provides a promising approach to identify intermediate endophenotypes, codetermined by genetic and epigenetic factors, which not only provide a way to conceptualize the overlap between many functional pain disorders and anxiety disorders, but also may reveal promising therapeutic targets. The interoceptive model [66] outlined above provides a plausible and testable biological framework that can explain the majority of shared findings and characteristics discussed for various functional pain syndromes in this volume, for several reasons: (1) The convergence of interoceptive signals not only from the viscera but from all bodily structures and systems within a single cortical region (e.g., the insula), and the convergence of cognitive and affective modulatory inputs to this region can explain the characteristic clinical phenomenon of comorbidity of different pain syndromes. (2) The ability of the model to provide a plausible framework for both anxiety and functional pain disorders is consistent with characteristically increased levels of anxiety in the majority of functional pain disorders, and with the frequent overlap of functional pain syndromes with disorders of mood and affect, including anxiety (Chapter 10), PTSD (Chapter 9), depression (Chapter 11), and somatization (Chapter 12). (3) The close interaction between the interoceptive cortex and limbic motor cortex (e.g., dACC) provides a neuroanatomical basis for observed changes in the output of the emotional motor system, such as sympathetic nervous system hyperactivity, reduced vagal tone, altered HPA axis function (Chapter 15) and compromised endogenous pain modulation (Chapters 18, 19). (4) The effectiveness of cognitive-behavioral therapy in the majority of functional pain syndromes as well as in anxiety disorders is consistent with the prominent role of maladaptive cognitive and attentional mechanisms in interoceptive modulation (Chapter 24).

   With all the unifying mechanisms outlined above, the skeptic rightly will ask the question: Why do the majority of patients refer their primary complaint to a single body region or organ? A related important question is: Can all syndromes be fully explained by altered CNS processes modulating an essentially normal interoceptive signal, or is there an important role for the "body" in this model? Even though we cannot definitely answer these questions, there are several plausible answers. As outlined above, in the intricate interplay between interoceptive processing in the insula and dACC and emotional motor responses, the resulting "body loops" may play an essential role in maintaining the chronicity of the syndromes (discussed in Chapter 14) (Fig. 3B). For example, chronically enhanced activity of the skeletomotor system and muscle spasms can result in sensitization of somatic afferents, which could play a role in chronic symptom generation in FM, low back pain, TMJD, and IC/PBS.

There are several mechanisms by which altered activity of the sympathetic nervous system and the HPA axis could result in secondary end-organ changes. Neuroplastic changes in primary afferent neurons have been reported in a chronic stress model, demonstrating that chronically increased sympathetic nervous system activity can produce a direct responsiveness of primary afferent neurons to stress mediators [45]. Stress induces a switch of intracellular signaling in sensory neurons in a model of generalized pain.

Chronically altered autonomic and HPA axis output have been shown to change the responsiveness of the immune system [30], and pro-inflammatory mediators associated with such centrally induced immune activation could, in turn, sensitize primary afferents. Such top-down mechanisms can increase gut permeability, increasing the access of the intestinal microflora to the gut-associated immune system (Chapter 17). Chronic activity of the sympathetic nervous system or HPA axis may also play a role in the activation of microglia in the spinal cord and produce a long-lasting state of sensitization [11] (Chapter 16). Such centrally induced changes in peripheral transducing systems (including mast cells, enterochromaffin cells in the gut, and primary afferent terminals) could then provide altered interoceptive positive feedback to the brain, further exacerbating symptoms of pain and discomfort. While HPA-axis and sympathoadrenally mediated effects obviously could not explain end-organ selectivity, the sympathetic nervous system has unique target selectivity and would therefore be an attractive candidate to mediate a certain degree of end-organ selectivity superimposed on generalized alterations in homeostatic function (Chapter 14).

Conversely, infection or injury to a particular organ or body part could initiate a period of enhanced interoceptive processing, associated with peripheral and central sensitization. While such sensitization is generally self-limited and counter-regulated by endogenous pain inhibition systems in the majority of patients, in a patient with vulnerability factors for chronic pain (alterations in attentional or affective modulation of interoceptive signals and compromised endogenous pain inhibition systems), such peripherally triggered symptoms could develop into a chronic pain syndrome. In this case, the vicious cycle initiated by a specific lesion to a peripheral target could continue even after complete resolution of the initial insult, in a process largely driven by the central mechanisms discussed above.

In the proposed body loop model, the peripheral (e.g., end-organ) versus central etiology of functional pain syndromes is no longer mutually exclusive. Symptom onset may arise in response to either peripheral injuries or psychological stressors. Similarly, while in some patients a body loop may be required to maintain the chronicity of symptoms, in others, symptoms could arise solely from central representations, and even removal of the end organ may not result in symptom improvement.

Conclusion

It is hoped that the proposed model will help to transcend several barriers that stand in the way of progress toward the development of better treatment strategies for patients with functional pain syndromes. It can transcend the traditional controversies between protagonists of a peripheral, "organic" etiology of symptoms and those in favor of a top-down model of CNS-driven abnormalities. It provides a plausible biological model to understand the etiology of multiple physical and mental symptoms so characteristic of functional pain syndromes. Finally, it can provide an attractive concept for government funding agencies and for the pharmaceutical industry to abandon the paradigm of the "silo" funding of research projects and to contemplate a more unified approach for drug development.

Acknowledgment

Dr. Mayer acknowledges National Institutes of Health grants DK48351, DK64530, and AT00268.

References

[1]   Apkarian AV, Sosa Y, Krauss BR, Thomas PS, Fredrickson BE, Levy RE, Harden RN, Chialvo DR. Chronic pain patients are impaired on an emotional decision-making task. Pain 2004;108:129–36.
[2]   Baliki MN, Chialvo DR, Geha PY, Levy RM, Harden RN, Parrish TB, Apkarian AV. Chronic pain and the emotional brain: specific brain activity associated with spontaneous fluctuations of intensity of chronic back pain. J Neurosci 2006;26:12165–73.

[3]   Barsky AJ, Borus JF. Somatization and medicalization in the era of managed care. JAMA 1995;274:1931–4.
[4]   Berman SM, Naliboff BD, Suyenobu B, Labus JS, Stains J, Ohning G, Kilpatrick L, Bueller JA, Ruby K, Jarcho J, Mayer EA. Reduced brainstem inhibition during anticipated pelvic visceral pain correlates with enhanced brain response to the visceral stimulus in women with irritable bowel syndrome. J Neurosci 2008;28:349–59.
[5]   Bilder RM. Psychiatry grand rounds. Los Angeles: UCLA; 2008.
[6]   Bishop SJ. Neurocognitive mechanisms of anxiety: an integrative account. Trends Cogn Sci 2007;11:307–16.
[7]   Bishop SJ. Trait anxiety and impoverished prefrontal control of attention. Nat Neurosci 2009;12:92–8.
[8]   Borkovec TD, Roemer L. Perceived functions of worry among generalized anxiety disorder subjects: distraction from more emotionally distressing topics? J Behav Ther Exp Psychiatry 1995;26:25–30.
[9]   Botvinick MM, Cohen JD, Carter CS. Conflict monitoring and anterior cingulate cortex: an update. Trends Cogn Sci 2004;8:539–46.
[10] Bouton ME, Mineka S, Barlow DH. A modern learning theory perspective on the etiology of panic disorder. Psychol Rev 2001;108:4–32.
[11] Bradesi S, Martinez V, Lao L, Larsson H, Mayer EA. Involvement of vasopressin 3 receptors in chronic psychological stress-induced visceral hyperalgesia in rats. Am J Physiol Gastrointest Liver Physiol 2009;296:G302–9.
[12] Braff DL, Freedman R, Schork NJ, Gottesman, II. Deconstructing schizophrenia: an overview of the use of endophenotypes in order to understand a complex disorder. Schizophr Bull 2007;33:21–32.
[13] Bremner JD, Elzinga B, Schmahl C, Vermetten E. Structural and functional plasticity of the human brain in posttraumatic stress disorder. Prog Brain Res 2008;167:171–86.
[14] Campo JV, Bridge J, Ehmann M, Altman S, Lucas A, Birmaher B, Di Lorenzo C, Iyengar S, Brent DA. Recurrent abdominal pain, anxiety, and depression in primary care. Pediatrics 2004;113:817–24.
[15] Cannon TD, Keller MC. Endophenotypes in the genetic analyses of mental disorders. Annu Rev Clin Psychol 2006;2:267–90.
[16] Chang L, Mayer EA, Johnson T, FitzGerald L, Naliboff B. Differences in somatic perception in female patients with irritable bowel syndrome with and without fibromyalgia. Pain 2000;84:297–307.
[17] Chang L, Sundaresh S, Elliott J, Anton PA, Baldi P, Licudine A, Mayer M, Vuong T, Hirano M, Naliboff BD, Ameen VZ, Mayer EA. Dysregulation of the hypothalamic-pituitary-adrenal (HPA) axis in irritable bowel syndrome. Neurogastroenterol Motil 2008; Epub Aug 5.
[18] Chrousos GP, Gold PW. The concepts of stress and stress system disorders. Overview of physical and behavioral homeostasis. JAMA 1992;267:1244–52.
[19] Clauw DJ, Engel CC Jr, Aronowitz R, Jones E, Kipen HM, Kroenke K, Ratzan S, Sharpe M, Wessely S. Unexplained symptoms after terrorism and war: an expert consensus statement. J Occup Environ Med 2003;45:1040–8.
[20] Craig A. Interoception and emotion: a neuroanatomical perspective. In: Lewis M, Haviland-Jones JM, Barrett LF, editors. Handbook of emotions, 3rd ed. New York: Guilford Press; 2008.
[21] Craig A. How do you feel—now? The anterior insula and human awareness. Nat Rev Neurosci 2009;10:59–70.
[22] Craig AD. How do you feel? Interoception: the sense of the physiological condition of the body. Nat Rev Neurosci 2002;3:655–66.
[23] Craske MG, Waters AM. Panic disorder, phobias, and generalized anxiety disorder. Annu Rev Clin Psychol 2005;1:197–225.
[24] Critchley HD. The human cortex responds to an interoceptive challenge. Proc Natl Acad Sci USA 2004;101:6333–4.
[25] Critchley HD, Corfield DR, Chandler MP, Mathias CJ, Dolan RJ. Cerebral correlates of autonomic cardiovascular arousal: a functional neuroimaging investigation in humans. J Physiol 2000;523:259–70.

[26] Critchley HD, Mathias CJ, Josephs O, O'Doherty J, Zanini S, Dewar BK, Cipolotti L, Shallice T, Dolan RJ. Human cingulate cortex and autonomic control: Converging neuroimaging and clinical evidence. Brain 2003;126:2139–52.

[27] Crombez G, Eccleston C, van den BA, Goubert L, Van Houdenhove B. Hypervigilance to pain in fibromyalgia: the mediating role of pain intensity and catastrophic thinking about pain. Clin J Pain 2004;20:98–102.

[28] Dancey CP, Attree EA, Stuart G, Wilson C, Sonnet A. Words fail me: the verbal IQ deficit in inflammatory bowel disease and irritable bowel syndrome. Inflamm Bowel Dis 2009; Epub Jan 7.

[29] Drossman DA. Do psychosocial factors define symptom severity and patient status in irritable bowel syndrome? Am J Med 1999;107:41S–50S.

[30] Elenkov IJ, Wilder RL, Chrousos GP, Vizi ES. The sympathetic nerve: an integrative interface between two supersystems: the brain and the immune system. Pharmacol Rev 2000;52:585–638.

[31] Geisser ME, Glass JM, Rajcevska LD, Clauw DJ, Williams DA, Kileny PR, Gracely RH. A psychophysical study of auditory and pressure sensitivity in patients with fibromyalgia and healthy controls. J Pain 2008;9:417–22.

[32] Geisser ME, Strader DC, Petzke F, Gracely RH, Clauw DJ, Williams DA. Comorbid somatic symptoms and functional status in patients with fibromyalgia and chronic fatigue syndrome: sensory amplification as a common mechanism. Psychosomatics 2008;49:235–42.

[33] Giesecke T, Gracely RH, Grant MA, Nachemson A, Petzke F, Williams DA, Clauw DJ. Evidence of augmented central pain processing in idiopathic chronic low back pain. Arthritis Rheum 2004;50:613–23.

[34] Glass JM, Park DC. Cognitive dysfunction in fibromyalgia. Curr Rheumatol Rep 2001;3:123–7.

[35] Gracely RH, Geisser ME, Giesecke T, Grant MA, Petzke F, Williams DA, Clauw DJ. Pain catastrophizing and neural responses to pain among persons with fibromyalgia. Brain 2004;127:835–43.

[36] Gracely RH, Petzke F, Wolf JM, Clauw DJ. Functional magnetic resonance imaging evidence of augmented pain processing in fibromyalgia. Arthritis Rheum 2002;46:1333–43.

[37] Hagelberg N, Forssell H, Rinne JO, Scheinin H, Taiminen T, Aalto S, Luutonen S, Nagren K, Jaaskelainen S. Striatal dopamine D1 and D2 receptors in burning mouth syndrome. Pain 2003;101:149–54.

[38] Halder SL, Locke GR 3rd, Schleck CD, Zinsmeister AR, Melton LJ 3rd, Talley NJ. Natural history of functional gastrointestinal disorders: a 12-year longitudinal population-based study. Gastroenterology 2007;133:799–807.

[39] Hanno PM, Wein AJ, Kavoussi LR, Novick AC, Partin AW, Peters CA. Painful bladder syndrome/interstitial cystitis and related disorders. In: Campbell MF, editor. Campbell-Walsh urology. Philadelphia: W.B. Saunders; 2007.

[40] Harris RE, Clauw DJ, Scott DJ, McLean SA, Gracely RH, Zubieta JK. Decreased central mu-opioid receptor availability in fibromyalgia. J Neurosci 2007;27:10000–6.

[41] Hart J Jr, Kimbrell T, Fauver P, Cherry BJ, Pitcock J, Booe LQ, Tillman G, Freeman TW. Cognitive dysfunctions associated with PTSD: evidence from World War II prisoners of war. J Neuropsychiatry Clin Neurosci 2008;20:309–16.

[42] Holstege G, Bandler R, Saper CB, Holstege G, Bandler R, Saper CB. The emotional motor system. Prog Brain Res 1996;107:3–6.

[43] Johannesson U, de Boussard CN, Brodda JG, Bohm-Starke N. Evidence of diffuse noxious inhibitory controls (DNIC) elicited by cold noxious stimulation in patients with provoked vestibulodynia. Pain 2007;130:31–9.

[44] Johansen JP, Fields HL, Manning BH. The affective component of pain in rodents: direct evidence for a contribution of the anterior cingulate cortex. Proc Natl Acad Sci USA 2001;98:8077–82.

[45] Khasar SG, Burkham J, Dina OA, Brown AS, Bogen O, Alessandri-Haber N, Green PG, Reichling DB, Levine JD. Stress induces a switch of intracellular signaling in sensory neurons in a model of generalized pain. J Neurosci 2008;28:5721–30.

[46] Kitayama N, Vaccarino V, Kutner M, Weiss P, Bremner JD. Magnetic resonance imaging (MRI) measurement of hippocampal volume in posttraumatic stress disorder: a meta-analysis. J Affect Disord 2005;88:79–86.

[47] Klauenberg S, Maier C, Assion HJ, Hoffmann A, Krumova EK, Magerl W, Scherens A, Treede RD, Juckel G. Depression and changed pain perception: hints for a central disinhibition mechanism. Pain 2008;140:332–43.

[48] Kosek E, Hansson P. Modulatory influence on somatosensory perception from vibration and heterotopic noxious conditioning stimulation (HNCS) in fibromyalgia patients and healthy subjects. Pain 1997;70:41–51.

[49] Lautenbacher S, Rollman GB. Possible deficiencies of pain modulation in fibromyalgia. Clin J Pain 1997;13:189–96.

[50] Leavitt F, Katz RS, Mills M, Heard AR. Cognitive and dissociative manifestations in fibromyalgia. J Clin Rheumatol 2002;8:77–84.

[51] Luerding R, Weigand T, Bogdahn U, Schmidt-Wilcke T. Working memory performance is correlated with local brain morphology in the medial frontal and anterior cingulate cortex in fibromyalgia patients: structural correlates of pain-cognition interaction. Brain 2008;131:3222–31.

[52] Maixner W, Fillingim RB, Sigurdsson A, Kincaid S, Silva S. Sensitivity of patients with painful temporomandibular disorders to experimentally evoked pain: evidence for altered temporal summation of pain. Pain 1998;76:71–81.

[53] Martinez V, Tach Y. CRF1 receptors as a therapeutic target for irritable bowel syndrome. Curr Pharm Des 2006;12:4071–88.

[54] May A. Chronic pain may change the structure of the brain. Pain 2008;137:7–15.

[55] Mayer EA, Berman S, Suyenobu B, Labus J, Mandelkern MA, Naliboff BD, Chang L. Differences in brain responses to visceral pain between patients with irritable bowel syndrome and ulcerative colitis. Pain 2005;115:398–409.

[56] Mayer EA, Bradesi S, Chang L, Spiegel BM, Bueller JA, Naliboff BD. Functional GI disorders: from animal models to drug development. Gut 2008;57:384–404.

[57] Mayer EA, Labus JS, Berkley K. Sex differences in pain. In: Becker JB, Berkley KJ, Geary N, Hampson E, Herman JP, Young E, editors. Sex differences in the brain: from genes to behavior. New York: Oxford University Press; 2007. p. 371–96.

[58] Mayer EA, Naliboff BD, Craig AD. Neuroimaging of the brain-gut axis: from basic understanding to treatment of functional GI disorders. Gastroenterology 2006;131:1925–42.

[59] Mertz H, Naliboff B, Munakata J, Niazi N, Mayer EA. Altered rectal perception is a biological marker of patients with irritable bowel syndrome. Gastroenterology 1995;109:40–52.

[60] Meyer-Lindenberg A, Weinberger DR. Intermediate phenotypes and genetic mechanisms of psychiatric disorders. Nat Rev Neurosci 2006;7:818–27.

[61] Millan MJ. Descending control of pain. Prog Neurobiol 2002;66:355–474.

[62] Moynihan R, Heath I, Henry D. Selling sickness: the pharmaceutical industry and disease mongering. BMJ 2002;324:886–90.

[63] Murphy DL, Lesch KP. Targeting the murine serotonin transporter: insights into human neurobiology. Nat Rev Neurosci 2008;9:85–96.

[64] Naliboff BD, Lackner JM, Mayer EA. Psychosocial factors in the care of patients with functional gastrointestinal disorders. In: Yamada T, Alpers DH, Kaplowitz N, Kalloo A, Owyang C, Powell DW, editors. Principles of clinical gastroenterology. Oxford: Wiley-Blackwell; 2009; in press. p. 20–37.

[65] Park DC, Glass JM, Minear M, Crofford LJ. Cognitive function in fibromyalgia patients. Arthritis Rheum 2001;44:2125–33.

[66] Paulus MP, Stein MB. An insular view of anxiety. Biol Psychiatry 2006;60:383–7.

[67] Ploghaus A, Tracey I, Gati JS, Clare S, Menon RS, Matthews PM, Rawlins JNP. Dissociating pain from its anticipation in the human brain. Science 1999;284:1979–81.

[68] Porreca F, Ossipov MH, Gebhart GF. Chronic pain and medullary descending facilitation. Trends Neurosci 2002;25:319–25.

[69] Posner MI, Rothbart MK. Research on attention networks as a model for the integration of psychological science. Annu Rev Psychol 2007;58:1–23.

[70] Pukall CF, Binik YM, Khalife S, Amsel R, Abbott FV. Vestibular tactile and pain thresholds in women with vulvar vestibulitis syndrome. Pain 2002;96:163–75.

[71] Pukall CF, Strigo IA, Binik YM, Amsel R, Khalife S, Bushnell MC. Neural correlates of painful genital touch in women with vulvar vestibulitis syndrome. Pain 2005;115:118–27.

[72] Rainville P, Duncan GH, Price DD, Carrier B, Bushnell MC. Pain affect encoded in human anterior cingulate but not somatosensory cortex. Science 1997;277:968–71.

[73] Reiss S, Peterson RA, Gursky DM, McNally RJ. Anxiety sensitivity, anxiety frequency and the predictions of fearfulness. Behav Res Ther 1986;24:1–8.

[74] Ringel Y, Whitehead WE, Toner BB, Diamant NE, Hu Y, Jia H, Bangdiwala SI, Drossman DA. Sexual and physical abuse are not associated with rectal hypersensitivity in patients with irritable bowel syndrome. Gut 2004;53:838–42.

[75] Rodrigues AC, Nicholas VG, Schmidt S, Mauderli AP. Hypersensitivity to cutaneous thermal nociceptive stimuli in irritable bowel syndrome. Pain 2005;115:5–11.

[76] Roy-Byrne PP, Davidson KW, Kessler RC, Asmundson GJ, Goodwin RD, Kubzansky L, Lydiard RB, Massie MJ, Katon W, Laden SK, Stein MB. Anxiety disorders and comorbid medical illness. Gen Hosp Psychiatry 2008;30:208–25.

[77] Sabb FW, Bearden CE, Glahn DC, Parker DS, Freimer N, Bilder RM. A collaborative knowledge base for cognitive phenomics. Mol Psychiatry 2008;13:350–60.

[78] Schultz W, Dayan P, Montague PR. A neural substrate of prediction and reward. Science 1997;275:1593–9.

[79] Schweinhardt P, Sauro KM, Bushnell MC. Fibromyalgia: a disorder of the brain? Neuroscientist 2008;

[80] Silverman DH, Munakata JA, Ennes H, Mandelkern MA, Hoh CK, Mayer EA. Regional cerebral activity in normal and pathological perception of visceral pain. Gastroenterology 1997;112:64–72.

[81] Small DM, Apkarian AV. Increased taste intensity perception exhibited by patients with chronic back pain. Pain 2006;120:124–30.

[82] Staud R. Treatment of fibromyalgia and its symptoms. Expert Opin Pharmacother 2007;8:1629–42.

[83] Staud R, Robinson ME, Vierck CJ Jr, Price DD. Diffuse noxious inhibitory controls (DNIC) attenuate temporal summation of second pain in normal males but not in normal females or fibromyalgia patients. Pain 2003;101:167–74.

[84] Strigo IA, Simmons AN, Matthews SC, Craig AD, Paulus MP. Association of major depressive disorder with altered functional brain response during anticipation and processing of heat pain. Arch Gen Psychiatry 2008;65:1275–84.

[85] Vasic N, Walter H, Hose A, Wolf RC. Gray matter reduction associated with psychopathology and cognitive dysfunction in unipolar depression: a voxel-based morphometry study. J Affect Disord 2008;109:107–16.

[86] Vogt BA. Pain and emotion interactions in subregions of the cingulate gyrus. Nat Rev Neurosci 2005;6:533–44.

[87] Wilder-Smith CH, Robert-Yap J. Abnormal endogenous pain modulation and somatic and visceral hypersensitivity in female patients with irritable bowel syndrome. World J Gastroenterol 2007;13:3699–704.

[88] Wood PB, Patterson JC, Sunderland JJ, Tainter KH, Glabus MF, Lilien DL. Reduced presynaptic dopamine activity in fibromyalgia syndrome demonstrated with positron emission tomography: a pilot study. J Pain 2007;8:51–8.

[89] Wood PB, Schweinhardt P, Jaeger E, Dagher A, Hakyemez H, Rabiner EA, Bushnell MC, Chizh BA. Fibromyalgia patients show an abnormal dopamine response to pain. Eur J Neurosci 2007;25:3576–82.

[90] Zubieta JK, Ketter TA, Bueller JA, Xu Y, Kilbourn MR, Young EA, Koeppe RA. Regulation of human affective responses by anterior cingulate and limbic mu-opioid neurotransmission. Arch Gen Psychiatry 2003;60:1145–53.

Correspondence to: Emeran A. Mayer, MD, Center for Neurobiology of Stress, Suite 2338F, 10945 Le Conte Avenue, Los Angeles, CA 90095, USA. Email: emayer@ucla.edu.

Index

Page numbers followed by f refer to figures; page numbers followed by t refer to tables.

Q

R